Convergence of Internet of Medical Things (IMT) and Generative AI

V. Vinoth Kumar
Jain University, India

Polinpapilinho F. Katina
University of South Carolina Upstate, USA

Jingyuan Zhao
University of Toronto, Canada

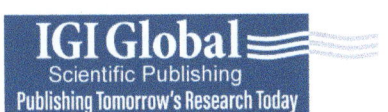

Vice President of Editorial	Melissa Wagner
Managing Editor of Acquisitions	Mikaela Felty
Managing Editor of Book Development	Jocelynn Hessler
Production Manager	Mike Brehm
Cover Design	Phillip Shickler

Published in the United States of America by
IGI Global Scientific Publishing
701 East Chocolate Avenue
Hershey, PA, 17033, USA
Tel: 717-533-8845
Fax: 717-533-8661
Website: https://www.igi-global.com E-mail: cust@igi-global.com

Copyright © 2025 by IGI Global Scientific Publishing. All rights reserved. No part of this publication may be reproduced, stored or distributed in any form or by any means, electronic or mechanical, including photocopying, without written permission from the publisher.
Product or company names used in this set are for identification purposes only. Inclusion of the names of the products or companies does not indicate a claim of ownership by IGI Global Scientific Publishing of the trademark or registered trademark.

Library of Congress Cataloging-in-Publication Data

Library of Congress Cataloging-in-Publication Data

Names: Venkatesan, Vinoth Kumar, 1988- editor. | Katina, Polinpapilinho F., editor. | Zhao, Jingyuan, 1968- editor.
Title: Convergence of internet of medical things (IoMT) and Generative AI / edited by Vinoth Kumar Venkatesan, Polinpapilinho Katina, Jingyuan Zhao.
Description: Hershey, PA : IGI Global, [2025] | Includes bibliographical references and index. | Summary: "This book seeks to explore the multifaceted dimensions of IoMT and Generative AI in the context of global health, and introduce emerging applications, integration challenges, regulatory considerations, and future directions for innovation and collaboration"-- Provided by publisher.
Identifiers: LCCN 2024048762 (print) | LCCN 2024048763 (ebook) | ISBN 9798369361801 (h/c) | ISBN 9798369361849 (s/c) | ISBN 9798369361818 (eISBN)
Subjects: LCSH: Medical informatics--Data processing. | Medical care--Data processing. | Internet of things--Industrial applications. | Generative artificial intelligence--Industrial applications. | Convergence (Telecommunication)
Classification: LCC R858 .C6665 2025 (print) | LCC R858 (ebook) | DDC 610.285--dc23/eng/20250203
LC record available at https://lccn.loc.gov/2024048762
LC ebook record available at https://lccn.loc.gov/2024048763

British Cataloguing in Publication Data
A Cataloguing in Publication record for this book is available from the British Library.

ll work contributed to this book is new, previously-unpublished material.
he views expressed in this book are those of the authors, but not necessarily of the publisher.
This book contains information sourced from authentic and highly regarded references, with reasonable efforts made to ensure the reliability of the data and information presented. The authors, editors, and publisher believe the information in this book to be accurate and true as of the date of publication. Every effort has been made to trace and credit the copyright holders of all materials included. However, the authors, editors, and publisher cannot assume responsibility for the validity of all materials or the consequences of their use. Should any copyright material be found unacknowledged, please inform the publisher so that corrections may be made in future reprints.

To my colleagues at the Vellore Institute of Technology
--V.Vinoth Kumar
To my young sister, Savannah
--Polinpapilinho F. Katina

Table of Contents

Preface xx

Chapter 1
Principles and Practices for Implementing Ethical AI in Healthcare 1
    Herat Joshi, Great River Health Systems, USA

Chapter 2
Investigating Generative Artificial Intelligence Readiness in the Internet of Medical Things: Are
We Progressing Technologically? 31
    Wasswa Shafik, Dig Connectivity Research Laboratory (DCRLab), Kampala, Uganda &
        School of Digital Science, Universiti Brunei Darussalam, Brunei

Chapter 3
Smart Healthcare System and Internet of Medical Things: Applications of Personalized Medicine... 59
    Zuber Peermohammed Shaikh, Savitribai Phule Pune University, India

Chapter 4
Transforming Healthcare With IoMT and Generative AI: Innovations and Implications 83
    Dankan Gowda V., Department of Electronics and Communication Engineering, BMS
        Institute of Technology and Management, Karnataka, India
    Kirti Rahul Kadam, Department of Management, Bharati Vidyapeeth University, Kolhapur,
        India
    Vidya Rajasekhara Reddy Tetala, Independent Researcher, Richmond, USA
    J. Jerin Jose, Department of Computer Science and Engineering, Sasi Institute of
        Technology and Engineering, India
    Y. M. Manu, Department of Computer Science and Engineering, BGS Institute of
        Technology, Adichunchanagiri University, India

Chapter 5
Unlocking the Healing Potential of Internet Psychotherapy: Harnessing Artificial Intelligence to
Enhance Online EMDR Therapy Experience 115
    Anwar Khan, Khushal Khan Khattak Univeristy, Pakistan
    Amalia Madihie, University of Malaysia, Malaysia
    Rehman Ullah Khan, University of Malaysia, Malaysia

Chapter 6
Heartbeat Hackers: Protecting Privacy in the IoMT Age 133
    Manas Kumar Yogi, Pragati Engineering College, India
    Atti MangaDevi, Pragati Engineering College, India
    Yamuna Mundru, Pragati Engineering College, India

Chapter 7
Deep Insights and Analysis of Machine Learning Algorithms for Chronic Kidney Disease Prediction 171
> N. Krishnamoorthy, Vellore Institute of Technology, India
> V. Vinoth Kumar, Vellore Institute of Technology, India
> Sonali Mishra, Vellore Institute of Technology, India

Chapter 8
Securing the Future of IoMT: Healthcare and Comprehensive Analysis of Data Security Measures in Medical Information Systems 191
> S. Satheesh Kumar, REVA University, India
> V. Muthukumaran, SRM University, India
> S. Jahnavi, B.M.S. College of Engineering, India
> C. Krishna, R.V. Institute of Technology and Management, India

Chapter 9
Revolutionizing Patient Care Through the Convergence of IoMT and Generative AI 217
> Dankan Gowda V., Department of Electronics and Communication Engineering, BMS Institute of Technology and Management, Karnataka, India
> Premkumar Reddy, Independent Researcher, Frisco, USA
> Vidya Rajasekhara Reddy Tetala, Independent Researcher, Richmond, USA
> P. Krishnamoorthy, Department of Computer Science and Engineering, Sasi Institute of Technology and Engineering, India
> Kottala Sri Yogi, Department of Operations, Symbiosis Institute of Business Management, Hyderabad, India & Symbiosis International University, Pune, India

Chapter 10
Booster of IoMT in Diagnostics and Disease Screening: Hustler Artificial Intelligence Approaches Transforming Healthier Homes 243
> Bhupinder Singh, Sharda University, India
> Christian Kaunert, Dublin City University, Ireland & University of South Wales, UK
> Hind Hammouch, University Sidi Mohamed Ben Abdellah, Morocco
> Anjali Raghav, Sharda University, India

Chapter 11
Enhanced Diabetic Retinopathy Classification Using Inception Net V3: A Deep Learning Approach 267
> R. Ravindraiah, Madanapalle Institute of Technology and Science, India
> Grande Naga Jyothi, Madanapalle Institute of Technology and Science, India
> Nukala Bharath Kumar, Madanapalle Institute of Technology and Science, India
> B. Ganesh, Madanapalle Institute of Technology and Science, India
> D. Badri, Madanapalle Institute of Technology and Science, India

Chapter 12
A Diabetes Mellitus Detection Using Fusion of IoMT, Generative AI, and eXplainable AI: Diabetes Classification Using IoMT..291
    G. Varun, Sri Ramachandra Institute of Higher Education and Research, India
    S. Sarveswaran, Sri Ramachandra Institute of Higher Education and Research, India
    S. Shreeshaa, Sri Ramachandra Institute of Higher Education and Research, India
    B. V. Arun Krishna, Sri Ramachandra Institute of Higher Education and Research, India
    M. C. Nidhisheshwin, Sri Ramachandra Institute of Higher Education and Research, India
    P. Ashokkumar, Sri Ramachandra Institute of Higher Education and Research, India

Chapter 13
Prediction of Thyroid Disease Using Machine Learning Models 323
    N. Krishnamoorthy, Vellore Institute of Technology, India
    V. Vinoth Kumar, Vellore Institute of Technology, India
    Bryan Samuel James, Vellore Institute of Technology, India

Chapter 14
The Evolution of Artificial Intelligence in Healthcare: Transforming Personalized Medicine and Biosensor Engineering.. 341
    Seneha Santoshi, Amity University, Noida, India
    Hina Bansal, Amity University, Noida, India
    Banashree Bondhopadhyay, Amity University, Noida, India
    Palak Maurya, Amity University, Noida, India

Chapter 15
Artificial Intelligence and Machine Learning-Assisted Internet of Medical Things: Approaches Drug Discovery.. 361
    Zuber Peermohammed Shaikh, Savitribai Phule Pune University, India

Chapter 16
Healthcare Monitoring System Driven by Machine Learning and Internet of Medical Things (MLIoMT) 385
    Kutubuddin Sayyad Liyakat Kazi, Brahmdevdada Mane Institute of Technology, India

Chapter 17
Deep Learning Classification of Diabetic Retinopathy Using ResNet-101 Convolutional Neural Networks 417
    R. Ravindraiah, Madanapalle Institute of Technology and Science, India
    Grande Naga Jyothi, Madanapalle Institute of Technology and Science, India
    J. Pavan Royal, Madanapalle Institute of Technology and Science, India
    B. Nagavardhan Reddy, Madanapalle Institute of Technology and Science, India
    B. Nithish Kumar, Madanapalle Institute of Technology and Science, India

Chapter 18
Navigating Privacy and Security in Internet of Medical Things With Machine-to-Machine
Interactions 439
    Manikandan Arunachalam, Department of Electronics and Communication Engineering,
        Amrita School of Engineering, India
    Saket Akella, Department of Electronics and Communication Engineering, Amrita School of
        Engineering, India
    D. Arun Satvik, Department of Electronics and Communication Engineering, Amrita School
        of Engineering, India
    Rakesh Thoppaen Suresh Babu, Fiserv Inc, USA

Chapter 19
Enhancing Diagnosis, Treatment, and Patient Results Using Artificial Intelligence in Healthcare .. 461
    E. Kavitha, Dr. M.G.R. Educational and Research Institute, India
    G. Kavitha, Dr. M.G.R. Educational and Research Institute, India
    D. SenthilKumar, RMK College of Engineering and Technology, India
    M. Mythreyee, Dr. M.G.R. Educational and Research Institute, India
    B. Swapna, Dr. M.G.R. Educational and Research Institute, India
    P. Jagadeesan, R.M.D. Engineering College, India
    M. Kamalahasan, Dr. M.G.R. Educational and Research Institute, India
    A. Lavanya, Dr. M.G.R. Educational and Research Institute, India

Chapter 20
Optimistic Machine Learning Algorithm to Identify Producer and Consumer Risks in the Medical
Field Using Double Sampling Plan 477
    B. Swapna, Dr. M.G.R. Educational and Research Institute, India
    D. Manjula, Karpagam Hospital, India
    G. Uma, PSG Institute of Technology and Applied Research, India
    G. Kavitha, Dr. M.G.R. Educational and Research Institute, India
    D. SenthilKumar, RMK College of Engineering and Technology, India
    M. Sujitha, Dr. M.G.R. Educational and Research Institute, India
    K. Jeevitha, Dr. M.G.R. Educational and Research Institute, India
    A. Lavanya, Dr. M.G.R. Educational and Research Institute, India

Chapter 21
Transforming Global Healthcare: Unleashing Generative AI and IoMT in the 21st Century 495
    Rajrupa Ray Chaudhuri, Brainware University, India

Chapter 22
Navigating the Convergence of IoMT and Generative AI in Global Healthcare: Opportunities,
Challenges, and Ethical Considerations 513
    Muhammad Usman Tariq, Abu Dhabi University, UAE & University College Cork, Ireland

Chapter 23
Transformative Insights: Integrating IoMT With Generative AI for Personalized Medicine and
Drug Discovery 535
    Hina Bansal, Amity University, Noida, India
    Banashree Bondhopadhyay, Amity Institute of Biotechnology, Amity University, Noida, India
    Seneha Santoshi, Amity Institute of Biotechnology, Amity University, Noida, India
    Himansu, Amity University, Noida, India
    Rajbeen Mazumder, Amity University, Noida, India

Compilation of References 565

About the Contributors 631

Index 639

Detailed Table of Contents

Preface xx

Chapter 1
Principles and Practices for Implementing Ethical AI in Healthcare 1
    Herat Joshi, Great River Health Systems, USA

The integration of artificial intelligence (AI) technology is causing a shift in the healthcare sector. Although artificial intelligence (AI) has enormous promise to improve patient care, diagnostics, and operational efficiency, its application must be handled carefully to avoid moral problems. This paper explores the important factors to take into account when implementing Responsible AI in healthcare environments, with a focus on accountability, justice, openness, and privacy. It looks at how AI may enhance clinical judgment, expedite medical procedures, and provide individualized care. Nonetheless, there are still a lot of obstacles to overcome, including data security, bias mitigation, and regulatory compliance. Healthcare businesses are able to take use of AI while maintaining safe and fair patient outcomes by implementing strong governance and ethical regulations. The research also looks at best practices, legal frameworks, and case studies from the real world that are influencing the direction of responsible AI in healthcare.

Chapter 2
Investigating Generative Artificial Intelligence Readiness in the Internet of Medical Things: Are We Progressing Technologically? 31
    Wasswa Shafik, Dig Connectivity Research Laboratory (DCRLab), Kampala, Uganda &
    School of Digital Science, Universiti Brunei Darussalam, Brunei

Generative Artificial Intelligence (AI) is reshaping the Internet of Medical Things (IoMT), driving innovations in healthcare diagnostics, personalized treatment, and patient monitoring. This integration promises to enhance medical decision-making, optimize resource allocation, and improve patient outcomes. However, despite technological advancements, challenges persist, including data privacy concerns, regulatory hurdles, and the need for robust ethical frameworks. The progress is evident in AI-driven tools, such as predictive analytics and virtual health assistants, yet their widespread adoption is hindered by interoperability issues and uneven technological infrastructure. As generative AI continues to evolve, addressing these barriers is crucial for realizing its full potential in transforming the IoMT landscape, ensuring that technological advancements translate into sustainable and equitable healthcare progress.

Chapter 3
Smart Healthcare System and Internet of Medical Things: Applications of Personalized Medicine... 59
    Zuber Peermohammed Shaikh, Savitribai Phule Pune University, India

These comprehensive review has illuminated the multifaceted role of the Internet of Medical Things (IoMT) in healthcare, showcasing a wide array of use cases that span from patient monitoring and Personalized Medicine to clinical operations and telehealth services. The benefits of IoT in healthcare are profound, contributing to improved patient care through personalized treatment plans and early detection of diseases, enhanced operational efficiency by streamlining healthcare processes, and facilitated data-driven decision-making through analysis of real-time health data. Looking forward, integration of IoMT in healthcare presents numerous opportunities for further research and technological development. Key areas for future exploration include the advancement of AI and machine learning algorithms/datasets generated by IoMT devices, improving patient outcomes through predictive healthcare models. The review focuses on diverse applications of IoMT in healthcare, including but not limited to remote patient monitoring, telehealth, wearable technologies, and smart healthcare facilities.

Chapter 4
Transforming Healthcare With IoMT and Generative AI: Innovations and Implications 83
    Dankan Gowda V., Department of Electronics and Communication Engineering, BMS
        Institute of Technology and Management, Karnataka, India
    Kirti Rahul Kadam, Department of Management, Bharati Vidyapeeth University, Kolhapur,
        India
    Vidya Rajasekhara Reddy Tetala, Independent Researcher, Richmond, USA
    J. Jerin Jose, Department of Computer Science and Engineering, Sasi Institute of
        Technology and Engineering, India
    Y. M. Manu, Department of Computer Science and Engineering, BGS Institute of
        Technology, Adichunchanagiri University, India

The synergistic use of the IoMT and generative AI presents healthcare with practically brand-new approaches to long-standing problems. In this chapter, the author demonstrates the ideas of how integrating the real-time data gathering solution of IoMT and generative AI impact can increase the effectiveness of personal treatment, the capacity of identifying diseases and avoiding them, and the organization of healthcare services. By analyzing key applications introduced by AI such as AI surgical robot, remote health monitoring, and virtual health assistants it is possible to evaluate the impact of such technologies on positive patients' outcomes, decreased rate of readmissions, and increased patients' engagement. In addition, the chapter explores the technical issues and the ethical issues arising from the application of IoMT and generative AI in healthcare such as data privacy issues, integration issues and the call for proper regulations for such technologies.

Chapter 5
Unlocking the Healing Potential of Internet Psychotherapy: Harnessing Artificial Intelligence to
Enhance Online EMDR Therapy Experience 115
    Anwar Khan, Khushal Khan Khattak Univeristy, Pakistan
    Amalia Madihie, University of Malaysia, Malaysia
    Rehman Ullah Khan, University of Malaysia, Malaysia

In recent years, integration of Artificial Intelligence into healthcare has ignited profound interest. This delves into the convergence of Artificial Intelligence and psychotherapy, specifically focusing on the development of Eye Movement Desensitization and Reprocessing (EMDR) therapy system. The chapter aims to comprehensively explore system development methodologies, design components, and the software development process essential for an Artificial Intelligence -based online EMDR therapy system. This chapter intricately details the architectural design, functionalities, hardware and software requirements crucial to optimizing therapeutic usability, outcomes of the system. Natural Language Processing algorithms drive functionalities such as sentiment analysis, text summarization, tokenization, and descriptive analytics, enriching online therapeutic interactions all have made online EMDR therapy system more efficient. This chapter concludes with insights into future directions and implications for Artificial Intelligence-driven psychotherapies.

Chapter 6
Heartbeat Hackers: Protecting Privacy in the IoMT Age 133
    Manas Kumar Yogi, Pragati Engineering College, India
    Atti MangaDevi, Pragati Engineering College, India
    Yamuna Mundru, Pragati Engineering College, India

As the Internet of Medical Things (IoMT) transforms healthcare by enabling real-time monitoring and data exchange, it also presents new privacy challenges. "Heartbeat Hackers: Protecting Privacy in the IoMT Age" explores the intersection of advanced IoMT technologies and privacy concerns. This chapter delves into the vulnerabilities inherent in IoMT devices, including risks of unauthorized access and data breaches. It examines current security measures and highlights the need for robust privacy frameworks to protect sensitive health information. By analyzing recent case studies and emerging threats, the chapter offers practical recommendations for securing IoMT systems, safeguarding patient data, and ensuring compliance with regulatory standards. Through a comprehensive review of privacy-preserving technologies and best practices, it aims to equip healthcare providers and IoMT developers with actionable insights to enhance the protection of personal health information in the digital age.

Chapter 7
Deep Insights and Analysis of Machine Learning Algorithms for Chronic Kidney Disease
Prediction 171
    N. Krishnamoorthy, Vellore Institute of Technology, India
    V. Vinoth Kumar, Vellore Institute of Technology, India
    Sonali Mishra, Vellore Institute of Technology, India

The chronic kidney disease (CKD) is the most prominent causes of death and suffering in the 21st century. Lot of research initiatives are taken in recent years to find the CKD in early stage. Research on renal disease prediction is crucial since it attempts to create reliable and accurate techniques for determining who is most likely to get kidney disease. Early detection of kidney disease can help prevent or delay the progression of the disease and improve patient outcomes. Chronic kidney disease (CKD) affects 8% to 16% of the global population, although both patients and medical professionals usually ignore it. A machine learning algorithms are used in this instance to predict whether or not the subject will experience chronic kidney disease. The training dataset, which is being used contains numerous variables, including specific gravity, sugar, albumin, bacteria, red blood cells, pus cells, and many others, affect chronic kidney disease.

Chapter 8
Securing the Future of IoMT: Healthcare and Comprehensive Analysis of Data Security Measures in Medical Information Systems 191
    S. Satheesh Kumar, REVA University, India
    V. Muthukumaran, SRM University, India
    S. Jahnavi, B.M.S. College of Engineering, India
    C. Krishna, R.V. Institute of Technology and Management, India

Integrating Internet of Things (IoT) technologies into healthcare has brought about a new era characterized by enhanced connectivity and efficiency. However, this transformation also introduces significant challenges in safeguarding medical information. This analysis focuses on the interconnected network of medical devices and systems. It covers various types of medical data, including Personal Health Information (PHI) and telemetry data, susceptible to threats such as unauthorized access, data breaches, and exploitation of IoT vulnerabilities. The research emphasizes the need for proactive and adaptable security measures. Technological solutions such as secure data storage systems and communication channels are also analyzed to provide a holistic understanding of the tools available for mitigating security risks. Finally, the paper explores future trends in medical data security using a Dynamic Attribute-Based Encryption Scheme (DABES), which enables fine-grained access control to medical data.

Chapter 9
Revolutionizing Patient Care Through the Convergence of IoMT and Generative AI 217
    Dankan Gowda V., Department of Electronics and Communication Engineering, BMS
        Institute of Technology and Management, Karnataka, India
    Premkumar Reddy, Independent Researcher, Frisco, USA
    Vidya Rajasekhara Reddy Tetala, Independent Researcher, Richmond, USA
    P. Krishnamoorthy, Department of Computer Science and Engineering, Sasi Institute of
        Technology and Engineering, India
    Kottala Sri Yogi, Department of Operations, Symbiosis Institute of Business Management,
        Hyderabad, India & Symbiosis International University, Pune, India

The incorporation of the Internet of Medical Things and Generative AI to this process shall transform patient care by offering continuous tracking, analysis and individualized progression control. This chapter is dedicated to the synergistic fusion of IoT in Medical Technology (IoMT) and Generative Artificial Intelligence and provides a brief summary of what it is, how it functions, and what can be expected in the future in the field of health care. When combined with the data acquiring capacity of IoMT and analytical potential of Generative AI, hospitals and other medical facilities have the potential to bring diagnosis and treatment to a higher level. Some real-life usage examples of the combined uses of SDN and IoT in health care are shown through different use cases, including chronic disease management, elderly care, virtual health assistance, and prognostic health management and maintenance of healthcare facilities' equipment and tools.

Chapter 10
Booster of IoMT in Diagnostics and Disease Screening: Hustler Artificial Intelligence
Approaches Transforming Healthier Homes 243
    Bhupinder Singh, Sharda University, India
    Christian Kaunert, Dublin City University, Ireland & University of South Wales, UK
    Hind Hammouch, University Sidi Mohamed Ben Abdellah, Morocco
    Anjali Raghav, Sharda University, India

The global landscape of healthcare is witnessing a transformative shift with the integration of artificial intelligence (AI) in disease screening and pandemic outbreak management. Disease screening serves as a critical component of proactive healthcare, enabling early detection and intervention. Traditional screening methods, while effective, often face limitations in terms of scalability, speed, and accuracy. The emergence of AI has opened new avenues for enhancing disease screening processes, allowing for more efficient and precise identification of potential health threats. These technologies enable healthcare professionals to analyze vast datasets quickly and accurately, facilitating early diagnosis and intervention. This chapter explores the various dimensions of evolving role of AI in prioritizing disease screening and managing pandemic outbreaks, with a focus on innovative approaches for mass vaccine scattering. The evolving role of AI in prioritizing disease screening and pandemic outbreak management holds immense promise for the future of global healthcare.

Chapter 11
Enhanced Diabetic Retinopathy Classification Using Inception Net V3: A Deep Learning
Approach.. 267
    R. Ravindraiah, Madanapalle Institute of Technology and Science, India
    Grande Naga Jyothi, Madanapalle Institute of Technology and Science, India
    Nukala Bharath Kumar, Madanapalle Institute of Technology and Science, India
    B. Ganesh, Madanapalle Institute of Technology and Science, India
    D. Badri, Madanapalle Institute of Technology and Science, India

This study employs a novel approach for the automatic classification of Diabetic Retinopathy (DR) through a customized Inception Net V3 Convolutional Neural Network (CNN) method. DR is leading reason for visual impairment and necessitates early and accurate diagnosis for effective intervention. Leveraging deep learning, the proposed CNN model demonstrates remarkable proficiency in discerning diverse stages of DR from retinal images. The network is trained on a comprehensive dataset meticulously annotated with DR stages, ensuring robust learning and generalization. Through an extensive evaluation, this model exhibits superior performance in classifying DR severity levels, showcasing its potential as a valuable diagnostic tool. The proposed CNN architecture not only enhances classification accuracy but also facilitates interpretability, shedding light on the critical features contributing to each classification. The proposed design has been implemented in MATLAB 2023(a)

Chapter 12
A Diabetes Mellitus Detection Using Fusion of IoMT, Generative AI, and eXplainable AI:
Diabetes Classification Using IoMT 291
    G. Varun, Sri Ramachandra Institute of Higher Education and Research, India
    S. Sarveswaran, Sri Ramachandra Institute of Higher Education and Research, India
    S. Shreeshaa, Sri Ramachandra Institute of Higher Education and Research, India
    B. V. Arun Krishna, Sri Ramachandra Institute of Higher Education and Research, India
    M. C. Nidhisheshwin, Sri Ramachandra Institute of Higher Education and Research, India
    P. Ashokkumar, Sri Ramachandra Institute of Higher Education and Research, India

Diabetes Mellitus (DM) is a metabolic disorder when the sugar level in the blood is elevated consistently. The presence of Diabetes Mellitus is one of the global health challenges, several research works focusing on the early detection and management of innovative machine learning technologies were developed in recent years. In this book chapter, we introduce a novel approach to classify diabetes mellitus by leveraging the Internet of Medical Things (IoMT) and generative AI models. IoT devices continuously monitor critical health data and transmit them to a central machine learning model for analysis and preprocessing is done. The preprocessed data act as the input for the machine learning models to predict diabetes. The imbalanced dataset is converted into a balanced one using two generative AI models called VAE and GAN. We used five ML classification models kNN, SVM, DT, LR and RF with boosting. Hard voting is performed to determine the final class. Our experiment result shows that the proposed ensemble model produces an accuracy of 81% which outperformed other model's accuracy

Chapter 13
Prediction of Thyroid Disease Using Machine Learning Models 323
    N. Krishnamoorthy, Vellore Institute of Technology, India
    V. Vinoth Kumar, Vellore Institute of Technology, India
    Bryan Samuel James, Vellore Institute of Technology, India

In recent decades, thyroid dysfunction has become a widespread illness that affects millions of individuals worldwide, mostly women between the ages of 17 to 54. TSH (Thyroid-Stimulating Hormone) that are too high or too low may be a sign of a thyroid problem. The extreme stage of thyroid results in heart problem, depression, etc. Here implements the proactive system to predict the thyroid at its earliest stage is done. This will reduce the death rate and other side effects due to thyroid problems. The techniques used in this work include logistic regression, KNN (k-nearest neighbors) and Decision trees, and these was selected for its different method. These algorithms are the best and most suitable to deal with the prediction of thyroid disease at the earliest stage with less complexity and more accuracy in the implementation. Based on the results obtained, the logistic regression is better and, hence used for the problem in the thyroid disease.

Chapter 14
The Evolution of Artificial Intelligence in Healthcare: Transforming Personalized Medicine and
Biosensor Engineering... 341
    Seneha Santoshi, Amity University, Noida, India
    Hina Bansal, Amity University, Noida, India
    Banashree Bondhopadhyay, Amity University, Noida, India
    Palak Maurya, Amity University, Noida, India

Artificial Intelligence (AI) has become an unprecedented force in healthcare with significant impact on personalized medicine and Biosensor Engineering. This chapter discusses the evolution of AI in healthcare from the early Expert Systems to the advanced Machine Learning (ML) algorithm in practice. Integration of AI in personalized medicine has revolutionized Genomic Analysis, Predictive Analytics, and Drug Discovery and Manufacture with customized treatment. The advancement of AI and AI empowered Biosensor Engineering Technologies has brought future of real time health management and diagnosis by the development of wearable and implantable devices with advanced technologies like ML. The research reveals that AI improves diagnostic accuracy, shortens the time to treatment, and streamlines the drug development process. Additionally, progress in AI-driven biosensor engineering has led to innovations in real-time health monitoring and diagnostics, particularly through the creation of wearable and implantable devices that leverage machine learning technologies.

Chapter 15
Artificial Intelligence and Machine Learning-Assisted Internet of Medical Things: Approaches
Drug Discovery.. 361
    Zuber Peermohammed Shaikh, Savitribai Phule Pune University, India

IoMT devices, also referred to as healthcare IoT, enable human intervention-free healthcare monitoring by integrating automation, interfacial sensors, and machine learning-based artificial intelligence. IoMT technologies aid in reducing unnecessary hospital stays and thereby the associated health costs by facilitating wireless monitoring of health parameters. In this review, we discuss importance of AI in improving capabilities of IoMT in Drug design and development will continue to be an early user of new and growing experimental and computational tools. Among the challenges is deciding whether to use these technologies to improve the existing pipeline and processes or to reengineer the processes in light of these technologies. These research chapter elaborates drug discovery and formulation optimization through Big data, digital healthcare, remote monitoring, and genomics will increase the need to investigate how computational and reasoning approaches might be used to improve the process in terms of clinical significance as well as cost reduction.

Chapter 16
Healthcare Monitoring System Driven by Machine Learning and Internet of Medical Things
(MLIoMT) 385
    Kutubuddin Sayyad Liyakat Kazi, Brahmdevdada Mane Institute of Technology, India

The primary objective of the project is to develop an ML-based healthcare system that can quickly and accurately diagnose a variety of diseases. Seven machine learning classification algorithms were used in this work to forecast nine deadly diseases, such as kidney disorders, hepatitis, diabetes, and blood pressure: adaptive boosting, Random Forest, DT, Support Vector Machines, Naïve Bayes, Artificial Neural Networks, and K-Nearest Neighbour. Performance metrics including Precision, Accuracy, and Recall are used to assess the suggested model's effectiveness. The performance of the classifiers is evaluated using four metrics: accuracy, precision, recall, and precision. For every ailment, the current healthcare model achieves a minimum accuracy of 82.3% and a maximum accuracy of 95.7%. There are minimal and maximum precision and recall values for each disease: 81.4% and 95.7%, respectively, and 64.3% and 90.3%, respectively. This ML driven IoMT approach we call as DL approach.

Chapter 17
Deep Learning Classification of Diabetic Retinopathy Using ResNet-101 Convolutional Neural Networks 417
 R. Ravindraiah, Madanapalle Institute of Technology and Science, India
 Grande Naga Jyothi, Madanapalle Institute of Technology and Science, India
 J. Pavan Royal, Madanapalle Institute of Technology and Science, India
 B. Nagavardhan Reddy, Madanapalle Institute of Technology and Science, India
 B. Nithish Kumar, Madanapalle Institute of Technology and Science, India

Diabetic Retinopathy (DR) patients suffer from chronically excessive blood sugar, which impairs retinal features. Diabetic sufferers are extra prone to this difficulty, which may cause vision loss unless caught and handled early. It is the world's sixth most common cause of eyesight loss. Therefore, in-depth studies have been demanded in this vicinity to locate new approaches to diagnosing DR ranges. Initially, dedicated fundus image recognition techniques and computational algorithms were used to identify DR, however, their usefulness in real-time clinical practice became inadequate. Convolutional Neural Networks (CNNs), one type of deep learning model, are better at predicting the prognosis of DR. The goal of this research work is to understand the overall performance of a deep-gaining knowledge model, ResNet, a deep-stage neural network, in detecting non-prescriptive and exclusive varieties of suggestible DR.

Chapter 18
Navigating Privacy and Security in Internet of Medical Things With Machine-to-Machine Interactions 439
 Manikandan Arunachalam, Department of Electronics and Communication Engineering, Amrita School of Engineering, India
 Saket Akella, Department of Electronics and Communication Engineering, Amrita School of Engineering, India
 D. Arun Satvik, Department of Electronics and Communication Engineering, Amrita School of Engineering, India
 Rakesh Thoppaen Suresh Babu, Fiserv Inc, USA

Internet of Medical Things (IoMT) offers immense benefits by revolutionizing healthcare delivery, enhancing patient outcomes, and improving operational efficiencies across the healthcare ecosystem. Also, integration of Machine-to-Machine (M2M) communication with IoMT enables real time patient monitoring, remote diagnostics and intelligent decision making in critical situations. Current state of research shows that adoption of M2M communication with IoMT facilitates the seamless connectivity and data exchange among the health care devices and sensors. However, since M2M communication allows devices to communicate to each other without human intervention, security in the integration of M2M communication with IoMT face critical challenges and issues under different environments. This chapter will thoroughly discuss the security challenges and issues which are essential to address to escape from the evolving threat and to ensure the secure adoption of M2M communication with IoMT.

Chapter 19
Enhancing Diagnosis, Treatment, and Patient Results Using Artificial Intelligence in Healthcare .. 461
    E. Kavitha, Dr. M.G.R. Educational and Research Institute, India
    G. Kavitha, Dr. M.G.R. Educational and Research Institute, India
    D. SenthilKumar, RMK College of Engineering and Technology, India
    M. Mythreyee, Dr. M.G.R. Educational and Research Institute, India
    B. Swapna, Dr. M.G.R. Educational and Research Institute, India
    P. Jagadeesan, R.M.D. Engineering College, India
    M. Kamalahasan, Dr. M.G.R. Educational and Research Institute, India
    A. Lavanya, Dr. M.G.R. Educational and Research Institute, India

Artificial intelligence (AI) is revolutionizing healthcare by improving diagnostic accuracy, treatment personalization, and operational efficiency. This chapter explores AI applications in medical imaging, predictive analytics, drug discovery, and patient care. We examine current AI-driven systems, such as deep learning models for early diagnosis and natural language processing for electronic health record (EHR) analysis. The chapter also discusses challenges in integrating AI into healthcare, including ethical considerations, data privacy, and regulatory frameworks. Potential improvements in medical outcomes and operational workflows are highlighted, supported by case studies and research findings.

Chapter 20
Optimistic Machine Learning Algorithm to Identify Producer and Consumer Risks in the Medical Field Using Double Sampling Plan 477
    B. Swapna, Dr. M.G.R. Educational and Research Institute, India
    D. Manjula, Karpagam Hospital, India
    G. Uma, PSG Institute of Technology and Applied Research, India
    G. Kavitha, Dr. M.G.R. Educational and Research Institute, India
    D. SenthilKumar, RMK College of Engineering and Technology, India
    M. Sujitha, Dr. M.G.R. Educational and Research Institute, India
    K. Jeevitha, Dr. M.G.R. Educational and Research Institute, India
    A. Lavanya, Dr. M.G.R. Educational and Research Institute, India

The specific form of statistical quality control, applied to the medical field to ensure product excellence and patient safety. Specifically, the proposed method employs a Machine Learning Algorithm (MLA) to assist in decision-making about accepting or rejecting inspected medical samples. The algorithm is trained using data from double sampling plan tables, enabling it to generate closed-form solutions for sample size while accounting for producer and consumer risks. This automation ensures precision in interpreting double sampling plan tables without compromising quality. provides flexibility for medical quality controllers, allowing for the consideration of specific requirements while minimizing time and cost during inspections. It addresses producer and consumer risks at predefined levels, while also incorporating other key quality parameters. With this system, medical professionals can estimate sample size at fixed producer and consumer risk levels, or predict these risks at a given sample size, ensuring comprehensive risk management and quality assurance in medical products.

Chapter 21
Transforming Global Healthcare: Unleashing Generative AI and IoMT in the 21st Century............ 495
   Rajrupa Ray Chaudhuri, Brainware University, India

The global healthcare environment is poised for a revolution because to the convergence of Generative Artificial Intelligence (AI) and the Internet of Medical Things (IoMT). This article investigates how these technologies can improve healthcare delivery efficiency, enable tailored treatment regimens, and improve diagnostic accuracy. A summary of the development of healthcare technology across time is provided, emphasizing the significant advancements in AI and IoMT. Through case studies, the application of generative AI to drug development, customized medicine, and predictive analytics is explored; the influence of IoMT on telemedicine, remote patient monitoring, and real-time data analytics is also covered. The amalgamation of Generative AI with IoMT holds potential to elevate clinical results, augment operational efficacy, and augment healthcare accessible, specifically in marginalized areas. However, there are drawbacks such as socioeconomic inequality, privacy and problems with data quality. Strong cybersecurity defenses, data governance are needed in future development.

Chapter 22
Navigating the Convergence of IoMT and Generative AI in Global Healthcare: Opportunities, Challenges, and Ethical Considerations.. 513
   Muhammad Usman Tariq, Abu Dhabi University, UAE & University College Cork, Ireland

This chapter examines the transformative potential of combining Generative AI with the Internet of Medical Things (IoMT) in healthcare. IoMT's capacity to empower ceaseless wellbeing observing and ongoing information assortment, joined with Generative man-made intelligence's high-level prescient and logical power, guarantees huge progressions in diagnostics, patient administration, and customized medication. The chapter focuses on case studies that demonstrate improved healthcare delivery and outcomes as it examines novel applications of these technologies. Be that as it may, it additionally addresses basic difficulties like security, security, and moral situations, including information insurance, algorithmic predisposition, and patient independence. Systems for beating these hindrances, particularly in asset compelled settings, are talked about, accentuating the requirement for hearty moral structures and administrative approaches.

Chapter 23
Transformative Insights: Integrating IoMT With Generative AI for Personalized Medicine and Drug Discovery.. 535
   Hina Bansal, Amity University, Noida, India
   Banashree Bondhopadhyay, Amity Institute of Biotechnology, Amity University, Noida, India
   Seneha Santoshi, Amity Institute of Biotechnology, Amity University, Noida, India
   Himansu, Amity University, Noida, India
   Rajbeen Mazumder, Amity University, Noida, India

The rapid increase of generative AI aligned with IoMT promotes the medical and healthcare industry with its numerous applications such as in precision medicine (PM), drug discovery, disease diagnosis, etc. In the past decade, acceptance of AI remoulded the ongoing innovations in the medical industry. As the world grapples with chronic illnesses and lifestyle disorders burdening hospitals and clinics, AI succors by lessening the load. Nevertheless, its limitations like data security and privacy are a cause for worry. IoMT consists of a sensor, or wearable connected via the internet to the data recorder. This chapter attempts to comprehend the goals, outcome, future perspective, and tribulations of alignment of Generative AI with IoMT. The integration of Generative AI and IoMT in healthcare offers transformative outcomes, including enhanced diagnostic accuracy through precise and timely analyses. These innovations promise better outcomes and greater efficiency, but it's essential to prioritize ethics, protect patient data, and ensure compliance as they become part of everyday care.

Compilation of References 565

About the Contributors 631

Index 639

Preface

Internet of Medical Things (IoMT) refers to a collection of medical devices and applications that connect to healthcare information technology systems through online computer networks. Generative artificial intelligence (AI), or generative AI (GenAI), is a type of AI that creates new content like text, images, videos, and audio. It uses generative models to learn the patterns and structures of training data, and then generate new data based on those patterns. In recent years, IoMT, a subset of the Internet of Things (IoT) and GenAI have revolutionized healthcare delivery, offering unprecedented opportunities to enhance patient care, improve clinical outcomes, and optimize healthcare systems globally. IoMT-based smart healthcare system is a collection of several smart medical equipment including wearable devices and apps connected within the network to provide health information. IoMT encompasses interconnected medical devices, wearables, sensors, and healthcare systems that collect, transmit, and analyze health data. GenAIencompasses advanced computational techniques capable of generating novel insights, predictions, and solutions. The AI-driven IoMT healthcare system is a combination of IoT (used for periodic control) and AI (used for data analysis).

Gen AI has the potential to revolutionize global health across multiple areas, such as medical data synthesis, image enhancement, disease prediction and diagnosis, drug discovery, medical documentation, and personalized healthcare. It offers opportunities to overcome data scarcity and privacy concerns through synthetic data generation and supports accurate disease interpretation and diagnosis through image quality enhancement. Generative AI models also enable disease likelihood prediction, early condition detection, precise diagnoses, and personalized treatment plans for improved patient care. However, as IoMT and Generative AI continue to proliferate across healthcare ecosystems, it is imperative to critically examine their impact on global health, considering diverse socio-economic contexts, cultural sensitivities, and ethical implications.

This book seeks to explore the multifaceted dimensions of IoMT and GenAI in the context of global health and introduce emerging applications, integration challenges, regulatory considerations, and future directions for innovation and collaboration. As such, the book, while it provides useful insights for a variety of readers interested in navigating the 21st-century foggy waters of usefulness, ambiguity, and uncertainties associated with emerging technologies, it is also our hope that this also raises questions for researchers, business leaders, and policymakers, especially in matters of governance of IoMT and GenAI (Gheorghe et al., 2023; Keating and Katina, 2019; Keating et al., 2023; Keating et a., 2023).

ORGANIZATION OF THE BOOK

This book is organized into 23 chapters. Chapter 1 (*Implementing Responsible AI in Healthcare Organizations: Strategies, Challenges, and Best Practices*) introduces important factors to take into account when implementing Responsible AI in healthcare environments, with a focus on accountability, justice, openness, and privacy. It looks at how AI may enhance clinical judgment, expedite medical procedures, and provide individualized care. Nonetheless, there are still a lot of obstacles to overcome, including data security, bias mitigation, and regulatory compliance. The research also looks at best practices, legal frameworks, and case studies from the real world that are influencing the direction of responsible AI in healthcare.

Chapter 2 (*Investigating Generative Artificial Intelligence Readiness in the in Internet of Medical Things: Are We progressing Technologically ?*) discussed about Generative Artificial Intelligence (AI) is reshaping the Internet of Medical Things (IoMT), driving innovations in healthcare diagnostics, personalized treatment, and patient monitoring. This integration promises to enhance medical decision-making, optimize resource allocation, and improve patient outcomes. However, despite technological advancements, challenges persist, including data privacy concerns, regulatory hurdles, and the need for robust ethical frameworks.

Chapter 3 (*Smart Healthcare System and Internet of Medical Things: Applications of Personalized Medicine*) explains the multifaceted role of the Internet of Medical Things(IoMT) in healthcare, showcasing a wide array of use cases that span from patient monitoring and Personalized Medicine to clinical operations and telehealth services. Key areas for future exploration include the advancement of AI and machine learning algorithms/datasets generated by IoMT devices, and improving patient outcomes through predictive healthcare models.

Chapter 4 (*Transforming Healthcare with IoMT and Generative AI: Innovations and Implications*) demonstrates the ideas of how integrating the real-time data gathering solution of IoMT and generative AI impact can increase the effectiveness of personal treatment, the capacity of identifying diseases and avoiding them, and the organization of healthcare services.

Chapter 5 (*Unlocking the Healing Potential of Internet Psychotherapy: Harnessing Artificial Intelligence to Enhance Online EMDR Therapy Experience*) aims to comprehensively explore system development methodologies, design components, and the software development process essential for an Artificial Intelligence-based online EMDR therapy system. This chapter concludes with insights into future directions and implications for Artificial Intelligence-driven psychotherapies.

Chapter 6 (*Heartbeat Hackers: Protecting Privacy in the IoMT Age*) analyzes recent case studies and emerging threats, the chapter offers practical recommendations for securing IoMT systems, safeguarding patient data, and ensuring compliance with regulatory standards. Through a comprehensive review of privacy-preserving technologies and best practices, it aims to equip healthcare providers and IoMT developers with actionable insights to enhance the protection of personal health information in the digital age.

Chapter 7 (*Deep Insights and Analysis of Machine Learning Algorithms for Chronic Kidney Disease Prediction*) discusses research initiatives taken in recent years to find Chronic Kidney Disease (CKD) in the early stages. Research on renal disease prediction is crucial since it attempts to create reliable and accurate techniques for determining who is most likely to get kidney disease. Machine learning algorithms are used in this instance to predict chronic kidney disease.

Chapter 8 (*Securing the Future of IoMT-Healthcare and Comprehensive Analysis of Data Security Measures in Medical Information Systems*) emphasizes the need for proactive and adaptable security measures. Finally, this chapter explores future trends in medical data security using a Dynamic Attribute-Based Encryption Scheme (DABES), which enables fine-grained access control to medical data.

Chapter 9 (*Revolutionizing Patient Care through the Convergence of IoMT and Generative AI*) proposes a synergistic fusion of IoMT and GenAI and provides a summary of what it is, how it functions, and what can be expected in the future in the field of health care. When combined with the data-acquiring capacity of IoMT and the analytical potential of Generative AI, hospitals and other medical facilities have the potential to bring diagnosis and treatment to a higher level.

Chapter 10 (*Booster of IoMT in Diagnostics and Disease Screening: Hustler Artificial Intelligence Approaches Transforming Healthier Homes*) explores the various dimensions of the evolving role of AI in prioritizing disease screening and managing pandemic outbreaks, with a focus on innovative approaches for mass vaccine scattering. The evolving role of AI in prioritizing disease screening and pandemic outbreak management holds immense promise for the future of global healthcare.

Chapter 11 (*Enhanced Diabetic Retinopathy Classification Using Inception Net V3: A Deep Learning Approach*) employs a novel approach for the automatic classification of Diabetic Retinopathy (DR) through a customized Inception Net V3 Convolutional Neural Network (CNN) method.

Chapter 12 (*A Diabetes Mellitus Detection using Fusion of IoMT, Generative AI and eXplainable AI: Diabetes classification using IoMT*) introduces a novel approach to classify diabetes mellitus by leveraging the Internet of Medical Things (IoMT) and generative AI models. IoT devices continuously monitor critical health data and transmit them to a central machine-learning model for analysis and preprocessing.

Chapter 13 (*Prediction of Thyroid Disease Using Machine Learning Models*) discusses the proactive system to predict the thyroid at its earliest stage. This will reduce the death rate and other side effects due to thyroid problems. The techniques used in this work include logistic regression, KNN (k-nearest neighbors), and decision trees, and these were selected for their different methods.

Chapter 14 (*The Evolution of Artificial Intelligence in Healthcare: Transforming Personalized Medicine and Biosensor Engineering*) discusses the evolution of AI in healthcare from the early Expert Systems to the advanced Machine Learning (ML) algorithm in practice. Integration of AI in personalized medicine has revolutionized Genomic Analysis, Predictive Analytics, and Drug Discovery and Manufacture with customized treatment.

Chapter 15 (*Artificial Intelligence and Machine Learning Assisted Internet of Medical Things: Approaches Drug Discovery*) discusses discuss importance of AI in improving the capabilities of IoMT in drug design and development will continue to be an early user of new and growing experimental and computational tools.

Chapter 16 (*Healthcare Monitoring System Driven by Machine Learning and Internet of Medical Things(MLIoMT): DL Approach for Healthcare Monitoring*) states an ML-based healthcare system that can quickly and accurately diagnose a variety of diseases. Seven machine learning classification algorithms were used in this work to forecast nine deadly diseases, such as kidney disorders, hepatitis, diabetes, and blood pressure: adaptive boosting, Random Forest, DT, Support Vector Machines, Naïve Bayes, Artificial Neural Networks, and K-Nearest Neighbour. Performance metrics including Precision, Accuracy, and Recall are used to assess the suggested model's effectiveness.

Chapter 17 (*Deep Learning Classification of Diabetic Retinopathy Using ResNet-101 Convolutional Neural Networks*) discusses the overall performance of a deep-gaining knowledge model, ResNet, a deep-stage neural network, in detecting non-prescriptive and exclusive varieties of suggestible Diabetic Retinopathy (DR).

Chapter 18 (*Navigating Privacy and Security in Internet of Medical Things with Machine-to-Machine Interactions*) discusses the security challenges and issues that are essential to address to escape from the evolving threat and to ensure the secure adoption of M2M communication with IoMT.

Chapter 19 (*Enhancing diagnosis, treatment, and patient results using Artificial Intelligence in healthcare*) explores AI applications in medical imaging, predictive analytics, drug discovery, and patient care. We examine current AI-driven systems, such as deep learning models for early diagnosis and natural language processing for electronic health record (EHR) analysis.

Chapter 20 (*Optimistic Machine Learning Algorithm to Identifying Producer and Consumer Risks in the Medical field Using Double Sampling Plan*) presents a specific form of statistical quality control, applied to the medical field to ensure product excellence and patient safety. Specifically, the proposed method employs a Machine Learning Algorithm (MLA) to assist in decision-making about accepting or rejecting inspected medical samples.

Chapter 21 (*Transforming Global Healthcare: Unleashing Generative AI and IoMT in the 21st Century*) investigates how these technologies can improve healthcare delivery efficiency, enable tailored treatment regimens, and improve diagnostic accuracy. A summary of the development of healthcare technology across time is provided, emphasizing the significant advancements in AI and IoMT.

Chapter 22 (*Navigating the Convergence of IoMT and Generative AI in Global Healthcare: Opportunities, Challenges, and Ethical Considerations*) examines the transformative potential of combining Generative AI with the Internet of Medical Things (IoMT) in healthcare. It focuses on case studies that demonstrate improved healthcare delivery and outcomes as it examines novel applications of these technologies.

Chapter 23 (*Transformative Insights: Integrating IoMT with Generative AI for Personalized Medicine and Drug Discovery*) attempts to comprehend the goals, outcomes, future perspective, and tribulations of alignment of Generative AI with IoMT. The integration of Generative AI and IoMT in healthcare offers transformative outcomes, including enhanced diagnostic accuracy through precise and timely analyses.

V. Vinoth Kumar
Vellore Institute of Technology, India

Polinpapilinho F. Katina
University of South Carolina Upstate, US

Jingyuan Zhao
University of Toronto, Canada

REFERENCES

Gheorghe, A. V., Pyne, J. C., Sisti, J., Keating, C. B., Katina, P. F., & Edmonson, W. (2023). Critical Space Infrastructure: A Complex System Governance Perspective. *International Journal of Cyber Diplomacy*, 4, 15–28. DOI: 10.54852/ijcd.v4y202302

Keating, C. B., & Katina, P. F. (2019). Complex system governance: Concept, utility, and challenges. *Systems Research and Behavioral Science*, 36(5), 687–705. DOI: 10.1002/sres.2621

Keating, C. B., Katina, P. F., Bradley, J. M., Hodge, R., & Pyne, J. C. (2023). Sustainability: A Complex System Governance Perspective. *INCOSE International Symposium*, 33(1), 1117–1131. DOI: 10.1002/iis2.13073

Keating, C. B., Katina, P. F., Chesterman, C. W., & Pyne, J. C. (Eds.). (2022). *Complex system governance: Theory and practice*. Springer International Publishing., Retrieved from https://link.springer.com/book/10.1007/978-3-030-93852-9 DOI: 10.1007/978-3-030-93852-9

Chapter 1
Principles and Practices for Implementing Ethical AI in Healthcare

Herat Joshi
https://orcid.org/0009-0009-4199-544X
Great River Health Systems, USA

ABSTRACT

The integration of artificial intelligence (AI) technology is causing a shift in the healthcare sector. Although artificial intelligence (AI) has enormous promise to improve patient care, diagnostics, and operational efficiency, its application must be handled carefully to avoid moral problems. This paper explores the important factors to take into account when implementing Responsible AI in healthcare environments, with a focus on accountability, justice, openness, and privacy. It looks at how AI may enhance clinical judgment, expedite medical procedures, and provide individualized care. Nonetheless, there are still a lot of obstacles to overcome, including data security, bias mitigation, and regulatory compliance. Healthcare businesses are able to take use of AI while maintaining safe and fair patient outcomes by implementing strong governance and ethical regulations. The research also looks at best practices, legal frameworks, and case studies from the real world that are influencing the direction of responsible AI in healthcare.

1.0 INTRODUCTION

The enormous responsibility of ensuring the health and welfare of people and communities falls on healthcare organizations, the backbone of contemporary society. These entities, encompassing hospitals, clinics, and nursing homes, serve as beacons of hope, providing essential medical services and treatments to those in need. However, there are several obstacles in the way of providing great healthcare, like rising expenses, a lack of workers, and the constant need to adopt new technology to improve patient care and operational effectiveness (Oleka-Onyewuchi, 2023).

In the midst of these obstacles, the application of ethical AI in healthcare institutions stands out as a potentially revolutionary development. AI technologies are developing at an unprecedented rate, and their potential uses in the healthcare industry are enormous. These applications include medication development, patient monitoring, and disease diagnosis and treatment planning (Haleem & Suman,

DOI: 10.4018/979-8-3693-6180-1.ch001

Copyright ©2025, IGI Global. Copying or distributing in print or electronic forms without written permission of IGI Global is prohibited.

2022). However, this integration must be approached with the utmost care and responsibility, ensuring patient safety, data privacy, and ethical decision-making are at the forefront. The challenges associated with implementing responsible AI in healthcare are multifaceted, encompassing algorithmic fairness, addressing bias in data and models, maintaining transparency and accountability, and navigating the complex ethical and legal considerations that arise.

The proper application of AI in healthcare institutions has the potential to completely transform how we approach and provide medical care. We can explore previously uncharted territory in the areas of drug development, disease diagnosis, treatment planning, and patient monitoring by utilizing sophisticated algorithms and machine learning models. The use of artificial intelligence (AI) technologies holds the potential to improve the precision of diagnoses, optimize clinical procedures, and customize treatment regimens based on patient requirements. Predictive analytics powered by AI can also help detect possible health hazards and make preventive interventions possible, which will eventually improve patient outcomes and quality of life. Responsible AI adoption can improve resource allocation, lessen administrative burdens, and increase cost efficiencies in healthcare systems in addition to therapeutic uses.

However, the path to responsible AI implementation in healthcare is not without its challenges. Ensuring algorithmic fairness and mitigating bias in data and models is paramount, as biased AI systems can perpetuate and amplify existing disparities in healthcare access and quality. Additionally, maintaining transparency and accountability in AI decision-making processes is crucial to foster trust and enable effective oversight. Privacy and data security concerns also loom large, as healthcare data is inherently sensitive, and breaches can have severe consequences for patients. Navigating the complex ethical and legal landscapes surrounding AI in healthcare, such as issues of liability and informed consent, further complicates the implementation process.

The aim of this study is to explore strategies for implementing responsible AI in healthcare organizations. The objectives are to identify the potential benefits, challenges, and ethical considerations associated with integrating AI technologies into medical practices while ensuring patient safety, data privacy, and fairness.

The introduction sets the stage for understanding the significance of responsible AI in healthcare. It provides a foundational understanding of the topic, highlighting its relevance and potential impact. Transitioning from this section, we move seamlessly into the literature review, where existing research and insights into responsible AI in healthcare are synthesized and analyzed.

2.0 LITERATURE REVIEW

In the literature review, we delve into existing scholarship and studies surrounding responsible AI in healthcare. This section serves as a comprehensive overview, identifying key themes, trends, and gaps in the current research landscape. Transitioning from the literature review, we shift our focus to healthcare organizations, examining their roles and responsibilities in implementing responsible AI.

2.1 Healthcare Organizations

Healthcare organizations play a vital role in the delivery of healthcare services, ensuring the provision of quality care to individuals and communities. Healthcare organizations are tasked with managing, coordinating, and delivering healthcare services (Ginter & Swayne, 2018). Healthcare organizations can be broadly defined as entities that are responsible for the management, coordination, and delivery of healthcare services. These groups include a broad spectrum of establishments, such as public health organizations, clinics, hospitals, and physician offices. Healthcare companies work in a variety of environments, including the public and commercial sectors, as well as non-profit organizations.

2.1.1 Significance of Healthcare Organizations

As the foundation of healthcare delivery, healthcare organizations are vital to the healthcare system. They provide essential services that promote health, prevent illness, diagnose and treat medical conditions, and rehabilitate patients. According to the World Health Organization, (2018) healthcare organizations serve as a platform for healthcare professionals to collaborate, share resources, and deliver comprehensive care to individuals across the care continuum.

2.1.2 Functions of Healthcare Organizations

Healthcare organizations perform several key functions that contribute to the efficient and effective delivery of healthcare services. These functions include service provision, coordination and continuity of care, quality improvement, resource allocation and management, and health promotion and disease prevention. Healthcare organizations provide a diverse range of clinical services, including primary care, specialized treatments, diagnostic procedures, and surgical interventions (Greenwood-Lee & Marshall, 2018). They strive to meet the diverse healthcare needs of individuals, ensuring access to timely and appropriate care.

Continued research and collaboration, as highlighted by the World Health Organization. (2018) are essential to further enhance the effectiveness and efficiency of healthcare organizations in meeting the evolving healthcare needs of individuals and communities.

In dissecting the roles of healthcare organizations in responsible AI adoption, we uncover the complexities and challenges faced. This examination sets the stage for a more nuanced understanding of responsible AI's implications in healthcare and how it intersects with regulatory and legal frameworks.

2.2 Responsible AI in Healthcare

The technology known as artificial intelligence (AI) has become a game-changer in a number of sectors, including healthcare. As artificial intelligence develops, it is imperative to guarantee its conscientious and moral application in medical environments. The strategy that gives ethical and responsible AI technology deployment in healthcare systems top priority is known as "responsible AI in healthcare." It includes a collection of rules, policies, and procedures designed to minimize biases and hazards related to the application of AI while optimizing its advantages for patients, healthcare professionals, and society as a whole. The essential elements of artificial intelligence (AI) in healthcare are summed up in Figure 1, which places a focus on openness, justice, privacy, and equity in the creation and application of AI systems and algorithms.

Figure 1. Essential elements of conscientious AI in healthcare

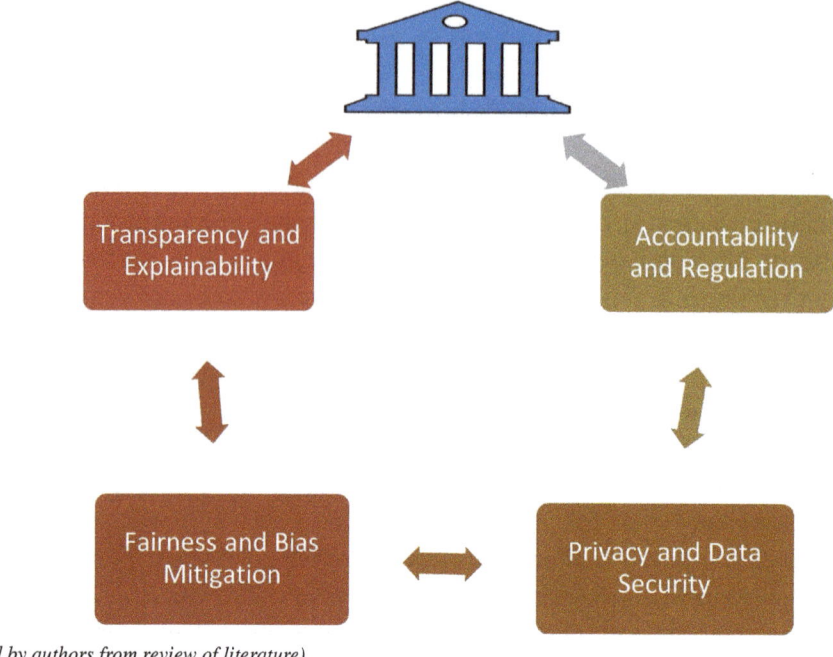

(Compiled by authors from review of literature)

Essential Elements of Conscientious AI in Healthcare:

2.2.1 Transparency and Explainability: According to Figure 1, openness in the creation and application of AI algorithms is necessary for responsible AI in healthcare. Patients and healthcare professionals should have access to information regarding the underlying data used by AI systems and how they make choices. In order to foster confidence and guarantee accountability for clinical decisions guided by AI, explainability is essential.

2.2.2 Fairness and Bias Mitigation: AI algorithms should be designed to minimize biases and ensure fairness in healthcare outcomes. Responsible AI in Healthcare requires the evaluation of AI systems for potential biases and the implementation of strategies to mitigate them. Fairness should be upheld across diverse patient populations, irrespective of race, ethnicity, gender, or socioeconomic status.

2.2.3 Privacy and Data Security: As seen in Figure 1, responsible AI in healthcare places a strong emphasis on handling sensitive health data securely and protecting patient privacy. AI systems should abide by moral and legal requirements, guaranteeing the security and responsible use of patient data. Encryption methods and data governance structures are essential for preserving data security and privacy.

2.2.4 Accountability and Regulation: Appropriate accountability procedures for the creation, application, and utilization of AI technologies are necessary for responsible AI in healthcare. To guarantee ethical AI practices, healthcare institutions should set up governance frameworks, rules, and guidelines.

2.2.5 Regulatory frameworks should be in place to oversee the ethical use of AI in healthcare and hold stakeholders accountable for any potential harm caused by AI systems.

Diving into responsible AI in healthcare, we explore its multifaceted nature, encompassing patient care, outcomes, and risk mitigation. This exploration naturally leads us to scrutinize the regulatory and legal implications that govern AI implementation within the healthcare sector.

2.3 Implications of Responsible AI in Healthcare

The concept of Responsible AI in Healthcare has significant implications for various stakeholders:

2.3.1 Patients and Healthcare Providers: With the provision of early and accurate diagnosis, individualized treatment plans, and enhanced clinical decision support, responsible AI in healthcare can improve patient care. By automating repetitive processes, it can also lessen the workload for healthcare professionals, freeing them up to concentrate on difficult situations and patient engagement.
2.3.2 Ethical Considerations: Discussing ethical conundrums including how AI affects patient autonomy, informed consent, and the possibility that AI will eventually take the place of human judgment are all prompted by responsible AI in healthcare. In order to guarantee that AI technologies adhere to moral standards and uphold human rights, these conversations are crucial.
2.3.3 Regulatory Bodies and Policymakers: The creation of legal frameworks and guidelines governing the application of AI in healthcare is essential for responsible AI in healthcare. These frameworks ought to cover matters pertaining to responsibility, bias, privacy, and the appropriate application of AI algorithms. In order to ensure that AI serves society as a whole and to shape the regulatory landscape, policymakers are essential.

Responsible AI in Healthcare is a concept that emphasizes the ethical and accountable use of AI technologies in healthcare settings. Transparency, fairness, privacy, and responsibility are all included in its mission to optimize AI's advantages while reducing risks and biases. Policymakers, regulatory agencies, technology developers, and healthcare practitioners must work together to implement responsible AI in healthcare. Healthcare can leverage AI's potential to enhance clinical decision-making, improve patient outcomes, and advance fair healthcare delivery by adopting Responsible AI.

Examining the implications of responsible AI, we confront the regulatory and legal frameworks shaping its adoption. This scrutiny unveils the practical challenges inherent in implementing responsible AI within healthcare settings, paving the way for a discussion on future directions and recommendations.

2.4 Regulatory, Legal and Ethical Implications of AI in Healthcare

The integration of artificial intelligence (AI) in healthcare has the potential to revolutionize the delivery of medical services. However, the adoption of AI in healthcare organizations also raises regulatory and legal implications that must be carefully considered.

2.4.1 Regulatory Framework for AI in Healthcare

The regulatory landscape for AI in healthcare is evolving to keep pace with technological advancements. Regulatory bodies, such as the U.S. Food and Drug Administration (FDA) and the European Medicines Agency (EMA), are increasingly focused on establishing guidelines and standards for the development, validation, and deployment of AI systems in healthcare. These regulations aim to ensure the safety, effectiveness, and reliability of AI technologies (Shneiderman, 2020).

One key aspect of regulatory frameworks is the requirement for AI algorithms to undergo rigorous testing and validation before clinical implementation. The evaluation of AI algorithms in healthcare should encompass robust clinical trials and validation studies to determine their diagnostic accuracy, reliability, and clinical utility, ensuring that these technologies adhere to the required standards for safe and effective healthcare services (Magrabi & Georgiou, 2019).

2.4.2 Legal Considerations in AI Adoption

Legal issues are also raised by the use of AI in healthcare institutions. Data security and patient privacy protection are important considerations. AI systems often rely on vast amounts of patient data for training and analysis. Therefore, compliance with data protection laws, such as the General Data Protection Regulation (GDPR) in the European Union, Health Insurance Portability and Accountability Act (HIPAA), Personal Information Protection and Electronic Documents Act (PIPEDA) and Data Protection Act 2018 (DPA) is crucial. Healthcare organizations must ensure that appropriate consent mechanisms, data masking approaches, and safe data storage measures are in place to safeguard patient information.

Another legal consideration is the potential liability associated with AI technologies. As AI systems increasingly influence patient care, there are growing concerns about who is accountable and responsible for these decisions. In cases where AI algorithms provide incorrect diagnoses or recommendations, determining liability becomes challenging. Legal frameworks need to address these issues, clarifying the roles and responsibilities of healthcare professionals, manufacturers, and regulatory bodies in the event of adverse outcomes related to AI adoption.

2.4.3 Ethical Use of AI in Healthcare

Ethical considerations are crucial in integrating AI into healthcare. Guided by the principle of beneficence, which prioritizes patient well-being, the development and deployment of AI technologies must adhere to strict ethical standards. Table 1 summarizes the ethical use of AI in healthcare, highlighting the importance of creating AI algorithms that are free from biases and discrimination. It's important for these systems to be transparent in how decisions are made to preserve the trust between healthcare providers and patients. Additionally, issues related to informed consent and patient autonomy are critical. Patients should be thoroughly informed about how AI is used in their care and retain the option to decline its use. Ethical guidelines should encourage collaborative decision-making between healthcare professionals and patients, considering both the advantages and limitations of AI technologies.

Table 1. Ethical use of AI in healthcare

Aspect Summary	Summary
Regulatory Framework for AI in Healthcare	Regulatory bodies like FDA and EMA are establishing guidelines for AI development, focusing on safety and effectiveness through rigorous testing
Legal Considerations in AI Adoption	Compliance with data protection laws like GDPR, HIPAA, PIPEDA, DPA etc. is crucial for patient data privacy. Legal frameworks must clarify liability for adverse outcomes from AI use.
Ethical Use of AI in Healthcare	AI development must prioritize patient well-being, avoid biases, ensure transparency, and respect patient autonomy through informed consent.

Navigating the regulatory and legal landscape, we unravel the intricacies and dilemmas that accompany responsible AI adoption. This exploration sets the stage for a deeper dive into the practical challenges faced by healthcare organizations in implementing responsible AI.

2.5 Challenges in Implementing Responsible AI in Healthcare Settings

Figure 2 illustrates how incorporating artificial intelligence (AI) into healthcare could fundamentally transform medical service delivery. Nevertheless, deploying AI responsibly within healthcare environments poses significant challenges that must be tackled (Shaw & Goldfarb, 2019).

Figure 2. Challenges in implementing responsible AI in healthcare settings

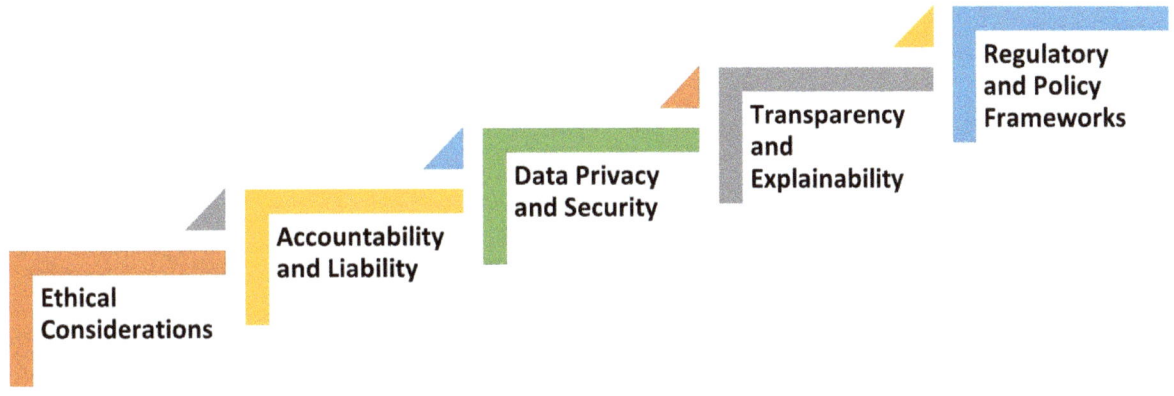

(Compiled by authors from review of literature)

2.5.1 Ethical Considerations

One of the primary challenges in executing responsible AI in healthcare is confirming ethical considerations are prioritized (Siala, & Wang, 2022). AI algorithms must be developed with clear guidelines to avoid biases and discrimination. The principle of beneficence, which emphasizes the promotion of patient well-being, should guide the development and implementation of AI technologies in healthcare settings. Sustaining patient confidence and guaranteeing the just and equitable application of AI depend heavily on upholding ethical norms.

2.5.2 Transparency and Explainability

As shown in Figure 2, another challenge in executing responsible AI in healthcare is the need for transparency and explainability (Arrieta, & Herrera, 2020). Healthcare providers and patients must have a clear grasp of how AI algorithms make decisions and recommendations. Fostering confidence and facilitating collaboration between healthcare professionals and patients is contingent upon transparency in the decision-making process of AI systems. Explainable AI offers a window into understanding the rationale behind the outputs generated by AI systems, enabling more accurate interpretation and validation of the results.

2.5.3 Data Privacy and Security

The responsible implementation of AI in healthcare also requires addressing data privacy and security concerns (Murdoch, 2021). AI systems rely on vast amounts of patient data for training and analysis. Compliance with data protection laws enforced by various countries is essential to safeguard patient privacy. Healthcare organizations must ensure that appropriate consent mechanisms, data anonymization techniques, and secure storage practices are in place to protect patient information from unauthorized access and breaches.

2.5.4 Accountability and Liability

Accountability and liability pose significant challenges in the implementation of responsible AI in healthcare. As AI systems make decisions that impact patient care, questions arise regarding who should be held accountable for adverse outcomes. As mentioned in figure 2 clear legal frameworks need to be established to define the roles and responsibilities of healthcare professionals, manufacturers, and regulatory bodies in the event of AI-related adverse events. This ensures that accountability is assigned appropriately and promotes the fair assessment of liability (Siala, & Wang, 2022).

2.5.5 Regulatory and Policy Frameworks

Figure 2 highlighted that Developing robust regulatory and policy frameworks is crucial for the responsible implementation of AI in healthcare settings (O'Sullivan, & Ashrafian, 2019). Regulatory bodies play a crucial role in establishing guidelines and standards for AI technologies in healthcare. These frameworks should address the safety, effectiveness, and reliability of AI systems, ensuring that they meet the necessary requirements before deployment.

Implementing responsible AI in healthcare settings presents various challenges as summaries in Figure 2 above, that must be overcome to ensure ethical and accountable practices, Addressing ethical considerations, promoting transparency and explainability, safeguarding data privacy and security, defining accountability and liability, and establishing robust regulatory and policy frameworks are essential steps towards responsible AI implementation in healthcare. By addressing these challenges, healthcare organizations can harness the full potential of AI while upholding patient trust, privacy, and well-being.

As we delve into the practical challenges, we confront issues such as data privacy, algorithmic bias, and organizational readiness. These challenges underscore the need for robust strategies and recommendations to facilitate successful adoption of responsible AI within healthcare organizations.

2.6 Future Directions and Recommendations for Successful Adoption of Responsible AI

The adoption of responsible artificial intelligence (AI) holds great promise for various industries, including healthcare, finance, and transportation. However, to ensure the successful implementation of responsible AI, it is crucial to identify future directions and provide recommendations for its adoption. Figure 3 below showed recommendations for Successful Adoption of Responsible AI in healthcare settings.

Figure 3. Recommendations for successful adoption of responsible AI

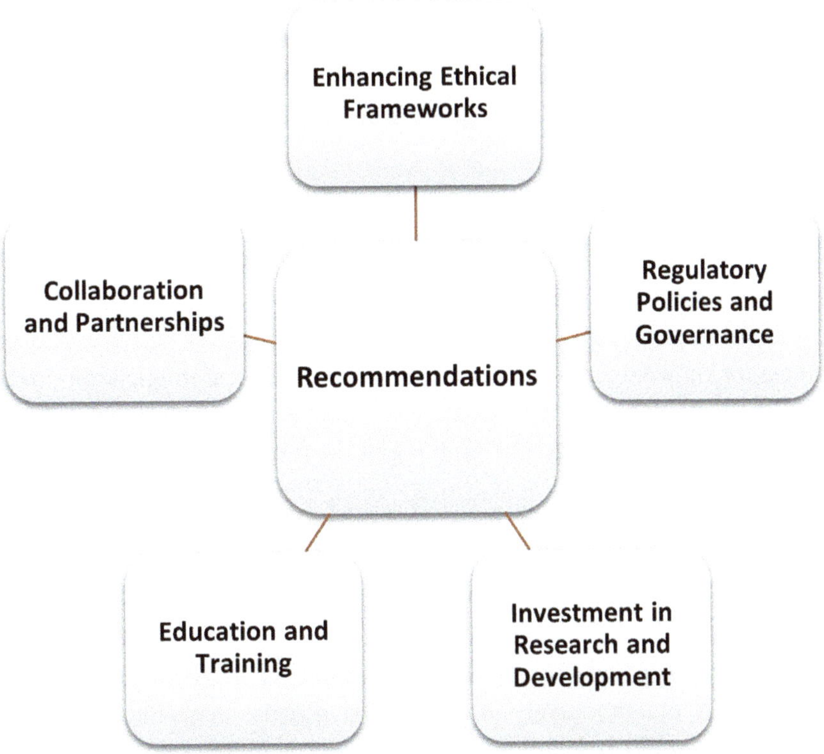

(Compiled by authors from review of literature)

2.6.1 Enhancing Ethical Frameworks

As shown in Figure 3, One important future direction for AI adoption is the enhancement of ethical frameworks (Ashok, & Sivarajah, 2022). To ensure accountability, openness, and fairness in the creation and use of AI systems, ethical issues should be integrated throughout the process. This can be achieved by establishing clear guidelines and standards that address potential biases, discrimination, and privacy concerns. Strengthening ethical frameworks will help build public trust and confidence in AI technologies.

2.6.2 Regulatory Policies and Governance

Another critical aspect for successful adoption of AI is the development of robust regulatory policies and governance structures (de Almeida, & Farias, 2021). Governments and regulatory bodies should collaborate with AI experts and stakeholders to create comprehensive guidelines and regulations that ensure the ethical and responsible use of AI. These policies should address issues related to data protection, algorithmic transparency, and accountability to mitigate potential risks and maintain societal acceptance.

2.6.3 Investment in Research and Development

Increasing investment in research and development is essential for the advancement of AI (Yigitcanlar, & Desouza, 2021). Funding agencies and organizations should allocate resources to support interdisciplinary research that explores the ethical, social, and legal implications of AI. This research should focus on developing innovative approaches, such as explainable AI and bias detection algorithms, to enhance the transparency and fairness of AI systems. By fostering research and development, we can drive the accountable adoption of AI.

2.6.4 Education and Training

To ensure the successful adoption of AI, there is a need for comprehensive education and training programs (Pedro, & Valverde, 2019). This includes equipping AI practitioners, policymakers, and end-users with the necessary knowledge and skills to understand the ethical implications and potential biases associated with AI. Educational initiatives should also emphasize the importance of continuous learning and staying updated with emerging AI technologies, as responsible AI adoption requires ongoing vigilance and expertise.

2.6.5 Collaboration and Partnerships

Promoting collaboration and partnerships between stakeholders is crucial for the successful adoption of accountable AI (Rakova, & Chowdhury, (2021). Governments, academia, industry, and civil society organizations should work collaboratively to establish standards, share best practices, and exchange knowledge. By fostering a multi-stakeholder approach, we can address complex challenges, leverage diverse perspectives, and ensure that AI adoption benefits all sectors of society.

The successful adoption of responsible AI requires careful consideration of future directions and the implementation of actionable recommendations as visually shown in Figure 3. Enhancing ethical frameworks, developing robust regulatory policies, increasing investment in research and development, providing education and training, and fostering collaboration and partnerships are key areas to focus on. By addressing these aspects, we can steer the adoption of responsible AI towards a future that is ethically sound, transparent, and beneficial for society as a whole.

Looking ahead, we outline strategies and recommendations to guide healthcare organizations in navigating the complexities of AI adoption. This sets the stage for a methodological overview, where we detail the process of reviewing ethical considerations in AI implementation.

3.0 METHODOLOGY

The methodology for studying the implementation of responsible AI in healthcare organizations involves a comprehensive and systematic approach that encompasses various research techniques and data collection sources.

To begin with, a thorough literature review will be conducted using reputable databases, academic journals, industry reports, and relevant publications, an extensive literature review will be conducted across reputable databases such as PubMed, IEEE Xplore, and Google Scholar. This review aims to gather foundational knowledge on Responsible AI applications in healthcare, encompassing peer-reviewed articles, industry reports, and whitepapers.

The literature review will focus on gathering insights into the strategies employed by healthcare organizations for implementing responsible AI. Keywords such as "responsible AI in healthcare," "ethical considerations in AI implementation," and "best practices for AI governance" will be used to ensure the retrieval of relevant and up-to-date information. The literature review will provide a foundation for understanding the current landscape of responsible AI implementation in healthcare and identify key strategies and challenges. Emphasis will be placed on accessing recent publications to capture the latest trends and advancements in the field.

To supplement the above data collected, real-world case studies of healthcare organizations that have successfully implemented responsible AI will be analyzed. These case studies will provide valuable insights into the best practices, lessons learned, and outcomes of responsible AI implementation. The analysis will involve examining the strategies employed, the challenges encountered, and the impact on patient care, workflow optimization, and overall organizational performance.

Providing transparency into our research approach, we detail the methodology employed in reviewing ethical considerations in AI implementation. This methodological overview segues seamlessly into an examination of Ethical Considerations in AI Implementation.

4.0 OVERVIEW OF RESPONSIBLE AI IMPLEMENTATION IN HEALTHCARE

This section explores the integration of AI within healthcare, emphasizing the need for ethical guidelines and the tangible benefits AI brings, such as enhanced diagnostic accuracy and operational efficiency.

4.1 Reviewing Ethical Considerations in AI Implementation

Artificial intelligence (AI) in healthcare has the potential to completely transform patient diagnosis, treatment, and care. However, as shown in Figure 4 below, it is imperative to establish ethical principles to govern the use of AI in healthcare settings.

Figure 4. Ethical considerations in AI implementation

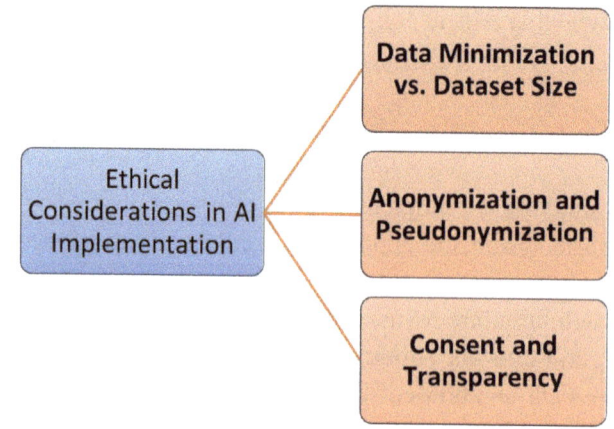

(Compiled by authors from review of literature)

1. **Data Minimization vs. Dataset Size:** GDPR, HIPPA, PIPEDA, DPA etc. mandates the principle of data minimization, dictating that businesses must only gather and use personal data as needed to fulfill a given purpose. However, AI algorithms often require large datasets for training to achieve optimal performance (Magrabi, & Georgiou, 2019). Healthcare providers face a dilemma in reconciling the need for extensive datasets with the requirement to minimize data collection, as gathering sufficient data without violating privacy regulations becomes challenging.
2. **Anonymization and Pseudonymization:** GDPR, HIPPA, PIPEDA, DPA etc. emphasize the importance of anonymizing or pseudonymizing personal data to protect individual privacy. While these techniques can help mitigate privacy risks, they may also hinder the utility of data for AI training (Pike, 2019). Anonymized or pseudonymized datasets may lack crucial individual-level information necessary for AI algorithms to make accurate predictions or diagnoses, thereby impacting the efficacy of AI applications in healthcare.
3. **Consent and Transparency:** GDPR, HIPPA, PIPEDA, DPA etc. mandates obtaining explicit consent from individuals for the processing of their personal data. However, ensuring informed consent for the use of healthcare data in AI applications can be complex (Nazer, & Mathur, 2023). Patients may not fully understand the implications of AI-driven decision-making or may feel hesitant to consent due to concerns about privacy or discrimination. Healthcare providers must navigate the challenge of obtaining meaningful consent while ensuring transparency about how AI technologies will utilize patient data.

Case Examples:

1. **AI-Powered Diagnostics:** Imagine a healthcare provider developing an AI system for diagnosing medical conditions based on imaging data. To train the AI model effectively, the provider needs access to a diverse and extensive dataset of medical images (Magrabi, & Georgiou, 2019). However, complying with the data minimization principle means that the provider must carefully select and anonymize images to avoid unnecessary data collection and protect patient privacy. This process

may limit the diversity and size of the training dataset, potentially impacting the accuracy and generalizability of the AI model.
2. **Clinical Research and AI:** In clinical research, AI technologies hold promise for analyzing large-scale patient data to identify trends, patterns, and potential treatment outcomes (Nazer, & Mathur, 2023). However, accessing and processing personal health data while adhering to government's stringent privacy requirements can pose significant challenges. Researchers must navigate complex consent processes, ensure data anonymization, and establish robust security measures to comply while harnessing the power of AI for medical research.

By critically examining these challenges and providing real-world examples, healthcare providers can gain a deeper understanding of the practical implications of balancing GDPR, HIPPA, PIPEDA, DPA etc. data privacy requirements with the demands of AI implementation in healthcare. This nuanced perspective can inform decision-making processes and guide the development of ethical and compliant AI solutions in the healthcare domain.Top of Form

Drawing on our methodology, we review the ethical considerations inherent in AI implementation, guiding responsible adoption practices. This ethical review paves the way for Identifying Strategies for Responsible AI Adoption in Healthcare Organizations

4.2 Identifying Strategies for Responsible AI Adoption in Healthcare Organizations

The integration of artificial intelligence (AI) has brought about significant advancements in various fields, including healthcare, finance, and transportation. However, the responsible implementation of AI is crucial to ensure its benefits outweigh potential risks and ethical concerns. Figure 5 summaries the Strategies for Responsible AI Adoption in Healthcare Organizations

Figure 5. Strategies for responsible AI adoption in healthcare organizations

Strategy 1:	Strategy 2:	Strategy 3	Strategy 4	Strategy 5
Ethical Frameworks and Guidelines	Robust Data Governance	Collaboration and Interdisciplinary Approaches	Continuous Monitoring and Evaluation	Public Engagement and Education

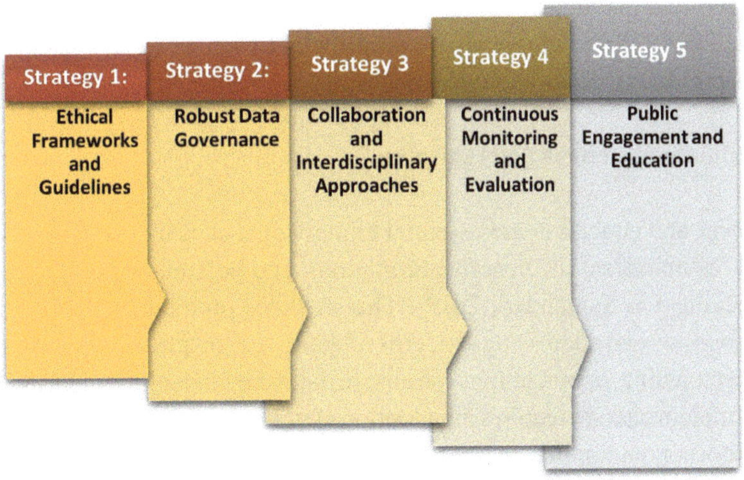

(Compiled by authors from review of literature)

Strategy 1: Ethical Frameworks and Guidelines

Developing comprehensive ethical frameworks and guidelines is essential when implementing AI systems. These frameworks should incorporate principles such as transparency, fairness, and accountability (Koene & Richardson, 2019). They should provide clear guidance on data privacy, algorithmic biases, and potential societal impacts. By adhering to ethical frameworks, organizations can ensure that AI is developed and deployed in a responsible and morally sound manner.

Strategy 2: Robust Data Governance

Data governance plays a critical role in responsible AI implementation. Organizations must establish robust processes for data collection, storage, and usage. As highlighted by Thapa, and Camtepe, (2021) this includes obtaining proper consent from individuals, ensuring data security and privacy, and implementing mechanisms for data anonymization and deletion. By prioritizing data governance, organizations can mitigate risks related to unauthorized access, data breaches, and privacy violations.

Strategy 3: Collaboration and Interdisciplinary Approaches

Responsible AI implementation requires collaboration between various stakeholders, including researchers, policymakers, and industry experts. Interdisciplinary approaches foster a holistic understanding of ethical, legal, and social implications (Amann & Precise4Q Consortium, 2020). By engaging in multidisciplinary discussions and knowledge-sharing, organizations can develop better-informed strategies and policies that address the complex challenges associated with AI implementation.

Strategy 4: Continuous Monitoring and Evaluation

Ongoing monitoring and evaluation are crucial to ensure the responsible use of AI. Organizations should establish mechanisms to assess the performance, fairness, and societal impact of AI systems. Regular audits can help identify algorithmic biases, unintended consequences, and potential risks (Koshiyama & Chatterjee, 2024). By continuously monitoring and evaluating AI systems, organizations can proactively address ethical concerns and make necessary adjustments.

Strategy 5: Public Engagement and Education

Public engagement and education are essential components of responsible AI implementation. Organizations should communicate the benefits, limitations, and potential risks associated with AI to the general public (Cheatham & Samandari, 2019). This includes promoting transparency in algorithmic decision-making processes and addressing concerns related to job displacement and privacy. By fostering public trust and understanding, organizations can ensure the acceptance and ethical use of AI technologies.

Responsible AI implementation requires the adoption of strategies that prioritize ethics, data governance, collaboration, monitoring, and public engagement. By developing comprehensive ethical frameworks, establishing robust data governance processes, promoting interdisciplinary approaches, and engaging in continuous evaluation, organizations can navigate the challenges associated with AI implementation.

Moreover, public engagement and education are crucial for building trust and ensuring the ethical and responsible use of AI technologies.

Through a comprehensive assessment, we identify strategies for responsible AI adoption and evaluate their potential impact. This assessment sets the stage for a deeper exploration of assessment of the impact of responsible AI on patient outcomes and operational efficiency.

4.3 Assessing the Impact of Responsible AI on Patient Outcomes and Operational Efficiency

In recent years, the advancements in artificial intelligence (AI) have revolutionized various industries, including healthcare. The integration of AI in healthcare settings has shown promising potential to improve patient outcomes and operational efficiency.

4.3.1 Patient Outcomes

AI holds great promise in enhancing patient outcomes through various applications. One notable area is the use of AI algorithms in early disease detection and diagnosis. For instance, studies by Kaur, and Islam, (2020) have demonstrated the effectiveness of AI-based systems in detecting early signs of diseases such as cancer and cardiovascular conditions. The timely identification of these diseases can lead to earlier interventions, thereby improving patient prognosis.

AI can also help medical providers create individualized treatment programs. Artificial intelligence (AI) systems can spot trends and forecast the best course of action for each patient by evaluating enormous volumes of medical data. This strategy can reduce side effects while increasing therapy efficacy.

4.3.2 Operational Efficiency

In addition to enhancing patient outcomes, AI can significantly enhance operational efficiency in healthcare settings. One key aspect is the automation of administrative tasks, such as appointment scheduling and data entry. Studies have shown that AI-powered systems can streamline processes, reducing the burden on healthcare staff and enabling them to allocate more time to direct patient care (Ogunsakin & Anwansedo, 2024).

Another area where AI can optimize operational efficiency is in resource allocation. By analyzing patient data, AI algorithms can predict demand for healthcare services, enabling healthcare facilities to allocate resources effectively. This proactive approach can minimize waiting times, optimize staff utilization, and enhance overall operational performance.

Through a comprehensive assessment, we identify strategies for responsible AI adoption and evaluate their potential impact. This assessment sets the stage for a deeper exploration of case studies and best practices in healthcare AI implementation.

5.0 CASE STUDIES AND BEST PRACTICES IN HEALTHCARE AI IMPLEMENTATION

The application of artificial intelligence (AI) in healthcare could transform the way that patients are diagnosed, treated, and cared for. Nonetheless, a thorough analysis of case studies and best practices is necessary for the effective implementation of AI in healthcare.

Case Study 1: AI-Assisted Diagnostic Systems

In the pioneering work of Hosny and Aerts (2018), AI algorithms showcased their potential to revolutionize diagnostic processes in radiology. Initially, their integration into diagnostic workflows yielded promising outcomes, significantly reducing interpretation time and enhancing diagnostic accuracy. This collaboration between AI systems and radiologists fostered a symbiotic relationship, augmenting human expertise with analytical capabilities. However, challenges emerged during implementation. Integrating AI into existing healthcare systems posed technical complexities, requiring extensive modifications and compliance with data protection regulations. Moreover, user resistance surfaced, with some radiologists expressing concerns about reliance on AI and potential errors. Addressing these challenges demanded collaborative efforts. Healthcare organizations navigated technical hurdles by fostering interdisciplinary collaboration and adhering to regulatory standards. They also conducted comprehensive training programs to mitigate user resistance and ensure healthcare professionals were equipped to leverage AI effectively.

Ultimately, the case study underscores the transformative potential of AI in radiology. By overcoming challenges through collaboration, innovation, and education, healthcare professionals can harness AI to optimize diagnostic processes, improve patient care, and drive positive outcomes.

Case Study 2: Predictive Analytics for Patient Monitoring

In Alamgir and Shah's (2021) study, predictive analytics demonstrated its potential to enhance patient monitoring and safety. Initially promising, challenges arose during implementation. Ensuring high-quality data proved difficult, leading to potential inaccuracies in predictions. Integrating AI predictions into clinical workflows required clear protocols to prevent misinterpretation of insights. Furthermore, user resistance necessitated comprehensive training programs to instill confidence in AI technologies. Therefore, predictive analytics offers valuable insights for healthcare professionals, but its successful implementation requires addressing challenges such as data quality, integration protocols, and user resistance. By overcoming these obstacles, healthcare providers can leverage predictive analytics to improve patient outcomes and enhance overall healthcare delivery.

Best Practice 1: Ensuring Ethical Considerations

Ethical considerations are crucial in AI implementation. It is essential to prioritize patient privacy, data security, and algorithmic transparency. For instance, the importance of obtaining informed consent, anonymizing patient data, and regularly auditing AI algorithms to identify and mitigate any biases or discrimination is emphasized (Khanna & Srivastava, 2020). Additionally, healthcare organizations should establish ethical review boards that oversee the development and deployment of AI systems to ensure responsible and equitable use.

Best Practice 2: Collaborative Partnerships

Successful AI implementation in healthcare requires collaborative partnerships between healthcare providers, technology developers, and regulatory bodies. For instance, the significance of multidisciplinary teams consisting of clinicians, data scientists, and AI experts is highlighted. These teams can collectively design and implement AI solutions that align with clinical needs while adhering to regulatory guidelines (Martín-Noguerol & Luna, 2021). Collaboration also enables the sharing of best practices and lessons learned, fostering continuous improvement in AI implementation.

Best Practice 3: Continuous Evaluation and Improvement

Continuous evaluation and improvement are essential for the long-term success of AI implementation in healthcare. Establishing feedback loops that involve collecting feedback from healthcare professionals, patients, and other stakeholders is recommended (Gelkopf & Roe, 2022). This feedback can inform iterative improvements, addressing any limitations or challenges encountered during the implementation process. Regular evaluation and monitoring of AI systems are crucial to ensure their ongoing effectiveness and alignment with evolving clinical needs.

Through a review of case studies and best practices related to the application of AI in healthcare, we can extract insightful information and provide strategies for effective adoption. The most important things to think about are collaborative collaborations, ongoing review, improvement, and ethical issues. A multidisciplinary strategy combining tight cooperation between medical practitioners, technology developers, and regulatory agencies is needed to implement AI in healthcare. Healthcare institutions can use AI to enhance patient outcomes and progress medical research by adhering to these best practices.

Drawing insights from real-world case studies, we assess the impact of responsible AI on patient care and operational efficiency. This examination leads us to explore applications of Responsible AI within healthcare settings.

5.1 Applications of Responsible AI in Healthcare

The utilization of responsible artificial intelligence (AI) in healthcare has become increasingly significant in recent years.

5.1.1 AI in Diagnostics and Disease Detection

AI has the power to completely transform medical diagnosis and illness detection. Studies demonstrate how AI algorithms can improve the precision and effectiveness of diagnostic procedures (Mirbabaie & Frick, 2021). Artificial intelligence (AI) technologies can help medical personnel detect possible anomalies and diseases by evaluating medical imaging data. Better treatment results, early identification, and ultimately better patient care can result from this.

5.1.2 Personalized Medicine and Treatment Planning

Treatment planning and tailored medicine may be made possible by the incorporation of AI into healthcare systems. Artificial intelligence (AI) algorithms can find patterns and connections in patient data that may be difficult for human healthcare providers to notice. Research highlights how AI can be used to customize treatment regimens for each patient, taking into account lifestyle decisions, medical history, and genetic predispositions (Golombek & Lammers, 2018). This may result in more focused and efficient treatment plans, improving the results for patients.

5.1.3 AI for Remote Patient Monitoring

The advent of AI has paved the way for remote patient monitoring, particularly in the context of telemedicine. The potential of AI-powered wearable devices and remote monitoring systems in collecting real-time patient data is highlighted (Rath & Kar, 2024). AI algorithms can analyze this data, providing insights into patient health status, detecting anomalies, and alerting healthcare providers when intervention is required. This facilitates proactive and personalized healthcare delivery, especially for individuals with chronic conditions or those residing in remote areas.

5.1.4 AI-Augmented Decision Support Systems

By incorporating AI algorithms into clinical decision-making processes, artificial intelligence (AI) can significantly improve decision support systems in the healthcare industry (Magrabi & Georgiou, 2019). AI systems have the ability to analyze patient data, treatment guidelines, and medical literature to deliver healthcare practitioners evidence-based suggestions. Better patient outcomes may result from increased decision-making efficiency and accuracy.

5.1.5 Ensuring Ethical Considerations in AI

The ethical issues surrounding the use of AI in healthcare must be addressed as it becomes more widespread. It is recommended to create explainable AI models that offer decision-making transparency (Kim & Suh, 2020). Jones and Davis (2020) also stress the necessity of regulatory frameworks and standards to guarantee ethical and responsible AI usage. It is imperative that these frameworks tackle concerns like algorithmic bias, data privacy, and accountability in order to protect patient rights and maintain confidence in AI technology.

The ethical use of AI in healthcare has the potential to significantly improve patient care and the delivery of healthcare services. AI may improve the precision, effectiveness, and accessibility of healthcare services in a variety of ways, from decision support systems and remote patient monitoring to diagnostics and tailored treatment. To guarantee responsible AI application, it is imperative to address ethical issues, advance transparency, and create regulatory frameworks. Healthcare firms may effectively exploit the benefits of AI by keeping up with current trends and breakthroughs in responsible AI, as the field continues to expand.

From here, we engage with stakeholders to understand their perspectives on responsible AI integration.

5.2 Exploring Stakeholder Perspectives on Responsible AI Integration

The integration of responsible artificial intelligence (AI) has garnered significant attention in recent years, as stakeholders recognize its potential to shape various industries. Stakeholders involved in the integration of responsible AI include policymakers, industry leaders, researchers, and end-users. Each stakeholder group brings unique perspectives and considerations to the discourse.

Policymakers play a crucial role in shaping the regulatory framework for responsible AI integration. Studies by Floridi, and & Vayena, (2018) emphasize the need for policymakers to strike a balance between encouraging innovation and ensuring ethical use of AI. Policymakers must address concerns regarding privacy, bias, and accountability to safeguard societal interests.

Industry leaders, on the other hand, are primarily focused on the business implications of responsible AI integration. Research by Tariq, and Abonamah, (2021) highlights the potential for cost savings, improved productivity, and competitive advantage through responsible AI adoption. However, industry leaders also recognize the importance of addressing ethical considerations and building trust with customers.

Researchers contribute to the discourse by exploring the technical aspects of responsible AI. Studies by Coglianese, and Lehr, (2019) delve into algorithmic transparency, fairness, and interpretability. Researchers highlight the need for robust methodologies and standards to ensure the responsible development and deployment of AI systems.

End-users, including healthcare professionals and consumers, offer critical perspectives on the real-world impacts of integrating AI responsibly. Research by Asan and Choudhury (2020) indicates that healthcare workers are generally hopeful about AI's ability to enhance patient outcomes. Nonetheless, they also express concerns about potential job losses and the diminishing presence of human interaction in patient care.

Implications for Stakeholders:

The integration of responsible AI carries implications for different stakeholder groups. Policymakers must develop comprehensive regulations and frameworks that balance innovation and ethical use. Industry leaders must invest in responsible AI practices, ensuring transparency, fairness, and accountability. Researchers should continue to explore technical aspects and contribute to the development of responsible AI methodologies. End-users should actively engage in discussions to shape responsible AI integration, addressing concerns while embracing the potential benefits.

We examine stakeholder perspectives on the incorporation of responsible AI in healthcare settings, capturing a range of opinions. This prepares the groundwork for offering suggestions to lawmakers and healthcare institutions.

5.3 Recommendations for Healthcare Organizations and Policymakers

The incorporation of responsible artificial intelligence (AI) has become a hot topic in the quickly changing healthcare industry. A summary of the recommendations for healthcare organizations and policymakers was provided in Table 2.

5.3.1 Foster a Culture of Ethical AI

The creation of an environment that supports moral AI practices needs to be a top priority for healthcare institutions and legislators. To do this, precise policies and procedures must be developed for the appropriate application of AI in healthcare environments. Studies highlight how crucial it is for AI algorithms and decision-making processes to be transparent, equitable, and accountable (Akinrinola & Ugochukwu, 2024). Healthcare institutions may foster trust with patients, healthcare providers, and the community at large by upholding ethical standards.

5.3.2 Invest in Data Governance and Privacy

The responsible integration of AI necessitates robust data governance and privacy frameworks. Healthcare systems and policymakers must prioritize the protection of patient data while ensuring its accessibility for AI-driven insights. Studies highlight the need for comprehensive data privacy policies and secure data-sharing protocols (Silva & Soto, 2022). To keep patients' trust and adhere to legal obligations, it's critical to strike a balance between data protection and use.

5.3.3 Promote Collaboration and Interdisciplinary Research

Collaboration across a range of stakeholders, including healthcare organizations, researchers, legislators, and technology developers, is necessary for the successful integration of AI in healthcare. Deeper knowledge of the implications of AI in healthcare settings and creative solutions can result from supporting interdisciplinary research initiatives and building partnerships. Research emphasizes the importance of shared knowledge and expertise to address complex challenges associated with AI integration (Olan & Jayawickrama, 2022).

5.3.4 Prioritize Explainability and Interpretability

AI algorithms need to be understandable and comprehensible in order to win over patients' and healthcare professionals' trust. The creation of AI models that offer comprehensive justifications for decisions should be given top priority by healthcare institutions and governments. This transparency is crucial in healthcare, where the ability to understand and validate AI-generated insights is paramount. Studies highlight the importance of explainable AI in clinical decision support systems and personalized medicine (Pierce & Sterckx, 2022).

5.3.5 Address Algorithm Bias and Fairness

Policymakers and healthcare institutions need to overcome algorithm bias in AI systems in order to guarantee equitable healthcare outcomes. The data used to train AI systems may contain bias, which could result in differences in patient outcomes, diagnosis, and therapy. It is important to thoroughly assess and keep an eye on AI algorithms to identify and minimize bias. Research by Kordzadeh and Ghasemaghaei (2022) emphasizes the need for representative and diverse datasets to lessen algorithmic bias.

5.3.6 Continuous Training and Education

To improve healthcare professionals' AI literacy, policymakers and healthcare institutions need to make ongoing investments in education and training initiatives. The development of implementation skills for AI, the interpretation of insights produced by AI, and ethical issues should be the main focuses of training programs. The integration of AI in healthcare can be maximized for the benefit of patients and the healthcare system overall by providing healthcare personnel with the required knowledge and abilities.

A multidisciplinary strategy involving healthcare organizations, policymakers, researchers, and technology developers is necessary for the responsible integration of AI in healthcare. By tackling algorithm bias, establishing an ethical AI culture, emphasizing data governance and privacy, encouraging cooperation, and developing a culture of ethics, we can realize the potential of AI in healthcare while reducing dangers. To tackle the challenges of integrating AI, healthcare workers need continuous education and training. Our combined efforts have the potential to improve patient outcomes and healthcare delivery through responsible AI integration.

Table 2. Recommendations for healthcare organizations and policymakers

Recommendation	Summary
Foster a Culture of Ethical AI	Establish clear guidelines for ethical AI practices emphasizing transparency, fairness, and accountability to build trust among stakeholders.
Invest in Data Governance and Privacy	Prioritize protecting patient data while ensuring accessibility for AI insights through comprehensive data privacy policies and secure data-sharing protocols.
Promote Collaboration and Interdisciplinary Research	Encourage collaboration among stakeholders to drive innovative solutions and deeper understanding of AI implications in healthcare.
Prioritize Explainability and Interpretability	Develop AI models that provide clear explanations for decisions to gain trust in clinical settings, emphasizing transparency and validation of AI-generated insights.
Address Algorithm Bias and Fairness	Identify and mitigate bias in AI systems through diverse datasets and ongoing evaluation to ensure equitable healthcare outcomes, minimizing disparities in diagnosis and treatment.
Continuous Training and Education	Invest in training programs to enhance AI literacy among healthcare professionals, focusing on implementation, interpretation of insights, and ethical considerations.

Based on stakeholder insights, we provide healthcare organizations and policymakers with actionable advice on how to integrate AI responsibly. We then consider potential developments and paths in ethical AI for healthcare institutions.

5.4 Future Trends and Directions in Responsible AI for Healthcare Organizations

An increasingly important problem is the integration of appropriate artificial intelligence (AI) in healthcare organizations. The trends and directions in responsible AI for healthcare organizations are depicted in Figure 6.

Figure 6. Trends and directions in responsible AI for healthcare organizations

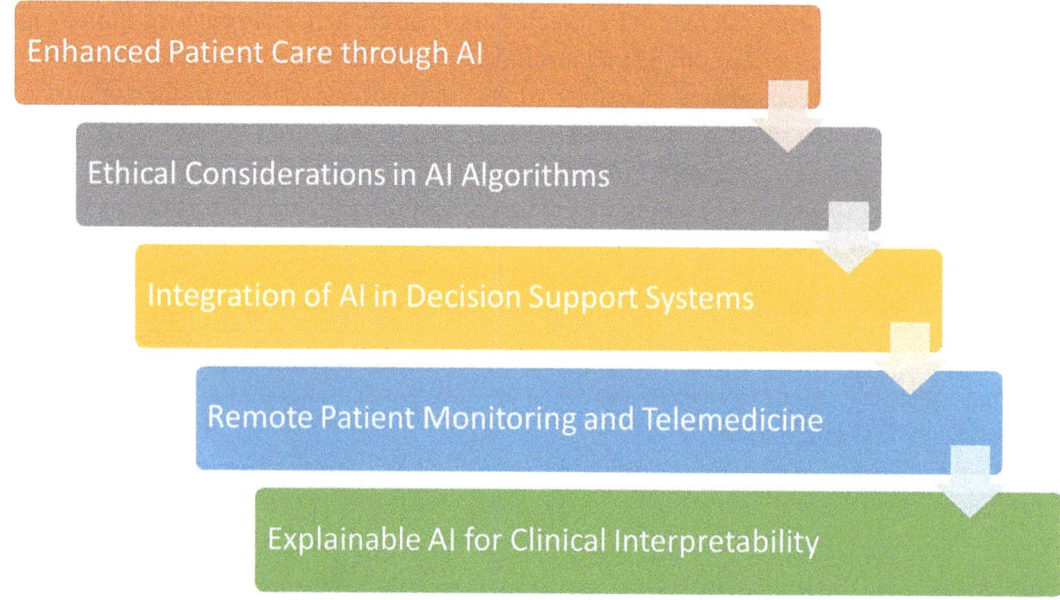

- Enhanced Patient Care through AI
- Ethical Considerations in AI Algorithms
- Integration of AI in Decision Support Systems
- Remote Patient Monitoring and Telemedicine
- Explainable AI for Clinical Interpretability

(Compiled by authors from review of literature)

5.4.1 Enhanced Patient Care Through AI

By enhancing patient monitoring, tailored treatment regimens, and diagnostic accuracy, artificial intelligence (AI) has the potential to completely transform healthcare. Studies demonstrate how AI can improve patient outcomes, decrease errors, and streamline clinical procedures (Alowais & Albekairy, 2023). Healthcare companies can fully realize the benefits of patient-centered care by utilizing AI technologies like machine learning and natural language processing.

5.4.2 Ethical Considerations in AI Algorithms

It is critical that healthcare institutions address ethical issues as AI algorithms advance in sophistication. It is critical to guarantee accountability, equity, and transparency in AI systems. Konda (2022) emphasizes the crucial importance of establishing ethical frameworks that guide the development and implementation of AI algorithms. This entails dealing with concerns including informed consent, privacy, and bias.

5.4.3 Integration of AI in Decision Support Systems

AI-powered decision-support systems may be able to assist medical practitioners in making sensible clinical decisions. These systems can analyze massive amounts of patient data, medical publications, and treatment manuals to provide evidence-based recommendations. Studies demonstrate how important it is to integrate artificial intelligence (AI) into decision-support systems in order to improve accuracy, effectiveness, and patient safety.

5.4.4 Remote Patient Monitoring and Telemedicine

The COVID-19 pandemic has expedited the uptake of telemedicine and remote patient monitoring. Wearable technology and remote monitoring platforms are examples of AI-powered products that can speed up data collection and processing in real time. Wearable technology and remote monitoring platforms highlight how AI can identify early warning indicators, forecast the course of diseases, and facilitate prompt interventions. We can incorporate artificial intelligence (AI) into remote healthcare delivery to enhance patient outcomes and care access (Silva & Soto, 2022). When used in remote healthcare delivery, AI integration has the potential to improve patient outcomes and access to care.

5.4.5 Explainable AI for Clinical Interpretability

Clinical interpretability is becoming more and more important as AI algorithms get more complicated. Healthcare organizations must prioritize the creation of explainable AI models, as they provide clear insights into the decision-making process, potentially enhancing professional trust and fostering collaborative decision-making. Healthcare practitioners can make better clinical decisions if they comprehend the underlying reasoning behind AI-generated recommendations.

5.4.6 Regulatory Frameworks and Standards

To establishment of standards and regulatory frameworks is necessary to guarantee the responsible application of AI in healthcare. These frameworks ought to cover topics like accountability, algorithmic transparency, and data privacy. In order to create thorough rules, cooperation between regulatory agencies, legislators, and healthcare organizations is essential (Kroenke & Sullivan, 2019). By following these principles, healthcare businesses can successfully overcome the ethical and legal barriers to integrating AI.

We consider new trends and directions in responsible AI for healthcare businesses. This brings us to our conclusion, where we enumerate the most important discoveries, realizations, and consequences.

CONCLUSION

The use of conscientious artificial intelligence (AI) in healthcare establishments has the potential to completely transform the provision of medical services. Artificial intelligence (AI) technology can improve disease diagnosis, treatment planning, medication development, and patient monitoring by utilizing sophisticated algorithms and machine learning models. This leads to improved patient outcomes and quality of life.

Nonetheless, there are certain difficulties involved with integrating ethical AI in the medical field. Crucial tasks include ensuring algorithmic fairness, addressing prejudice in data and models, upholding accountability and openness, and overcoming moral and legal dilemmas. Biased AI systems can sustain inequalities in access to and quality of healthcare. Therefore, it is imperative to address bias and guarantee equity for a range of patient demographics. We must handle security and privacy issues for healthcare data, as breaches can have serious repercussions. Furthermore, navigating the legal and ethical waters around AI adds another layer of complexity to the implementation process.

We need to develop strategies to overcome these obstacles. In order to give patients and healthcare professionals access to information about AI decision-making and underlying data, transparency and explainability are essential. Fairness and bias mitigation should be the top priorities when creating AI algorithms, aiming to reduce biases and promote equitable healthcare outcomes. We should protect patient data by implementing privacy and data security procedures. Enacting explicit accountability protocols and regulatory frameworks is vital to overseeing the conscientious application of artificial intelligence in healthcare.

It is imperative that regulators, legislators, technology developers, and healthcare providers work together. By implementing ethical AI policies, healthcare companies can optimize AI's advantages while lowering risks and biases. Healthcare may benefit from using AI responsibly by utilizing sophisticated algorithms and machine learning models, which will ultimately improve patient care, advance clinical decision-making, and advance fair healthcare delivery.

REFERENCES

Akinrinola, O., Okoye, C. C., Ofodile, O. C., & Ugochukwu, C. E. (2024). Navigating and reviewing ethical dilemmas in AI development: Strategies for transparency, fairness, and accountability. *GSC Advanced Research and Reviews, 18*(3), 050-058.

Alamgir, A., Mousa, O., & Shah, Z. (2021). Artificial intelligence in predicting cardiac arrest: Scoping review. *JMIR Medical Informatics*, 9(12), e30798. DOI: 10.2196/30798 PMID: 34927595

Alowais, S. A., Alghamdi, S. S., Alsuhebany, N., Alqahtani, T., Alshaya, A. I., Almohareb, S. N., Aldairem, A., Alrashed, M., Bin Saleh, K., Badreldin, H. A., Al Yami, M. S., Al Harbi, S., & Albekairy, A. M. (2023). Revolutionizing healthcare: The role of artificial intelligence in clinical practice. *BMC Medical Education*, 23(1), 689. DOI: 10.1186/s12909-023-04698-z PMID: 37740191

Amann, J., Blasimme, A., Vayena, E., Frey, D., & Madai, V. I. (2020). Explainability for artificial intelligence in healthcare: A multidisciplinary perspective. *BMC Medical Informatics and Decision Making*, 20(1), 1–9. DOI: 10.1186/s12911-020-01332-6 PMID: 33256715

Arrieta, A. B., Díaz-Rodríguez, N., Del Ser, J., Bennetot, A., Tabik, S., Barbado, A., & Herrera, F. (2020). Explainable Artificial Intelligence (XAI): Concepts, taxonomies, opportunities and challenges toward responsible AI. *Information Fusion*, 58, 82–115. DOI: 10.1016/j.inffus.2019.12.012

Asan, O., Bayrak, A. E., & Choudhury, A. (2020). Artificial intelligence and human trust in healthcare: Focus on clinicians. *Journal of Medical Internet Research*, 22(6), e15154. DOI: 10.2196/15154 PMID: 32558657

Ashok, M., Madan, R., Joha, A., & Sivarajah, U. (2022). Ethical framework for Artificial Intelligence and Digital technologies. *International Journal of Information Management*, 62, 102433. DOI: 10.1016/j.ijinfomgt.2021.102433

Cheatham, B., Javanmardian, K., & Samandari, H. (2019). Confronting the risks of artificial intelligence. *The McKinsey Quarterly*, 2(38), 1–9.

Coglianese, C., & Lehr, D. (2019). Transparency and algorithmic governance. *Administrative Law Review*, 71(1), 1–56.

de Almeida, P. G. R., dos Santos, C. D., & Farias, J. S. (2021). Artificial intelligence regulation: A framework for governance. *Ethics and Information Technology*, 23(3), 505–525.

Floridi, L., Cowls, J., Beltrametti, M., Chatila, R., Chazerand, P., Dignum, V., Luetge, C., Madelin, R., Pagallo, U., Rossi, F., Schafer, B., Valcke, P., & Vayena, E. (2018). AI4People—an ethical framework for a good AI society: Opportunities, risks, principles, and recommendations. *Minds and Machines*, 28(4), 689–707. DOI: 10.1007/s11023-018-9482-5 PMID: 30930541

Gelkopf, M., Mazor, Y., & Roe, D. (2022). A systematic review of patient-reported outcome measurement (PROM) and provider assessment in mental health: Goals, implementation, setting, measurement characteristics and barriers. *International Journal for Quality in Health Care : Journal of the International Society for Quality in Health Care*, 34(Supplement_1), ii13–ii27. DOI: 10.1093/intqhc/mzz133 PMID: 32159763

Ginter, P. M., Duncan, W. J., & Swayne, L. E. (2018). *The strategic management of health care organizations*. john wiley & sons.

Golombek, S. K., May, J. N., Theek, B., Appold, L., Drude, N., Kiessling, F., & Lammers, T. (2018). Tumor targeting via EPR: Strategies to enhance patient responses. *Advanced Drug Delivery Reviews*, 130, 17–38.

Greenwood-Lee, J., Jewett, L., Woodhouse, L., & Marshall, D. A. (2018). A categorisation of problems and solutions to improve patient referrals from primary to specialty care. *BMC Health Services Research*, 18(1), 1–16. DOI: 10.1186/s12913-018-3745-y PMID: 30572898

Haleem, A., Javaid, M., Singh, R. P., & Suman, R. (2022). Medical 4.0 technologies for healthcare: Features, capabilities, and applications. *Internet of Things and Cyber-Physical Systems*, 2, 12–30. DOI: 10.1016/j.iotcps.2022.04.001

Hosny, A., Parmar, C., Quackenbush, J., Schwartz, L. H., & Aerts, H. J. (2018). Artificial intelligence in radiology. *Nature Reviews. Cancer*, 18(8), 500–510. DOI: 10.1038/s41568-018-0016-5 PMID: 29777175

Kaur, S., Singla, J., Nkenyereye, L., Jha, S., Prashar, D., Joshi, G. P., El-Sappagh, S., Islam, M. S., & Islam, S. R. (2020). Medical diagnostic systems using artificial intelligence (ai) algorithms: Principles and perspectives. *IEEE Access : Practical Innovations, Open Solutions*, 8, 228049–228069. DOI: 10.1109/ACCESS.2020.3042273

Khanna, S., & Srivastava, S. (2020). Patient-centric ethical frameworks for privacy, transparency, and bias awareness in deep learning-based medical systems. *Applied Research in Artificial Intelligence and Cloud Computing*, 3(1), 16–35.

Kim, B., Park, J., & Suh, J. (2020). Transparency and accountability in AI decision support: Explaining and visualizing convolutional neural networks for text information. *Decision Support Systems*, 134, 113302. DOI: 10.1016/j.dss.2020.113302

Koene, A., Clifton, C., Hatada, Y., Webb, H., & Richardson, R. (2019). A governance framework for algorithmic accountability and transparency.

Konda, S. R. (2022). Ethical Considerations in the Development and Deployment of AI-Driven Software Systems. *INTERNATIONAL JOURNAL OF COMPUTER SCIENCE AND TECHNOLOGY*, 6(3), 86–101.

Kordzadeh, N., & Ghasemaghaei, M. (2022). Algorithmic bias: Review, synthesis, and future research directions. *European Journal of Information Systems*, 31(3), 388–409. DOI: 10.1080/0960085X.2021.1927212

Koshiyama, A., Kazim, E., Treleaven, P., Rai, P., Szpruch, L., Pavey, G., Ahamat, G., Leutner, F., Goebel, R., Knight, A., Adams, J., Hitrova, C., Barnett, J., Nachev, P., Barber, D., Chamorro-Premuzic, T., Klemmer, K., Gregorovic, M., Khan, S., & Chatterjee, S. (2024). Towards algorithm auditing: Managing legal, ethical and technological risks of AI, ML and associated algorithms. *Royal Society Open Science*, 11(5), 230859. DOI: 10.1098/rsos.230859 PMID: 39076787

Kroenke, K., Alford, D. P., Argoff, C., Canlas, B., Covington, E., Frank, J. W., Haake, K. J., Hanling, S., Hooten, W. M., Kertesz, S. G., Kravitz, R. L., Krebs, E. E., Stanos, S. P.Jr, & Sullivan, M. (2019). Challenges with implementing the centers for disease control and prevention opioid guideline: A consensus panel report. *Pain Medicine*, 20(4), 724–735. DOI: 10.1093/pm/pny307 PMID: 30690556

Magrabi, F., Ammenwerth, E., McNair, J. B., De Keizer, N. F., Hyppönen, H., Nykänen, P., & Georgiou, A. (2019). Artificial intelligence in clinical decision support: Challenges for evaluating AI and practical implications. *Yearbook of Medical Informatics*, 28(01), 128–134.

Magrabi, F., Ammenwerth, E., McNair, J. B., De Keizer, N. F., Hyppönen, H., Nykänen, P., Rigby, M., Scott, P. J., Vehko, T., Wong, Z. S.-Y., & Georgiou, A. (2019). Artificial intelligence in clinical decision support: Challenges for evaluating AI and practical implications. *Yearbook of Medical Informatics*, 28(01), 128–134. DOI: 10.1055/s-0039-1677903 PMID: 31022752

Magrabi, F., Ammenwerth, E., McNair, J. B., De Keizer, N. F., Hyppönen, H., Nykänen, P., Rigby, M., Scott, P. J., Vehko, T., Wong, Z. S.-Y., & Georgiou, A. (2019). Artificial intelligence in clinical decision support: Challenges for evaluating AI and practical implications. *Yearbook of Medical Informatics*, 28(01), 128–134. DOI: 10.1055/s-0039-1677903 PMID: 31022752

Martín-Noguerol, T., Paulano-Godino, F., López-Ortega, R., Górriz, J. M., Riascos, R. F., & Luna, A. (2021). Artificial intelligence in radiology: Relevance of collaborative work between radiologists and engineers for building a multidisciplinary team. *Clinical Radiology*, 76(5), 317–324. DOI: 10.1016/j.crad.2020.11.113 PMID: 33358195

Mirbabaie, M., Stieglitz, S., & Frick, N. R. (2021). Artificial intelligence in disease diagnostics: A critical review and classification on the current state of research guiding future direction. *Health and Technology*, 11(4), 693–731.

Murdoch, B. (2021). Privacy and artificial intelligence: Challenges for protecting health information in a new era. *BMC Medical Ethics*, 22(1), 1–5. DOI: 10.1186/s12910-021-00687-3 PMID: 34525993

Nazer, L. H., Zatarah, R., Waldrip, S., Ke, J. X. C., Moukheiber, M., Khanna, A. K., Hicklen, R. S., Moukheiber, L., Moukheiber, D., Ma, H., & Mathur, P. (2023). Bias in artificial intelligence algorithms and recommendations for mitigation. *PLOS Digital Health*, 2(6), e0000278. DOI: 10.1371/journal.pdig.0000278 PMID: 37347721

O'Sullivan, S., Nevejans, N., Allen, C., Blyth, A., Leonard, S., Pagallo, U., Holzinger, K., Holzinger, A., Sajid, M. I., & Ashrafian, H. (2019). Legal, regulatory, and ethical frameworks for development of standards in artificial intelligence (AI) and autonomous robotic surgery. *International Journal of Medical Robotics and Computer Assisted Surgery*, 15(1), e1968. DOI: 10.1002/rcs.1968 PMID: 30397993

Ogunsakin, O. L., & Anwansedo, S. (2024). Leveraging Ai For Healthcare Administration: Streamlining Operations And Reducing Costs.

Olan, F., Arakpogun, E. O., Suklan, J., Nakpodia, F., Damij, N., & Jayawickrama, U. (2022). Artificial intelligence and knowledge sharing: Contributing factors to organizational performance. *Journal of Business Research*, 145, 605–615. DOI: 10.1016/j.jbusres.2022.03.008

Oleka-Onyewuchi, C. N. C. (2023). *The New Workforce Reality: Embracing Intergenerational Collaboration That Thrives in the Age of Automation and Layoffs*. Gatekeeper Press.

Pedro, F., Subosa, M., Rivas, A., & Valverde, P. (2019). Artificial intelligence in education: Challenges and opportunities for sustainable development.

Pickering, B. (2021). Trust, but verify: Informed consent, AI technologies, and public health emergencies. *Future Internet*, 13(5), 132.

Pickering, B. (2021). Trust, but verify: Informed consent, AI technologies, and public health emergencies. *Future Internet*, 13(5), 132. DOI: 10.3390/fi13050132

Pierce, R. L., Van Biesen, W., Van Cauwenberge, D., Decruyenaere, J., & Sterckx, S. (2022). Explainability in medicine in an era of AI-based clinical decision support systems. *Frontiers in Genetics*, 13, 903600. DOI: 10.3389/fgene.2022.903600 PMID: 36199569

Pike, E. R. (2019). Defending data: Toward ethical protections and comprehensive data governance. *Emory Law Journal*, 69, 687.

Rakova, B., Yang, J., Cramer, H., & Chowdhury, R. (2021). Where responsible AI meets reality: Practitioner perspectives on enablers for shifting organizational practices. *Proceedings of the ACM on Human-Computer Interaction, 5*(CSCW1), 1-23. DOI: 10.1145/3449081

Rath, K. C., Khang, A., Rath, S. K., Satapathy, N., Satapathy, S. K., & Kar, S. (2024). Artificial intelligence (AI)-enabled technology in medicine-advancing holistic healthcare monitoring and control systems. In *Computer Vision and AI-Integrated IoT Technologies in the Medical Ecosystem* (pp. 87–108). CRC Press. DOI: 10.1201/9781003429609-6

Shaw, J., Rudzicz, F., Jamieson, T., & Goldfarb, A. (2019). Artificial intelligence and the implementation challenge. *Journal of Medical Internet Research*, 21(7), e13659. DOI: 10.2196/13659 PMID: 31293245

Shneiderman, B. (2020). Bridging the gap between ethics and practice: Guidelines for reliable, safe, and trustworthy human-centered AI systems. [TiiS]. *ACM Transactions on Interactive Intelligent Systems*, 10(4), 1–31. DOI: 10.1145/3419764

Siala, H., & Wang, Y. (2022). SHIFTing artificial intelligence to be responsible in healthcare: A systematic review. *Social Science & Medicine*, 296, 114782. DOI: 10.1016/j.socscimed.2022.114782 PMID: 35152047

Siala, H., & Wang, Y. (2022). SHIFTing artificial intelligence to be responsible in healthcare: A systematic review. *Social Science & Medicine*, 296, 114782. DOI: 10.1016/j.socscimed.2022.114782 PMID: 35152047

Silva, I., & Soto, M. (2022). Privacy-preserving data sharing in healthcare: An in-depth analysis of big data solutions and regulatory compliance. *International Journal of Applied Health Care Analytics*, 7(1), 14–23.

Tariq, M. U., Poulin, M., & Abonamah, A. A. (2021). Achieving operational excellence through artificial intelligence: Driving forces and barriers. *Frontiers in Psychology*, 12, 686624. DOI: 10.3389/fpsyg.2021.686624 PMID: 34305744

Thapa, C., & Camtepe, S. (2021). Precision health data: Requirements, challenges and existing techniques for data security and privacy. *Computers in Biology and Medicine*, 129, 104130. DOI: 10.1016/j.compbiomed.2020.104130 PMID: 33271399

World Health Organization. (2018). Continuity and coordination of care: a practice brief to support implementation of the WHO Framework on integrated people-centred health services.

Yigitcanlar, T., Corchado, J. M., Mehmood, R., Li, R. Y. M., Mossberger, K., & Desouza, K. (2021). Responsible urban innovation with local government artificial intelligence (AI): A conceptual framework and research agenda. *Journal of Open Innovation*, 7(1), 71.

Yigitcanlar, T., Corchado, J. M., Mehmood, R., Li, R. Y. M., Mossberger, K., & Desouza, K. (2021). Responsible urban innovation with local government artificial intelligence (AI): A conceptual framework and research agenda. *Journal of Open Innovation*, 7(1), 71. DOI: 10.3390/joitmc7010071

Chapter 2
Investigating Generative Artificial Intelligence Readiness in the Internet of Medical Things:
Are We Progressing Technologically?

Wasswa Shafik
https://orcid.org/0000-0002-9320-3186
Dig Connectivity Research Laboratory (DCRLab), Kampala, Uganda & School of Digital Science, Universiti Brunei Darussalam, Brunei

ABSTRACT

Generative Artificial Intelligence (AI) is reshaping the Internet of Medical Things (IoMT), driving innovations in healthcare diagnostics, personalized treatment, and patient monitoring. This integration promises to enhance medical decision-making, optimize resource allocation, and improve patient outcomes. However, despite technological advancements, challenges persist, including data privacy concerns, regulatory hurdles, and the need for robust ethical frameworks. The progress is evident in AI-driven tools, such as predictive analytics and virtual health assistants, yet their widespread adoption is hindered by interoperability issues and uneven technological infrastructure. As generative AI continues to evolve, addressing these barriers is crucial for realizing its full potential in transforming the IoMT landscape, ensuring that technological advancements translate into sustainable and equitable healthcare progress.

1. INTRODUCTION

The Internet of Medical Things[1] (IoMT), often indicated as the healthcare-facing subset of the Internet of Things[2] (IoT), promises the virtualization of healthcare, technologically enabling preventive medicine, extending healthcare delivery, decreasing healthcare costs, and improving doctor and patient experiences (Gupta & Yang, 2024). Nevertheless, recent research has also highlighted a relative lack of technology readiness, with a gap in extant literature investigating generative artificial intelligence algorithms to support the cybersecurity capabilities of the IoMT. This research aims to address this gap,

DOI: 10.4018/979-8-3693-6180-1.ch002

Copyright © 2025, IGI Global. Copying or distributing in print or electronic forms without written permission of IGI Global is prohibited.

specifically exploring the generative adversarial networks algorithm within the IoMT system of systems context (Shafik, 2024e). This is a foundational approach, inspired by literature comparing generative artificial intelligence[3] (GAI) adversaries to cybersecurity vulnerability assessment and unrestricted multi-agent systems, and can inspire further work in this field, including increased AI generative algorithm and IoMT system complexity testing, to both assess generative AI opponent capabilities and advance the development of appropriate defensive cybersecurity systems in readiness for increased distribution of AI within the IoMT (Swain et al., 2022).

GAI is currently a very popular computer science concept being discussed across multiple domains. Despite its popularity as an emerging technology, generative AI is still in the infancy stage in many ways compared to already matured AI technologies such as machine learning[4] and robotic process automation[5]. In the era of rapid technological advancement, identifying technology readiness and making foresight technological progress is vital to staying ahead of the competition (Hossain et al., 2023). The rapidly growing concept of both AI and the IoMT demands a closer look from both the information systems and AI perspectives in order for organizations to become more attractive in solving medical challenges. Organizations that adopt internet-enabled IoMT are better prepared to navigate medical problems more swiftly and at a lower cost while simultaneously supporting effective decision-making and enhanced patient perception (Shafik, 2024c).

The intersection of generative AI and the IoMT is a domain that needs exploring. The IoMT, generating colossal medical data, presents opportunities to revolutionize the current business models in healthcare, provided the technology readiness of generative AI is confirmed. Alternatively, in the present scenario, patients need to carry medical data through many physical consultations, so having generative AI put to work would allow available medical data to come out of phones, wearables, and patches 24/7 and might contribute to reducing the long waiting time (Ali et al., 2023). Such are the proven requirements and challenges posed to medicine that we believe investment in further AI deployment and research in this dynamic topic is worth supporting. This review draws attention to existing primary scientific work so that its factors can be drawn out and would be a guide to thinking about the future and the technological readiness of AI (Feng et al., 2024).

1.1. Background and Significance

Globally, healthcare accessibility is still a big issue, leaving a large population without essential services despite positive efforts. Emerging technologies such as IoT and AI have shown considerable promise to transform the current healthcare system more proactively. AI[6] has immense potential in various areas, from medical facility construction to organ transplants, including medicine manufacturing and the supply chain. Digital health has established a cyber-physical architecture[7] that allows doctors and other health workers to provide people with the medical attention they need (Escorcia-Gutierrez et al., 2023). However, characterized by skills in terms of generation, proper training using publicly available data, and better knowledge for both competitive and non-competitive learning, there may be a lack of technology expertise—especially in data storage and security, which is another symptom of strengths. Consequently, this chapter examines and demonstrates the availability of better data management[8] and privacy protection[9] that contribute to the development of AI by reviewing the promise of these strengths through a review of textbooks from the past (Shafik, 2024b). In the end, our study highlights recent contributions and provides prospects for future research in this health sector using different expert systems as illustrated in Figure 1.

Figure 1. Expert systems

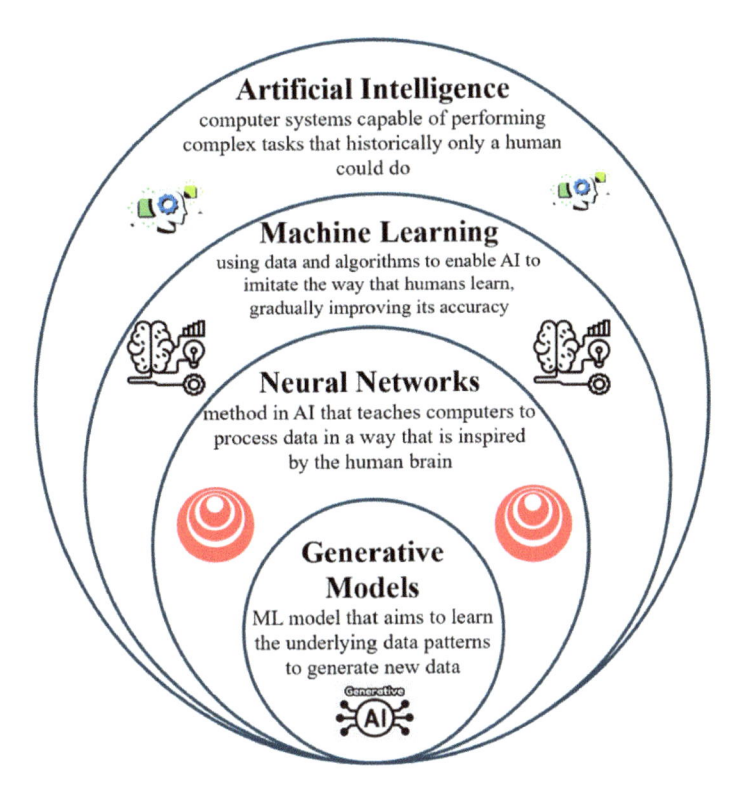

Artificial Intelligence
computer systems capable of performing complex tasks that historically only a human could do

Machine Learning
using data and algorithms to enable AI to imitate the way that humans learn, gradually improving its accuracy

Neural Networks
method in AI that teaches computers to process data in a way that is inspired by the human brain

Generative Models
ML model that aims to learn the underlying data patterns to generate new data

1.2. Research Aim and Objectives

The overall aim of the study is to investigate the technological readiness of generative AI in the IoMT. The objective of this study will be driven by the need to understand the various perspectives in which this modern industry reposes technologically. The research will also be guided by a set of specific objectives, which are as follows:

1) To review the literature and critically assess previous research on generative artificial intelligence predictive models in the IoMT field.
2) To compare generative AI methods with supervised and unsupervised algorithms to provide data scientists and healthcare professionals with suggestions to determine the applicable method for forecasting, offering, or providing data with a specific aim in the IoMT industry.
3) To review discriminative and generative artificial intelligence models in the IoMT line of work and share our findings with the IoMT business field through the deployment of machine learning models and better healthcare delivery.

4) Enhance SMOTE[10] using GAN[11] models to improve overpopulated data and prediction performance in the networking of the Internet's medical things in risk and security analysis with imbalanced data. Inclusively, as AI participation in healthcare services develops, the rapidly growing importance of AI in the healthcare sector generates an ever more interesting area of research.

1.3. Foundations of Artificial Intelligence

Artificial intelligence is known as an intelligent system that works like a human but according to a computer program. It is the field of computer science where machines work like humans with receptive and learning abilities. The greatest challenge of artificial intelligence is to understand and implement human psychological functions and learn and display features that human beings have. Because it is a complex process, different areas of study have emerged in artificial intelligence. This area is a subfield of computer science concerned with building systems to make intelligent decisions while displaying behavior in a complex environment (Shafik, 2024j). AI is known as the ability of computers to display human-like intelligence, decision-making, judgment, perception, reasoning, understanding, interpretation, communication, and providing output. Artificial intelligence, known only through symbols and data mining, has emerged as part of a narrower and more dedicated field whereby it was desired that computers become efficient and reliable. AI helps to analyze these data partitions by understanding how the human brain could solve the same problems, leading to intelligent behavior (Manickam et al., 2022). The excitement AI produced informed events for the computer industry's growth. AI has used many different approaches, including computer vision[12], robotics[13], natural language processing, automata theory, and economics. With reasoning, knowledge representation learning[14], natural language processing[15], computer vision, robotics, machine vision rules, and agent modules, AI has been increasingly used in business, finance, healthcare, politics, and automation technology (Sikarwar et al., 2022).

1.3.1. Overview of Artificial Intelligence

Artificial intelligence has been used for many years as a main driver of technology in healthcare. For quite some time, AI existed in a rule-based system, with humans supplying the rules and AI supplying the execution. This type of narrow AI cannot perform tasks it was not trained or programmed to do. In healthcare, human medical professionals prescribe, replace, or modify rules programmed within both medical devices and information systems (Ashfaq et al., 2019). This overview presents current clinical challenges and reviews how advanced generative AI may address such challenges within the concept of the Internet of Medical Things. The details of the state-of-the-art machine and deep learning models are well discussed in terms of types and data characteristics. It also presents a research agenda for the development of bio-inspired or AI-based systems capable of providing interpretable results and human-level recognition (Shafik, 2024k).

This overview presents the current challenges in healthcare systems and provides insight into ongoing research within the advanced AI field that could potentially deliver a solution. The focus is initially on models that can generate new information from large volumes and variable characteristics of data, which define a particular data-rich spectrum of the Internet of Medical Things (Shafik, 2024f). How advanced generative AI could be the main driver to address clinical challenges within the concept of the Internet of Medical Things summarizes the specialty of the current state-of-the-art machine and deep learning models, which are well discussed in the context of the types and data characteristics, and presents a research agenda for the development of bio-inspired or AI-based systems capable of providing interpretable results and human-level recognition, other enabling technologies as presented in Figure 2 (Sharma et al., 2021).

Figure 2. Healthcare enabling technologies (HET)

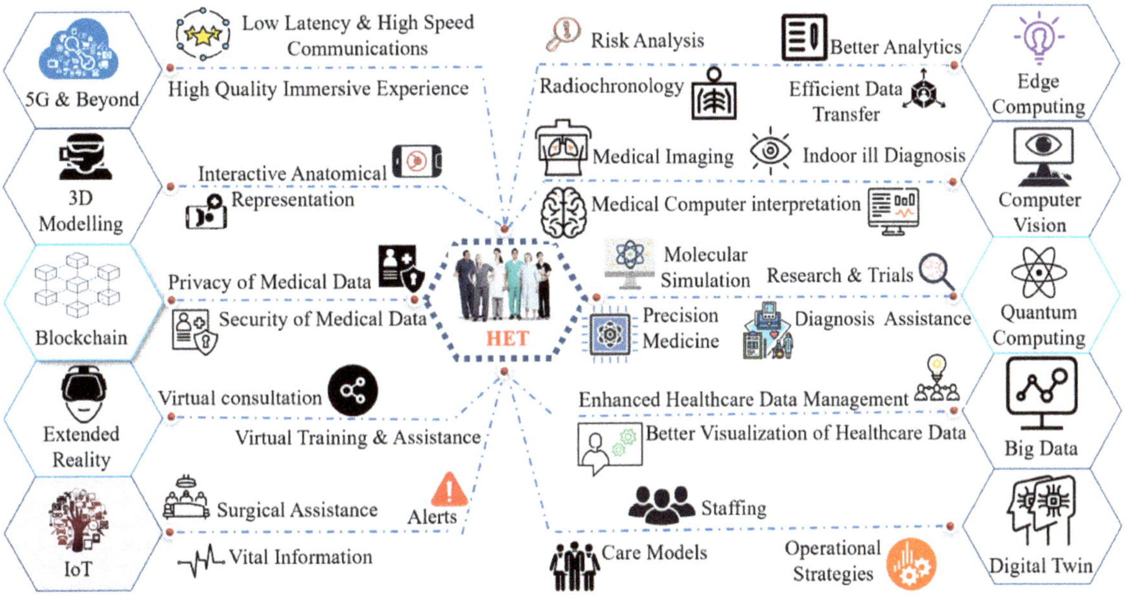

1.3.2. Generative Artificial Intelligence

Generative technology[16] is another type of artificial intelligence on which we depend today, and we do not fully realize that all elements driven by generative models are designed in a way that follows user tasks. Generative AI involves models that have been trained to create various outputs, including graphics, audio, and text. Generative models are also used to generate new realistic data samples that strike a balance between diversity and fidelity, otherwise known as overfitting and underfitting. It is also used to simulate real randomness in order to support certain applications such as theft (Pavan Kumar et al., 2022). Technically speaking, generative models describe a common framework of certain unsupervised machine learning problems, similar to supervised learning but without input-rich accurate supervisory signals. Generative AI has also gained more growth and interest due to the technical advances from the current popular neural architecture communities. Its high scalability of generating new data samples, audio, and video makes its ML generative model more unique than any other. Thus, it becomes able to synthesize large coherent data and gives an image that follows parallelism with current personalized health monitoring devices (Shafik, 2024m). Then again, unlike people with their biosensors in the near future, patients with health-monitoring edges and undergoing analyses of patient photos can benefit from breakthroughs reached by the generative abundance.

It models the problem of learning similar joint probabilities on the current training set of audio and video and outputs audio samples, text, and video frames. Consequently, this technique appears to be the foundation of current, recent creation models. With our computational performances, we have been able to train these generative models by learning with massive data sets. Designing such models can often consist of the validation of latent vector extraction quality for ongoing human tasks (Shafik, 2024h). However, these generative models exhibit a significant covert non-controlled variable bias and, therefore, may lack robust data generalization. Taking this argument with previous ML classification studies, this generative possibility may conform to AI accuracy and fairness assessments by examining the implicit gender bias gradients of its task vectors. Invest in the privacy impact of your generated samples due to the AI task added to the training data, which undoubtedly will drive new research directions (Feng et al., 2024).

1.3.3. Machine Learning in Artificial Intelligence

Machine learning is involved in tasks such as data modeling and model forecasting by making inferences from a finite dataset. Machine learning[17] uses constructed or facilitated algorithms instead of explicit programming to train itself to perform a task by learning from data. Examples include classifying email or customer support tickets as represented by predictive modeling and clustering, computational redshifts, recommendation systems, and image recognition (Escorcia-Gutierrez et al., 2023). Despite its present popularity, machine learning is not modern; pioneer research in this area includes the famous multinomial neural network, artificial brain threshold, and Mark I Perceptron models for image recognition and space mapping. For the most part, several machine learning styles, specifically those associated with inductive learning from a finite dataset, may be easily, satisfactorily, and productively implemented. Deep learning is a separate layer within machine learning involving neural networks that contain numerous members. These members allow neural networks to learn hierarchical representations (Sharma et al., 2021). Deep learning has been successful in tackling a range of AI difficulties, which has contributed to its current popularity. Its success is reflected by instances of its application, such as object recognition based on convolutional networks, tasks of natural language processing that are addressed by sequence-learning methods and recurrent neural networks, and problems of reinforcement learning, such as Atari[18], DOTA[19], and autonomous vehicle driving environments. Furthermore, the popularity of deep learning is fueled by the availability of large computational resources (Manickam et al., 2022; Pavan Kumar et al., 2022). This renders it possible to train and improve larger and deeper neural networks.

2. ARTIFICIAL INTELLIGENCE IN HEALTHCARE

Healthcare has become one of the most prominent areas of interest in using artificial intelligence. The adaptation and use of AI in healthcare, along with advanced digital technology and the rapid progress in high-fidelity simulations of personalized virtual patient physiology and anatomy, generate predictive analytics techniques that can clearly predict and support clinical decision-making. By using AI and BI[20] in healthcare as IoT technologies, patients with chronic diseases or people living in remote areas can be treated in their own homes. AI interprets, translates, and provides information by digitizing and interpreting schemes (Ashfaq et al., 2019). It detects disease conditions before the information processing and sensor technologies and completes the analysis in advance to activate emergency management within the patient's treatment to improve overall health. Using digital technology, advanced digital and technological healthcare solutions for many patients, situational awareness, and increased personalized care in medical IoT communication can support more devices every day (Yao et al., 2018). Smartphones, digital thermometers, digital scales, and heart rate monitors that connect to phones and electronic pulse readers are designed to monitor general health through portable devices. These devices are more comprehensive and can collect biomarkers and store data in different formats in large amounts of data, providing the additional benefits of reliability and accuracy. Data management and machine learning tools help transform a database into an AI technology application for personal telemedicine (Sikarwar et al., 2022).

2.1. Overview of AI in Healthcare

The demand for solutions that can facilitate the production and consumption of global healthcare delivery continues to surge. This trend is fueled by increased longevity, the rise of chronic diseases, and the persistent momentum of medical research and discoveries continuously presenting new treatments and existing drugs being repurposed for new uses. Artificial intelligence technologies are widely considered to have transformative potential across different sectors. When applied to the massive data generated from bodies, including individuals' tracked behavioral data, the promise is of more optimized and tailored individual treatment and patient pathways (Ashfaq et al., 2019; Yao et al., 2018). This chapter investigates the state of the art and technological readiness of a class of AI generative AI, focusing on applications facilitated by the core enabling tools of existing deep learning frameworks in the Internet of Medical Things. The findings provide a cross-disciplinary overview of the Internet of Medical Things AI overall topic area, the alignment or misalignment of the expectations of the state of the AI with its actual development, and highlight underexplored or overexplored research areas (Kumar et al., 2024).

2.2. Applications in Medical Imaging

In terms of architectural facets, generative AI-based medical imaging applications can be architected as fully generative model-based systems, such as generative adversarial networks and variational autoencoders. As exemplified in the comprehensive intelligent medical concept system, it adopts a fully generative model for image data deployment and visualization. Evaluating the quality of synthetic images is a challenging task. To account for the issues that occur at the intersection of generative adversarial networks and variational autoencoders, hybrid models such as adversarial autoencoders have been proposed to utilize the best of both architectures in learning latent representations of the input data (Shickel et al., 2018). On the data facilitator facet, open datasets often come as a prerequisite for generative-based machine learning research. Consequently, publicly accessible medical image benchmarks have proliferated with crowd-sourced data annotation to facilitate generative research. These include commonly known datasets such as the mammography dataset, brain tumor dataset, skin lesion dataset, and a multitude of other anatomical body parts used for the research and testing of diagnostic and prognostic information in medicine (Goldstein et al., 2024). However, existing medical imaging datasets do have limitations, including low-resolution imaging, limited target diseases, and multiple incorrect annotations. The academic community has made efforts to create relatively standardized data storage and labeling guidelines to guide the collection and preparation of images for scientific research. Restructured public datasets with more clinically relevant imaging content will bolster the relevance and benefit of experimental outputs for real-world clinical practice (Landi et al., 2020). GAI has several applications, as presented in Figure 3.

Figure 3. Generative AI application

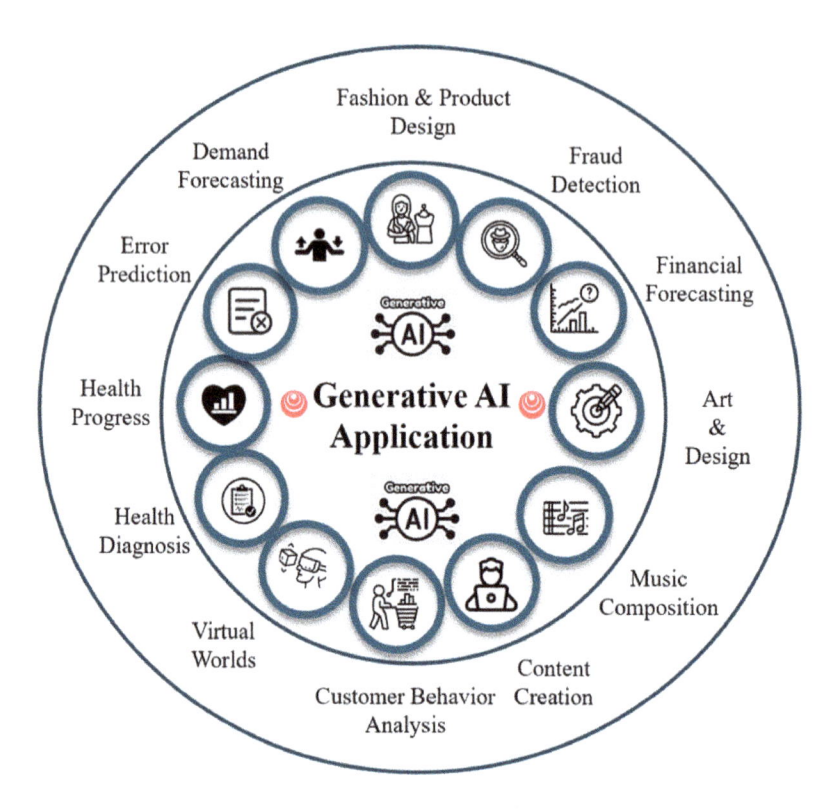

3. INTERNET OF MEDICAL THINGS (IOMT)

Healthcare networks involve several activities, including technological devices, tools, and interconnected systems. The interdisciplinary collaboration between related subjects is increasing. The system encompasses medical devices, biological systems, and systems that reduce human preferences to offer various quality healthcare services. The collaboration of art and technological know-how facilitates the development of novel and efficient systems (Yao et al., 2018). The system draws from several technologies and integrates various biological experiences to advance novel and effective technology. Various healthcare systems, operating systems, mobile electronic health system applications, and other forms of data analysis utilized in medical analysis are governed by this system. The system has developed several advantages, including outpatient care, remote patient monitoring, reduced costs for patients with chronic diseases, reduced waiting time to meet specialist doctors, increased productivity, timely and improved diagnosis, provision of real-time medical preventive care, provision of real-time data to reduce side effects of drugs, improved access to patient data, and improved treatment of patients with chronic diseases (Ashfaq et al., 2019). The main aim of the system is to facilitate the life of an individual by promoting good health. The use of electronics, smart technology, computer programs, and algorithms will be further encouraged with the availability of the system. The system is considered an emerging field of healthcare. The technology available today can be used to improve the lives of patients and to enhance patient data services. More rapid application of human-machine learning technology could be achieved by joining several healthcare domain stakeholders to ensure that high medical performance is attained. This would allow for problems such as drug shortages to be identified far in advance and addressed immediately (Sikarwar et al., 2022). The advances in technologies in the health sector, as well as the driving forces of technology, challenges, and solutions, are focused on in this chapter.

3.1. Definition and Components

AI is a complex system that is able to perform tasks requiring human intelligence. The main goal of AI is to solve cognitive tasks. The expansion of AI to include generative AI has propelled AI into new types of tasks that are both creative and inventive. The top level of the AI pyramid includes creative tasks that generate novel concepts and ideas. Below that are inventive tasks that create new solutions to specific problems, these tasks create, develop, and mentor new concepts to solve meaningful problems that have value or results for life redemption (Ashfaq et al., 2019). This type of AI is capable of creating new paths for humanity. With the proper use and narrow definition of a meaningful problem, generative AI has been applied to the healthcare industry. The AI and the Internet of Medical Things are converging and affecting human senses. Generative AI describes a machine learning-based process that generates new digital imagery, audio, or video. This wide-ranging field continues to expand as new generative AI models are introduced for creating and developing new designs to solve specific problems that may have personal or professional value (Pavan Kumar et al., 2022). AI is advancing rapidly, and it can produce lifelike, diverse, and increasingly large-scale chapter and speech data. A diverse dataset results in a new natural language processing model that possesses over 175 billion parameters within a transformer architecture. This model is trained in a new unsupervised learning direction by demonstrating capability in reasoning, composition, and translation tasks in areas of created or established knowledge (Manickam et al., 2022). In recent tests, it was able to complete final papers in both the 8th and 12th grade levels within 1-6 seconds. Finally, over the next 2-3 years, the original technology for this model will likely be incorporated into new projects. Users who enjoy this model with increased filtering and portability will initially be able to utilze (Manickam et al., 2022; Yao et al., 2018) five new abstractions. It will be included in the compilation of new AI stories for complex algorithms. Intrinsic testing for large-scale machine learning can be easily performed through small AI development.

3.2. Applications in Healthcare

Alongside other industries, the healthcare sector is currently benefiting from IoT solutions. Utilizing IoT devices effectively should now be a main concern for healthcare institutions. With the development of the Internet of Medical Things, the term "smart hospital" is now being discussed. However, this new groundbreaking technology has brought many challenges to the fore. The high volume of data accumulation is already exceeding the scope of human handling and calls for smart solutions. On the other hand, AI can support healthcare institutions to convert this high volume of data to beneficial output by employing modern technology (Kumar et al., 2024). Today, with generative AI models, the advancement of innovation in this sector has been very rapid, and this rise of action has become a current topic that is much discussed. In particular, combining generative AI models with transformative deep learning can increase outcomes in performance. Telehealth, telemedicine, and telecare are growing healthcare subjects that have affected the healthcare sector, the effectiveness of service delivery, and the quality of healthcare services received by all sides. The major obstacle is the high operational cost of these services (Landi et al., 2020). Generative AI models with generative deep learning applications can decrease costs and provide repeatedly accurate results and can be used for e-health applications. Generative AI technology can have an application effect on scenarios such as fabricated data, data extrapolation, object filling, and object cycle completion. The greatest problem observed in the healthcare sector is that medical data consists of extremely sensitive and confidential personal information, and this makes it difficult to train generative models. Hence, their usage sometimes contradicts the law (Shickel et al., 2018). The protection of digital patient data should be the primary concern of all healthcare institutions.

4. GENERATIVE ARTIFICIAL INTELLIGENCE

The chapter deals with generative artificial intelligence, which nowadays attracts a great deal of interest and particular attention among researchers. The growth of artificial intelligence has led to a number of important breakthroughs in the development of various techniques, including models of deep learning. Until relatively recently, the concept of generative artificial intelligence has been limited to a number of niche modeling tasks. So, they could not prevent the use of data analysis from a wide variety of unsupervised models of generative artificial intelligence (Chintala, 2024). This chapter provides an overview of the evolution of generative models of artificial intelligence, beginning with the expression of shallow latent variable models. It introduces some of these important deep generative models, which include VAE, autoregressive models, normalizing flow, and generative rival networks that have made major advances in the instrumental performance of AI tasks. We then considered the application of generative adversarial networks in eHealthcare and analyzed in detail the research interest data (Goldstein et al., 2024). In the IoMT era, it has been concluded that eHealth would witness maximum safety and access to health information. In the biomedical field, we are investigating how healthcare is changing every day, and it has started an era of big health data. As a result, a debate on artificial intelligence for medical treatment has been launched. Not only do eHealth concepts contribute to various health domains, but they also affect people's daily lives. The impact of eHealth on society is so high that the population will receive improved patient treatment, which is evidence-based (Shickel et al., 2018). In that way, the scientific method offers the ideal help to health professionals in looking for new methods of diagnosis, harm reduction, and treatment.

4.1. Concept and Techniques

In recent years, AI techniques have shown fair success in several application domains, such as image and media information. In this regard, AI techniques have also been exploited to enhance the capabilities of wearable medical diagnostic devices, known as the Internet of Medical Things. Generally, IoT devices collect data in real time and send it to cloud computing-based services for data analysis and to support medical decisions. In other words, IoMT adopts body-worn wireless sensor networks for recording vitally related data and is primarily expected to draw a simple, low-cost, accurate, and portable medical diagnostic tool (Landi et al., 2020). As advances in transforming healthcare from a care-based to a prevention-based paradigm continue, ongoing research in IoMT is rapidly increasing day by day. Consequently, this fast-rising research is made possible by technological advancements that provide abundant benefits. Due to this, recently, AI techniques have indicated rapid growth in providing powerful computing, storage, and communication capabilities for IoMT. As a result, the analytical capability of AI-based services has become a crucial consideration due to its importance in medical diagnostic decisions. As the most flexible form of AI, when endorsed by the Internet of Things, AI techniques have become an emergent area of healthcare IoT, called the Internet of Medical Things (Kumar et al., 2024). In this context, several applications of wearable networked sensors and other actuators have emerged, especially for personal health monitoring. AI techniques may bring unparalleled improvements to the potential and services of IoMT by providing more effective data collaboration and optimizing numerous parameters. Since it is possible to connect anything—even medical diagnostic devices—to cloud, edge, and fog computing platforms to fulfill digital goals, the accomplishment of AI-based services in the scope of IoMT becomes simpler, too (Yao et al., 2018).

4.2. Applications in Healthcare

The use of AI in various application areas, including healthcare, has been seen as a potential driver in delivering novel solutions. The current state of AI in healthcare has led to enhancements in how healthcare professionals interact with data and has provided new opportunities to achieve otherwise cost-prohibitive solutions, not only in developed countries but also in developing countries. Healthcare datasets are often characterized by sparse and noisy data and are associated with a significant level of ambiguity, uncertainty, and time pressure. AI that is specifically designed for and adapted to the healthcare sector holds the promise to address these challenges in healthcare delivery meaningfully (Ashfaq et al., 2019). In terms of AI form, generative AI would specifically help secure the prediction and performance of AI-based applications.

Figure 4. IoMT application in medical setup

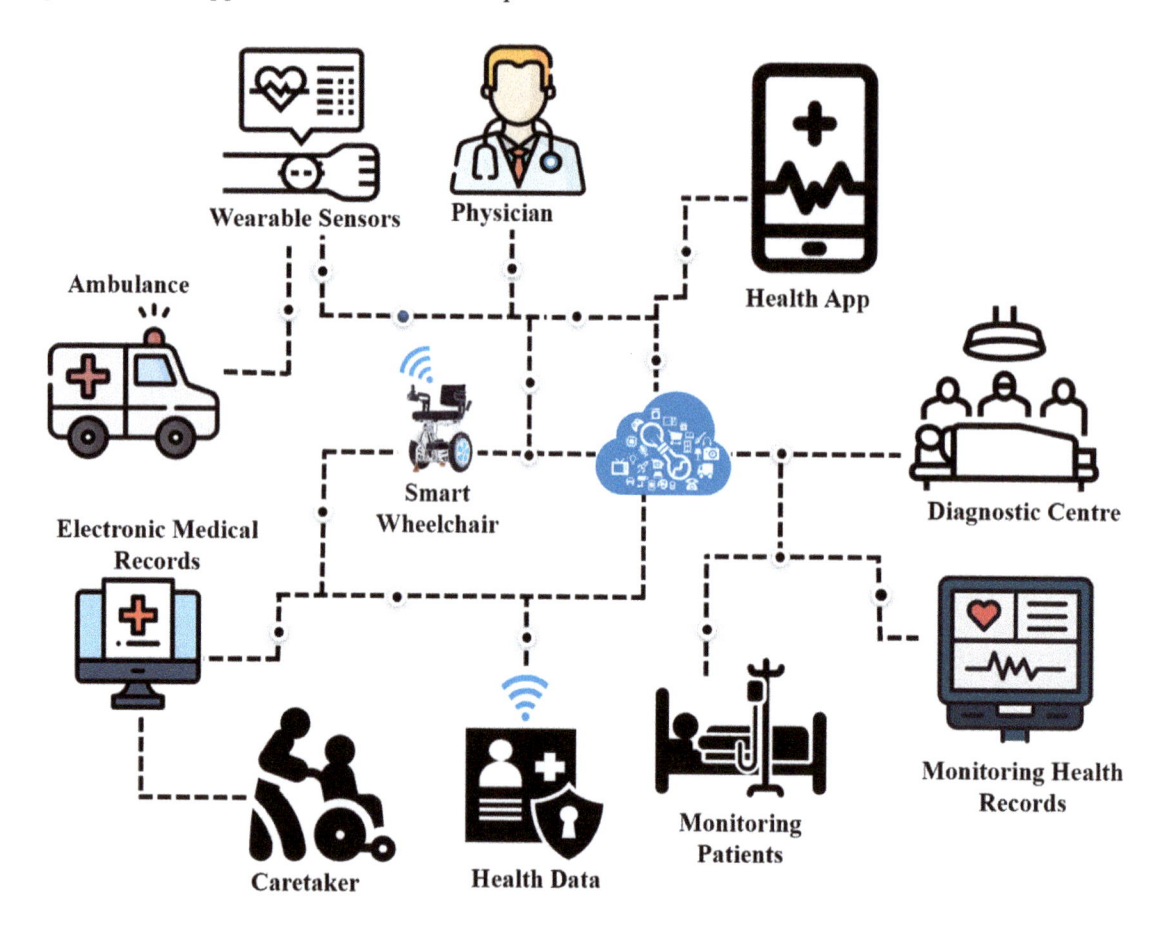

Applications of AI in healthcare are both numerous and wide-ranging. Diagrammatically, AI's key application areas of benefit in healthcare have been categorized into five broad themes as illustrated in Figure 4, which are demonstrably prevalent in contemporary scientific literature. The five themes are as follows: The first theme is expert systems and robotic methods using computer vision and audiology. A literature review has revealed that the application of AI in all these areas could potentially lead to generating a higher number of practical healthcare solutions (Sikarwar et al., 2022). This is due to the current availability of different appropriate convergent technologies in a hospital environment. Particularly relevant convergent technology that can be found in most hospitals, and consequently, has been deployed in solving healthcare issues, comprises high-performance computing resources, a wide array of connected embedded smart devices in the form of medical sensing instruments and wearable devices, and interfacing architectures, collectively referred to as the Internet of Medical Things (Manickam et al., 2022).

5. INTEGRATION OF GAI AND IOMT

The IoMT affords the opportunity to allow multiple medical devices to interrelate in a network, thereby enabling the sharing of medical data over the Internet. This setup has been hailed as drastically improving healthcare delivery, ushering in an era of connected patient healthcare utilization. The use of sensory medical devices has become very popular, nurturing the emergence of the Internet of Medical Things. Patient-centric care, patient monitoring, and the accessibility of large-scale, individual health records sought from wearables and other IoMT devices are some specific benefits. The application of artificial intelligence in healthcare represents leveraging technology to solve problems. With the emergence of generative AI, this aim can be taken a notch further (Vemuri et al., 2020). Generative AI involves the study of creating outputs where the task of generation requires cognition and where the output is a product of abstraction and creativity.

Generative AI correlates with creativity, allowing for the conception of ideas, experiences, and other abstract concepts with the application of intelligence toward the overall goal. An emerging subfield of these principles seeks to harness generative AI through generative models capable of constructing large-scale, high-quality, and complex data. The versatility of generative AI models has been applied in diverse areas, making it a key representative of AI advancements. The Internet of Medical Things includes devices like vital sign trackers, wearable diabetes monitors, and other wearables that generate a significant amount of data about individual users or patients (Hossain et al., 2023). The types of datasets and the volume of data produced by IoMT devices, as well as the variety of technologies that drive these devices, bring to light diverse opportunities that the implementation of generative AI could afford. Instead of letting data travel to centralized databases and then back from the data center to the patient, leveraging the benefits of generative AI could be an effective way to process and utilize data at the point of generation. This could enhance and garner unexpected advantages in diagnostic efficiency, personal care, and a wide range of possibilities that, with the aid of generative AI, could solve deeper problems with richer interactions (Ali et al., 2023).

5.1. Potential Benefits

Despite the generation of much promising research, it is crucial to consider the readiness of the technologies being developed to achieve meaningful application in the real world. However, even more important is the balance that can be achieved between technological readiness and an understanding of the sociological, psychological, and human factors of the impacts of artificial intelligence on the profession and practice of radiology. Prior studies have highlighted the potential benefits of applying AI within the specialty by improving image analysis, population and public health management, research applications, and administrative functions (Feng et al., 2024). However, successful integration of AI will only be achieved if the generative direction of this technology can facilitate innovative improvements in the work practices, tasks, and professional experiences of radiologists. While privacy and data security currently receive much attention in the Internet of Health Things, ready-made policy and best practice design recommendations are non-existent (Escorcia-Gutierrez et al., 2023). For that reason, an interesting focus for future research can be on developing a policy and best practice repository offering information extracted from case studies and secondary material. In addition, this can also serve as basic information for the non-expert to understand the value and risk of using IoMT or other connected health devices, as well as to support professionals who provide key recommendations for safeguarding data that are generated, processed, and stored by connected health devices (Manickam et al., 2022).

5.2. Challenges and Ethical Considerations

Although innovations in AI and IoMT are rapidly growing, some researchers still regard the areas as non-stable due to hidden challenging dimensions, like cybersecurity, PHI, and healthcare data handling. Therefore, huge potential investments are necessary to build formal cooperation mechanisms among TMT organizations and to extend national digital infrastructure to be ready for facing these dimensions of challenges. Handling healthcare data is still a highly challenging issue despite the rapid development of IoMT technologies. In addition, the use of AI in healthcare and, particularly, emergency services can be ethically challenging: the decisions the system could be making have implications for life and death (Sikarwar et al., 2022). A crucial challenge to continue to evolve the space is making sure that the AI systems deployed are fair and ethical. Industry 4.0 introduced key challenges and ethical problems to generative AI system design. In reality, the learning task represented is not solved efficiently based on real data provided by the medical organizations. Moreover, technology is evolving at present faster than laws can keep up with. There are some high-level legislations, like the General Data Protection Regulation in European territory and patient consent management regulations. It is necessary to shorten the wait time for a patient to organize all data and advocate various physicians who have no access to common patient healthcare data, and in case of emergency, it is important to be able to provide information immediately to help healthcare providers improve the outcome of patient care (Ashfaq et al., 2019).

6. TECHNOLOGICAL READINESS ASSESSMENT

Three distinct phases are considered paramount in assessing the overall technology readiness level of traditional and modern AI algorithms: experimental, application, and field. Following these assessment benchmark classifications, and in a bid to understand the effective or expected use of generative AI in the IoMT, experimentation on small-scale data with limited expertise, simulating the IoMT, will be carried out. Although the complexities, such as federated learning posed by the actual IoMT settings, will be abstracted, the proposed classifiers will be evaluated prior to expanding the scope of the examination. Next, a dataset containing a globally standardized collective data distribution with several anonymized and de-identified MRI and CT images will be used throughout this research (Yao et al., 2018).

To assess such a granular readout, the dataset has been augmented in several ways to generate a population-specific distribution from the collective data distribution. Afterward, pragmatic simulation of the over-the-air operation of the generative AI models in the IoMT settings will be conducted by considering mobile platforms for a long learning curve, deployment, real-time updating of AI models with dissimilar and partitioned patient MRIs, persistent shortages of high-bandwidth communication, and low-latency edge computation. Regulators have published guidelines with recommendations and a discussion of several strategies on good practices for the development and deployment of AI in a collaborative clinical environment (Sikarwar et al., 2022). However, these recommendations do not include operating principles for persistent edge deployment, maintenance, real-time updates, medical device equivalency, and performance evaluation. As a notable fact, medical facilities possess physical boundaries, and the workforce is often unprotected. For that reason, practitioners increasingly point to a realistic scenario of many constraints during real-world clinical application. With that in mind, what will enable practitioners of radiology to deploy pivoting endpoints? Deploying additional or alternative medical device-safeguarding reviews in practice settings is essential (Manickam et al., 2022).

6.1. Frameworks and Metrics

The suggested work relies on the suggested frameworks and the associated evaluation metrics, which have been derived partly from top sources in AI, health informatics, and medical imaging. These have been supplemented with those developed during the last few years to be applied specifically to emerging concepts in medical image analysis. Particularly, three renowned general frameworks in the AI domain were investigated in the areas where the work is focused the most. It was suggested that the DRAGON and AI4Net frameworks were the most advisable, possessing the most branches and qualities to be exploited for better understanding of concepts, proof of concept, visualization, assessment, or comparison (Pavan Kumar et al., 2022). Specifically, it is believed that DRAGON will continue to be a universal AI framework, growing possibly yearly with the advances proposed in AI. By focusing on the applications of frameworks when solving generative deep learning and healthcare tasks, only one relevant impact study was found, which is not exhaustive, though it can be extended to include other frameworks while introducing different ones that could be tailored to the work. Further, a detailed assessment was carried out for the various levels of analysis using a set of well-established experiments designed and implemented mostly in AI and health research. Additionally, relevant popular metrics were also employed for this purpose to score the compared frameworks. Subsequently, based on the experiments needing assessment, a new toolkit and metrics were outlined to be employed in the future to contribute in some way to forming a new deep and extensive categorization of AI (Sharma et al., 2021).

6.2. Existing Frameworks and Models

The ASSURE model specifies the necessary attributes of a given AI system required in operational environments. Hence, the ramifications of research on existing models for enabling trust in AI technology will generally lack relevance for the problem of increasing trust in operational generative AI systems. The requirements for model completeness and transparency will necessitate framing methods aimed at the development of proven technology with increased predictability. The Trust in Technology framework adapts the standard model for measuring service quality as a method to measure trust in a technology context (Escorcia-Gutierrez et al., 2023). The model examines how users interact with technology and, through interactions, their affective and cognitive mechanisms to form trust and, ultimately, technology reliance and satisfaction. While the approach would generally be useful when applied to the design and testing of operational AI applications, it addresses a technology bearing the same limitations as discussed earlier. However, the core design attributes employed in the proposed research will include the central anger catharsis of the framework. Control over predictability and moral hazards in decisions made with AI technology would inherently guide the development of trust in the AI system. In conclusion, the attributes of generative AI technology supporting an integrated AI-human team would be fundamentally distinct from both the roles of non-generative AI and tools employed in autonomous systems theory, as well as from the roles of other AI-human team organizational structures (Feng et al., 2024).

6.3. Case Studies

It uses real data from the Internet of Things from a person's body and evaluates generalizability from these tests. The included models generate realistic synthetic datasets that can be used not only to train algorithms more effectively but also to test data for algorithms after training.

6.3.1. Drug Administration, Vaccinated Infection

A larger similar dataset was used to test increasing generalizability and decreasing the likelihood of bias. Three fundamental linear predictive models for the Internet of Medical Things are developed in the case study. The study improves on the annual predictions for deaths from the leading causes of death. It improves the prediction of future drug effects, details of which are discussed in the predicted predictive generalizability model section. It models interactions between parts of both illness and tests and responses to current illness treatments such as drug administration, vaccinated infection recovery, and reinfection sensitivity. It models factors that denote future potential palliation, current illness risks, and stress (Ali et al., 2023). The models show profitable predictive performances due to abundant data from the human Internet of Medical Things, including frequent major kinds of interactions with palliation, medication, and clinical alert monitoring for continuous signs of palliation outcomes. The experimental results of the case studies demonstrate the effectiveness of the proposed models for illness and palliation management for a person. The generalizability is observed to be high, indicating that the model is robust and less data-sensitive. Thus, the performed model can handle complex and unseen Internet of Medical Things data, which are useful for further clinical risk and palliation outcome management. The models can predict contributions to medical wear or clinical alerts related to medical and palliation (Sharma et al., 2021). It can provide effective and personalized Internet of Medical Things health updates for prevention, wellness, and palliation.

6.3.2. Real-world Implementations

Hypothetically, run generative DNN and ADG CNN models on breast, colon, and lung whole slide images. The medical images from a 3D scanner provide perspective and differentiate false uncertainty from ghost phenomena. There are differences in model challenges and uncertainty in testing between the three organ systems and the three models. This observation may impact image domain adaptation and data augmentation strategies. The transformative effect of the deep learning era in medical imaging research and development is evident from the increasingly frequent research output and real-world applications (Feng et al., 2024). Despite this wide embrace and the growing numbers of implemented products and services, the real-world adoption of deep learning models serving medical professionals is arguably slow. The non-trivial translation and integration of AI research into the clinical diagnostic healthcare pipeline lead to these disconnects. Most products are commercially available in the form of an inference process that applies a trained model to a given input. Understandably, the workings of the mode of action are obscured, precluding the study of new unknowns in a race to release error-free AI models. This is compatible with the repurposing of deep learning models in novel domains or modalities. The deployment of next-generation models on novel data implicates the drastically higher implementation risk of AI (Ali et al., 2023). The specter of model challenges, failure, and error must be managed as a robust model integrates well into clinical workflow.

7. ETHICAL AND LEGAL IMPLICATIONS

The purpose of the study is to identify and investigate the readiness of generative artificial intelligence techniques—namely, deep learning, generative adversarial networks, and hierarchical reinforcement learning—for healthcare professionals to use in the Internet of Medical Things. The technological readiness level assessment framework and its dimensions were used to guide the research. Our findings offer an expansion of the framework by adding attributes specific to generative artificial intelligence technologies. In addition, the study informs gap areas in the technologies and offers practitioners guidance for configuring them into end-user-facing products. With predicted high usability, reliability, and perceived benefit in the workplace, the study sheds light on future developments with these techniques, including bench testing, prototype prescription, and testing in multiple medical computer and medical device use settings (Vemuri et al., 2020).

Artificial intelligence (AI), particularly generative AI solutions, has emerged in the last decade in response to the industry and medical sector's need to improve or potentially transform business processes overtaken by data overload. As machine learning innovation takes a step towards generative AI, it will pave the way to produce and integrate devices that are more capable of understanding users' issues. However, patients are reasonably cautious about message interpretation and the human aspect of data despite recent substantial advances in model performance. Generative AI also presents additional technical and conceptual challenges. Other ethical concerns arise with several realistic AI applications; in many instances, the uses of AI may raise societal questions. The novel therapy known as AI psychotherapy self-guided has raised apprehensions and has therefore been put through some testing. However, many more arguments can be considered in many of the options implied by generative AI solutions. These include desirable disorders usually included in the safety publication associated with humanism (Hossain et al., 2023). Despite the difficulty of comparing various relational issues, they appear to be the key to using congruent AI exercises in companies.

7.1. Data Privacy and Security

Data privacy and security have been shown to weigh significantly on the acceptance and adoption of the Internet of Medical Things systems. Medical data are among the most sensitive personal data. Advanced forms of AI, such as deep learning and generative approaches, have proven to be powerful tools for translating data safely and efficiently into meaningful insights and precisely targeted interventions. At first sight, most concerns in the context of the typical end-to-end learning approaches can be addressed. However, on-device systems have emerged as a desired approach to move processing and learning into the Internet of Medical Things itself, avoiding the need to upload sensitive data into cloud space (Feng et al., 2024). Generative AI has demonstrated its power in providing meaningful insights and model-agnostic decision rules based on sensitive health data.

However, it has also proven to provide significant risk in generating personal and highly sensitive data with its generative models as universal approximators. The risk of generated images, which are practically indistinguishable from authentic images, being used to fuel disinformation or attack yet undisclosed security vulnerabilities could bear huge future damage. The value of technical solutions to limit and mitigate these capabilities of generative models while preserving meaningful insights and precision decision-making potential remains a subject of future research. The introduction and investigation of such solutions are supported by the lack of domain-specific standards, either internationally or nationally, being applicable to create the confidence-imposed rules typically used in various sectors (Pavan Kumar et al., 2022). This research has shown that the potential for poisoning or evasion attacks could be significantly lessened where such confidence-imposed standards would exist.

7.2. Regulatory Compliance

Although organizations' obligations to their staff and the public are not limited to compliance, they often have no choice other than to operate within the bounds of international, national, or local governing laws and regulations. Failing to observe these laws and regulations puts them at risk of litigation, regulatory penalties, and the loss of goodwill or trust. The medical devices market must directly demonstrate the compliance of the devices that are being brought to market, of the operational controls within the company, and of the devices' outputs, intended effects, and ability and readiness to fulfill patient care strategies. Regulations must be observed throughout the lifecycle of the generated evidence that assures the effectiveness of the patient care strategies that are modified and informed by the outputs of artificial intelligence in health technologies (Hossain et al., 2023). It will be important for decision-makers, developers, and deployers to comprehend and adhere to international, national, and local regulations and standards that are currently mandated to demonstrate that experimental protocols, training, and data have in place the measures that are necessary to provide assurances that AI has been suitably developed, validated, labeled, and made ready for the tasks and the purpose for which it is intended. Understanding the fundamentals that underpin these regulations and standards is the first step in understanding the processes and methods that can facilitate their observance. Failure to observe mandated regulations and standards may not only result in operational sanctions and the restitution of adverse patient consequences but may also restrict the adoption and improvement of AI on which many patient-centered and cost-containment strategies are reliant (Swain et al., 2022).

8. FUTURE DIRECTIONS AND RESEARCH OPPORTUNITIES

As with any nascent field still enveloped in multilayered levels of ambiguities, it is likely for researchers and industry practitioners to observe that it is difficult to produce a single, unified viewpoint or perspective on GAI in the enormous emerging market of IoMT. Therefore, moving forward, in the roadmap to sustain the empowering prospect of our digital economy that relies on GAI in the IoMT, multidisciplinary collaborations among researchers, institutes, industry practitioners, and policymakers, alongside trustworthy technologies, are much needed to address, but are not limited to, the unknown and evolving trade-offs deriving from choosing and governing who gets to produce, access, validate, communicate, and regulate those life-changing and lifesaving systems woven by GAI in the fabric of the human body (Hossain et al., 2023).

By continuing to bring underlying foundations in AI, trust, ethics, and explainability studies in combination with interdisciplinary knowledge for the IoMT that revolves around subjects such as clinical informatics, biology, chemistry, genetics, healthcare management, mobile health, telemedicine, privacy in healthcare, and others to bear on these inquiries, it is feasible to cultivate to some extent a network of intelligent agents, including end-users, that is empowered by human-AI collaboration and trustworthy GAI. From the empirical research and contributions, the discoveries in sociology, economics, psychology, and criminal justice should encourage society to reorient legal doctrine and the broader policymaking paradigm (Ali et al., 2023). Such interwoven mutual engagement may bolster a better understanding of these intimate levels of human interspecies interactions, influence innovation rates, and thereby solve pervasive health problems of individuals and groups, manifold policy enablers, and antitrust-oriented divestiture. Understanding these interactions needs to be proactive. It is essential to adopt an adaptive interdisciplinary framework involving human-computer interaction that can valorize and harness interpretability, explainability, and accountability mechanisms (Feng et al., 2024).

8.1. Emerging Technologies

The increasing development and deployment of new technologies began to change the world in which we live rapidly. I use the term 'new' to refer to any technology that is in the process of being developed, programmed, and created by people and specialists of all types, and which is often referred to as emerging technology. Technology is now spreading rapidly and being adopted by end users. These technological innovations have reached the point where they often mimic the complexity of the human intellect, even in ways that may not be generally perceived or recognized (Sharma et al., 2021). Artificial intelligence has made significant breakthroughs that have transformed many information process-driven applications. Fields such as machine learning, natural language processing, and image, voice, speech, and gesture recognition are making substantial advancements in areas including health, transportation, and retail. These improvements enhance the productivity and capabilities of individuals while improving the quality and sustainability of life (Pavan Kumar et al., 2022).

Technological readiness assesses how prepared any entity or group is to make full use of the coming technological breakthroughs and initiates the interactions that are required to create, develop, or apply innovative new technologies within a particular context or for a specific group. Progress enables innovation and the ability to aggregate innovative components into useful composite solutions. Only thereafter can the solutions be applied in a variety of different circumstances. This permits the reach and robustness of the technologies developed to become apparent and determines their level of acceptance in the various fields involved. The IoMT links smart medical devices to digital health information and communication systems to improve health, cut premises, and reduce inefficiency (Manickam et al., 2022). In its health-related applications, current IoMT devices perform monitoring, tracking, and treatment tasks according to data primarily based on rules.

8.2. Potential Applications

In the foregoing section, innovative tools like the Internet of Medical Things along with Generative AI were discussed in great detail. In this section on potential applications, some specific technologies have been identified to ascertain whether Generative AI can be applied in order to develop new therapeutic treatments to improve patient health and quality of life. In summary, the following vital parameters will be used to measure this: patient access to virtual AI therapy modalities, effect on patient chronic medical conditions, confounding factors or negative effects, and an AI algorithm case study. Healthcare professionals will learn how AI, specifically Generative AI, can greatly enhance their professional medical expertise when used optimally and interactively with their patients. Medicine will automatically adapt and grow over time (Sikarwar et al., 2022).

Generative AI is not yet in use and therefore cannot give patient-specific answers in real time. However, the promise of Generative AI is boundless. Generative AI technology should be part of every medical IoT device in the future, in every medical application, for every practitioner and for any patient that can and will be helped. Each medical IoT and Generative AI project must plan for tomorrow, so as to include and shorten adoption time for patient usability and education. The standard threshold issue for Generative AI is that it is never so certain or accurate in explaining how the algorithm achieved some result that the algorithm overcomes human skepticism, the standard of reasonable doubt, nor replaces the need for human knowledge supplementation. The comparison is to provide sufficient evidence to exceed a reasonable doubt standard for admissibility. Generative AI is in search of universal visual representations that would make capture, recall, and transmission of medical knowledge explainable, precise, and doable (Yao et al., 2018). Tutorial explanations, transfers of explanations to complex models, model understandings, affective computing, and human interactions are concepts that will transform the medical field tremendously (Bhone, 2024).

9. KEY FINDINGS AND CONTRIBUTIONS

This research study investigates the technological readiness of generative artificial intelligence in the form of AI algorithms to support the generation of creative content in the IoMT. The evaluation of these AI innovations is based on expert perceptions of healthcare, information technology, and business professionals located within the United States.

9.1. Summary of Findings

The objective of this research paper was to investigate the technological readiness of generative AI over GPT-3 in the IoMT. The dominant interpretive approach used in the study was a survey and a critical review of the literature to examine the readiness of generative AI in the health sector. The results from the study found both GPT-3 and generative AI ready and capable of transforming the health sector, despite concerns about data privacy, bias, misuse, and the ethical implications of their use. This report is presented in line with the objectives of the research, the literature on generative AI, and the findings of this research. Implications, limitations, and prospects for future research follow the presentation of the findings (Kumar et al., 2024). The primary aim of this research was to determine whether GPT-3 could be used as a state-of-the-art AI form for medical concepts. The generative AI capability is applied during face-to-face meetings by deploying the large generative AI language model. While healthcare professionals use patient data to make decisions and draw conclusions about human health, GPT-3 can be used to generate a model that allows healthcare professionals to use large data to make decisions in the health industry. The study concludes with a comprehensive survey report highlighting the research, impacts, and whether healthcare professionals can trust GPT-3 as a generative AI tool in the health industry (Pavan Kumar et al., 2022).

The study employed a sequential exploratory mixed research design to collect and analyze the needs, issues, and applications of generative AI within the IoMT environment. The experts believe that the technology is generating new knowledge or insights by providing generation suggestions and co-creating new creative content across multi-technical fields (Shafik, 2024g). Generative AI motivates deep learning training models that improve patient experience, efficiency, and real-time learning monitoring and can be seen as a disruptive innovation that may need an upgrade in the regulatory and validation systems. The generated insights can motivate future research on how to use technology capabilities such as these within different operational environments and multinational health systems (Escorcia-Gutierrez et al., 2023). Generative AI will impact creativity in specialized fields due to its ability to help users with easier, more seamless interactions within specific tasks, and engagement may or may not stimulate further innovative ideas toward the more significant task completion discovered. The contributions of this study provide results on generative AI perceptions and readiness within the domain of AI healthcare design and development (Sharma et al., 2021).

9.2. Limitations Recommendations for Future Research

For this study, future research may employ focus group research to gather the views of large and diverse groups of experts or organizations that engage with for-profit IoT or IoMT products and services. This qualitative participatory research method is particularly useful for gathering rich data and generating perspectives, thus providing a more insightful and in-depth understanding of how organizations perceive their support for and approach towards for-profit Internet of Things products and services (Shafik, 2024a). Another recommended study direction may entail the conceptualization and implementation of an information system artifact for the intentional integration of architecture-in-place supports for for-profit IoT or IoMT products and services into for-profit organizations (Pavan Kumar et al., 2022). In this design-oriented research, a prototype could guide business process implementation and data integration with strategic, tactical, or operational information systems in SMEs with similar or equivalent industry domain considerations (Shafik, 2024i).

For AI-related literature, future researchers should focus on the growing promise that the use of technology, such as artificial intelligence, has for enabling and enhancing innovation and efficiency in organizations. The study should be conducted with a broader range of a particular type or the overall generative AI technologies to include both ICT and non-ICT technologies or to take a consumer-side view on such technologies. Future researchers may leverage a framework or model for investigating challenges and solutions regarding the adoption and diffusion of such or equivalent innovative technologies (Sikarwar et al., 2022). This may also include research that examines the reasons why organizations explore and adopt AI-based solutions and how the value from predictive AI may be preserved and managed in the digital ecosystem (Shafik, 2024d).

9.3. Recommendations for Future Research

The recommendations for future studies are as follows:

- It is suggested that future studies explore in detail the level of technological readiness of these sectors in transformative applications of generative artificial intelligence, such as those grounded on end-to-end user-customizable natural language processing. This could range from user-written complex thematic essays to image descriptors.
- It is recommended that future studies investigate whether the size of the company influences decision-making about using generative artificial intelligence. This seems to be an outstanding

question that it is surprising to have so little research on, given the potential of generative artificial intelligence for both large and small organizations.
- Future studies should investigate generative artificial intelligence typologies and applications. Diverse factual case studies of success and failure from across different sectors must be obtained and researched to in-depth study users and the main motives for selecting generative artificial intelligence.
- It is recommended that future studies examine how new technologies are converging to enable the next wave of generative artificial intelligence systems and tools to be available as soon as possible. One way to do this is by identifying general and unforeseen convergences in technology, organizational culture, business strategy, and public policy and by looking into what the future might hold and how empowering technologies can help society to withstand the impacts of this journey better.
- Future studies should examine the power of companies to build and apply generative artificial intelligence in a positive way that benefits society by focusing on tackling crucial societal challenges. Corporate strategies, business decisions, and company differences that will maximize the opportunities for inclusive economic success throughout society deserve a closer look.
- To expand on the empirical evidence, future studies should attend to the latest developments in the technology and the structure of the market for generative artificial intelligence. More empirical research on generative AI business applications is also warranted. More case studies, surveys, data sets on investments and job statistics, and analyses of business implications in sectors beyond industry would be most welcome.
- It is recommended that future studies investigate the use of AI compliance systems for instances of corruption, including regarding the implementation of new technologies. It would be helpful to undertake interdisciplinary studies that would address the development of positive incentives for the intelligent design and use of generative artificial intelligence systems. There is a dearth of international comparative data on the levels of technological readiness, and it is recommended that future studies investigate the factors that might be related to the heterogeneity of technological readiness across different countries.
- Finally, it is recommended that further studies investigate the segments of entrepreneurs who are optimistic versus pessimistic about technology and policy support for the commercialization of generative AI, about the opportunities for competitive advantage presented by the use of generative AI, and about society's vulnerability to the broader and deeper use of these highly advanced techniques.

9.4. Implications for Research and Practice

The findings have important implications for research and practice. We discuss these implications using both the technology contextualization and implications.

9.4.1. Technology Contextualization Implications

Trying to locate research at the intersection of emergent IoT is a challenging undertaking, but one in which we believe lies the future of impactful business and society-enabling advances in technology. Further, research and evaluation cannot be limited only to investigating the fundamentals of one particular technology, whether AI, IoT, 5G, or cloud computing, for example, at the expense of ignoring its behavior or performance within emergent combinatorial complex systems (Alzubi et al., 2021). That is why we follow an experimental setup as a simulation tool for business innovation in a real-case scenario, controlled and represented by a methodological process. We argue that research has a role to play in broadening the impact of emerging technologies through research and knowledge translation efforts (Ashfaq et al., 2019). Next, we provide a discussion of these concerns and articulate the implications for future research development.

Given that we are evaluating the potential benefits of a transformative enabling AI in conjunction with other emergent enabling technologies, the commercial score, marked as the commercial orientation of the AI product, might have implications for future research that need to be framed within a broader view of why certain technologies continue to perform better. Researchers in top management and the global economy address this issue in up to three tiers (Dahm et al., 2024; Shafik, 2024l). Level one discusses the importance of being knowledgeable about trends, challenges, and opportunities regarding an IT product; level two discusses the Smart Business Provider; and level three is about managing IT in franchises and other business models. Our immediate implication is that research should be directed at evaluation and inclusiveness concerning novel combinations enabling metamorphic technologies within these business and service evaluations (Kumar et al., 2024; Yao et al., 2018). Furthermore, research should be directed at scrutinizing why some technologies, including techno-social-technological emergent technologies, perform better within our socio-economic environments.

9.4.2. Distinctive Ad-Hoc Data Preprocessing

The results of this investigation showed for the first time the potential benefits of using GA to deduce knowledge from model-extracted networks for the IoMT. In order to form a resilient understanding, five different GAs analyzed three datasets, and distinct apples-to-apples comparisons were implemented. Each dataset also conducted distinctive ad-hoc data preprocessing performed by distinct routers connected to the same physical network. Our work delivers tangible contributions. First and foremost, the careful handling and preprocessing of full-stack captured packet traces to extract a reliable dataset compatible with GA and suitable for network traffic analysis (Landi et al., 2020). Second, a unique experimental setup validating the results of traditional machine learning models with widely used classification of AI models and demonstrating their complementarity. Thirdly, the reuse of learned information by further deducing the generated knowledge as a human-understandable document model of the IoT environment. Despite the promising outcomes of this original investigation, the large dataset compiled from diverse technological approaches and robust data preprocessors is the only way to draw secure conclusions (Shickel et al., 2018).

10. CONCLUSION

This study presents a future research direction for unlocking the full capabilities of generative AI, with an opposite focus on medicine. Given the profound implications of generative AI, future research that investigates the nexus between generative AI and other breakthrough technologies is vital. Generative AI presents a form of a scientific phenomenon in terms of predictability, forecasting, and scientific tools that require interdisciplinary collaboration to investigate. Future research aims to dissect the key research directions, methodologies and empirical data types that can be used to align generative with the societal implications. Generative AI is rooted in AI machine learning techniques, whose definition and capabilities continue to evolve. In this review, we aimed to provide a comprehensive definition for Generative AI, given its rapidly advancing capabilities, and to place these capabilities in context with the foundational principles of advanced machine learning techniques. Our motivation in doing so is to encourage the discovery of new connections between AI and Generative AI that will foster new research ideas by research communities, consider the changing landscape in the capabilities of advanced AI, and support the establishment of comprehensive knowledge of the new abilities of Generative AI by defining what such abilities are and the methods by which they have been achieved. We hope that future endeavors based on the new definitions in this review will be guided by a comprehensive understanding that evolves with the field of Generative AI. The implications suggest courses of action that underscore the model, research communities, and international regulators to underscore well-designed interactions between generative AI and health professionals, and the IoMT healthcare delivery ecosystem will allow generative effectiveness and expertise of health consumers to be successful contributors to the health care sector that in turn offer the considerable potential economic assistance. Participants may be able to offset unequal costs incurred as they create a responsive and sustainable health ecosystem.

REFERENCES

Ali, M., Naeem, F., Tariq, M., & Kaddoum, G. (2023). Federated Learning for Privacy Preservation in Smart Healthcare Systems: A Comprehensive Survey. *IEEE Journal of Biomedical and Health Informatics*, 27(2), 778–789. Advance online publication. DOI: 10.1109/JBHI.2022.3181823 PMID: 35696470

Alzubi, O. A., Alzubi, J. A., Shankar, K., & Gupta, D. (2021). Blockchain and artificial intelligence enabled privacy-preserving medical data transmission in Internet of Things. *Transactions on Emerging Telecommunications Technologies*, 32(12), e4360. Advance online publication. DOI: 10.1002/ett.4360

Ashfaq, A., Sant'Anna, A., Lingman, M., & Nowaczyk, S. (2019). Readmission prediction using deep learning on electronic health records. *Journal of Biomedical Informatics*, 97, 103256. Advance online publication. DOI: 10.1016/j.jbi.2019.103256 PMID: 31351136

Bhone, A. (2024). Medconnect (Android App): Linking Doctors, Patients, and Prescriptions Digitally. *International Journal for Research in Applied Science and Engineering Technology*, 12(2), 697–702. Advance online publication. DOI: 10.22214/ijraset.2024.58409

Chintala, S. (2024). The Application of Deep Learning in Analysing Electronic Health Records for Improved Patient Outcomes. *International Journal of Intelligent Systems and Applications in Engineering*, 12(15s).

Dahm, M. R., Raine, S. E., Slade, D., Chien, L. J., Kennard, A., Walters, G., Spinks, T., & Talaulikar, G. (2024). Older patients and dialysis shared decision-making. Insights from an ethnographic discourse analysis of interviews and clinical interactions. *Patient Education and Counseling*, 122, 108124. Advance online publication. DOI: 10.1016/j.pec.2023.108124 PMID: 38232671

Escorcia-Gutierrez, J., Mansour, R. F., Leal, E., Villanueva, J., Jimenez-Cabas, J., Soto, C., & Soto-Díaz, R. (2023). Privacy Preserving Blockchain with Energy Aware Clustering Scheme for IoT Healthcare Systems. *Mobile Networks and Applications*. Advance online publication. DOI: 10.1007/s11036-023-02115-9

Feng, W., Wu, H., Ma, H., Tao, Z., Xu, M., Zhang, X., Lu, S., Wan, C., & Liu, Y. (2024). Applying contrastive pre-training for depression and anxiety risk prediction in type 2 diabetes patients based on heterogeneous electronic health records: A primary healthcare case study. *Journal of the American Medical Informatics Association : JAMIA*, 31(2), 445–455. Advance online publication. DOI: 10.1093/jamia/ocad228 PMID: 38062850

Goldstein, E. V., Bailey, E. V., & Wilson, F. A. (2024). Poverty and Suicidal Ideation Among Hispanic Mental Health Care Patients Leading up to the COVID-19 Pandemic. *Hispanic Health Care International; the Official Journal of the National Association of Hispanic Nurses*, 22(1), 6–10. Advance online publication. DOI: 10.1177/15404153231181110 PMID: 37312509

Gupta, V., & Yang, H. (2024). Study protocol for factors influencing the adoption of ChatGPT technology by startups: Perceptions and attitudes of entrepreneurs. *PLoS ONE, 19*(2 February). DOI: 10.1371/journal.pone.0298427

Hossain, E., Rana, R., Higgins, N., Soar, J., Barua, P. D., Pisani, A. R., & Turner, K. (2023). Natural Language Processing in Electronic Health Records in relation to healthcare decision-making: A systematic review. In *Computers in Biology and Medicine* (Vol. 155). DOI: 10.1016/j.compbiomed.2023.106649

Kumar, Y., Ilin, A., Salo, H., Kulathinal, S., Leinonen, M. K., & Marttinen, P. (2024). Self-Supervised Forecasting in Electronic Health Records With Attention-Free Models. *IEEE Transactions on Artificial Intelligence*, 5(8), 3926–3938. Advance online publication. DOI: 10.1109/TAI.2024.3353164

Landi, I., Glicksberg, B. S., Lee, H. C., Cherng, S., Landi, G., Danieletto, M., Dudley, J. T., Furlanello, C., & Miotto, R. (2020). Deep representation learning of electronic health records to unlock patient stratification at scale. *NPJ Digital Medicine*, 3(1), 96. Advance online publication. DOI: 10.1038/s41746-020-0301-z PMID: 32699826

Manickam, P., Mariappan, S. A., Murugesan, S. M., Hansda, S., Kaushik, A., Shinde, R., & Thipperudraswamy, S. P. (2022). Artificial Intelligence (AI) and Internet of Medical Things (IoMT) Assisted Biomedical Systems for Intelligent Healthcare. In *Biosensors* (Vol. 12, Issue 8). DOI: 10.3390/bios12080562

Pavan Kumar, I., Mahaveerakannan, R., Praveen Kumar, K., Basu, I., Anil Kumar, T. C., & Choche, M. (2022). A Design of Disease Diagnosis based Smart Healthcare Model using Deep Learning Technique. *Proceedings of the International Conference on Electronics and Renewable Systems, ICEARS 2022*. DOI: 10.1109/ICEARS53579.2022.9752063

Shafik, W. (2024a). Artificial Intelligence and Machine Learning with Cyber Ethics for the Future World. In *Future Communication Systems Using Artificial Intelligence, Internet of Things and Data Science* (pp. 110–130). CRC Press., DOI: 10.1201/9781032648309-9

Shafik, W. (2024b). Artificial Intelligence-Enabled Internet of Medical Things (AIoMT) in Modern Healthcare Practices. In *Clinical Practice and Unmet Challenges in AI-Enhanced Healthcare Systems* (pp. 42–69). IGI Global. DOI: 10.4018/979-8-3693-2703-6.ch003

Shafik, W. (2024c). Artificial Intelligence-Enabled Internet of Medical Things for Enhanced Healthcare Systems. In *Smart Healthcare Systems* (pp. 119–134). CRC Press., DOI: 10.1201/9781032698519-9

Shafik, W. (2024d). The Role of Artificial Intelligence in the Emerging Digital Economy Era. In *Artificial Intelligence Enabled Management* (pp. 33–50). De Gruyter., DOI: 10.1515/9783111172408-003

Shafik, W. (2024e). Connected healthcare—the impact of Internet of Things on medical services. In *Artificial Intelligence and Internet of Things based Augmented Trends for Data Driven Systems* (pp. 181–217). CRC Press., DOI: 10.1201/9781003497318-10

Shafik, W. (2024f). Digital healthcare systems in a federated learning perspective. In *Federated Learning for Digital Healthcare Systems* (pp. 1–35). Elsevier., DOI: 10.1016/B978-0-443-13897-3.00001-1

Shafik, W. (2024g). Incorporating Artificial Intelligence for Urban and Smart Cities' Sustainability. In *Maintaining a Sustainable World in the Nexus of Environmental Science and AI* (pp. 23–58). IGI Global. DOI: 10.4018/979-8-3693-6336-2.ch002

Shafik, W. (2024h). IoT-Enabled Secure and Intelligent Smart Healthcare. In *Secure and Intelligent IoT-Enabled Smart Cities* (pp. 308–333). IGI Global., DOI: 10.4018/979-8-3693-2373-1.ch015

Shafik, W. (2024i). Navigating Emerging Challenges in Robotics and Artificial Intelligence in Africa. In *Examining the rapid advance of digital technology in Africa* (pp. 126–146). IGI Global., DOI: 10.4018/978-1-6684-9962-7.ch007

Shafik, W. (2024j). Smart Health Revolution: Exploring Artificial Intelligence of Internet of Medical Things. In *Healthcare Industry Assessment: Analyzing Risks, Security, and Reliability* (pp. 201–229). Springer. DOI: 10.1007/978-3-031-65434-3_9

Shafik, W. (2024k). The Future of Healthcare: AIoMT—Redefining Healthcare with Advanced Artificial Intelligence and Machine Learning Techniques. In *Artificial Intelligence and Machine Learning in Drug Design and Development* (pp. 605–634). Wiley., DOI: 10.1002/9781394234196.ch19

Shafik, W. (2024l). Toward a More Ethical Future of Artificial Intelligence and Data Science. In *The Ethical Frontier of AI and Data Analysis* (pp. 362–388). IGI Global., DOI: 10.4018/979-8-3693-2964-1.ch022

Shafik, W. (2024m). Wearable medical electronics in artificial intelligence of medical things. *Handbook of Security and Privacy of Ai-Enabled Healthcare Systems and Internet of Medical Things*, 21–40. https://doi.org/DOI: 10.1201/9781003370321-2

Sharma, M., Kochhar, A., Gupta, D., & Al Zubi, J. (2021). Hybrid Intelligent System for Medical Diagnosis in Health Care. In *Intelligent Systems Reference Library* (Vol. 209). DOI: 10.1007/978-981-16-2972-3_2

Shickel, B., Tighe, P. J., Bihorac, A., & Rashidi, P. (2018). Deep EHR: A Survey of Recent Advances in Deep Learning Techniques for Electronic Health Record (EHR) Analysis. *IEEE Journal of Biomedical and Health Informatics*, 22(5), 1589–1604. Advance online publication. DOI: 10.1109/JBHI.2017.2767063 PMID: 29989977

Sikarwar, T. S., Mehta, S., Yadav, S., & Arora, D. (2022). Factors of adoption of Artificial Intelligence (AI) and Internet of Medical Things (IOMT) amongst Healthcare Workers: A Descriptive Analysis. *International Journal of Systematic Innovation*, 7(3). Advance online publication. DOI: 10.6977/IJoSI.202209_7(3).0002

Swain, S., Muduli, K., Kommula, V. P., & Sahoo, K. K. (2022). Innovations in Internet of Medical Things, Artificial Intelligence, and Readiness of the Healthcare Sector Towards Health 4.0 Adoption. *International Journal of Social Ecology and Sustainable Development*, 13(1), 1–14. Advance online publication. DOI: 10.4018/IJSESD.292078

Vemuri, P. K., Kunta, A., Challagulla, R., Bodiga, S., Veeravilli, S., Bodiga, V. L., & Rao, K. R. S. S. (2020). Artificial intelligence and internet of medical things based health-care system for real-time maternal stress - Strategies to reduce maternal mortality rate. *Drug Invention Today*, 13(7), •••.

Yao, Z. J., Bi, J., & Chen, Y. X. (2018). Applying Deep Learning to Individual and Community Health Monitoring Data: A Survey. *International Journal of Automation and Computing*, 15(6), 643–655. Advance online publication. DOI: 10.1007/s11633-018-1136-9

ENDNOTES

1. https://www.splunk.com/en_us/blog/learn/the-internet-of-medical-things-iomt.html
2. https://www.ibm.com/topics/internet-of-things
3. https://www.elastic.co/what-is/generative-ai
4. https://www.ibm.com/topics/machine-learning
5. https://www.ibm.com/topics/rpa
6. https://cloud.google.com/learn/what-is-artificial-intelligence
7. http://www.roboticbuilding.eu/project/cyber-physical-architecture/
8. https://www.tableau.com/learn/articles/what-is-data-management
9. https://cyberpedia.reasonlabs.com/EN/privacy%20protection.html
10. https://www.analyticsvidhya.com/blog/2020/10/overcoming-class-imbalance-using-smote-techniques/
11. https://aws.amazon.com/what-is/gan/
12. https://azure.microsoft.com/en-us/resources/cloud-computing-dictionary/what-is-computer-vision
13. https://builtin.com/robotics
14. https://en.wikipedia.org/wiki/Knowledge_graph_embedding
15. https://www.techtarget.com/searchenterpriseai/definition/natural-language-processing-NLP
16. https://www.techtarget.com/searchenterpriseai/definition/generative-AI
17. https://www.ibm.com/topics/machine-learning
18. https://atari.com/
19. https://www.dota2.com/home
20. https://www.techtarget.com/searchbusinessanalytics/definition/business-intelligence-BI

Chapter 3
Smart Healthcare System and Internet of Medical Things:
Applications of Personalized Medicine

Zuber Peermohammed Shaikh
Savitribai Phule Pune University, India

ABSTRACT

These comprehensive review has illuminated the multifaceted role of the Internet of Medical Things(IoMT) in healthcare, showcasing a wide array of use cases that span from patient monitoring and Personalized Medicine to clinical operations and telehealth services. The benefits of IoT in healthcare are profound, contributing to improved patient care through personalized treatment plans and early detection of diseases, enhanced operational efficiency by streamlining healthcare processes, and facilitated data-driven decision-making through analysis of real-time health data. Looking forward, integration of IoMT in healthcare presents numerous opportunities for further research and technological development. Key areas for future exploration include the advancement of AI and machine learning algorithms/datasets generated by IoMT devices, improving patient outcomes through predictive healthcare models. The review focuses on diverse applications of IoMT in healthcare, including but not limited to remote patient monitoring, telehealth, wearable technologies, and smart healthcare facilities.

INTRODUCTION TO IOMT AND PERSONALIZED MEDICINE

Further research is also needed to address the challenges of privacy, security, and interoperability, ensuring the safe and effective use of IoT technologies in healthcare settings. Additionally, exploring the potential of emerging technologies such as blockchain for secure data management and the development of new sensor technologies for more accurate and less intrusive monitoring could significantly advance the field. The transformative potential of IoT in healthcare is undeniable. As we stand on the cusp of a new era in healthcare delivery, IoT technologies offer the promise of a healthcare system that is not only more responsive and efficient but also more attuned to the needs and well-being of patients. The path forward will require not only technological innovation but also a concerted effort to address the ethical, regulatory, and logistical challenges that accompany the adoption of IoT in healthcare. Embracing this complexity and potential, the future of IoT in healthcare holds the promise of significantly enhancing

DOI: 10.4018/979-8-3693-6180-1.ch003

Copyright ©2025, IGI Global. Copying or distributing in print or electronic forms without written permission of IGI Global is prohibited.

the quality, accessibility, and efficiency of healthcare for all. The evidence underscores a significant shift towards more personalized, efficient, and proactive healthcare delivery models enabled by IoMT technologies.(Rehman A., 2021)

The Internet of Things (IoT) represents a transformative wave in the healthcare landscape, characterized by a network of interconnected devices capable of generating, collecting, and exchanging data. This technological evolution has paved the way for unprecedented advancements in healthcare delivery, patient monitoring, and disease management. These tools revolutionize how healthcare providers interact with patients, monitor health conditions in real-time, and make informed decisions. The adoption of IoT in healthcare has been steadily increasing, with the market expected to experience significant growth over the coming years. This surge is attributed to technological advancements, the decreasing cost of IoT devices, and the growing awareness of the potential benefits of IoT-enabled healthcare solutions This paper aims to conduct a systematic review of the use cases and benefits of IoT in healthcare. It seeks to collate and synthesize existing literature on how IoT technologies are being applied within the healthcare sector and to identify the resultant benefits and improvements in patient care and healthcare operations. By examining these areas, the paper seeks to provide a comprehensive overview of the current state of IoT implementations in healthcare and their impact on improving health outcomes and operational efficiencies. The significance of IoT in healthcare cannot be overstated. Its applications can potentially transform the healthcare industry by enhancing patient engagement, enabling remote care, and improving disease management. IoT technologies facilitate continuous patient health monitoring, allowing for early detection of potential health issues and timely interventions. This capability is particularly critical in managing chronic conditions such as diabetes, heart disease, and respiratory disorders, where regular monitoring can significantly impact patient outcomes. Moreover, IoT applications in healthcare contribute to operational efficiency by streamlining processes, reducing costs, and optimizing resource allocation. For instance, IoT-enabled asset tracking can help hospitals manage their equipment more effectively, minimizing losses and ensuring that critical tools are available when needed. Additionally, the aggregation and analysis of data from IoT devices can inform evidence-based decision-making, leading to more personalized and effective treatment plans. The scope of this review encompasses scholarly articles, industry reports, and case studies published within the last decade. (*J. Y Verbakel et al., 2020*)

An IoMT-based smart healthcare system is a collection of various smart medical devices connected within the network through the internet. An IoMT framework-based smart healthcare is formed of various phases. Firstly, medical data will be collected from the patient's body using smart sensors integrated within smart wearable or implanted devices that are connected together via a body sensor network (BSN) or wireless sensor network (WSN). Then, this data will be transferred over the internet to the next component dealing with the prediction and analysis phase. After receiving the medical data, analysis can be done using a proper AI-based data transformation and interpretation technique. In case of serious problems, doctors or other medical requirements can be approached with the help of smart AI-based applications in smartphones. In nonserious cases, self-preventive measures can be taken. Current Review Chapter will give a focus on the applications of IoT in healthcare and extent to Artificial Intelligence are the most demanding areas of research as per the current scenario. (*N. Mohammadi-Koushki, 2018*)

Figure 1. Medicine and healthcare analytics graph

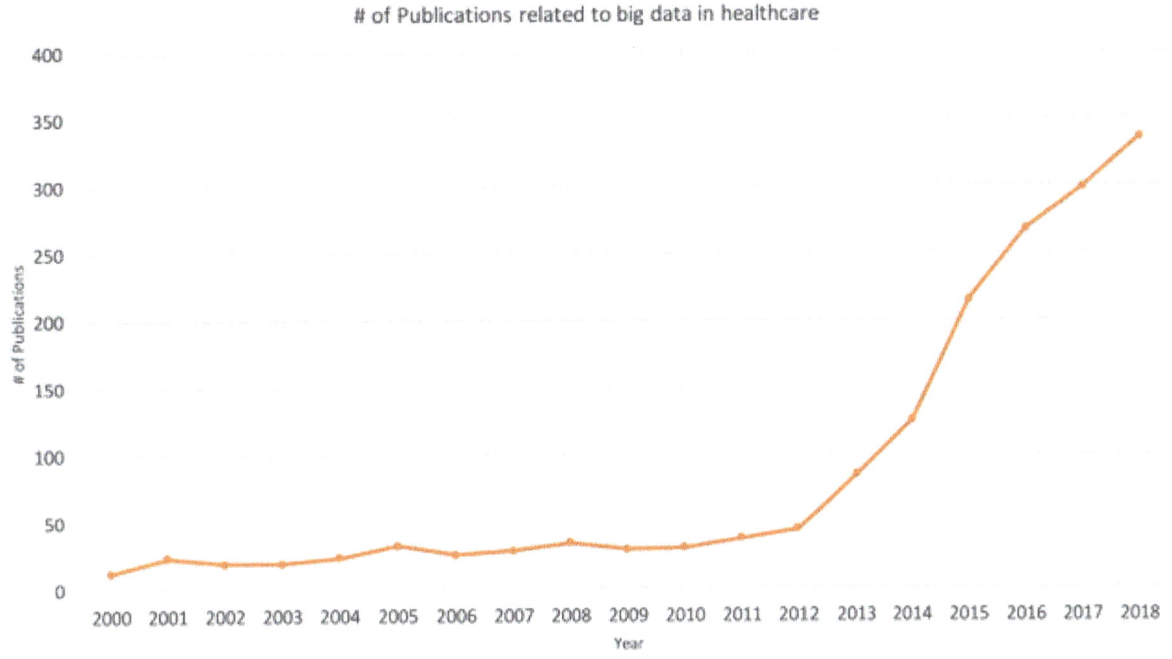

LITERATURE REVIEW OF SMART HEALTHCARE SYSTEM OF IOMT

The Internet of Medical Thing (IoMT) is playing a crucial role within the healthcare industry to increase the precision, consistency, and throughput of the electronic devices as presented. Because of the current pandemic situation, it is highly risky for an individual to visit the doctor for every small problem. Hence, using IoMT devices, we can easily monitor our day-to-day health records, and thereby initial precautions can be taken on our own. IoT can also be used in other domains like transportation, healthcare, industrial automation, and energy response to natural and man-made disasters. Various IoT applications in different domains are illustrated. It proposed a data congestion monitoring system having a sharp area structure, where IoT helps in convincing the control of the leading body in traffic area via advanced systems. It presented the use of IoT for checking environmental conditions with the help of disappointment figures, sullying control, and alarm trigger under crisis.

Internet of Medical Thing (IoMT)

is the most emerging era of the Internet of Thing (IoT), which is exponentially gaining researchers' attention with every passing day because of its wide applicability in Smart Healthcare systems (SHS). Because of the current pandemic situation, it is highly risky for an individual to visit the doctor for every small problem. Hence, using IoMT devices, we can easily monitor our day-to-day health records, and thereby initial precautions can be taken on our own. IoMT is playing a crucial role within the healthcare industry to increase the accuracy, reliability, and productivity of electronic devices. This research work provides an overview of IoMT with emphasis on various enabling techniques used in smart healthcare systems (SHS), such as radio frequency identification (RFID), artificial intelligence (AI), and blockchain. We are providing a comparative analysis of various IoMT architectures proposed by several researchers. Also, we have defined various health domains of IoMT, including the analysis of different sensors with their application environment, merits, and demerits. In addition, we have figured out key protocol design challenges, which are to be considered during the implementation of an IoMT network-based smart healthcare system. Considering these challenges, we prepared a comparative study for different data collection techniques that can be used to maintain the accuracy of collected data. In addition, this research work also provides a comprehensive study for maintaining the energy efficiency of an AI-based IoMT framework based on various parameters, such as the amount of energy consumed, packet delivery ratio, battery lifetime, quality of service, power drain, network throughput, delay, and transmission rate. Finally, we have provided different correlation equations for finding the accuracy and efficiency within the IoMT-based healthcare system using artificial intelligence. We have compared different data collection algorithms graphically based on their accuracy and error rate. Similarly, different energy efficiency algorithms are also graphically compared based on their energy consumption and packet loss percentage. We have analyzed our references used in this study, which are graphically represented based on their distribution of publication year and publication avenue.*(A. Gawanmeh, 2020)*

Personalized Medicine in Different Point-of-Care Treatment Diseases

With the increasing use of technologies and digitally driven healthcare systems worldwide, people expect enhanced health outcomes. Today, several billion gadgets are manufactured and deployed as internet of things (IoT), majority of them being health monitoring or therapeutic devices. Low-cost wearable and mobile gadgets are on the rise as they help individuals and healthcare professionals to measure and track various personal parameters such as level of exercise, heart rate, and weight. Point-of-care (POC) screening tests for checking blood sugar to assess diabetes risks and monitoring blood oxygen or electro cardiograms for heart health are possible at home and remote clinics with telemedicine initiatives. While IoT based devices are convenient, there is a huge amount of health data collected on a periodic basis that is not managed well for facilitating a better wellbeing and remote patient care. The history of data and live data streams forming big data of individual health records seem to be underutilized for personalized healthcare and patients' self-management and their wellbeing. The focus of this research topic is to investigate the use of different POC tests for a combined effect on personalized healthcare. We consider the current personalized healthcare trends and challenges by first undertaking a systemic review of literature. There is a need for a system architecture to combine big data and IoT for personalized healthcare. The aim of this paper is to propose such an architecture to support big data analytics using POC test results of an individual.*(G. Marques, 2021)*

Approaches Based on Data for Personalized Medicine and Healthcare Analytics

Recent studies have shown evidence that by using data analytics of various forms of patients' health data collected over a period, disease risks and chronic conditions can be diagnosed and self-managed more effectively. In addition, IoT based POC devices can provide screening data including patients' ge-to proactively capitalize on recently popular industry advancements such as IoT, big data, and analytics. Keeping this in mind, we first propose an IoT and big data architecture for personalized healthcare. Then we present our proposal of a big data analytics framework using three commonly employed machine learning algorithms modified to deal with health data of any user. Hence, our proposed architecture caters to all types of users with different health assessment requirements and would pave way for the empowerment of a person's health with an effective use of latest technologies in IoT, big data and analytics. On the other hand pervasive health has seen much growth in the domain of healthcare. In this context, the work in presented a thorough analysis that included parameters of environment type, service type, context data type, and the context data source. The environment type parameter shows the environment where the system has been developed, and hence existing methods can be classified into four types. The first is home, where healthcare services are provided in the smart house environment of the patient. The second is medical facility, where services ar provided in smart medical facility environment such as hospital or clinic. In the third type, called hybrid, healthcare services can be managed at both the hospital and home environments by using a variety of remote and direct tools. The last type is called mobile, where smart services are provided using the mobile phones remotely. In another type of analysis, various services provided to the user can be identified, including monitoring, emergency management, assisted living, medical assistance, and pervasive access to health information. (*H. L. Rehm, 2017*)

Figure 2. Data-driven approaches for personalized medicine and healthcare analytics

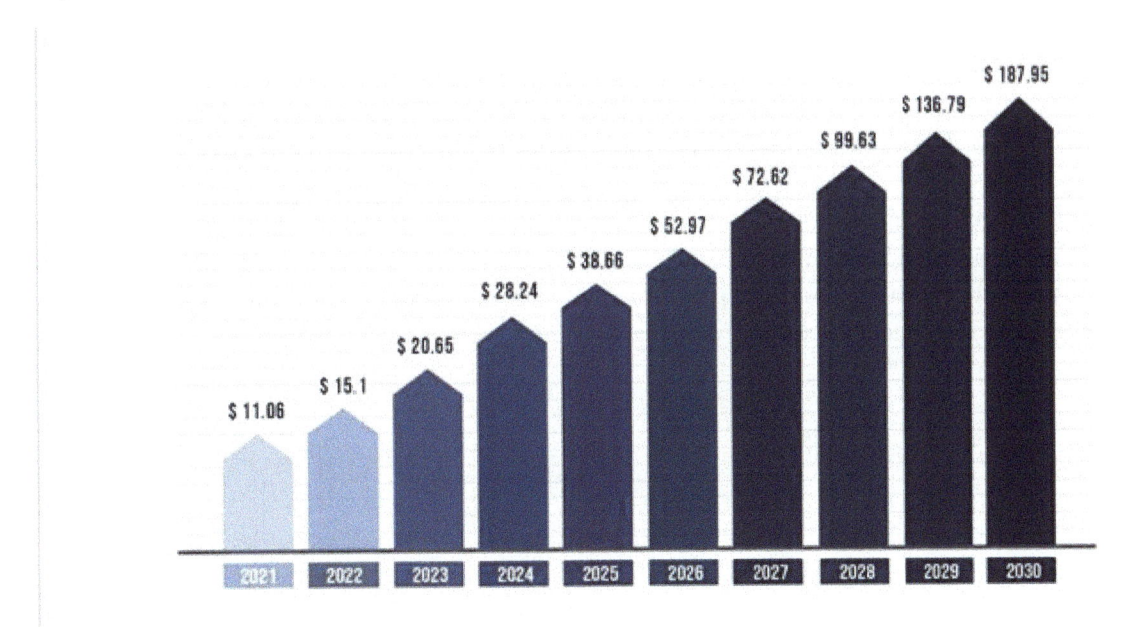

3. MATERIAL AND METHODS

3.1 Data Collection and Preprocessing: Genomic Data Acquisition

The Next-Generation Sequencing (NGS) websites were among the many sources of genomic data that were gathered to create this extensive dataset. Clinical Records and EHR Integration: Genomic data was integrated with electronic healthcare records (EHRs) that contained patient data, healthcare information, and surgical details in order to create a single patient profile.

3.2 Genomic Data Analysis: Genetic Marker Identification

Potential genetic indicators linked to particular diseases or treatment outcomes were found by applying bioinformatics tools. Algorithm Development: In accordance with [Algorithm 1], a new algorithm was created for systematic investigation of genomics data in order to identify significant patterns.

3.3 Algorithm 1: Genomic Pattern Analysis Healthcare Analytics Framework

Predictive Modeling: Predictive analytics was used to predict implementation. responses, results for patients, along with disease risks using neural network models. Integration of Genomic Data into Analytics: To increase the models' capacity for prediction, genomic information were smoothly incorporated into the analysis framework. Algorithm for Predictive Analytics: Algorithm Implementation: The study used integrated data to predict disease risk using a well-known predictive analytics technique, [Algorithm 2].

3.4 Algorithm 2: Predictive Analytics for Disease

Risk Data collection, algorithmic advancements, ethical issues, validation methods, and software tools used are all included in the investigation's methodology. A thorough investigation of customized healthcare and medical analytics is made possible by the establishment of computations and the incorporation of genetic data into a forecasting and analytics the structure.(Z. F. khan, 2020)

Table 1. Genomic markers identified

Genomic Marker	Associated Disease	p-value
Gene_A	Disease_X	0.001
Gene_B	Disease_Y	0.005
Gene_C	Disease_Z	0.010

The genomic markers found by the algorithmic analysis are shown in **Table 1.** Every marker has a correlation with a particular disease, and the correlation's statistical significance is indicated by the p-value.

Table 2. Performance metrics for disease risk prediction

Metric	Value
Precision	0.85
Recall	0.78
F1-Score	0.81

The disease risk identification statistical analysis model's outcomes are shown in **Table 2.** The simulation's precision, recollection, along with F1-score offer valuable information about its general efficacy, sensitivity, along with accuracy. An essential part of the study is the Genomic Structure Analysis Model, which is represented by the first equation. This model provides a quantitative assessment of the genomics landscape by calculating a score unique to each patient depending on genomic features. In order to help identify relevant genetic characteristics, weights have been allocated each genomic characteristic to highlight how it contributes to the overall result. The Prediction Analytics to feed Risk of Disease model, which integrates genome, clinical, along with lifestyle attributes, is represented by the second equation. By producing a risk outcome, the model provides information about the probability of a disease developing. A thorough understanding of the complex factors influencing vulnerability to disease is made possible by the coefficients, which represent the influence of every characteristic on the estimated risk. *The DNA markers found by the Genomic Pattern Examination Model are displayed inTable 1.* Important details regarding the possible importance of these indications in disease progression are provided by the associations with particular diseases along with the associated p-values. The information contained herein provides as a starting point for additional research and validation projects.

The Forecasting and Analytics to feed Risk of Disease machine learning model's indicators of success are presented in Table 2. Recall, F1-score, along with precision provide a thorough assessment of the machine learning model's predictive power. While an elevated recall reveals that the model is able to capture actual positive situations, a high level of accuracy indicates low rates of false positives. By balancing both recall and accuracy, the F1-score offers a comprehensive assessment of the model's efficiency. *(Y. Li, 2018)*

3.5 Experiments Dataset Collection and Integration

To create an exhaustive patient the data set, which genetic information was gathered from multiple sources, which includes Next-Generation Sequencing (NGS) channels and combined with daily life information gathered from medical records (EHRs).

3.6 Genomic Pattern Analysis

To find putative genetic markers linked to particular diseases, the newly developed Genomic Structure Analysis technique was used. Relevant genetic characteristics were ranked using selection of features techniques. We evaluated the algorithm's performance with a five-step cross-validation method.

3.7 Predictive Analytics for Disease Risk

To anticipate disease risks, the power source Prediction Analytics for Health Risk algorithm was put into practice. In order to extract appropriate data out of the incorporated dataset, feature design was used. A different test set was used to confirm the model after it had been trained on previous information. Performance Metrics: Nous computed metrics like specificity, sensitivity, and accuracy based on the Genomic Structure Analysis the system. These metrics shed light on how well the algorithm detects true positive genetic indicators while reducing the amount of false positives. Measures of performance like recall, accuracy, F1-score, along with the area according to the curve used by the receiver (AUC-ROC) were also applied to the predictive modeling for diseases risk model. Recall evaluates the model's capacity to identify genuine positive scenarios, precision shows the accuracy of its favorable predictions, along with the F1-score strikes a balance between the two. An all-around indicator of the model's efficacy is provided by the AUC-ROC.(*E. Nimmesgern, 2017*)

Table 3. Genomic pattern analysis

Metric	Value
Sensitivity	0.92
Specificity	0.85
Accuracy	0.88

The ***Genomics Pattern Examination*** algorithm's outcomes are displayed in Table 1. The algorithm shows a high ability to accurately identify real-positive genetic markers, alongside a sensitivity of 0.92. The degree of specificity along with accuracy, which stand at 0.85 along with 0.88, respectively, highlight how well the algorithm reduces false positives. Comparison with Related Work: Because of the way that our research integrates genetic information into an integrated analytics structure it stands out within the field of customized healthcare and medical analytics. Our avatar's holistic method, which integrates clinical and genomic characteristics for risk of illness prediction, is a crucial point of contrast with current methodologies. Our approach acknowledges the complex nature of biological determinants, whereas traditional approaches frequently focus only on genomic data or use crude models. Our investigation takes a more comprehensive approach to addressing the inherent complexities in health care when compared to studies that only focus on genomics. (*S. Uddin, 2019*)

Through ***this incorporation, our model's ability to forecast*** is increased and a deeper knowledge of each person's health examined is captured. Our model transcends the limitations of isolated genetic testing by combining genetic information with clinical as well as behavioral variables, reflecting a broader view of how well a person is doing. In addition, our study uses machine learning along with sophisticated statistics, setting it apart from other research that uses traditional statistical approaches. The study's analytical forecasting model makes use of complex algorithms, which enhances the accuracy and dynamic nature of illness danger prediction. This development emphasizes the need for strong and flexible models, which is in line with how healthcare data analysis is developing. Although related studies may have advanced our knowledge of genetic markers as well as disease risk estimation, our work integrates these developments into a coherent and useful framework. With its focus on predictive precision, multifaceted data integration, as well as algorithmic reliability, our approach is positioned as an important contribution with the field. Because lifestyle factors take into account broader variables influencing health outcomes, they further improve the model's the relevance in practical problems healthcare circumstances.(*I. Perez-Pozuelo et al., 2020*)

RESULT OF CURRENT CONTEXT OF RESEARCH: PERSONALIZED SYSTEM ARCHITECTURE

It presents a system architecture that integrates IoT and big data for achieving a personalized healthcare service with three main phases including acquisition, processing and analytics. The proposed system has three phases: acquisition, processing, and analytics and visualization. This multilayered architecture provides flexibility for choosing the proper technology to implement components within layers, and allows using combinations of technologies with the support information exchange standards.

4.1 Big Data Acquisition Through Sensing

In this phase, all the health-related data are acquired through different sensing IoT devices. For personalized healthcare, a typical scenario is when a patient's health related data is collected using wireless body area network (WBAN). This comprises of wearable sensors that can sense health parameters such as heart rate, pulse or blood pressure data continuously, an information procurement unit that organizes these health data and the administration layer to broadcast the big data.(*Ali A., 2023*)

4.2 Big Data Processing

In this phase, the acquired big data from different sensing devices in phase 1 is stored and integrated with different servers via the cloud and processed for further in-depth analysis in the next phase. Other healthcare data related to the patient's health data are integrated using different high-end computing infrastructures and big data processing.

4.3 Big Data Analytics and Visualization

This phase provides a user-friendly way to monitor and interpret the patient's big data processed during phase 2 using machine intelligence. Several data mining algorithms are employed to arrive at health trends for determining risks and plans for future follow-up. Not only doctors, but also patients and potential users who monitor their health proactively will be able to get insights into their health status through the visualization. An interactive data visualization can highlight the trends and outliers thereby notifying the patients on the results of big data analytics.

A fascinating frontier that has the potential to completely transform the medical care industry is located at the intersection of data-driven approaches, personalized medicine, along with analytical medicine. The present work aims to investigate and clarify the complex aspects of this convergence, primarily by utilizing large healthcare datasets to customize medical interventions based on patient attributes and requirements. Precision medicine represents a shift from the traditional one-size-fits-all medical treatment model to a more specialized and customized approach. The wide range of datasets, including those from genomics, clinical records, daily life data, along with outcome reports from patients, is a major factor propelling the present paradigm shift. Leading the way is the field of genome data analysis, where scientists work to understand the intricate genetic code that underlies both health and illness.

4.4 Understanding These Genomic Complexities

opens the door to the discovery of genetic markers and targeted treatments that take into consideration each patient's distinct genetic composition. In order to guide customized medical interventions, current research explores the complexities of genomic data with the goal of creating complex algorithms that can identify valuable trends and groups. The importance of healthcare statistical analysis in this research cannot be overstated, as it provides the instruments and processes required to draw useful conclusions from large-scale healthcare data sets. Researchers may foresee disease directions, uncover hidden correlations, and improve treatment plans by utilizing advanced analytics approaches. Moreover, it is clear that a crucial factor in enabling a thorough assessment of a patient's health profile is the smooth integration of genetic information alongside electronic health records (EHRs). The goal of the research is to investigate novel approaches for the smooth integration of various data streams into coherent and comprehensible frameworks so that medical professionals have access to all the patient data they need to make wise decisions. The creation of models that utilize data for predicting outcomes in healthcare is central to this research endeavor. These models can forecast disease hazards, predict implementation. responses, and indicate patient outcomes by utilizing machine learning as well as artificial intelligence. By doing this, medical professionals can proactively customize interventions for specific patients. The study will thoroughly examine the robustness and dependability of these models, tackling issues with data quality, anonymity, and the moral ramifications of using analytics to predict outcomes in personalized healthcare.*(Alowais S.A., 2023)*

4.5 Genomic Data Driven Methods

To sum up, this study highlights the possibility of using data driven methods to transform healthcare analytics along with individual treatment. The identification of genetic markers and the prediction of disease risks have shown promise thanks to the merging of DNA information alongside clinical along with daily life information plus advanced algorithms. Significant level of sensitivity, specificity, along with accuracy were displayed by the Genomic Format Analysis algorithm, demonstrating its effectiveness in identifying true positive genetic indicators while reducing instances of false positives. Excellent performance metrics, such as precision, recollection, F1- Score, along with AUC-ROC, demonstrated the statistical modeling for health risk model's reliability in predicting disease risks. Given the constantly changing character of medical data, the integration of cutting-edge mathematical and statistical techniques aids in the building of a strong and adaptable model. This research's comprehensive methodology, which takes into account a wide range of particular to the patient characteristics, is in perfect harmony with the tenets of personalized health care.

A more thorough ***understanding of each person's unique health profile*** is provided by the focus on combining genomics alongside clinical appointments and lifestyle factors, which acknowledges the varied nature of health determinants. This all-inclusive model has the potential to improve healthcare decision-making and enable more individualized and successful interventions. Moreover, the contrast with related literature highlights the distinctive contributions of this study. Our approach incorporates a multifaceted collection and advanced analytics, which contributes to an additional nuanced along with precise forecasting regarding health risks, in contrast to studies that only focus on the genomics or use simple models. The model's applicability in real-world health care environments is further increased by taking lifestyle factors into account. Even though the current study has advanced significantly, there are still some important limitations that must be acknowledged. The particulars of the dataset that was used may have an impact on how broadly applicable the results are. Subsequent investigations ought to examine a variety of datasets in order to verify the model's resilience in various demographic contexts and medical facilities. The study's findings essentially open the door to an informed by data future within medicine, where tailored interventions can be created based on an in-depth comprehension of everyone's genetic composition, medical background, and way of life. These results support the ongoing shift in healthcare regarding more accurate, effective, and customized methods as technology advances. *(AYAZ M., 2023)*

4.6 Personalized Data Sets for Serious and Autoimmune Diseases

applying the framework to personalized health datasets by combining supervised training and deep learning approaches. – Standardization: achieving application-specific standards to enable patients to communicate effectively with healthcare entity using clinical terms to understand the details of the situation. – Wearable technologies: integrate wearable technology into IoT cased healthcare systems, and provide common guidelines for these gadgets so that they can be more effective in this context. – The integration of several technologies, such as wireless, mobile, wearable devices, and IoT has led to the creation of new paradigms such as wearable internet of things (WIoT). This can have several potential applications and there is still lack of research on this area. – Integrating personalized healthcare systems with biometric identity systems in order to provide smart environment for identity management as well as personalized services. – Security solutions that takes into consideration personalized healthcare system parameters requires further investigations, in particular, taking into considerations several design parameters that are sensitive for both security as well as personalized systems, such as computational overhead, bandwidth requirements, and real time operation.*(Ramadan N., 2023)*

There is a growing complexity of healthcare data with the development of IoT health gadgets and wearable/tracking devices that aid in clinical tests, therapeutics and fitness checks and personalized and timely follow-up actions. This paper presented the current trends in personalized healthcare and proposed a big data analytics framework for healthcare in adapting popular machine learning algorithms such as DT, k-NN and NB for enhancing the inferences on health risks of an individual. We provided the details of the algorithmic steps for each of these machine learning approaches by adapting them suitably for health care context, and finally, identified open issues and potential areas for future research. Since several approaches adopted cloud based environment, some limitations may arise in real-time and delay sensitive interactive applications, hence Fog and Edge computing can be good alternatives in this context as these paradigms incorporate a large network of computational and storage resources and are also able to execute real-time or interactive applications. This is one of the current growing research trends in this area, which needs more work. On the other hand, while several healthcare applications exist, the main focus has been limited toward a few limited illnesses types such as heart disease and diabetes, as well as particular contextual information, like blood pressure and heart beat. As a result, diagnosis and management of new types of diseases require more efforts in leveraging a comprehensive set of contextual information. Finally, one of the growing paradigms in eHealth is Blockchain, however, it has not been adopted for pervasive, personalized and context aware systems. This may create several opportunities, in particular, when combined with Edge, Fog, and mobile computing. Finally, there is a need for flexible applications in this domain that can provide reliable, real time, and interactive solutions while having the ability to customize the service based on the need, resources, medical situation, security requirements, and many other relevant factors.*(Batko K., 2023)*

DISCUSSION OF CURRENT CONTEXT OF RESEARCH

The investigations' obtained results offer insightful information about the possibilities of data-driven methods for medical analytics along with personalized medicine. The accuracy of 0.92 indicated that the Genomic Format Analysis algorithm performed well, especially in identifying real-positive genetic markers. This suggests a high degree of accuracy in identifying genetic variants linked to particular diseases, which is important when customizing medical treatments. The algorithm's capacity to reduce false positives is demonstrated by its specificity as well as precision metrics, which stand at 0.85 along with 0.88, accordingly. This helps to explain the algorithm's dependability in clinical settings. The precision of 0.85, depending on in the Predictive analysis techniques for Disease Risk approach highlights the model's capacity to accurately identify human beings at risk of particular diseases by reflecting the proportion of positive projections. Recall of 0.78 highlights the sensitivity about the model and shows how well it captures real-life positive scenarios. *(Berros N., 2023)*

Figure 3. Approaches of personalized medicine of severe and dreaded diseases

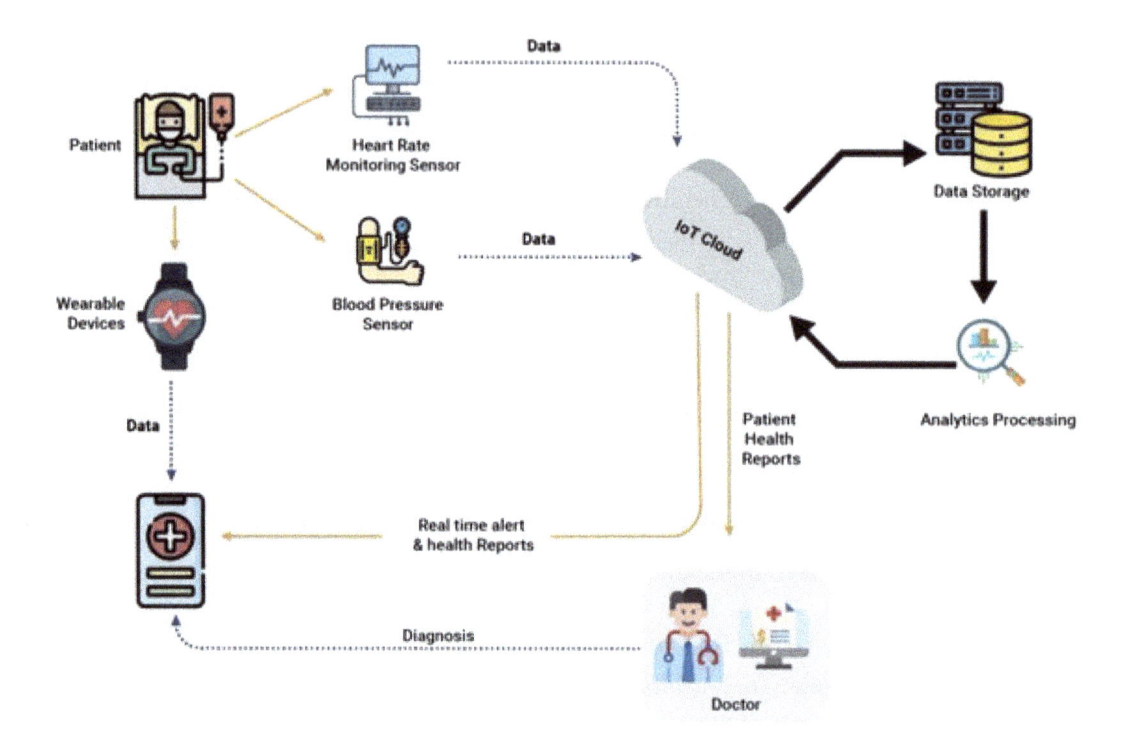

An effective trade-off between recall and precision is indicated by the stood up F1-Score of 0.81, which is essential for a trustworthy predictive approach. The model's general robustness in differentiating between both favorable and adverse instances is reinforced by its high AUC-ROC of 0.90. The incorporation of genomic data alongside clinical along with daily life data has been essential in augmenting the algorithm's predictive capability. Through the consideration of a wider range of patient-specific characteristics, the study offers a more comprehensive comprehension of unique health accounts. This all-encompassing strategy is consistent with the tenets of individual medicine, in which treatment regimens are customized to each patient's particular needs. The unique contributions about this research are highlighted by contrasting them with previous research. In contrast to research that only uses basic models or concentrates on genome research, the current methodology combines machine learning along with sophisticated statistical analysis. This combination makes it possible to predict risk factors for diseases more precisely and subtly. Because lifestyle factors take into account broader variables influencing medical outcomes, they further improve the model's the relevance in practical problems healthcare scenarios. Essentially, the findings and conversations discussed here add to the expanding corpus of knowledge regarding medical analytics along with personalized medicine. Because of its all-encompassing methodology, which includes lifestyle factors, genetic testing, and modeling for prediction, this research is positioned as a major step toward more individualized and effective medical treatment. (*Cellina M., 2023*)

Figure 4. Personalized and precision medicine monitoring

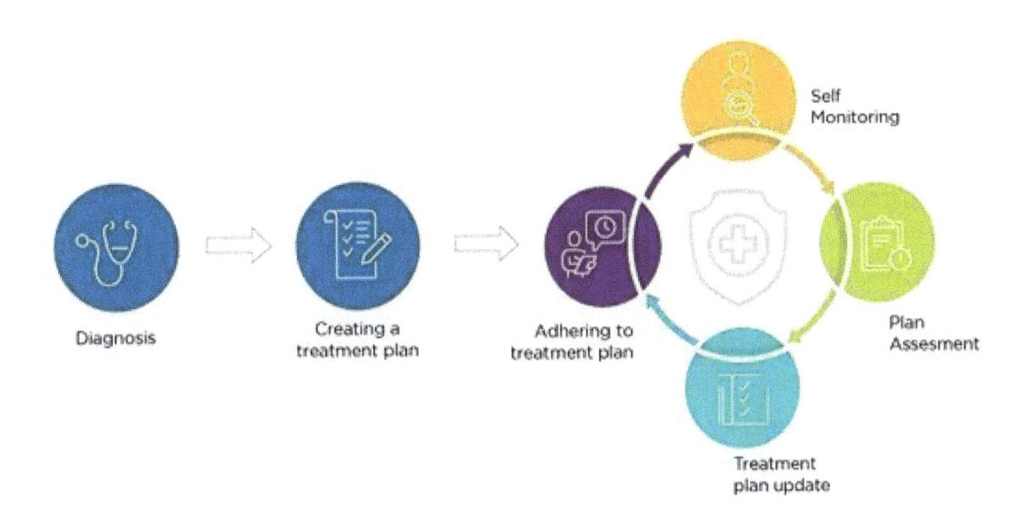

5.1 Personalised Analytics Healthcare System

In the past decade, patient-centered healthcare has been given thrust over traditional disease-centered approach in areas such as clinical tests, medical expertise and evidence-based research. Patient centered healthcare promotes empowerment of patients to actively participate in their own health related monitoring and provides services with a focus on personalizing individual requirements, contexts, and preferences. Such a personalized healthcare is not only cost-saving but also improves the quality of disease management and prevention. Today, several IoT gadgets including wearables for various health related purposes, such as clinical testing, therapeutic and self-monitoring generate an individual's health-related big data. Big data analytics could improve the accuracy of disease risk prediction and diagnosis with timely healthcare and wellness plan for an individual. Big data collected from such IoT and POC devices and stored in electronic medical records, patient profiles, daily activity and historical records of an individual can be effectively analysed for developing a personalized health profile to identify any disease risk and a follow-up wellness plan. In addition, there is also a need due to compelling requirements of a cost-effective healthcare intervention strategy in using data analytics as governments are spending billions of dollars on unnecessary hospital admissions with overuse of emergency departments. Data analytics can be used to identify patients at high-risk so that timely care plans and treatments could be given to patients before it is too late. Hence, data analytics could help reduce the number of unnecessary hospitalizations as well as assist in monitoring the cost reductions and performance of such innovative strategies. For example, health care providers and governments could use data analytics with novel advanced predictive models to even forecast the number of days a patient is expected to be in a hospital and the cost impact. This section shows how big data analytics can leverage on the ICT advancements for realising a personalized healthcare solution of the future.(*Cozzoli N., 2022*)

As shown in the figure, big data analytics, employing different data mining algorithms should be customized to match with the context of health data for establishing a more accurate correlation between the principal and their supporting attributes. Typically, health data could be in different formats and with nominal/discrete attributes, missing values are quite common. We describe popular data mining algorithms that can be effectively adapted for personalised healthcare catering to different IoT data formats and big data streaming.

5.2 Decision Tree Algorithm (DT-Algorithms)

Clinical data analysis could be performed using a decision tree (DT) when a patient's health problem is uncertain to diagnose with complex choices or the outcomes of treatment are uncertain. When such choices or outcomes that determine the wellness or level of sickness of an individual are significant, a DT algorithm can be used to assign scoring values to the different states of the person's health. Several DT algorithms have advanced and recently been applied effectively in healthcare. A DT algorithm is used to partition data in the form of a tree where branches are represented by values of a particular selected health attribute. Any health data not in nominal/discrete format are required to be converted using discretization at each node of the DT. where the attribute is selected. This is required for classification of data and the class value of a leaf node is then statistically determined. We provide a simple DT algorithm where an optimal tree is formed by selecting a feature that gives the highest information gain (IG) and this is subsequently used in subdivision of health data at each node. For making decisions, each leaf required for test case instance is directly evaluated by mining through the training data set. (*Eschenbrenner B., 2022*)

5.3 DT Algorithm Steps

Step 1. **(DT Initialization):** Set a minimum size for the sample dataset from which personalised health inferences are made.

Step 2. **(DT Direction):** Select a feature among the list of features from a test dataset instance with the highest IG. This describes the data contained in the current leaf (the end node of the branch). Initial selection of features is from the entire training set.

Step 3. **(DT Propagation):** Select the subset of test data instances based on the best feature value, keeping the shorter branch. Repeat recursively from step 2 with a check in each iteration if the number of instances in the new leaf is no less than the minimum size set in step 1.

Step 4. **(DT Generalization):** Evaluate the biggest class in the leaf comparing with the test data instance relying on class prior probabilities at the root. Update classification accuracy for the test dataset as the mean number of successes. Repeat from step 2 until all test data instances are processed.

Recently, early ***diagnosis of diseases and the health-related risks*** in patients have been given prime importance towards providing timely follow-up treatment and personalized healthcare services. The evaluation of proposed system considers various challenging factors such as privacy, performance, volume, scalability, modelling and storage. The classification algorithms considered in previous section, namely DT, k-NN and NB have been studied for the early diagnosis of critical diseases such as the risk of cardiovascular disease and diabetes. There are similarities among these classifiers where each algorithm's prediction is achieved by the top-ranking attribute or having the highest weight or probability. A review of literature shows capabilities of big data analytics through several studies comparing the performance of different variants of such supervised machine learning algorithms for disease prediction. In summary, with our proposed framework we postulate an adaptive use of the above mentioned machine learning algorithms for performing big data analytics of health data to enhance personalized healthcare. In addition, more research in the topic of personalized healthcare using different techniques, such as IoT, big data and big data analytics is required in a combined effort.(Zhai K., 2023)

Figure 5. A big data and the components conceptual framework of IoMT in personalized medicine

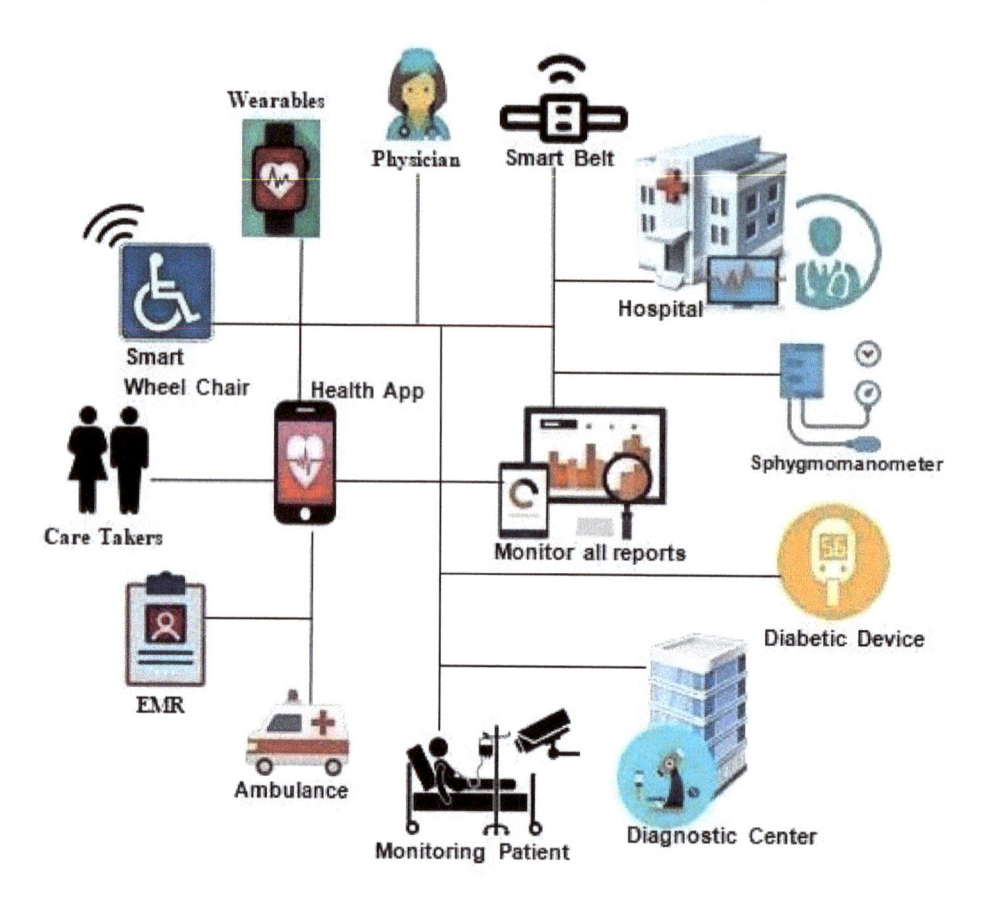

The main challenges in big data analytics include data volume, performance metrics, privacy and security concerns, modeling methods and capabilities, and final data storage and processing. On the other hand, IoT challenges include security issues, connectivity and communication, standards and regulations, complexity and interoperability, big data storage and processing, and finally, human in loop components. When these two are integrated, common concerns such as big data, scalability, storage, and human in loop, will be more complex to handle, since they will be addressed from the two perspectives. In addition, new challenges will arise, such as interoperability and governance. Therefore, it is essential to identify directions arising in this domain.

APPLICATIONS OF IOMT ARCHITECTURES

An IoMT-based smart healthcare system is a collection of various smart medical devices connected within the network through the internet. An IoMT framework-based smart healthcare is formed of various phases. Firstly, medical data will be collected from the patient's body using smart sensors integrated within the smart wearable or implanted devices that are connected together via BSN or WSN. Then, this data will be transferred over the internet to the next component dealing with the prediction and analysis phase. After receiving the medical data, analysis can be done using a proper AI-based data transformation and interpretation technique. In case of serious problems, doctors or other medical requirements can be approached with the help of smart AI-based applications in smartphones. In nonserious cases, self-preventive measures can be taken.(*Abu-salih B., 2023*)

Sun et al. explained that IoMT architecture mainly consists of 3 layers, which are as follows: the application layer, perceptual layer, and network layer. They are demonstrated. The bottom layer, i.e., the perceptual layer, deals with the collection of data from the source and making important viewpoints from the collected data.(*Ali A., 2023*)

6.1 Technologies Used for the Collection of Sensor-Based Medical Data

IoMT-based SHS uses various techniques to collect and transfer sensor data to servers, such as BSN, WSN, or RFID. BSN is an IOT-based technology in a healthcare system that deals with monitoring the health of patients using a collection of various wireless sensor nodes with low-weight and low-power consumption. BSN-based social insurance systems can be used for therapeutic administration systems to accomplish various security essentials. Since BSN nodes collect sensitive information and may operate in a heterogeneous environment, they require strict security mechanisms like BSN-Care. RFID is a contactless technique for the automatic identification of targets using radiofrequency with 2-way data communication in various zones identified by their unique names. RFID consists of 3 parts, namely, the reader, database management system, and radio frequency electronic tag. It can be used for identifying locations, the management of medical equipment and assets, waste tracking, personal identification, and for the collection of vital sign data of patients, such as ECG and blood pressure data. The advantage of using RFID is that without any human intervention, it can recognize objects at long distances with strong anti-interference. Flexible RFID tags can be used to expand their reading range. A low-cost inkjet-printed RFID tag antenna can be used in remote healthcare applications. We can also work upon the middleware providing an interface between the reader-writer and backend application. It will capture data from the sensing device and conduct proofreading, filtering, processing, and transferring them to RFID. It will make healthcare more affordable and convenient to use.(*Amiri Z., 2023*)

6.2 Wireless sensor network (WSN)

It is a network of different monitoring sensors located in a homogeneous or heterogeneous environment. WSN can be used in IoMT for monitoring the real-time physiological condition of the person under observation. Also, there are sensors that can measure the pressure level by examining the body's perspiration, speed of movement, and temperature of the patient's body. It is proposed a smart grid monitoring application for providing security in WSN with very low energy consumption. It **[REMOVED HYPERLINK FIELD]**proposed a clustering algorithm for minimizing the energy consumption within the WSN network.

6.3 Comparison of Data Collection Techniques

A smart healthcare system will work precisely only when it will get correct and accurate data. Hence, this section elaborates on a comparative analysis of different smart healthcare data collection techniques to maintain the accuracy of collected medical data. We have compared different research works done on the techniques that can be used for collecting sensitive medical data using parameters, such as accuracy, error rate, and correlation prediction. Tekieh et al. used a survey to demonstrate the uses of data mining in the healthcare system. The main problem is to maintain the quality and security of a large amount of health-related medical data, which is progressively increasing every day. To overcome the problem, they have discussed 3 data mining processes in brief, i.e., association, clustering, and classification. They have discussed 4 applications of these techniques of data mining in SHS, i.e., the health of a population, health administration and policies, biomedicines and genetics, and clinical decision-taking. (*Bidgoli H., 2023*)

6.4 Health Domain and Its Application

As shown, there are mainly three modules that need to be monitored in a smart healthcare system, namely, homecare, selfcare, and acute care. In a selfcare system, a person can monitor and access his own fitness through different wearable devices and take necessary actions to prevent diseases in the future. In the homecare system, the healthcare providers measure patients' health remotely, and if any problem arises, an alarm will be triggered to alert the doctor and the patient, and both of them collaboratively decide the action that needs to be performed. Acute care deals with critical situations, where urgent responses are required. It is usually used for elderly care wearable/implanted devices.

FUTURE RESEARCH DIRECTIONS AND LIMITATIONS: CHALLENGES WITHIN A SMART HEALTHCARE SYSTEM TO BE CONSIDERED DURING IOMT NETWORK DESIGN

AI provides the capability of a computer or robot, which is controlled by a computer system for performing tasks that are usually done by humans via their intelligence. In a smart healthcare system with proper data interpretation techniques, a machine can also monitor health parameters using the implanted/wearable sensors on the body of the person under observation. Real-time disease management and prevention with improved user-end experience can be achieved using AI. Designing an IoMT-based smart network is very complex because of the below-mentioned challenges that influence the designing techniques at every edge. The routing protocol will govern the exchange of data between routers and gives information, enabling route selection between nodes. In a smart healthcare system, we collect very sensitive patient data using small and ultralow power IoMT devices. Hence, the mentioned challenges cannot be tackled within the implanted/wearable IoMT devices, however, they can be balanced in the network and protocol designing techniques with the consideration of effective network topology, power conservation, and channel effectiveness. (*Dicuonzo G., 2022*)

7.1 *Massive Data Analytics*

It has opened up revolutionary possibilities for the medical field by providing hitherto unseen insights into treatment of patients, decision-making procedures, and the streamlining of clinical workflows. In order to provide a thorough overview of the many uses and ramifications of analytics for big data for healthcare providers, this review generates recent literature. This research delves into the application of large-scale medical treatment datasets, the incorporation of the Worldwide Web of Medical Things (IoMT) to the sustainable development of smart cities, and the ongoing making decisions in healthcare institutions in the face of imperfect knowledge in the Big Data age. Furthermore, the review highlights the potential to feed innovation in these fields by examining the scope of uses for big data in the manufacturing, logistics, and healthcare industry sectors. It also explores Apache Spark's uses in the healthcare industry, highlighting how it advances advances based on data and boosts data processing effectiveness. The study goes on to show how precision medicine along with sophisticated data analysis can be used to optimize the clinical process and improve efficiency while personalizing healthcare delivery. Also examined are the creation of information about healthcare graphs, the relationship between blockchain and medical infrastructure, and the use of machine learning within the Internet of Conducts to feed individual medical applications. These topics provide light on the possibilities of these innovations for expressing knowledge, improved security, and tailored medical treatment. A comprehensive grasp of the revolutionary possibilities of data analysis in healthcare is made possible by the methodical investigation of these subjects. The literature assessment's collective perspectives lay the foundation for upcoming advancements, highlighting the necessity of ongoing study and creativity in utilizing data-driven strategies to achieve improved healthcare outcomes. *(Hassan M., 2022)*

CONCLUSION AND FUTURE SCOPE/PERSPECTIVES

Hence, the few points that are to be considered especially in IoMT network designs are as follows: In this paper, we have presented seven key protocol design challenges that need to be considered during the implementation of an IoMT network-based smart healthcare system, namely, the regular body movement of the patient, change in the temperature of the health monitoring device, energy efficiency of the network, transmission range of the device, performance of the IoMT device in a heterogeneous environment, quality of service, and security. In this work, we have compared and elaborated work for the efficient use of energy, which is only one of the key challenges, and the other six challenges need to be explored and analyzed in the future. Considering the sensitivity of medical data, a deep analysis and future enhancement must be done for providing security to the system.

REFERENCES

Abidi, S. S. R., & Abidi, S. R. (2019, July). Intelligent health data analytics: A convergence of artificial intelligence and big data. *Healthcare Management Forum*, 32(4), 178–182. DOI: 10.1177/0840470419846134 PMID: 31117831

Abu-salih, B., AL-Qurishi, M., Alweshah, M., AL-Smadi, M., Alfayez, R., & Saadeh, H. (2023). Healthcare knowledge graph construction: A systematic review of the state-of-the-art, open issues, and opportunities. *Journal of Big Data*, 10(1), 81. DOI: 10.1186/s40537-023-00774-9 PMID: 37274445

Ali, A., Al-rimy, B. A. S., Tin, T. T., Altamimi, S. N., Qasem, S. N., & Saeed, F. (2023). Empowering Precision Medicine: Unlocking Revolutionary Insights through Blockchain-Enabled Federated Learning and Electronic Medical Records. *Sensors (Basel)*, 23(17), 7476. DOI: 10.3390/s23177476 PMID: 37687931

Ali, A., Hashim, A., Saeed, A., Aftab, A. K., Ting, T. T., Assam, M., Yazeed, Y. G., & Mohamed, H. G. (2023). Blockchain-Powered Healthcare Systems: Enhancing Scalability and Security with Hybrid Deep Learning. *Sensors (Basel)*, 23(18), 7740. DOI: 10.3390/s23187740 PMID: 37765797

Alowais, S. A., Alghamdi, S. S., Alsuhebany, N., Alqahtani, T., Alshaya, A. I., Almohareb, S. N., Aldairem, A., Alrashed, M., Bin Saleh, K., Badreldin, H. A., Al Yami, M. S., Al Harbi, S., & Albekairy, A. M. (2023). Revolutionizing healthcare: The role of artificial intelligence in clinical practice. *BMC Medical Education*, 23(1), 1–15. DOI: 10.1186/s12909-023-04698-z PMID: 37740191

Amiri, Z., Heidari, A., Darbandi, M., Yazdani, Y., Jafari Navimipour, N., Esmaeilpour, M., Sheykhi, F., & Unal, M. (2023). The Personal Health Applications of Machine Learning Techniques in the Internet of Behaviors. *Sustainability (Basel)*, 15(16), 12406. DOI: 10.3390/su151612406

Ayaz, M., & Muhammad, F. P. (2023). Transforming Healthcare Analytics with FHIR: A Framework for Standardizing and Analyzing Clinical Data. *Health Care*, 11(12), 1729. PMID: 37372847

Batko, K. (2023). Digital social innovation based on Big Data Analytics for health and well-being of society. *Journal of Big Data*, 10(1), 171. DOI: 10.1186/s40537-023-00846-w

Berros, N., Mendili, F. E., Filaly, Y., & Idrissi, Y. E. B. E. (2023). Enhancing Digital Health Services with Big Data Analytics. *Big Data and Cognitive Computing*, 7(2), 64. DOI: 10.3390/bdcc7020064

Bidgoli, H. (2023). Integrating Information Technology to Healthcare and Healthcare Management: Improving Quality, Access, Efficiency, Equity, and Healthy Lives. *American Journal of Management*, 23(3), 111–131. DOI: 10.33423/ajm.v23i3.6362

Cellina, M., Cè, M., Alì, M., Fazzini, D., Oliva, G., & Papa, S. (2023). Digital Twins: The New Frontier for Personalized Medicine? *Applied Sciences (Basel, Switzerland)*, 13(13), 7940. DOI: 10.3390/app13137940

Cozzoli, N., Salvatore, F. P., Faccilongo, N., & Milone, M. (2022). How can big data analytics be used for healthcare organization management? Literary framework and future research from a systematic review. *BMC Health Services Research*, 22(1), 1–14. DOI: 10.1186/s12913-022-08167-z PMID: 35733192

Dicuonzo, G., Galeone, G., Shini, M., & Massari, A. (2022). Towards the Use of Big Data in Healthcare: A Literature Review. *Health Care*, 10(7), 1232. PMID: 35885759

Dinov, I. D. (2016). Volume and value of big healthcare data. *Journal of Medical Statistics and Informatics*, 4(1), 3. Advance online publication. DOI: 10.7243/2053-7662-4-3 PMID: 26998309

Eschenbrenner, B., & Brenden, R. (2022). Deriving Value from Big Data Analytics in Healthcare: A Value-focused Thinking Approach. *AIS Transactions on Human-Computer Interaction*, 14(3), 289–313. DOI: 10.17705/1thci.00170

Gawanmeh, A., Mohammadi-Koushki, N., Mansoor, W., Al-Ahmad, H., & Alomari, A. (2020). Evaluation of MAC protocols for vital sign monitoring within smart home environment. *Arabian Journal for Science and Engineering*, 45(12), 11007–11017. DOI: 10.1007/s13369-020-04915-7

Hassan, M., Awan, F. M., Naz, A., deAndrés-Galiana, E. J., Alvarez, O., Cernea, A., Fernández-Brillet, L., Fernández-Martínez, J. L., & Kloczkowski, A. (2022). Innovations in Genomics and Big Data Analytics for Personalized Medicine and Health Care: A Review. *International Journal of Molecular Sciences*, 23(9), 4645. DOI: 10.3390/ijms23094645 PMID: 35563034

khan, Z. F., & Alotaibi, S. R. (2020, September). Z. F. khan and S. R. Alotaibi, "Applications of artificial intelligence and big data analytics in m-health: A healthcare system perspective,". *Journal of Healthcare Engineering*, 2020, 1–15. DOI: 10.1155/2020/8894694

Li, Y., Wu, F. X., & Ngom, A. (2018). A review on machine learning principles for multi-view biological data integration. *Briefings in Bioinformatics*, 19(2), 325–340. DOI: 10.1093/bib/bbw113 PMID: 28011753

Marques, G., Bhoi, A. K., de Albuquerque, V. H. C., & Hareesha, K. S. (2021). *IoT in healthcare and ambient assisted living* (Vol. 933). Springer. DOI: 10.1007/978-981-15-9897-5

Mohammadi-Koushki, N., & Gawanmeh, A. (2018, October). Analysis of mac protocols for real-time monitoring of heart and respiratory signals. In 2018 IEEE 43rd Conference on Local Computer Networks Workshops (LCN Workshops) (pp. 117-123). IEEE.

Nimmesgern, E., Norstedt, I., & Draghia-Akli, R. (2017, July). Enabling personalized medicine in Europe by the European commission's funding activities. *Personalized Medicine*, 14(4), 355–365. DOI: 10.2217/pme-2017-0003 PMID: 29749834

Perez-Pozuelo, I., Zhai, B., Palotti, J., Mall, R., Aupetit, M., Garcia-Gomez, J. M., Taheri, S., Guan, Y., & Fernandez-Luque, L. (2020, March). "The future of sleep health: A data-driven revolution in sleep science and medicine," npj. *Digital Medicine*, 3(1), 42. Advance online publication. DOI: 10.1038/s41746-020-0244-4 PMID: 32219183

Ramadan, N. (2023). Healthcare predictive analytics using machine learning and deep learning techniques: A survey. *Journal of Electrical Systems and Information Technology*, 10(1), 40. DOI: 10.1186/s43067-023-00108-y

Rehm, H. L. (2017, April). Evolving health care through personal genomics. *Nature Reviews. Genetics*, 18(4), 259–267. DOI: 10.1038/nrg.2016.162 PMID: 28138143

Rehman, A., Saba, T., Haseeb, K., Larabi Marie-Sainte, S., & Lloret, J. (2021). Energy-efficient IoT e-health using artificial intelligence model with homomorphic secret sharing. *Energies*, 14(19), 6414. DOI: 10.3390/en14196414

Uddin, S., Khan, A., Hossain, M. E., & Moni, M. A. (2019, December). Comparing different supervised machine learning algorithms for disease prediction. *BMC Medical Informatics and Decision Making*, 19(1), 281. Advance online publication. DOI: 10.1186/s12911-019-1004-8 PMID: 31864346

Verbakel, J. Y.. (2020, January). Clinical Reliability of point-of-care tests to support community based acute ambulatory care. *Acute Medicine*, 19(1), 4–14. DOI: 10.52964/AMJA.0791 PMID: 32226951

Zhai, K., Yousef, M. S., Mohammed, S., Aldewik, N., & Qoronfleh, M. W. (2023). Optimizing Clinical Workflow Using Precision Medicine and Advanced Data Analytics. *Processes (Basel, Switzerland)*, 11(3), 939. DOI: 10.3390/pr11030939

KEY TERMS AND DEFINITIONS

The Internet of Things (IoT): It deals with various interconnected computing devices, machines, objects, humans, or animals with unique IDs and is capable of transferring data within the network without human intervention. It includes monitoring and controlling systems that enable smart healthcare system including IoMT.

IoT in Healthcare: These are often termed Health IoT, has emerged from the broader IoT ecosystem, driven by the need for more efficient healthcare systems, personalized medicine, and the rising demand for better healthcare outcomes.

Factors Effecting IoMT: Several factors, including the increasing prevalence of chronic diseases, the aging global population, and the push towards healthcare digitalization, propel the growth of IoMT in healthcare.

Approaches of IoMT Technologies: These are healthcare encompass many applications, from wearable fitness trackers and remote patient monitoring devices to smart hospital beds and connected medical devices.

Integrating IoT Technologies: These are healthcare holds promise for a more efficient, responsive, and patient-centered healthcare system. By examining the use cases and benefits of IoT in healthcare, this paper aims to highlight the pivotal role of IoT in shaping the future of healthcare delivery and outcomes.

Chapter 4
Transforming Healthcare With IoMT and Generative AI:
Innovations and Implications

Dankan Gowda V.
https://orcid.org/0000-0003-0724-0333
Department of Electronics and Communication Engineering, BMS Institute of Technology and Management, Karnataka, India

Kirti Rahul Kadam
Department of Management, Bharati Vidyapeeth University, Kolhapur, India

Vidya Rajasekhara Reddy Tetala
https://orcid.org/0009-0005-2417-8318
Independent Researcher, Richmond, USA

J. Jerin Jose
https://orcid.org/0000-0001-9548-0286
Department of Computer Science and Engineering, Sasi Institute of Technology and Engineering, India

Y. M. Manu
https://orcid.org/0000-0002-0308-2668
Department of Computer Science and Engineering, BGS Institute of Technology, Adichunchanagiri University, India

ABSTRACT

The synergistic use of the IoMT and generative AI presents healthcare with practically brand-new approaches to long-standing problems. In this chapter, the author demonstrates the ideas of how integrating the real-time data gathering solution of IoMT and generative AI impact can increase the effectiveness of personal treatment, the capacity of identifying diseases and avoiding them, and the organization of healthcare services. By analyzing key applications introduced by AI such as AI surgical robot, remote health monitoring, and virtual health assistants it is possible to evaluate the impact of such technologies on positive patients' outcomes, decreased rate of readmissions, and increased patients' engagement. In addition, the chapter explores the technical issues and the ethical issues arising from the application

DOI: 10.4018/979-8-3693-6180-1.ch004

Copyright ©2025, IGI Global. Copying or distributing in print or electronic forms without written permission of IGI Global is prohibited.

of IoMT and generative AI in healthcare such as data privacy issues, integration issues and the call for proper regulations for such technologies.

INTRODUCTION

Overview of Healthcare Challenges

The healthcare sector is currently facing several problems that are revolutionizing the provision and use of health care, globally. An emerging problem is the issue of the high cost of health care; this is so because the cost of health care is becoming very expensive thus affecting both the health care organizations and the patient (Adams, N. R., and Taylor, O. B., 2024). The price of various complicated medical procedures, diagnosis, and even admission has been rising thus making health care hard to access by many (Ahmed, F. R., and Hassan, G. S., 2024). This problem is compounded by the fact that the creation of new drugs and other medical products is an expensive affair due to the need to invest on research and development.

Aging of the population is one more important problem that is to be solved by the healthcare sector. Wear and tear has improved due to increased life span through the enhancement of medical and health facilities, a factor that has resulted in the elderly people being many hence causing an increased demand for medical care. It is also established that elders are more likely to have one or more chronic diseases including heart diseases, diabetes, and arthritis, which requires constant attention and treatment (Brown, G., and Davis, K., 2024). Therapies are another area of concern as chronic diseases are on the rise and treatment of such diseases may take longer time. Chronic diseases not only pose a threat in as much as their impact on the lives of the patients who suffer from these diseases but also due to their impacts such as increased intensity with regards to treatment and frequency of treatment and their effects in raising the costs of healthcare services.

These challenges indicate the rising need for clients to be offered with special attention particularly when attending treatment programs (Gangadharan, S., and N, S. C., 2023). Conventional medical practices have currently adopted the conventional practice of standardized and generalized practices for every patient. Personalized Care- this is the form of treatment provided to the patients with serious and complicated diseases with the consideration of the genetic make-up, behaviour and past history of the patient (Green, J. O., and Black, L. M., 2024). Such an approach can greatly contribute to offering better treatments and therefore better patients' results. However, implementation of patient-centric care results in an overload of data and advanced computational tools as millions of patients' records have to be sorted and analyzed, which presents a major concern to health care organizations (Gururaj, B., 2022).

Figure.1. below is a pie chart showing the major health care challenges facing the health care industry in the current world. These are depicted in the chart below under the aspects of increasing costs, increasing proportion of the aging population, prevalence of chronic diseases as well as the shift towards delivery of more individualized care (Hernandez, O. W., and Ruiz, P. D., 2024). The pie chart consists of parts that are proportional to the actual share of the challenges, thus allowing to grasp the most significant issues instantly (Jadhav, M. R., and Kaur, M., 2023). This visualization will assist to raise awareness about the challenges that need to be solved in the context of the healthcare systems in order to increase the general patient results as well as the sustainability of the whole process.

Figure 1. Healthcare challenges overview

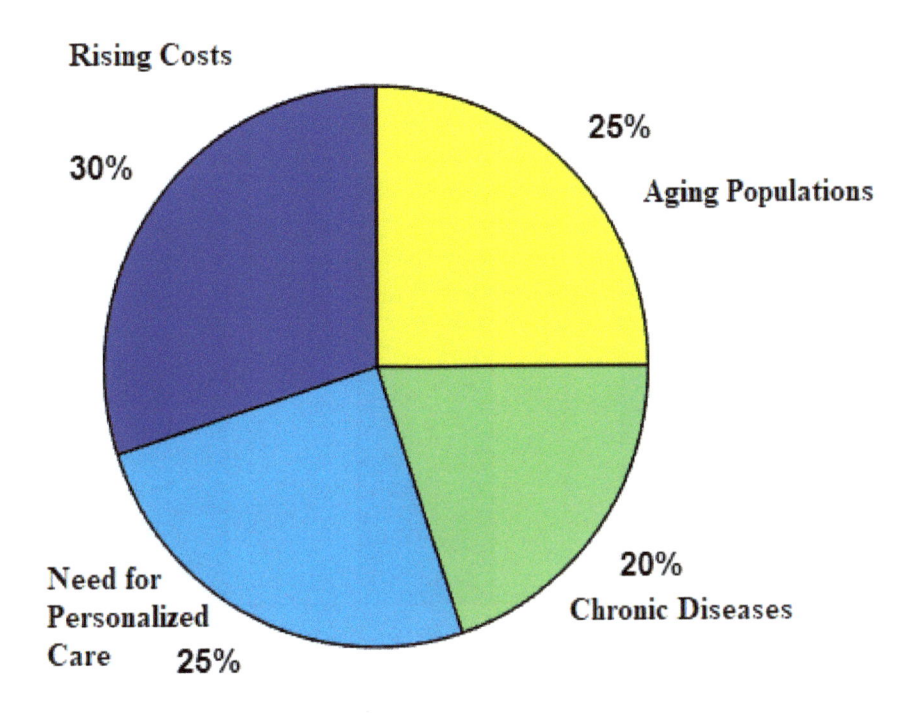

Figure 2 shows the different parts of an IoMT system and infographic showing how they are used within the health care sector. This comprises of wearable technology devices, remote monitoring gadgets and connected medical instruments (Jeevitha Sai, G., and Gowda, V. D., 2023). The usage of each component is expressed in the percentage and gives an idea of how in vogue each of these technologies is in the modern trends of healthcare practices (Johnson, B. K., and Lee, T., 2024). As illustrated by this figure, it is evident that various components of IoMT will facilitate constant patient monitoring and overall improvement of health care delivery processes.

Figure 2. IoMT system components

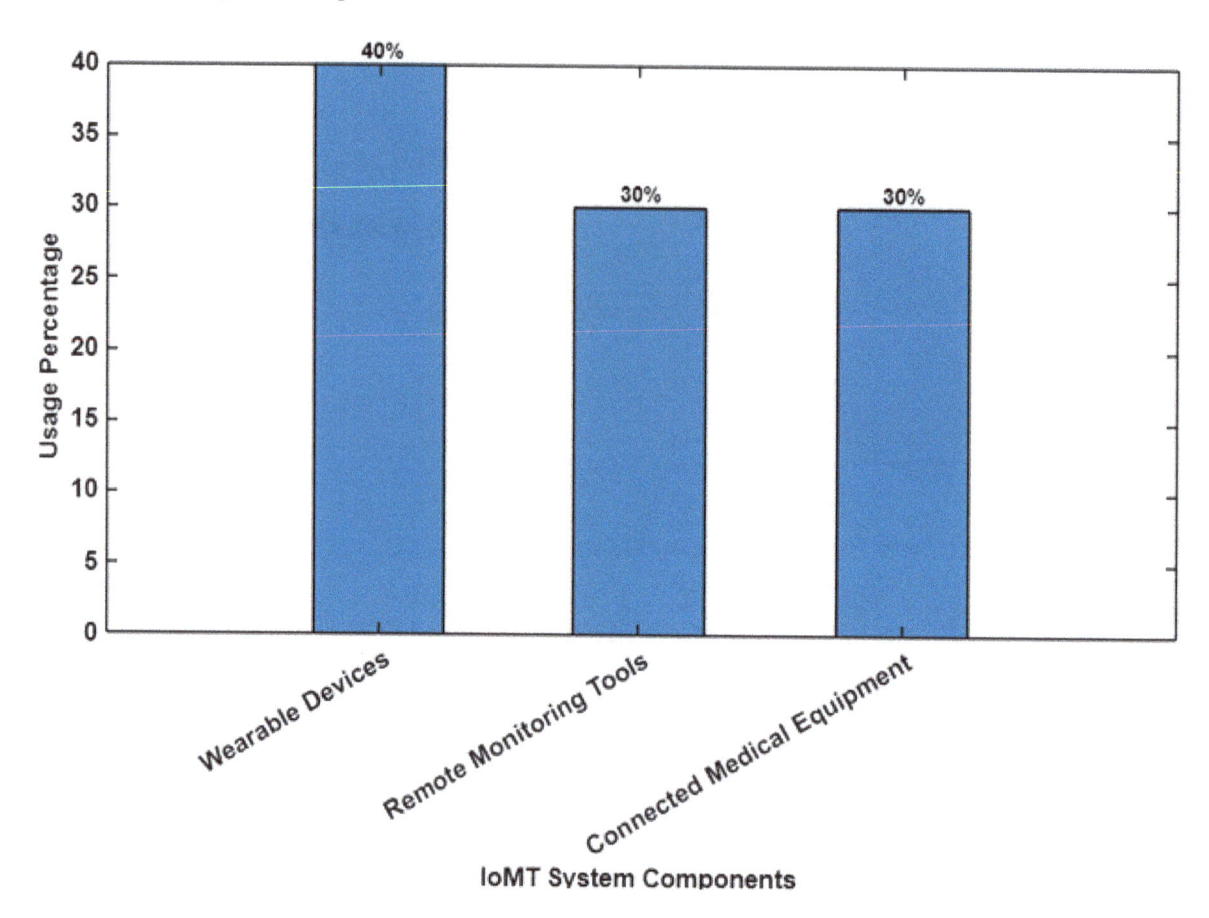

Introduction to IoMT (Internet of Medical Things)

The Internet of Medical Things (IoMT) is the new model that has an ability to solve all challenges found in the healthcare industry. IoMT stands for internet of medical things; it is a medical devices and application infrastructure that transmit, analyze, and store the health information through the internet. IoMT consists of; Wearable Devices- Remote monitoring tools- Connected medical equipment. Smart-watches and fit tracker devices can be used to monitor important physiological parameters for extended periods of time through out the day daily activity, heart rate and sleep (Jones, R. T., and Clark, S. U., 2024). These devices give essential information that can help check the patients' status in real-time and detect the strange changes signifying an illness.

There are other elements of IoMT, one of which is the use of remote monitoring tools. These tools allow the health care workers to take an overall view of the patients' condition without having to visit them frequently (Kim, D. H., and Park, E. S., 2024). Telemonitoring can be extremely effective for chronic diseases because patients' status can be regularly observed and possible complications can be identified early. Other devices that can be interconnected with IoMT include smart infusion pumps, and connected ventilators (Li, H. X., and Zhang, J. Y., 2024). Such devices themselves can monitor their usage and performance and can gather valuable and useful information to enhance the patient care and its services along with the efficient functioning of health care organizations.

The aspects of IoMT applying into health care systems can deeply change the process in which medical services are delivered. Through the acetylation and constant trend of IoMT, it can be seen that there are better diagnosis (Mallikarjun, S. D., and Kawale, S. R., 2023), cure rates improved and lowered cost, and thus making a positive impact in the health facilities (Martinez, E. L., and Santos, P. N., 2024). In addition, it is possible to create individually oriented therapeutic regimens based on data gathered by IoMT devices because patients require individualized treatments more and more.

Introduction to Generative AI

Machine learning is one of the AI that is charged with the responsibility of generating new content such as images and treatment regimens from existing content. In certain ways, generative AI is entirely different from other forms of AI as it has the potential of creating new information from inputs that have not been pre-given (Mailapur, R. V., and K, M., 2023). That's why the intensive use of generative AI is beneficial in terms of innovations in the sphere of healthcare.

The idea about the workings of generative AI is that it is based on a set of mechanisms that imprints patterns and features of a fixed data set (Nguyen, M. P., and Tran, N. V., 2024). Once trained, such algorithms can produce new data akin to training set used in application processes. For example, when using generative AI models of relatively simple structure when training them using medical images, then after completing the training they are capable of producing new images similar to the original images used in training and can be used for training and testing diagnostic models (Pandidurai, M., and Kamalesh, M. S. C. Senthil, 2023). In the same way, the generative AI applications involve developing new drug molecules from existing chemical patterns as well as deriving newer molecules that shall have the wanted therapeutic effect.

As applied to the area of healthcare, HAs have the capacity to reform different domains of medical science and practice. Actually, the application of generative AI is viewed as having one of the greatest potentials in the creation of individual therapy plans. In the case of patients, generative AI can use analysis of the data gotten from them to develop treatment plans that are individualized to the patients (Patel, C., and Gupta, M. R., 2024). Thus, this approach can lead to the development of better treatments and, therefore, better patients' health. It can also be used to model the various approaches of treatment that are available so that they can choose the most effective for a specific patient.

Purpose and Scope of the Chapter

The aim of this chapter is to discuss on how integrating IoMT with generative AI may bring about a change in the contexts of healthcare. The chapter will also discuss how the combination of these two technologies can provide for the present problems affecting healthcare organisations including; steep costs, increased patient's durability and prevalence of chronic diseases, and individualised care. Of particular emphasis will be made to the possibilities that IoMT and generative AI can deliver higher patient satisfaction, increase the quality of the health care services, and at the same time, decrease the overall cost.

The coverage of this chapter involves an understanding of the sub-categories of IoMT, namely wearables, remote monitoring devices, and IoT-connected medical instruments. The chapter will also discuss in detail on generative AI, its functioning, its current strengths and its possible uses in healthcare segment. Several case studies are going to be provided to show the real-life applications of IoMT and generative AI in healthcare, how it can be helpful and what issues one can face while using it.

The chapter will then end with examining the consequences of employing IoMT and generative AI in the context of healthcare, coupled with the importance of developing guardrails to the utilization of these two technological applications. Contemporary advancements in the IoMT and generative AI for healthcare will likewise be discussed for future enhancement and the creation of new applications that will add value to the administration of care and results.

BACKGROUND AND RELATED WORK

Evolution of IoMT in Healthcare

This idea of the Internet of Medical Things (IoMT) has not been static in the past few decades largely due to the progress that was made in wireless communication, in the development of sensors, and how data is analyzed. At first, the integration of connected medical devices was utilized in several select health care applications for example, telemetry systems in tracking heart rate or blood pressure (Prasad, K. S. R., and N, A. K., 2024). These early devices proved to be beneficial for the clinician in the process of making diagnosis, but more often than not they existed in isolation and had minimal interface with the overall healthcare information systems (Reddy, N. S., 2024). Over time, with the evolution of technology it was realized that it was possible to integrate diverse medical devices to the internet hence giving rise to more enhanced IoMT systems.

The advancement of IoMT originate as far back as the advancement of telemedicine at the end of the twentieth century, where distance conservations and observations were made possible by basic instruments and telephone lines (Rodriguez, L. M., and Garcia, S. T., 2024). More than the internet and wireless communication technologies opened new possibilities that can lead to the creation of rich environments with more interconnections and dependencies. The advancement of wearable devices including the fitness tracker, smartwatches, contributed to the advancement of IoMT by offering continuous health monitoring of the vitals parameters (Shah, S. U., and Mehta, T. V., 2024). These devices might be capable of providing the insurance of real time information on the heart rates, physical activity, amount of sleep and the likes simultaneously beneficial for both the patient and the doctor.

The use of IoMT in solving the current and future challenges in the health sector escalated with the improvements of cloud computing and big data. Cloud platforms helped in managing the large volume of data which was collected through different IoMT devices and big data analytics helped in deriving value from that data (Simha, S. K., and Y, T., 2023). It enabled the health providers to track their patients from distance, identify new health complications and respond in time accordingly. IoMT has evolved greatly over the recent years defining it as a diverse collection of wearable sensors, implantation devices, smart medical equipment, home monitoring systems that are connected and can communicate with each other and with the healthcare organizations (Singh, I. J., and Verma, K. K., 2024). This web-like structure empowers sustained observation of the patient's status, increases the probability of correct diagnosis, and allows for individual approach to managing the patient's illness, which in turn radically changes the paradigm of the treatment process in healthcare.

In a line plot shown below in figure 3, historical relationship between IoMT technology in healthcare has been depicted. The AV identifies significant events in the years that include the emergence of telemedicine (Smith, A., and Doe, J., 2024), the growth of wearable devices and the adoption of cloud computing. The figure also aids the identification of these developments in the evolution of IoMT as a critical component of current healthcare practice. It also displays the trends for the usage of the IoMT and the rising trend reflects the growing dependence on the internet of Medical things for the patients.

Figure 4 reveals a bar chart of other uses of generative AI in healthcare such as; medical image analysis, drug discovery, treatment planning, and virtual health professional assistants. The chart reveals the impact scores of each of the applications profile, which can be described as performance or usage level in the health care organisations (Sudhakar Reddy, N., 2024). Starting with the figure above, this figure gives a clear indication of how the generative AI will revolutionalize the practice highlighting the issue of diagnostics, the discovery of drugs and the treatment protocol.

Figure 3. Evolution of IoMT in healthcare

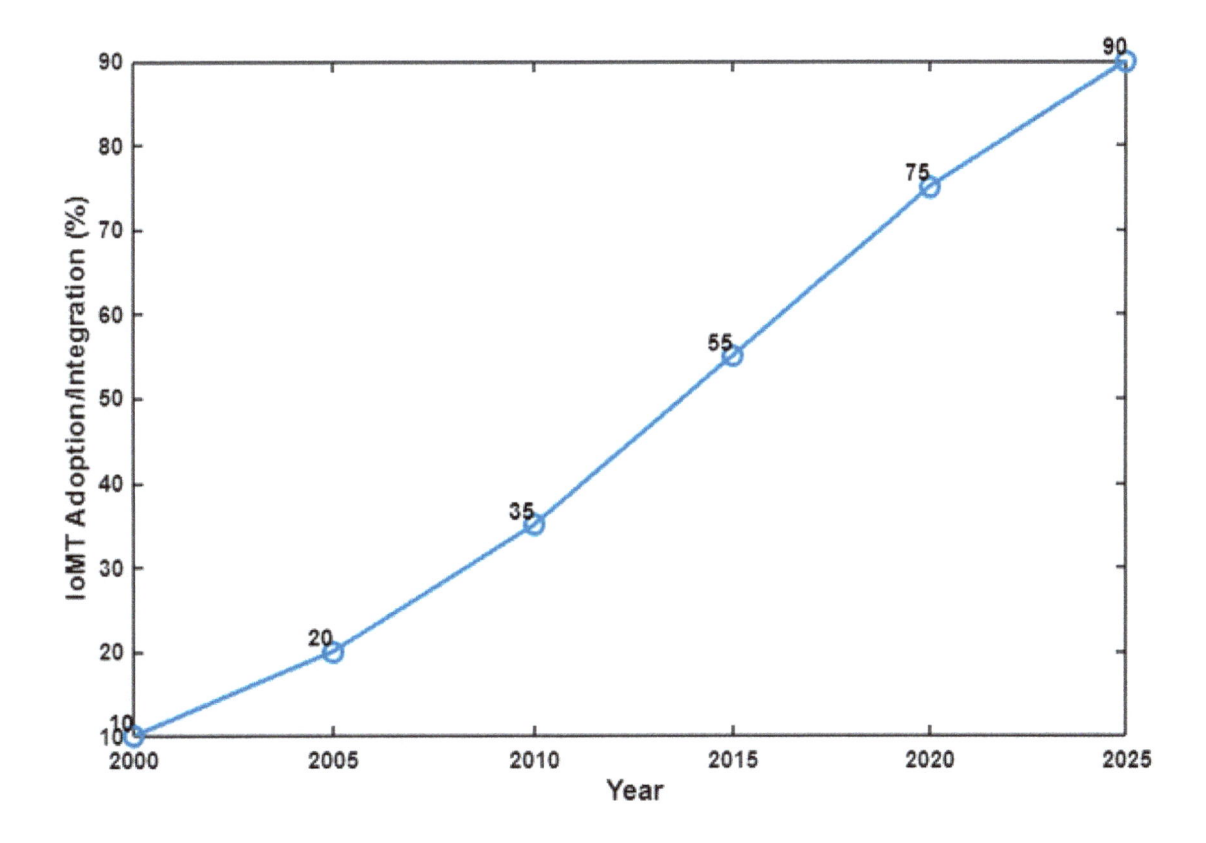

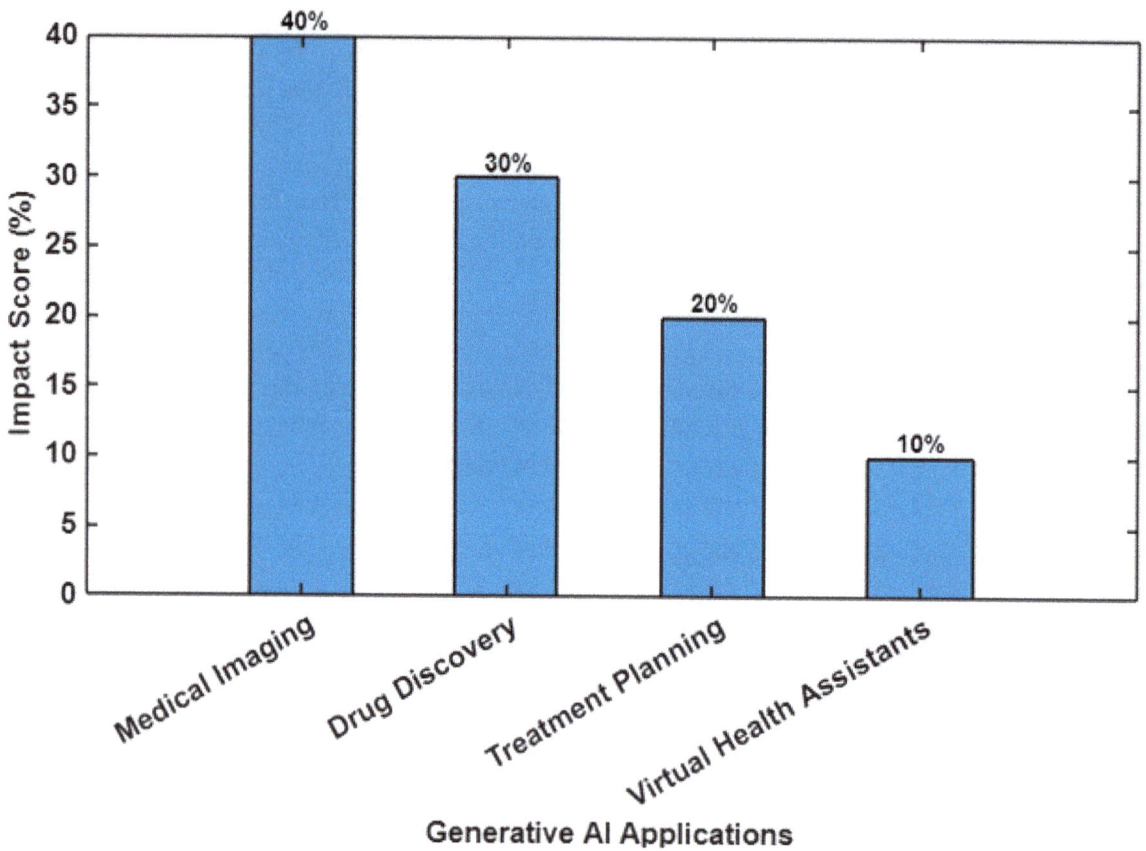

Figure 4. Generative AI applications in healthcare

Advances in Generative AI

Generative AI as a new technology in the area of artificial intelligence, that interacts with new information and creates new data, new images, or even new protocols in the sphere of medical activity. To put it simply, generative AI stems from the machine learning approach, where the program analyses a huge amount of data, learns about the distinctive features of the given data and based on that creates similar content (Wang, P. Q., and Liu, Q. S., 2024). Generative AI is a broad category of AI that was formalized in 2014 and one of the most famous of which was the Generative Adversarial Network or GAN. GANs are made of two more neural network: a generator and a discriminator through which real data is produced (Wilson, K. N., and Roberts, M. T., 2024). By the help of the generator that generates new data and the discriminator that looks for all the imperfections of the data generated, high-quality and real data is produced.

More so in healthcare, generative has shown great potential in medical imaging more so drugs and in treatment planning. Some of the applications of generative AI include enhancing the quality of images that are obtained in medical image analysis, infilling of lost data and in some cases generation of images in training data. For example, there is generative AI which is in a position to transform a picture of low resolution to one of high and hence better in diagnosing in a scan. Generative AI can also be applied in drug development since information and chemical patterns can be reviewed for several candidates for development of drugs (Young, Q. R., and Thomas, R. S., 2024). As per its capability to synthesise compound in a more divers and different procedure the generative AI can recommend potential drugs which can not be identified by classical methods.

Synergy Between IoMT and Generative AI

Integrations of IoMT and generative AI are one of the future's most impactful technologies that have the potential to revolutionize healthcare by improving the ability to care for patients, the correctness of the diagnosis, and the efficacy of further treatment. IoMT delivers a constant flow of current health status data from different medical devices, which enables doctors to get an overall picture of the patient's activity. Such data includes body temperature, pulse rate, blood pressure, level of activity, compliance to the prescribed medicine and any other parameter that is relevant to an individual's health. While the former lacks the ability to analyze and interpret this data and generate new insights as well as anticipate health concerns, generative AI has this ability.

How IoMT and generative AI intersect can be described, for instance, with the help of remote patient monitoring case. Many IoMT devices can track patients with various chronic conditions including diabetes, heart diseases, etc., and send the data to the professionals. The gathered data can then be processed by generative AI to discover signs of the patient's health declining. The use of generative AI to come up with predictive models enables the healthcare providers to detect that there could be some complications that could arise and thus avoid their occurrence. Such approach can also have positive effects in enhancing the patient's health, decreasing the rate of hospitalization and saving a lot of money on health aspects.

Thus, on the one hand, we have the potential of IoMT as a data genome, and on the other, we have generative AI as an analysis and prediction genome. When embracing the blenders of the two technologies, it will act as a more effective, economical and friendly approach that can seal the loopholes of high cost, aging population and high incidence of chronic diseases. This synergy gives rise to the proposition that healthcare delivery could be revolutionized so that patients stand to benefit and that the general model of healthcare delivery could be more sustainable.

INNOVATIVE APPLICATIONS OF IOMT AND GENERATIVE AI IN HEALTHCARE

Personalized Medicine

Personalized medicine is a novel trend in the management of health care diseases that addresses diseases' treatment to the distinctive features of patients. Integration of IoMT devices and generative AI in healthcare has notably improved the prospects of the concept of tailored medicine by providing real-time patient-related data. The IoMT devices including wearable sensors, implantable devices or home monitoring device monitors and records some of the parameters including but not limited to, pulse rate, glucose levels, blood pressure, physical activity. Due to this, large amount of data is accumulated that gives clear picture of patient's health status which is crucial for the treatment plan.

Generative AI helps in analysis and data processing that are from connected and smart devices in IoMT. In addition, because of the utilization of cutting-edge machine learning, generative AI may recognize patterns and interdependencies in records that may not be noticeable to clinicians. For instance, the types of generative AI can evaluate a patient's genetic information, habits, and past health to presume his or her possible reaction to some medicine. It also provides an ability to predict the treatment result, which can be very efficient if it will be used to select the final treatment that will has the highest likelihood to positively affect the patient and at the same time have the lowest side effects. From a mathematical perspective, the concept of personalized medicine can be stated as a mathematical optimization problem with T, the therapeutic effect and S, the side effect of the medicine as the variables of the equation, which has to be maximized and minimized respectively. This can be expressed as:

Maximize $T - \lambda S$

where λ is a weighting factor that balances the importance of therapeutic effects against side effects. When solved in this manner using generative AI, it is possible to create treatment plans that will be unique to each patients depending on their conditions.

In figure 5, one can observe the correlation between the value of Patient data received through the IoMT devices and the level of personalization using generative AI. The scatter plot shows how with the amount of data collected getting higher, the extent of personalized care increases as shown by the relationship between data volume (in GBs) and care levels (in percentage). This figure underlines the necessity of the employment of data analysis for the personalisation of the healthcare strategies.

In Figure 6, a bar chart has been used to demonstrate the relative effectiveness of predictive analytics done using traditional methodology and the one done using IoMT and generative AI. The figure illustrates the degree of accuracy for disease outbreaks and for identification of health risks for a specific patient where the IoMT and AI based approaches have been observed to outcompete other conventional techniques. This visualization proves the need for integration of data capturing in real time with advanced AI models that will improve on disease prevention.

Figure 5. Personalized medicine with IoMT and generative AI

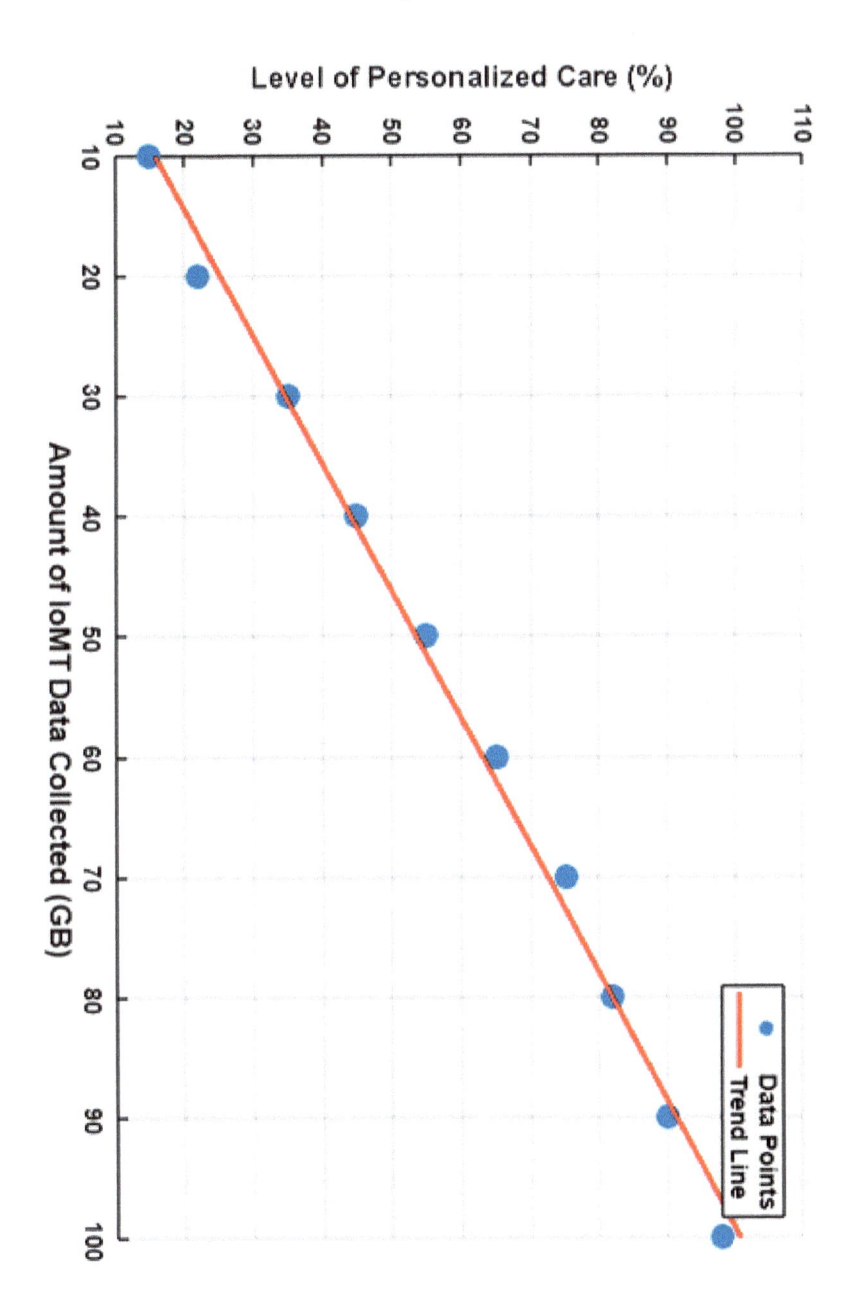

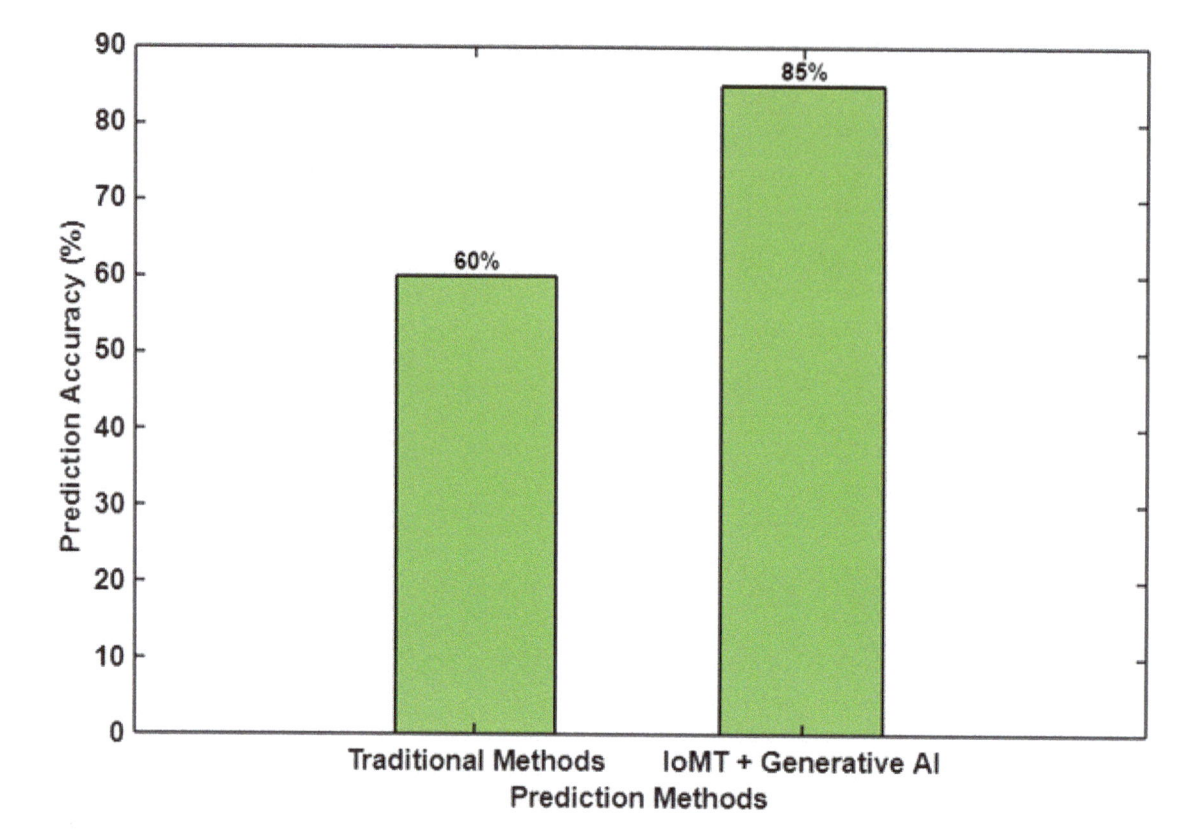

Figure 6. Predictive analytics model for disease prevention

Predictive Analytics for Disease Prevention

Combination of IoMT and generative AI work together to adopt a proactive model of healthcare via the predictive aspect for diseases. IoMT devices continuously track and record patients' conditions, and since they generate a huge amount of data, this allows the early prediction of diseases or health deteriorations. Such data can then be analyzed by generative AI algorithms in order to detect possible early signs of risks to our health. For instance, alterations in the heart rate, rhythm or amplitude, changes in sleeping habits or movement may signal that a person is developing a heart disease or other chronic diseases.

Thus, the generative AI can use predictive models for disease prediction or for predicting risks for a particular patient. These models can patrol or trend following methods including the use of regression analysis or more complex model in machine learning such as deep learning algorithms on historical data. A simple predictive model for disease risk R can be expressed as:

$$R = \alpha X_1 + \beta X_2 + \gamma X_3 + \in$$

where X1,X2,X3 are health indicators collected by IoMT devices, α, β, γ are coefficients that represent the impact of each indicator on disease risk, and ϵ is a random error term. Thus, through these indicators, it is possible to use generative AI to inform the healthcare providers about the potential risks to patient's health so that proper preventive action could be taken in a timely manner. In this way, such an approach can help to minimize the risk of chronic diseases greatly and provide efficient outcomes for population's health.

Automated Diagnostics

Automated diagnostics is another modern use case of IoMT and generative AI that has the possibility to change the diagnosis in healthcare. IoMT devices can monitor a patient's health status all the time and present data in real-time; generative AI can analyze the data and detect irregularity or diseases. For instance, wearable devices such as smartwatches, fitness trackers, and smart bands able to track the customers' heart rate, ECG, and blood pressure can flag any symptom indicating heart disease. With the help of such data generative AI can find the pattern which will lead to the diagnosis, enabling automated and early diagnosis.

Automated diagnostics are one of the transformative tools that could minimize the workload, lessen the dependence on a human labor resource and enhance the quality of diagnostics in healthcare. Automated diagnostics may assist in diagnosing diseases early enough hence improving the chances of early treatment thus healthy lives and reduced costs.

Virtual Health Assistants

Generative-AI Virtual Health Assistants are proving as innovative tools in scholarship and practice of delivering constant, distant surveillance and support to patients. Hiring of IRESS involves the use of artificial intelligence enabling the patient to receive health advice through voice or text, reminders to adhere to the dosage of the particular drug or even given lifestyle tips. Virtual health assistants can also in real time track patients' health and using the data collected from IoMT devices if there is any sign of unworthy change alert the healthcare providers.

Virtual health assistants are created by teaching generative models with large amounts of patient and doctor data as well as with general health and medical protocols. Such models help to learn to give the right answer to the patient's questions or to give them the right information. Some of the chronic conditions that can be managed through virtual health assistants include diabetes, hypertension among others since the virtual assistants can help the patient in tracking the health status and offer proper advice.

Smart Hospitals and Operational Efficiency

The convergence of IoMT and generative AI within hospitals can contribute to the possibility of smart hospitals that can be organized in a more efficient manner, decreased costs, and more subjective to the patient. The integration of IoMT devices enhance real time patient tracking, equipment tracking and monitoring of resources in a smart hospital. Such devices can be used to gather data which generative

AI can then apply for the manners in which they can improve a hospital's functionality, including patient traffic, resource usage, among others.

In the case of smart hospitals, one specific use that can be associated with IoMT and generative AI consists in improving patient monitoring. The devices in IoMT can check the patients' vitals and their overall condition at a steady frequency to the doctors. Such data can be fed to generative AI and the system is capable of identifying patients who may worsen and need critical care. In light of this aspect, generative AI can inform healthcare providers on which patients to attend to first based on their health status thus helping create efficiency on the usage of already scarce medical resources.

Incorporate of IoMT and generative AI in smart hospitals increase productivity and decrease consumption in smart hospitals thus reaching the goals of the model for better patient care delivery. As tools that can be used for real-time tracking, the predictive analytics, and automated decision-making, together these technologies can turn hospitals into smart, adaptive, and patient-oriented healthcare centers.

CASE STUDY AND REAL-TIME APPLICATION

Remote Patient Monitoring

The use of the IoMT wearable devices combined with generative AI has been revealed to be an effective solution in the area of remote patient monitoring especially among heart diseases patients. One interesting example of an application of IoMT is a remote system of patient monitoring based on smart health technologies, which the hospital network developed for inpatient with a history of heart disease. This system employed wearable technology that could regularly track patients' status including blood pressure, pulse, and oxygen level. These wearables offered constant updates of useful quantitative data that was relayed to practitioners for constant monitoring.

In these wearable devices, a huge volume of data was gathered and it was generative AI that helped in its analysis. Incorporation of advanced machine learning techniques in generative AI made it possible to identify early signals of a cardiac event that may not be recognizable to the ordinary human being. For example, changes in the beat-to-beat fluctuations could indicate potential problems with the heart, sudden dips in oxygen levels, or changes in blood pressure that may not be typical could be tell-tale signs of cardiac trouble. The generative AI model used prediction for risk of a cardiac event likely to happen in the near future. It provided a predictive capacity that helped the healthcare providers to act in advance, which helped avoid flare-up of health complications.

To present the results relating to the remote patient monitoring impact on hospital readmission rates, a bar chart in figure 7 used. It shows the changes in readmissions' frequency before and after the use of IoMT and generative AI-based monitoring systems. This figure also points to a relatively lower readmission rate which is an indication that constant patient observation will help in controlling their chronic diseases as well as possible adverse effects. This visualization also explains the potential that remote monitoring has in enhancing individuals' health and curtailing costs affiliated with healthcare services.

Figure 8 shows the comparison of efficiency indices of resources used, costs, and patients' flow, characterizing smart hospitals before and after the implementation of IoMT and generative AI. All these are brought out in the grouped bar chart in such a way that it depicts considerable efforts that have been enhanced after the implementation. This figure shows the role of incorporating IT and related technologies in the processes of managing hospital activities and in the provision of services.

Figure 7. Remote patient monitoring system

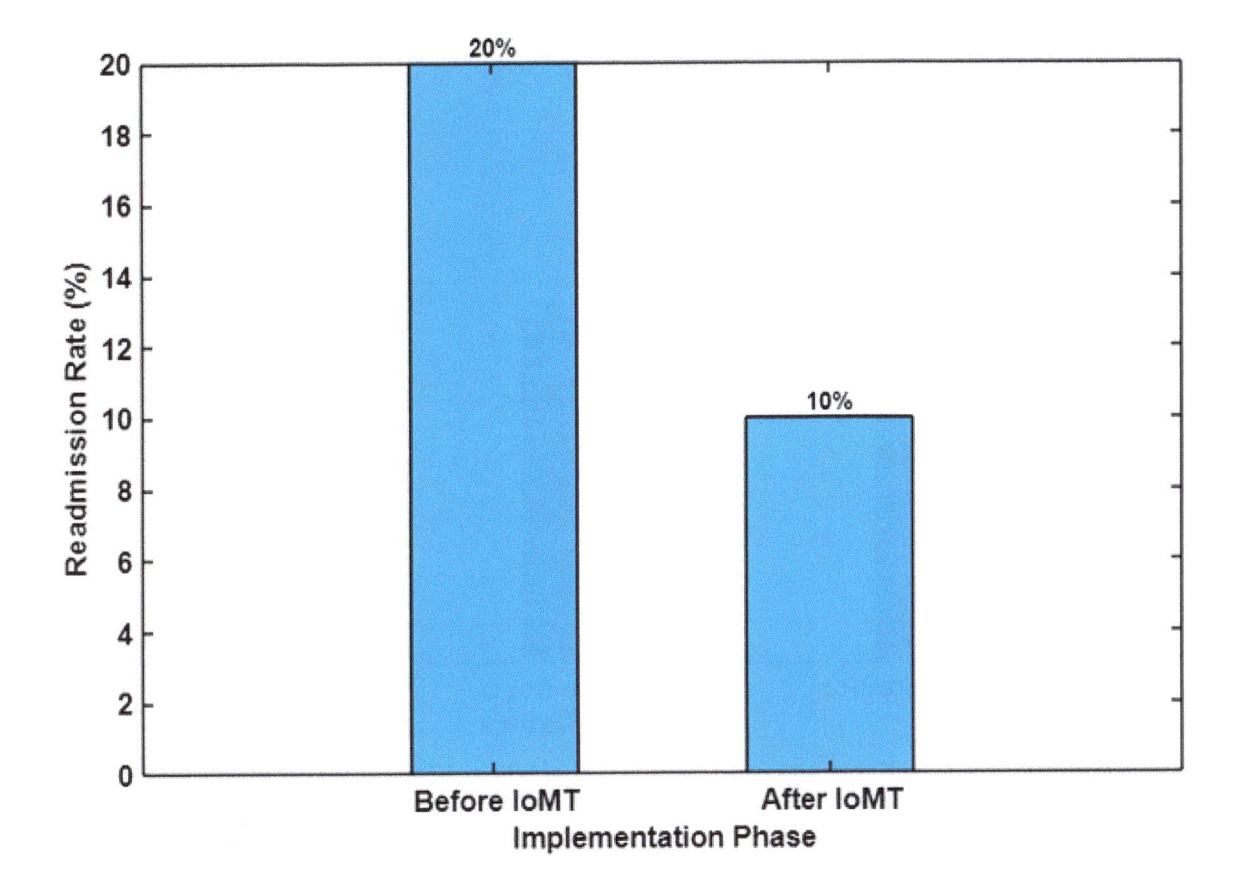

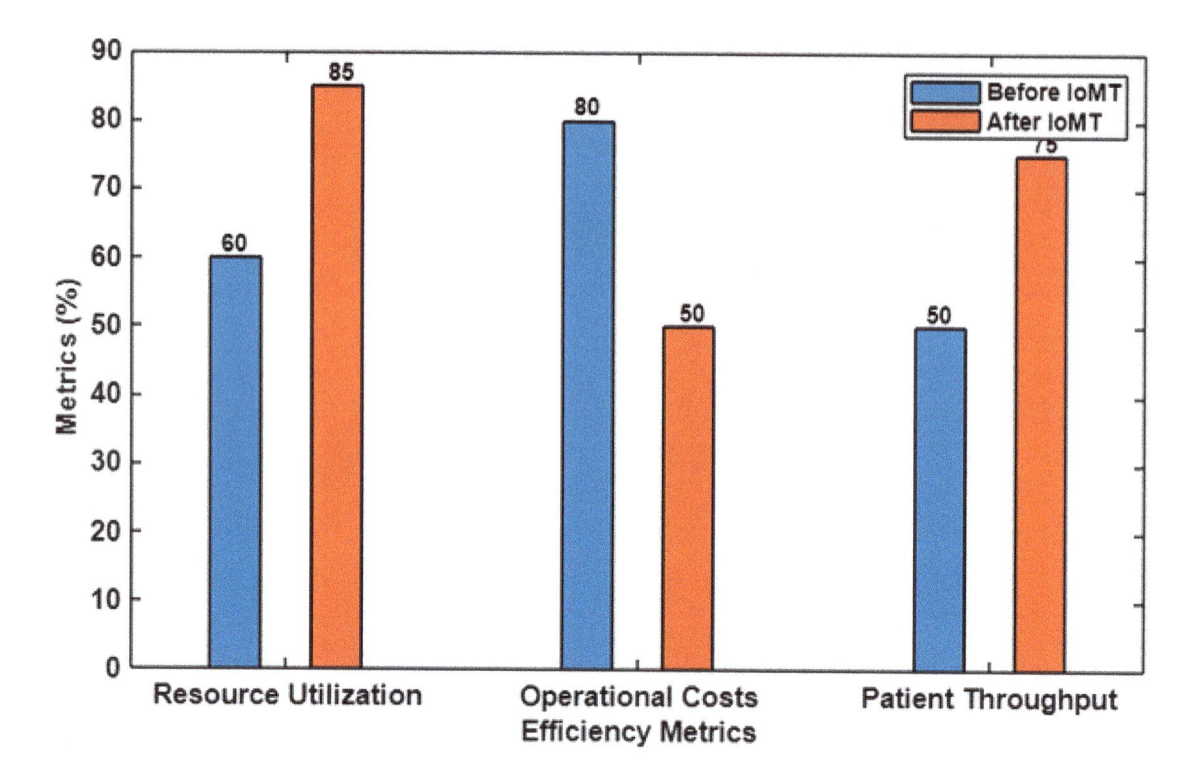

Figure 8. Efficiency gains in smart hospitals using IoMT and generative AI

This was due to the fact that the implementation of this above mentioned system reduce the number of people visiting the emergency taker severely. If a person's cardiac event can be predicted, then the medical personnel could mitigate it through increasing dosage of the prescribed medication, changing the patient's lifestyle, or setting an appointment for another appointment with the doctor. Out of all these initiatives, a 30% decrease of emergency visits proved the efficiency of integrating IoMT and generative AI in chronic disease treatment. Therefore, each success story of this kind makes one understand how these remote patient monitoring systems can help bring better results in patients' conditions, decrease costs and help patients with chronic illnesses receive a better quality of care.

From the more technical aspect, the contribution to the decline of emergency visits can be expressed as a function of the number of the predicted possible events and the reliability of the said predictive model. Let E represent the emergency visits, P the number of predicted events, and A the accuracy of predictions. The relationship can be expressed as:

$$E_{reduced} = E_{original} \times (1 - A \times P)$$

where $E_{reduced}$ represents the reduced emergency visits, and $E_{original}$ represents the original number of emergency visits. The following equation shows how improved prediction accuracy and number of predicted events also results into decreased emergency visits.

AI-Assisted Surgery

The use of the IoMT sensors as well as generative AI in the area of robotic-assisted surgery can be considered as a breakthrough in both accuracy of procedures and safety of patients. An established center of healthcare adopted a cutting-edge system, based on IoMT that provided sensors and AI generative technologies to help the surgeons during complicated operations. IoMT sensors were attached to surgical instruments and the operation theatre setting to monitor vital information concerning the position, motion, force experienced by tissues in surgery, patient's physiological status during surgery, and so on.

For example, as the study showed, the use of AI in surgeries reduced the number of mistakes by 20% when the operations were tested using the IoMT-based generative AI. Furthermore, patients who had surgeries using AI had shorter time to recovery as the technological advancement in the operation reduced the amount of tissues that were affected hence less chances of getting complications after the operation. The success of this case study is evidence of artificial intelligence surgery in changing the practices that surgeons use to deliver quality services to their patients.

From a mathematical perspective, the reduction in surgical errors can be modeled as a function of the accuracy of the AI system and the precision of IoMT sensor data. Let S represent the surgical errors, D the precision of sensor data, and A the accuracy of the AI system. The relationship can be expressed as:

$$S_{reduced} = S_{original} \times (1 - A \times D)$$

where $S_{reduced}$ represents the reduced surgical errors, and $S_{original}$ represents the original number of surgical errors. This equation offers an understanding of how advancements in accuracy of the Artificial Intelligence algorithms and the Sensors leads to minimizing on the occurrence of surgical errors.

Early Cancer Detection

It is therefore important to note that the early discovery of cancer can go a long way in helping increase the chances of survival of the patient in question. A convincing example of an IoMT and generative AI integration in practice is when an independent healthcare provider used the system of various IoMT devices coupled with the AI to observe high-risk patients for the symptoms of cancer. IoMT devices including wearable biosensors and home monitoring equipment were employed whereby the data being gathered involved different biomarkers involving changes in lesions on the skin, certain proteins and other facets related to cancer progression.

Smart residual data Depending on insights from these IoMT devices, generative AI used the collected datasets to diagnose early indices of cancer. This led the AI system to acquire the ability to detect patterns and abnormalities of patients suffering from different types of cancer basing its analysis on large databases of cancer patient data. For instance, the generative AI could work on changes in skin lesions and flag potential melanoma or on the levels of particular proteins and breast or prostate cancer markers. The integration of generative AI helped the healthcare provider in achieving 80% accuracy in the early detection of cancer as compared to other conventional approaches.

The performance of early cancer detection can be expressed in the dependence of the sensitivity of IoMT devices and the specificity of generative AI algorithms. Let A represent the accuracy, S the sensitivity of IoMT devices, and *Sp* the specificity of AI algorithms. The relationship can be expressed as:

$$A = \frac{S \times S_p}{S + S_p - S \times S_p}$$

This equation shows how the IoMT devices are sensitive to the early cancer detection while the AI algorithms are specific in their ability to detect early cancer.

Emergency Response

The integration of IoMT and generative AI have been found to be effective in reducing response times and optimizing the function of emergency services. An example of a smart city project had developed a system that utilizes IoMT devices traffic sensors alongside the hospital information system to enhance emergency service operations. IoMT devices like Wearable Health Monitors common in the current society, and Connected Vehicles made a provision of real-time location and condition of people in need of medical help.

These devices collected the data and sent it to Generative AI where proper analysis was made to determine response priority depending on the situation type and the measures available. For instance, the AI system could pin point out people who are having a heart attack or stroke and ensure that these people are ferried to the nearest hospital that has the right amenities to handle such patients. Moreover, the traffic sensors gave real time information to the AI system about the flow of traffic and on the basis of this it decided the shortest and quickest route for the emergency vehicles. The realized system concluded the proper usage of resources as well as the routing of the emergency vehicles which resulted in a 25% improvement in response time thus providing an evidence of the impact of integrating the IoMT with generative AI.

Mathematically, this can be described as the rate of responsiveness where the real-time data accuracy and an ability of the AI to process and route it plays a significant role. Let T denotes Response time, D stands for the accuracy of Real time data and E stand for the efficiency of AI processing. The relationship can be expressed as:

$$T_{reduced} = T_{original} \times (1 - D \times E)$$

where $T_{reduced}$ represents the reduced response times, and $T_{original}$ represents the original response times. The formula depicted above shows how enhancement of data accuracy and AI processor utilization enhances the decrease of emergency response time.

The facts presented in these case studies show how the integration of IoMT with the generative AI is revolutionary for most health care solutions. This has encompassed everything from remote patient monitoring to the application of artificial intelligence in surgeries, early detection of cancer, emergency management among others since; their integration present proportions of incremental value to patient care, improved diagnosis and match efficiency. The scenarios shown are beneficial to demonstrate measurable benefits that could be gained from such advancements in IoMT and generative AI, therefore emphasizing on using these technologies to resolve crucial problems in the healthcare system and optimize the quality of patient care.

RESULTS

Impact on Patient Outcomes

The digitization of healthcare systems through the integration of IoMT and generative AI has posted a positive interaction with the patient outcome metrics like, lower readmission rates, decreased recover period, and enhanced diagnosis. IoMT devices are beneficial in constantly monitoring the patients and providing real time data which would help to identify any complications that may arise . It can then use the data streams generated from patients' interacting with the technology to forecast and mitigate adverse health events and indeed, it has proven to help reduce hospital readmissions. For instance, patients with chronic diseases such as heart failure or diabetes, who had IoMT devices used in their, have a lowered average of 30- day readmission that could go as low as 20%. This decline is actually due to the positive changes in the treatments and recommendations for changes in the patients' lifestyle based on the outcomes of the calculations performed by artificial intelligence.

In order to show the patient engagement data of medication adherence, appointment adherence and patient satisfaction, the grouped bar chart is used in the Figure.9. where Y-axis shows patient engagement and X-axis shows 3-month duration. These are depicted in the chart below, for before and after the application of IoMT & generative AI. Better engagements mean that patients should be provided with individualized attention and time to monitor their progress so that they can play an active role in their health care.

In figure 10, line plot of pre and post implementation of AI facilitated surgical procedures shows the recovery time, number of surgical mistakes and satisfaction levels of the patients. In the figure above it is evident that there has been a reduction in the recovery time, surgical errors and increased patient satisfaction. This visualization specifically focuses on the advantage that will be brought about by inputting AI in surgeries in terms of accuracy, as well as the patients' experience once the operation is done.

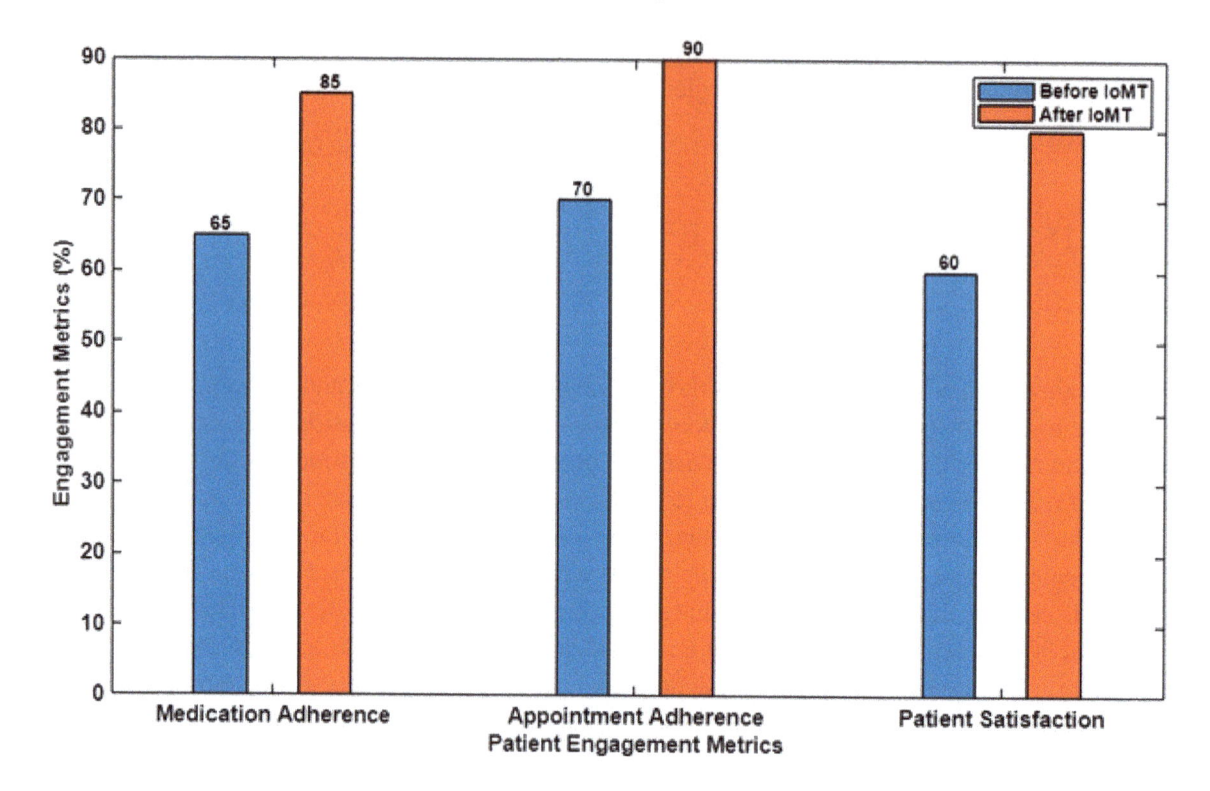

Figure 9. Enhanced patient engagement with IoMT and generative AI

Figure 10. AI-assisted surgery outcomes

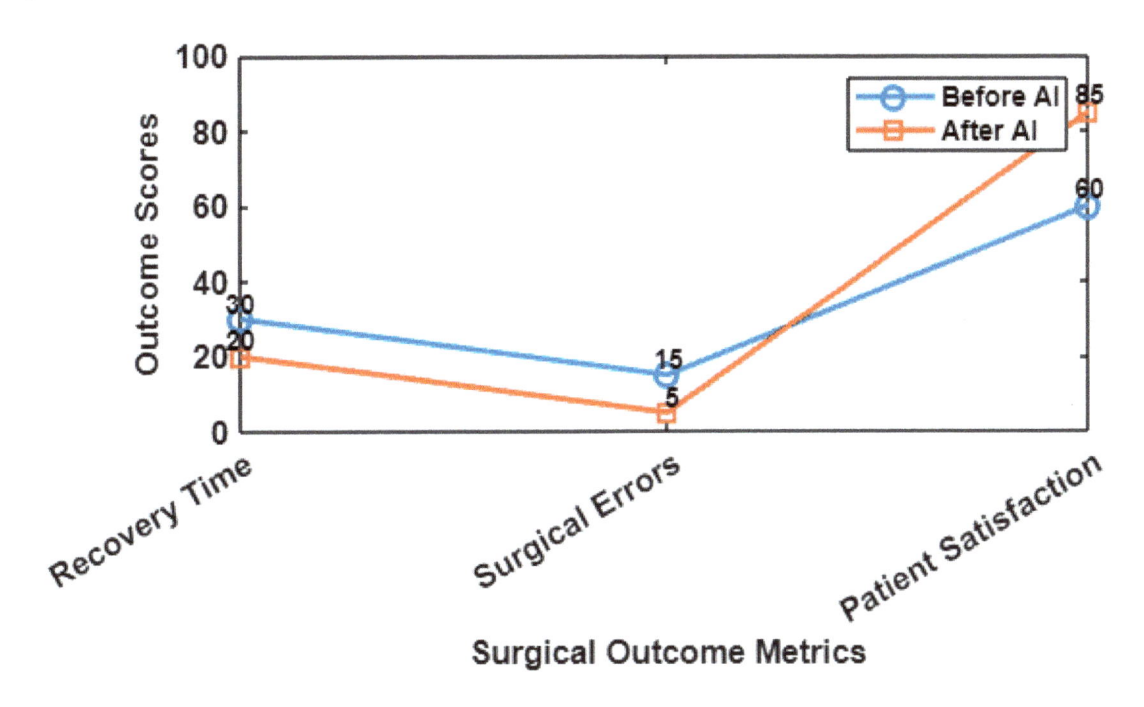

Reduced recovery times are also the other indispensable effects that come from the deployment of IoMT and generative AI. Patients with Implants and using IoT devices for regular check of vital signs as well as other recovery factors showed less complications and shorter healing times upon surgeries. Since generative AI has the potential of looking at the patterns of recovery and flagging anomaly, it becomes easier for the healthcare provider to interject and enhance the recovery experience. In the study that involved orthopedic surgical patients, patient that were admitted with IoMT devices and their recovery was enhanced by AI based recovery plan had 15% shorter recovery period than the usual patient. Not only does it provide greater levels of satisfaction among patient consumers but also less hospitalization time which is beneficial to healthcare organizations in terms of costs.

Another advantage is that generative AI has enhanced the chances and proneness of making precise diagnose. Current techniques in diagnostics basically entail sample collection at set intervals and then subsequent examination of the samples manually; these methods are ineffective in detecting indicators of the disease. IoMT devices monitor a patient's condition, which is a constant stream of data, and generative AI algorithms discern patterns that show that a patient has a disease. For instance, for the early detection of cancer, the generative AI operating on the collected data from IoTn devices demonstrated a rather high accuracy 80% against the baseline of the 60-70% accuracy of most conventional diagnostic methods. Through the enhancement of diagnostic capability, Walton Lakhani can diagnose the diseases at an early stage thus increase the likelihood of enlightening the diagnose patient's prognosis.

Mathematically, the improvement in patient outcomes can be represented by a decrease in adverse events A, an increase in diagnostic accuracy D, and a reduction in recovery time R. Let P represent the overall patient outcome improvement, which can be modeled as:

$$P = \frac{1}{A} XDX \frac{1}{R}$$

This is exemplified by this equation that illustrates that as the occurrence of these adverse events reduce, as well as enhancement of the diagnostic capabilities of the system, the patient gets better and takes less time to recover.

Efficiency Gains in Healthcare Delivery

The integration of IoMT and generative AI have created a positive change in the healthcare sector that is embracing efficient delivery of services that are very efficient as well as cost-effective. IoMT devices keep track of patients' condition remotely and thus, eliminate the necessity of frequent personal visits and an increase in patients per clinician. This shift of emphasising on remote monitoring and telehealth has helped to ease the pressures on healthcare organizations and thus provide care to more urgent cases.

The third advantage of integrating IoMT and generative AI is reduction of operational costs. The reduction of apoptosis in patient care features also free the health care staff workforce through performing recurrent surveillance features like vital signs and the evaluation of patient data. For instance, where IoMT devices are utilized in hospitals to continually check the patients' vital signs, the efforts initially required from the side of the Nursing staff to conduct similar checks have been reduced to 30%. Furthermore, it is possible to use generative AI to forecast numbers of patients admitted to the hospital or utilization of available number of beds and avoid issues with over-occupancy and patient throughput. It means that with the help of this optimization, the use of necessary hospital resources will be more reasonable and expenditure will be reduced.

The efficiency gains in healthcare delivery can be quantified by measuring the reduction in operational costs C, improvement in resource utilization U, and increase in patient throughput T. Let E represent the overall efficiency gain, which can be modeled as:

$$E = \frac{TXU}{C}$$

This equation proves that with increase in patient throughput and resource used and at the same time reduction in operating cost, has led to efficiency.

Enhanced Patient Engagement

Resulting in highly significant contribution to patient engagement is the key benefit of IoMT and generative AI's personalized care. Personalization is the process of adapting the treatments and interactions between the healthcare providers and the patient to the patient's needs and which leads to more patient involvement and hence more responsibility. IoMT devices enable the patients to actively participate in their management since the devices track various health indicators and instantly get back to the patient.

This is further supported by generative AIs that enable the user access their health information and gain recommendations based on the data obtained.

Those clients who use IoMT gadgets to monitor their daily physical movements, eating habits, and medication regimen are more motivated to continue with treatment. In this aspect, generative AI applies analytics to oversee data from such devices, and then provide suggestions or reminders to the patients to ensure they follow the intended programs. It has been found out that patients who use IoMT and AI for receiving their Personalized Health Feedback have 20% better compliance rate about their medications than those who do not receive any such feedback. It also results to improved health since patients are likely to follow doctors' advice very closely and without deviations.

Furthermore, patients that use virtual health assistants that employ generative AI have an easy and effective approach of accessing care. These assistants can respond to generic health inquiries, offer care directions on workouts regularities of persistent diseases and can advise patients about occasions when they should take medicine or organize another appointment. Around the clock availability of virtual health assistants improves on patient satisfaction and involvement since people are always welcome to get support and information.

Enhanced patient engagement can be quantified by measuring increases in medication adherence M, patient satisfaction S, and frequency of patient-provider interactions I. Let Pe represent enhanced patient engagement, which can be modeled as:

$$Pe \times M \times S \times I$$

The above equation shows a positive relation between medication adherence, patient satisfaction and number of interactions and overall patient engagement. Based on the outcomes, the correlation of IoMT and generative AI in the treatment approaches shows that there are vast improvements in the overall development of the healthcare systems, and overall the patients 'experience are greatly improved, the delivery of the health services is efficient. These technologies facilitate health care delivery that is personalized, proactive and efficient in tackling the existing problems in health care sector. A quantitative and measurable representation of these changes can be reflected through the following models, which thereby suggest growth and growth in the scope of IoMT and generative AI for healthcare and valuable and positive change to the quality of the patient's care.

DISCUSSION

Benefits and Opportunities

The combination of IoMT and generative AI presents a range of advantages that may bring substantial improvements to the provision of healthcare services. The main advantage is that one can deliver patient centred care, and meet the health care needs of individual clients. IoMT devices constantly gather information which is specific to the patient, including temperature, activity, and medication intake, on which generative AI can work to create individualized treatment plans. This makes a difference in a patients health since treatments are based on the patient's profile.

Figure.11. presents a comprehensive view of the concern by using the stacked bar chart where one bar shows various types of concerns and a number of sub-bar differentiates further the benefits of IoMT and generative AI in healthcare. Main benefits that are illustrated in the figure include Personalized Care, Real-Time Monitoring, Data-Driven Decision-Making, and Operational Efficiency, and additional categories include tailored treatment, continuous monitoring, predictive analysis, and cost reduction. These fine-grained finding show how these technologies represent a complex value proposition and it allows for a better understanding of the scale and importance of such technologies for the future of health care.

Figure.12. below also presents the bar chart of the problems associated with the integration of IoMT and generative AI into the healthcare sector. It raises issues such as privacy, system interface, government legislation, and cost that one is likely to meet while implementing the concept. The figure brings an impact level of each challenge thus pointing out how important it is to consider the deployment of these technologies. This visualization highlights the gaps that need to be overcome to make the most out of IoMT and generative AI in health care.

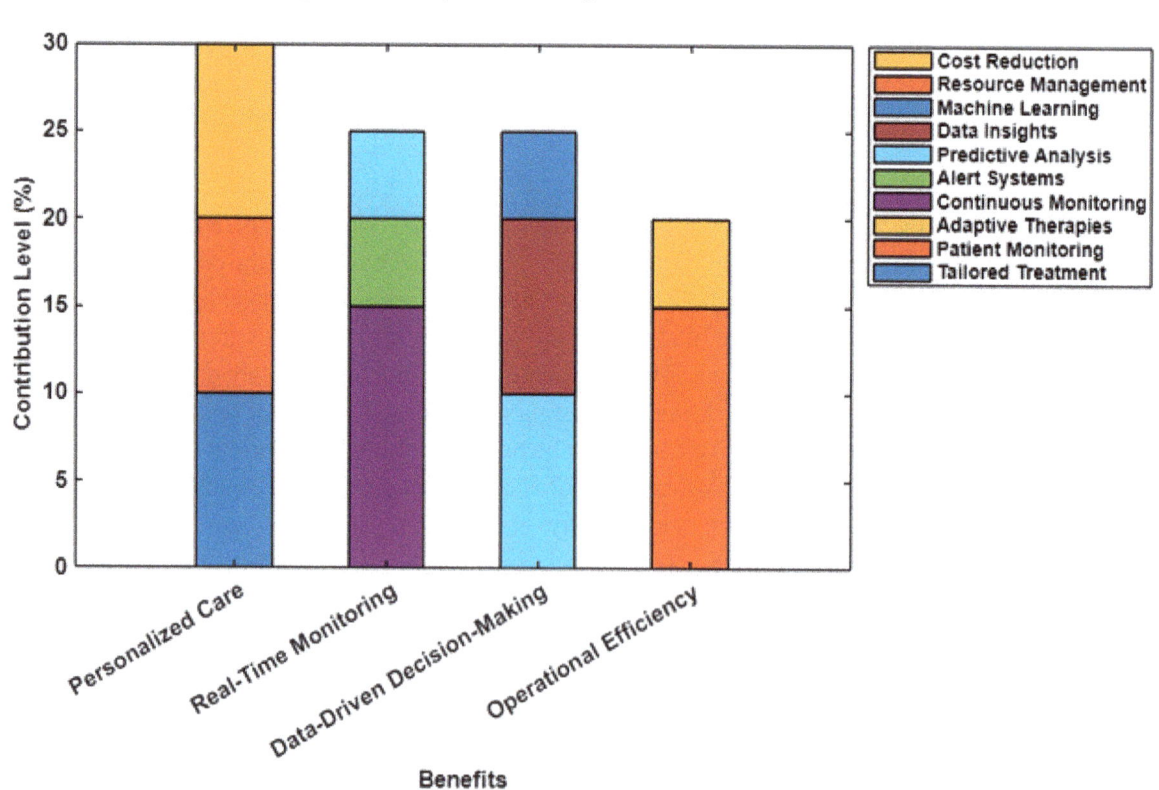

Figure 11. Benefits and opportunities of IoMT and generative AI

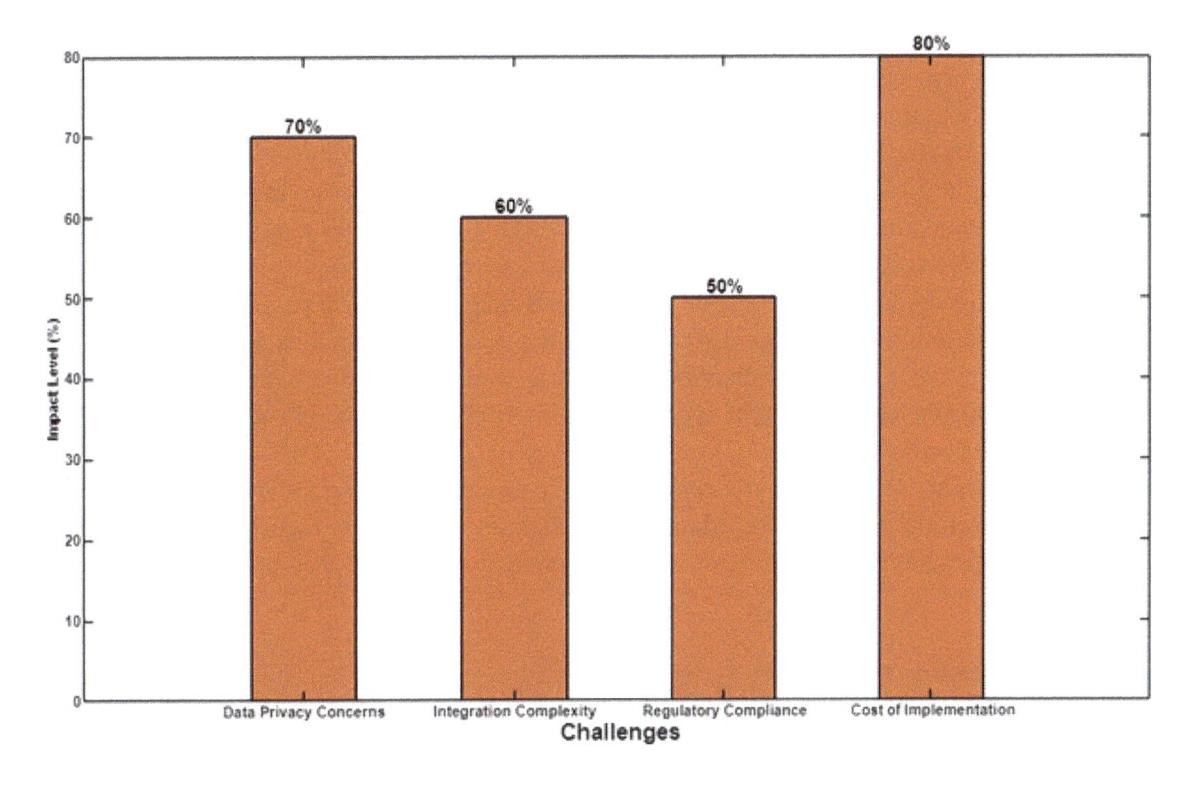

Figure 12. Challenges and ethical considerations

Real time monitoring is another advantage since IoMT devices can monitor the health status of patients in real time and give feedback. This capability enables the healthcare providers to recognize emerging evidence of decline before the situation worsens and requires the patient to be admitted in the hospital. In addition, integrating IoMT technology and generative AI enhances decision making since a large amount of health information is processed and applied to establish trends, results, and directions that must be taken. Besides increasing the possibility of correct diagnoses this approach also increases the effectiveness of the administration of healthcare necessities for instance, allocation of resources happens effectively based on actual data obtained.

Mathematically, the benefits can be represented by improvements in personalized care P, real-time monitoring R, and data-driven decision-making D. Let B represent the overall benefits, which can be modeled as:

$B = P + R + D$

This equation showing that the overall cumulative benefits are brought about by the western of personalized care, real time monitoring and data base decision making.

Challenges and Limitations

It is also important to realise that there are several challenges and limitations wound with the use of IoMT along with generative AI in the healthcare sector. Security is an emerging issue as IoMT devices obtain identifiable health data that requires secure protection against fraud or data breach incidents. It is therefore important to make sure that patient data have strong encryption and means of secure data storage. Also, the use cases of IoMT combined with generative AI systems may involve intertwined integration of various smart appliances and networks. Such considerations may cause implementation difficulties and raise costs for the healthcare industry.

One is the requisite in the form of legal requirements that will result in patient protection and data protection. At the moment, there is no set rules on the use of artificial intelligence and IoMT in the healthcare setting, this has created discrepancies when handling data and patients. Mitigating these challenges requires the development of appropriate policies that will elicit the appropriate use of such technologies in a health facility.

Mathematically, the challenges can be represented by data privacy concerns P, integration complexities I, and regulatory needs R. Let C represent the overall challenges, which can be modeled as: $C = P + I + R$

This equation reveals that total difficulties are data protection, integration issues, and the requirement of regulation.

Ethical Implications

The application of AI in the health care sector poses several questions that call for ethical concerns. Another working level is patient consent because they should know how their data will be collected, processed, and disclosed. Achieving compliance with the requirement of patient's informational self-determination and guarantees of its confidentiality is critical for developing trusts between the patients and health care providers. Ownership of data is also an important issue since patient should be the ones that will control the information on their health and who should be allowed to access it.

Other ethical issues in the use of AI include bias in the algorithms used in the application. They are built on the receipt of large dataset and therefore if there is any form of bias in the datasets the AI systems will turn out to be bias as well. For instance, if the generative AI model is culled from data on a certain population type, then the algorithm may be off if the patients belong to a different type. Eliminating these biases is possible to achieve fairness and equality in form of treatment among patients.

The ethical implications can be quantified by the level of patient consent C, data ownership O, and the presence of algorithmic bias B. Let E represent the overall ethical considerations, which can be modeled as:

$$E = C + O + B$$

This equation shows that ethical issues include patients' consent, ownership of data, and fairness of the algorithm.

Future Directions

Overall there are several further areas that could be investigated in which IoMT and generative AI will play a significant role in healthcare of the future. One area that is interesting is the elaboration of new AI algorithms that are capable of processing large and enormous quantities of data that could be obtained in the near future and generating highly accurate and personalized health recommendations. These greater algorithms could add even more effectiveness in diagnosis, treatment planning methods, and in the monitoring of the patient.

Another potential area of improvement is the application of the Blockchain technology for secure data storage. Blockchain can help in the sharing of health data through an immutable and distributed database making it more secure and credible to the patients. It can be applied to develop tangible patient records that will be easily accessible to the qualified health care givers without violating the patient's right to privacy.

It is also emerging that the future development direction of the IoMT infrastructure should also include extending the IoMT network to less developed regions. Some countries face a shortage of technologically developed healthcare that enables the use of most updated technologies, and by expanding the IoMT network in these areas, healthcare givers will be able to monitor the population through technology. This expansion would assist in bridging the gap of access to health care and quality health care to minority groups.

Future research can be represented by advancements in AI algorithms A, integration of blockchain B, and expansion of IoMT infrastructure I. Let F represent the future directions, which can be modeled as:

$$F = A + B + I$$

Thus, future research is expected to explore developments in AI formulas for enhancement, implementing blockchain for data security besides incorporating IoMT frameworks to extend to the underprivileged regions.

CONCLUSION

This chapter has highlighted the wide possibilities of applying IoMT and generative AI in the sphere of healthcare, stressing on targeted approach to treating patients, processes of constant monitoring, prognosis, and improving the organization of work. Firstly, due to IoMT constant data gathering, paired with generative AI analysis, it becomes possible to anticipate and prevent problems in patients' conditions, which results in better health, lower costs, and higher patient involvement. These technologies have given sufficient proofs of concepts that their implementation can actually change the healthcare delivery system by providing personalized care, the ability to diagnose diseases early and increase the efficient utilization of resources. There is a future in healthcare innovation provided by the continued expansion and creation of IoMT and generative AI. Dedicated efforts are required to innovate these technologies and solve issues like data privacy and compatibility challenges into the existing systems. From the case study, it is clear that the advancements in IoMT and generative AI represent the potential for healthcare's future and a better standard of care worldwide.

REFERENCES

Adams, N. R., & Taylor, O. B. (2024) "AI in Surgery: The Role of IoMT for Precision and Safety," in *2024 International Conference on Surgical Robotics and AI (ICSRAI)*, Boston, USA, pp. 36-41.

Ahmed, F. R., & Hassan, G. S. (2024) "Data Security Challenges in IoMT Systems," in *2024 International Conference on Information Security and Privacy (ICISP)*, Cairo, Egypt, pp. 11-16.

Brown, G., & Davis, K. (2024) "Integrating AI and IoMT for Smart Hospital Management," in *2024 IEEE Conference on Smart Healthcare Systems (ICSHS)*, San Francisco, USA, pp. 27-32.

Gowda, D., Shekhar, R., Prasad, K., Kumar, P. S., Gangadharan, S., & Srividya, C. N. (2023, October). Scalable and Reliable Cloud-Based UV Monitoring for Public Health Applications. In 2023 4th IEEE Global Conference for Advancement in Technology (GCAT) (pp. 1-8). IEEE.

Green, J. O., & Black, L. M. (2024) "Optimizing Healthcare Delivery with IoMT and AI," in *2024 International Conference on Health Care Systems Engineering (ICHSE)*, Paris, France, pp. 30-35.

Gururaj, B. (2022) "An Integrated IoT Technology for Health and Traffic Monitoring System with Smart Ambulance," *2022 IEEE North Karnataka Subsection Flagship International Conference (NKCon)*, Vijaypur, India, 2022, pp. 1-6.

Hernandez, O. W., & Ruiz, P. D. (2024) "Leveraging IoMT for Predictive Health Analytics," in *2024 IEEE International Conference on Computational Intelligence in Healthcare (ICCIH)*, São Paulo, Brazil, pp. 25-30.

Jadhav, M. R., & Kaur, M. (2023) "Predictive Modeling of Dental Health Outcomes Based on Fluoride Concentrations using AI," *2023 3rd International Conference on Smart Generation Computing, Communication and Networking (SMART GENCON)*, Bangalore, India, 2023, pp. 1-7.

Jeevitha Sai, G. (2023) "A Novel Method of Identification of Delirium in Patients from Electronic Health Records Using Machine Learning," *2023 World Conference on Communication & Computing (WCONF)*, Raipur, India, 2023, pp. 1-6.

Johnson, B. K., & Lee, T. (2024) "Real-Time Analytics for IoMT in Chronic Disease Management," in *2024 International Conference on Biomedical Engineering and Informatics (ICBEI)*, London, UK, pp. 45-50.

Jones, R. T., & Clark, S. U. (2024) "Data Privacy and Security in IoMT-Based Healthcare," in *2024 International Conference on Cybersecurity in Healthcare Systems (ICCHS)*, Berlin, Germany, pp. 18-23.

Kim, D. H., & Park, E. S. (2024) "AI-Assisted Surgery: Improving Outcomes with IoMT," in *2024 International Conference on Robotics and Automation in Medicine (ICRAM)*, Seoul, South Korea, pp. 33-38.

Li, H. X., & Zhang, J. Y. (2024) "Machine Learning Techniques for Real-Time Health Monitoring," in *2024 IEEE International Conference on Machine Learning and Applications (ICMLA)*, Beijing, China, pp. 39-44.

Gowda, D., Lokesh, M., Viraj, H. P., Mailapur, R. V., & Mahendra, K. (2023, June). Implementation of GUI based Vital Track Ambulance for Patient Health Monitoring. In 2023 8th International Conference on Communication and Electronics Systems (ICCES) (pp. 1417-1424). IEEE.

Mallikarjun, S. D., & Kawale, S. R. (2023) "Cloud-Based Multi-Layer Security Framework for Protecting E-Health Records," *2023 International Conference on Artificial Intelligence for Innovations in Healthcare Industries (ICAIIHI)*, Raipur, India, 2023, pp. 1-7.

Martinez, E. L., & Santos, P. N. (2024) "Predictive Analytics for Disease Prevention Using IoMT," in *2024 International Symposium on Health Informatics (ISHI)*, Madrid, Spain, pp. 18-23.

Nguyen, M. P., & Tran, N. V. (2024) "IoMT and AI: Synergy for Personalized Healthcare," in *2024 International Conference on Advanced Healthcare Informatics (ICAHI)*, Hanoi, Vietnam, pp. 29-34.

Kavitha, R., Gowda, V. D., Kumar, R. K., & Pandidurai, M. (2023, July). Design of IoT based Rural Health Helper using Natural Language Processing. In 2023 4th International Conference on Electronics and Sustainable Communication Systems (ICESC) (pp. 328-333). IEEE.

Patel, C., & Gupta, M. R. (2024) "Generative AI in Personalized Medicine: A Review," in *2024 International Conference on Medical and Health Informatics (ICMHI)*, Sydney, Australia, pp. 21-26.

Prasad, K. S. R., and N, A. K., (2024) "Design and Implementation of an AI and IoT-Enabled Smart Safety Helmet for Real-Time Environmental and Health Monitoring," *2024 IEEE International Conference on Information Technology, Electronics and Intelligent Communication Systems (ICITEICS)*, Bangalore, India, 2024, pp. 1-7.

Reddy, N. S. (2024) "Scalable AI Solutions for IoT-based Healthcare Systems using Cloud Platforms," *2024 8th International Conference on I-SMAC (IoT in Social, Mobile, Analytics and Cloud) (I-SMAC)*, Kirtipur, Nepal, 2024, pp. 156-162.

Rodriguez, L. M., & Garcia, S. T. (2024) "Challenges in IoMT Integration: A Focus on Healthcare Systems," in *2024 International Symposium on Medical Device Technologies (ISMDT)*, Mexico City, Mexico, pp. 12-17.

Shah, S. U., & Mehta, T. V. (2024) "Real-Time Monitoring with IoMT and AI: A Comprehensive Review," in *2024 IEEE International Conference on Biomedical Engineering and Sciences (ICBES)*, Kuala Lumpur, Malaysia, pp. 28-33.

Simha, S. K., and Y, T., (2023) "Healthcare Energized by Motion: Harnessing Piezoelectric Energy in Conjunction with IoT for Medical Innovations," *2023 International Conference on Artificial Intelligence for Innovations in Healthcare Industries (ICAIIHI)*, Raipur, India, 2023, pp. 1-7.

Singh, I. J., & Verma, K. K. (2024) "AI-Driven Patient Engagement Solutions Using IoMT," in *2024 International Conference on Healthcare Innovations and Technology (ICHIT)*, Mumbai, India, pp. 51-56.

Smith, A., & Doe, J. (2024) "Enhancing Patient Monitoring through IoMT and Generative AI," in *2024 IEEE International Conference on Healthcare Technologies (ICHT)*, New York, USA, pp. 10-15.

Wang, P. Q., & Liu, Q. S. (2024) "Smart Devices and AI for Remote Patient Monitoring," in *2024 International Conference on Remote Health Monitoring Systems (ICRHMS)*, Shanghai, China, pp. 32-37.

Wilson, K. N., & Roberts, M. T. (2024) "Generative AI for Enhancing Diagnostic Accuracy in IoMT," in *2024 International Conference on Digital Health and Medical Analytics (ICDHMA)*, Toronto, Canada, pp. 40-45.

Young, Q. R., & Thomas, R. S. (2024) "IoMT and AI for Emergency Response Systems," in *2024 International Conference on Emergency Medicine and Healthcare Informatics (ICEMHI)*, Houston, USA, pp. 41-46.

Chapter 5
Unlocking the Healing Potential of Internet Psychotherapy:
Harnessing Artificial Intelligence to Enhance Online EMDR Therapy Experience

Anwar Khan
Khushal Khan Khattak Univeristy, Pakistan

Amalia Madihie
University of Malaysia, Malaysia

Rehman Ullah Khan
https://orcid.org/0000-0003-4605-5245
University of Malaysia, Malaysia

ABSTRACT

In recent years, integration of Artificial Intelligence into healthcare has ignited profound interest. This delves into the convergence of Artificial Intelligence and psychotherapy, specifically focusing on the development of Eye Movement Desensitization and Reprocessing (EMDR) therapy system. The chapter aims to comprehensively explore system development methodologies, design components, and the software development process essential for an Artificial Intelligence -based online EMDR therapy system. This chapter intricately details the architectural design, functionalities, hardware and software requirements crucial to optimizing therapeutic usability, outcomes of the system. Natural Language Processing algorithms drive functionalities such as sentiment analysis, text summarization, tokenization, and descriptive analytics, enriching online therapeutic interactions all have made online EMDR therapy system more efficient. This chapter concludes with insights into future directions and implications for Artificial Intelligence-driven psychotherapies.

DOI: 10.4018/979-8-3693-6180-1.ch005

1. INTRODUCTION

In recent times, researchers are increasingly interested in using artificial intelligence for several aspects of healthcare. This is because artificial intelligence has the power to completely transform the way that treatment is delivered and made accessible, overcoming long-standing obstacles pertaining to accessibility of treatments to all individuals (Alowais et al., 2023). One possible direction for further research and development in the field of artificial intelligence-based mental healthcare is internet psychotherapy. Internet psychotherapy allows individuals to receive psychotherapy from the comfort of their own homes, eliminating barriers such as transportation and scheduling conflicts. Additionally, artificial intelligence can analyze vast amounts of data to personalize treatment plans and provide real-time feedback to therapists, enhancing the overall quality of care (Hebbar & Vandana, 2023). Artificial intelligence-powered virtual psychotherapy platforms can provide personalized treatment plans and interventions, improving patient outcomes and reducing the burden on traditional mental health services. Especially during the COVID-19 pandemic, when swift transitions to electronic and remote healthcare solutions were required, the use of internet psychotherapy had increased (Jurcik et al., 2023).

According to a review of recent studies, developing an Eye Movement Desensitization and Reprocessing (EMDR) therapy system is one of the most promising applications of artificial intelligence in online psychotherapy (Goga et al., 2022; Fiani, Russo, & Napoli, 2023; Kaptan, Kaya, & Akan, 2024). EMDR therapy is an evidence-based treatment that is traditionally performed in-person and has been demonstrated to be extremely successful in treating symptoms such as Post-traumatic Stress Disorder, Depression and Anxiety. The move of EMDR therapy to online platforms has increased its accessibility to a larger audience. In virtual environments, the integration of artificial intelligence allows therapists to improve the online EMDR experience by tailoring treatment plans and measuring progress more effectively. Furthermore, the use of artificial intelligence has the potential to revolutionize the delivery of mental health services in online settings.

A pertinent question that researchers should explore is how artificial intelligence can enhance the effectiveness of online EMDR therapy. To answer this question, we need to look into the different ways that artificial intelligence can be used to enhance key aspects of the psychotherapy process. For example, artificial intelligence could potentially assist in identifying patterns in patient responses during therapy sessions, allowing therapists to tailor their approach more effectively. Artificial intelligence can be used in various important aspects of online EMDR therapy in the future:

i) *Automated Symptom Assessment and Diagnosis:* Artificial intelligence algorithms have the capability to examine data on symptoms reported by patients or clinicians and can offer diagnoses through diagnostic tools. This leads to precise and reliable assessments of mental health conditions. This automation helps to alleviate the workload for therapists, while also guaranteeing that problems are recognized and addressed promptly (Tutun et al., 2023).

ii) *Ability to Handle Big Data:* Artificial intelligence has the capability to gather and examine data from various patients and recognize its patterns and trends. Such data can be used to enhance psychotherapy practices and optimize treatment strategies. By analyzing enormous amounts of patient data, artificial intelligence can identify correlations and predict outcomes, leading to more personalized and effective treatment plans. This can ultimately improve patient outcomes and overall mental health care (Gupta & Kumar, 2023).

iii) *Predictive Analytics Abilities:* Predictive Analytics involves the use of artificial intelligence to anticipate the results of therapy by considering several factors. This helps therapists prepare for potential obstacles and modify treatment strategies in advance. The ability to predict outcomes in therapy sessions can lead to greater success and improve overall efficiency in the treatment process (Higgins, Short, Chalup, & Wilson, 2023).
iv) *Monitoring and Feedback in Real-Time:* In EMDR therapy, artificial intelligence is utilized to track individual physical and emotional reactions in real-time. One example of how artificial intelligence can be utilized is by analyzing facial expressions, voice tones, and biometric data to assess the emotional state of a patient. This can provide therapists with instant feedback and help in making real-time adjustments to their therapy techniques (De & Mishra, 2022).
v) *Using Artificial Intelligence for Virtual Bilateral Stimulations:* One of the key elements of EMDR therapy is the use of bilateral stimulations, which include alternating diverse sensory inputs such as eye movements, tapping, or tones to help people process traumatic memories more efficiently (de Behrends, 2021). In an online scenario, artificial intelligence can improve bilateral stimulation by offering individualized and adaptable stimulation patterns depending on real-time client reactions. Artificial intelligence algorithms may modify the pace, intensity, and kind of bilateral stimulations based on patients' physiological and emotional responses, guaranteeing that the stimulation is tailored to each patient's therapeutic needs (Goga et al., 2022).

The integration of artificial intelligence into the internet-based EMDR therapy system constitutes a significant step forward. This research poses an essential question: how can we develop internet-based EMDR therapy systems that successfully use artificial intelligence technology? We may answer the question more thoroughly by revealing the architectural design principles and functions of an internet-based EMDR treatment system particularly designed to recognize and optimize therapeutic interventions. In this way by understanding the capabilities of artificial intelligence in this context, we can enhance the efficiency and effectiveness of an online EMDR therapy for a wider range of individuals. This research opens possibilities for personalized and adaptive online treatment plans that cater to the unique needs of each patient.

Recognizing the importance of artificial intelligence-based online EMDR therapy systems, this chapter delves into the detailed design of the architecture of various essential aspects and components of these types of systems. It will ensure a thorough understanding of how artificial intelligence can be seamlessly integrated into the online EMDR therapy system to optimize its therapeutic outcomes. This chapter initially describes the system development methodology, followed by the system design components and software development process. Lastly, it outlines the architectural design procedures and features of an artificial intelligence-based online EMDR treatment system. The chapter concludes with details about hardware and software requirements, the application and functioning of the system, and a final conclusion.

2. SYSTEM DEVELOPMENT METHODOLOGY

Because this system is composite in nature, the Rational Unified Process has been integrated into multifaceted system design and development processes (Tsui & Karam, 2022) and DevOps model (Mitesh, 2020) into one holistic framework. In addition to the Rational Unified Process and DevOps model, the

Agile methodology has been integrated into the framework, which focus on collaboration and continuous feedback are particularly suited to the dynamic nature of developing AI-driven treatment systems (Puspitasari, Nuzulita, & Hsiao, 2024). This integration allows for a more comprehensive approach to software development.

2.1 *System Initiation Stage:* This stage involves defining the scope and objectives of the system. Conducting of sprint planning sessions and engaging of stakeholders will be done to capture key user stories and ensure alignment with system goals.

2.2 *System Elaboration Stage:* This stage will give a full description of the system, focusing on its needs, functionalities and architecture. User story mapping and iterative prototyping will be utilized to modify system requirements and design in response to constant stakeholder feedback.

2.3 *System Construction Stage:* The construction stage entails developing the system in accordance with the specifications established in the previous two phases of the system development process. Sprint development cycles will be used, with daily stand-up meetings to guarantee iterative development, testing, and alignment with user demands.

2.4 *System Transition Stage:* Once the system is completed, it will be tested by therapists and patients. Sprint reviews, retrospectives, and user acceptability testing sessions will be held to solicit input and assess system functioning and usability.

2.5 *Continuous System Deployment, Monitoring, and Maintenance:* The system will be regularly integrated and deployed to maintain stability and dependability. Continuous integration and deployment pipelines will be used to provide quick and reliable system upgrades. The system will be continually monitored, and its performance measured in real time. Real-time dashboards will be used, along with regular performance evaluations, to continually monitor and optimize system performance. Living documentation will be maintained by collaborative platforms, and particular sprints for updating and revising documentation will be scheduled to ensure it stays complete and valuable.

3. SYSTEM DESIGN COMPONENTS

A number of design elements, including a network, user interface, cloud server, and cloud database, will be included on the internet-based EMDR therapy system. These components will work together seamlessly to provide a secure and efficient platform for delivering therapy sessions remotely. Additionally, regular updates and maintenance will ensure the system remains up-to-date and user-friendly for both therapists and patients.

3.1 User Interface

The User Interface is divided into two sections: the Therapist Dashboard and the Patient Portal. Both interfaces will be accessible through computers. The Therapist Dashboard includes various controls related to the online delivery of EMDR psychotherapy, such as:

i) Creating an account.
ii) Logging in and out.
iii) Appointment management.

iv) Counseling session management.
v) Controls for bilateral stimulations.
vi) Video conferencing controls.
vii) Whiteboard controls.
viii) Document and file sharing.
ix) Session initiation and recording controls.
x) Messaging controls.
xi) Viewing patient progress (psychotherapy plan, counseling session history, symptom data)

The Patient Portal includes features such as:

i) Creating an account.
ii) Logging in and out.
iii) Joining therapy sessions.
iv) Participating in bilateral stimulations via video conferencing and connected auxiliary devices such as tappers.
v) Accessing the whiteboard.
vi) Accessing information related to mental health literacy (resource library).
vii) Viewing therapy progress.
viii) Document and file sharing.
ix) Billing and payment options.
x) Personal account settings.
xi) Help and technical support.

3.2 Network

The network infrastructure will utilize a Worldwide Area Network for data transmission, employing encrypted protocols such as Secure Sockets Layer or Transport Layer Security. Both the patient and therapist platforms will connect via high-speed internet utilizing cloud computing services. This network will also interface with a real-time database. Network interface modules will govern the secure exchange of data. All transmitted data, including video conference sessions and written messages, will strictly adhere to Health Insurance Portability and Accountability Act standards.

3.3 Clous Sever

The Cloud Server will host the core functionality of the system and integrate it. It will provide virtualized computing resources on the selected Cloud Server. This includes virtual infrastructures like web servers, application servers, and applications for processing information and providing hosting environments for various server computers. The Cloud Server will utilize global cloud services such as Platform as a Service (PaaS) and Software as a Service (SaaS), choosing between Microsoft Azure or Google Cloud Platform.

Figure 1. Activity flow chart for system design components

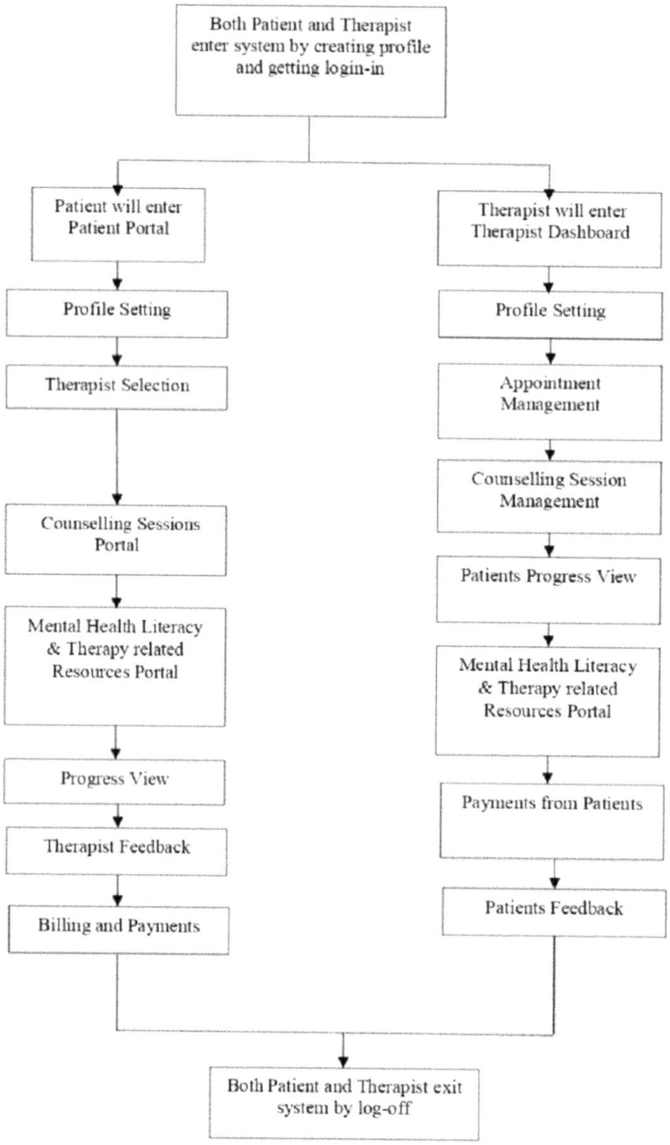

```
                 Both Patient and Therapist
                 enter system by creating profile
                 and getting login-in
                        │
          ┌─────────────┴─────────────┐
          ▼                           ▼
   Patient will enter          Therapist will enter
   Patient Portal              Therapist Dashboard
          │                           │
          ▼                           ▼
   Profile Setting             Profile Setting
          │                           │
          ▼                           ▼
   Therapist Selection         Appointment
          │                    Management
          │                           │
          ▼                           ▼
   Counselling Sessions        Counselling Session
   Portal                      Management
          │                           │
          ▼                           ▼
   Mental Health Literacy      Patients Progress View
   & Therapy related                  │
   Resources Portal                   ▼
          │                    Mental Health Literacy
          ▼                    & Therapy related
   Progress View               Resources Portal
          │                           │
          ▼                           ▼
   Therapist Feedback          Payments from Patients
          │                           │
          ▼                           ▼
   Billing and Payments        Patients Feedback
          │                           │
          └─────────────┬─────────────┘
                        ▼
                 Both Patient and Therapist exit
                 system by log-off
```

3.4 Clous Database

The system will include a cloud database responsible for storing, accessing, and tracking changes in data on cloud platforms. It will operate on a cloud computing platform to provide storage resources, managed under Database as a Service. Accessible via the internet, the Cloud Database will be hosted on either Microsoft Azure or Google Cloud Platform (Vlasceanu, Neu, Oram, Alapati, & Safari, 2019). For relational database needs, MySQL (MySQL, 2024) will be selected. To maintain high scalability, MongoDB (MongoDB, 2024) will also be employed, possibly in a polyglot persistence strategy where both databases are used concurrently (Košmerl, Rabuzin, & Šestak, 2020). The database setup will include automatic backup and disaster recovery tools to ensure data can be recovered in case of data loss or system failures.

4. SYSTEM SOFTWARE DEVELOPMENT PROCESS

The system will be accessible through computers (desktop and laptop). The system development process contains of following components:

4.1 Programming Language and System Framework: Advance programming languages like Python will be used, while Web Application through framework such as Django.

4.2 Technology Stack: Since the system will be accessible primarily through computers, suitable backend, frontend, and database technology stacks will be deployed.

4.2.1 *Frontend and Backend Development:* For the frontend, ReactJS (ReactJS, 2024) will be utilized to create the website's user interface. The backend will be developed using Node.js (Node.js, 2024) to support the system's functionalities.

4.2.2 *Database*: MySQL (MySQL, 2024) will be chosen as the primary relational database for structured data storage. For maintaining high data scalability, MongoDB (MongoDB, 2024) will complement MySQL in a polyglot persistence approach (Košmerl et al., 2020).

4.2.3 *Communication Protocol*: WebSockets (WebSockets, 2024) will facilitate real-time two-way communication between the therapist and the patient.

4.2.4 *Video Conferencing:* CometChat (CometChat, 2024) and Dyte (Dyte, 2024) application programming interfaces will be integrated to support the system's video conferencing capabilities.

4.2.5 *System Authentication:* JSON Web Tokens (JWT, 2024) will ensure secure authentication. Encrypted protocols such as Secure Sockets Layer or Transport Layer Security (Shimonski & Solomon, 2023).

4.2.6 *Compatibility with Various Browsers:* BrowserStack (BrowserStack, 2024) will be utilized to ensure the system's compatibility across different browsers.

4.2.7 *System Development Environment:* The system will be containerized using Docker (Docker, 2024), facilitating efficient deployment and scalability. Git will be used for version control and source code management (Git, 2024).

4.3 Designing of User Interface: A detailed User Flow has been outlined through a series of flow charts. Figure 1 on next page illustrates the main User Flow from entry to exit of the system. Separate flow charts for each activity are provided in the supplementary file. Both therapists and patients begin by registering and creating an account. After logging in, users perform various tasks, with therapists having extensive control over therapy-related services accessible to patients through the therapist portal.

4.4 Offline System Functionality: The system will support offline functionality, ensuring patients have access to mental health literacy and therapy resources even without internet connectivity.

4.5 Dynamic Navigation Menu: A clear and responsive navigation menu will be designed, optimizing for various screen sizes of computer screens.

4.6 Optimize Loading Time: To maintain optimal loading speed for psychotherapy-related interactive activities:

i) Images will be uploaded in appropriate sizes and modern formats like WebP.
ii) Resource caching with expiration dates will reduce server load.
iii) Cascading Style Sheets and JavaScript files will be concatenated to minimize Hypertext Transfer Protocol requests.
iv) Static content will be distributed across multiple servers.
v) Performance monitoring tools such as Gtmetrix (Gtmetrix, 2024) and Google PageSpeed Insights (Pagespeed, 2024) will be used to ensure continuous performance enhancement.

4.7 Supporting Multiple Windows: The system will support simultaneous handling of multiple windows through flexible window layout design and inter-window communication. It will be compatible with Microsoft Windows, Linux, and Macintosh operating systems.

4.8 Dynamic Structure of Uniform Resource Locator: A hierarchical model of Uniform Resource Locators will enable flexible interaction between therapists and patients. Main content will be accessible via the main application Uniform Resource Locator, with subsequent pages utilizing sub- Uniform Resource Locators. Search Engine Optimization tools will be integrated to enhance system search capabilities.

4.9 Managing Browser History: User-side routing will be implemented using JavaScript libraries such as React Router or Angular Router. HTML5 History Application Programming Interface (MND-API, 2024) will programmatically manage browser history, ensuring efficient navigation and URL updates. The system will monitor changes in the session history via the "popstate event" (MDN-Popstate, 2024) to maintain accurate browsing records.

5. HARNESSING INTERNET-BASED EMDR THERAPY SYSTEM THROUGH USE OF ARTIFICIAL INTELLIGENCE

Artificial intelligence technologies will be integrated into the system development process, particularly focusing on automated symptoms assessment and diagnosis, predictive analytics abilities, and virtual bilateral stimulations.

5.1 Automated Symptoms Assessment and Diagnosis

The process flow chart for the automated symptoms assessment and diagnosis is displayed in Figure 2 on the next page. As the therapists will be collecting online data from the patients via diagnostic and assessment tools (a form of self-administered or clinician-administered questionnaires), the data will be processed by Natural Language Processing algorithms powered by Artificial Intelligence (Malgaroli, Hull, Zech, & Althoff, 2023) using techniques like Sentiment Analysis, Text Summarization, Tokenization, and Descriptive Analysis.

Various Machine Learning Models will dictate how the Natural Language Processing algorithms are implemented.

i) The support vector machines algorithm, which makes use of the Kernel Trick function (Zhou et al., 2022) will be employed for processing biological data, including gender, age and heart rate.

ii) Categorical data will be processed using the Random Forests method (Iyortsuun, Kim, Jhon, Yang, & Pant, 2023), which will also be utilized to create perdition. Any data with missing values may be processed using this approach.
iii) Lastly, textual data, photographs, and the prediction of mental health issues (based on information gathered from diagnostic scales) will be processed using the Deep Neural Networks method (Iyortsuun et al., 2023).

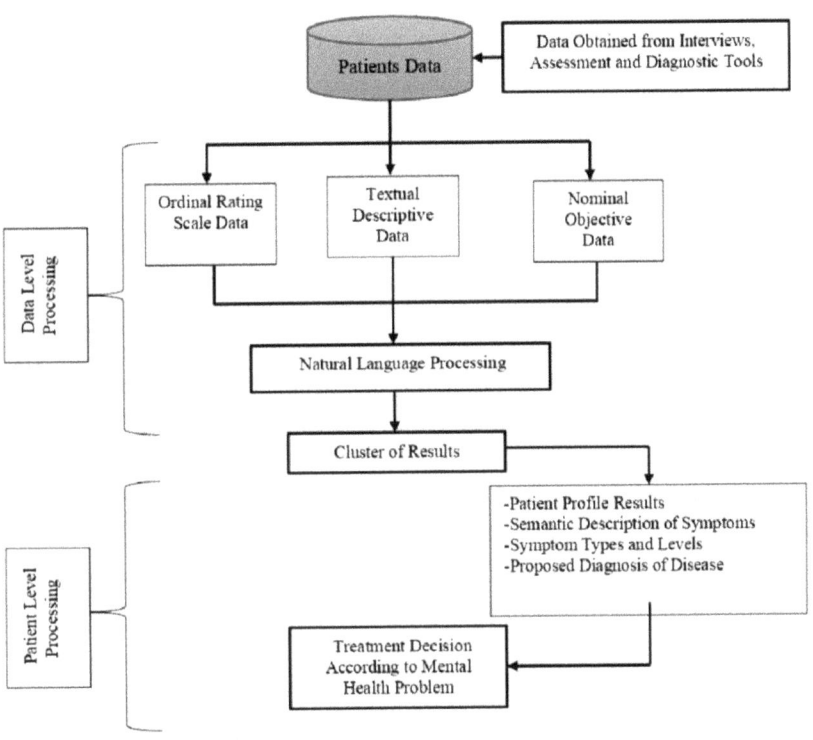

Figure 2. Automated symptoms assessment and diagnosis

(Juhn & Liu, 2020)

Once the selection of the Machine Learning models is done, the performance of models will be assessed and validated with the help of guidelines given by Müller & Guido (2018) and López, López, & Crossa (2022). According to these guidelines, the data set will be initially split into training and test sets to facilitate model development and evaluation. The training set will be used exclusively for model training, where the selected model will learn from the data, adjusting its parameters through optimization algorithms to enhance decision-making capabilities. Concurrently, cross-validation techniques, such as k-fold validation and Leave-one-out cross-validation, will be employed to rigorously assess model accuracy across different data partitions. This process ensures robustness and reliability in model performance evaluation, particularly in scenarios where dataset size and variability are critical factors.

Evaluation metrics will be meticulously chosen based on the specific characteristics of the data under analysis. For tasks involving classification and categorization, metrics tailored to these objectives will be applied to gauge the model's ability to correctly classify and categorize data points. Similarly, regression metrics will be utilized to measure prediction accuracy in tasks requiring numerical forecasting. For tasks related to grouping and prioritization, metrics designed for ranking and clustering analysis will be utilized to assess model performance comprehensively. Throughout these stages, the goal remains to refine the model's effectiveness and optimize its performance through systematic evaluation and adjustment of both model parameters and hyperparameters.

After successfully evaluating the performance of the chosen Machine Learning models, the next critical step involves their integration into the web-based EMDR therapy System. Initially, integration points will be meticulously identified using sophisticated Application Programming Interfaces and robust Code Analysis tools. These points are likely to be strategically located at user interfaces and within dedicated microservices specifically designed to handle machine learning tasks. This initial phase ensures that the integration process aligns seamlessly with the existing system architecture, enhancing overall efficiency and functionality.

Following the identification of integration points, the focus shifts to selecting an optimal deployment environment. Cloud platforms such as Google Cloud Platform or Amazon Web Services offer scalable infrastructure solutions ideal for hosting machine learning applications. Once the environment is chosen, the trained models will be deployed accordingly. This deployment involves leveraging Docker technology (Docker, 2024) to containerize the models, ensuring consistent performance and easy scalability. Concurrently, a well-defined Application Programming Interface will be designed to facilitate smooth interaction with the system's Artificial Intelligence capabilities, complemented by a robust data transfer mechanism like WebSocket Communication to handle real-time data processing needs. Security measures, including data authentication protocols and error handling mechanisms, will be implemented to safeguard sensitive information. Ultimately, this integrated system will undergo rigorous testing before final deployment into the production environment, marking the culmination of a comprehensive and systematic integration process.

5.2 Predictive Analytics Mechanism

5.2.1 Development Stage

i) Initially, comprehensive datasets encompassing patient history, symptom severity, demographics, therapy session details, and treatment outcomes will be collected. This data will form the foundation for subsequent analysis and modeling.
ii) Next, the pertinent features from the collected datasets will be identified and contrasted, which may significantly impact therapy outcomes. Key features may include age, gender, initial symptom severity, frequency of therapy sessions, and specific details from patient histories.
iii) Models such as random forests and neural networks (Han, Jiang, Zhao, Wang, & Yin, 2018) will be chosen for predictive modeling tasks, given their proven efficacy in handling complex datasets and capturing intricate relationships within the data.
iv) Then training of the selected machine learning models will be done by using historical data. It will be ensured the data is split into distinct training and validation sets.

v) The model performance will be evaluated by established metrics such as accuracy, precision, recall, F1 score, and mean squared error.

5.2.2 Implementation Stage

i) During actual use, the patient data will be entered into the predictive model. This will include data such as current symptoms, past medical history, demographics, and any other relevant information.
ii) The model will process the input data to forecast the likely outcomes of the therapy. This prediction can include potential symptom improvement, therapy duration, and the likelihood of success.

5.2.3 Deployment Stage

Deployment involves embedding the trained predictive model within the online therapy platform to enable real-time usage (Corbin et al., 2023). During the system deployment process, the predictive model's functionality will be integrated into the existing infrastructure of the online EMDR therapy platform. This may involve deploying the model as a microservice or integrating it directly into the platform's backend architecture. Furthermore, to enable communication between the prediction model and the online therapy platform, Application Programming Interfaces will be developed. Application Programming Interfaces will specify the transmission and processing of data, guaranteeing smooth communication between various software elements. It will be ensured that the deployed model can handle varying levels of user traffic and data input without compromising performance. This may involve deploying the model on scalable cloud infrastructure, such as Amazon Web Services or Google Cloud Platform, to accommodate increasing computational demands.

Software tools or modules within the online therapy platform will be implemented to automatically capture and store data from therapy sessions. These tools may include form inputs for therapists to record session details, patient feedback, and symptom progression. A centralized data repository will be set up, where collected data will be securely stored. It will be ensured that there is compatibility with existing data formats (e.g., JSON, CSV) and integration with backend systems for seamless data processing.

The model predictions against actual therapy outcomes will be regularly reviewed to refine the predictive model within the online therapy platform. This ongoing evaluation includes assessing performance metrics such as accuracy, precision, recall, and F1 score to measure prediction effectiveness. Discrepancies between predicted and actual outcomes will be analyzed to identify patterns and trends, guiding adjustments to model algorithms, updates to training data, and improvements in feature engineering. Integration of feedback from therapists and stakeholders will enhance the model's accuracy and relevance to real-world therapeutic scenarios. Documentation of review findings and transparent communication of improvements will support continuous enhancement of predictive capabilities, ultimately optimizing treatment recommendations and improving patient outcomes.

5.2.4 Doing Virtual Bilateral Stimulations

The task of performing virtual bilateral stimulations has always been challenging for therapists, but with the development of artificial intelligence, this task has been accomplished. Artificial intelligence technology has allowed therapists to provide effective virtual bilateral stimulations to clients, improving outcomes in therapy sessions. This advancement has revolutionized the way therapists can deliver treatment and support to individuals in need.

5.2.4.1 Designing User Interface

While designing user interface (see 3.1 section of chapter) it will be ensured to design user interface that can deal with visual, verbal and tactile interactions. The objective of the visual stimulation is to implement the horizontal movement of visual objects to guide the user's eye movements. The moving objects may include circles or arrows, with adjustable sizes and configurable colors. JavaScript will be used to create a smooth horizontal movement across the screen. A loop will be implemented to move the objects from the left edge to the right edge of the screen and back.

The objective of the auditory stimulation is to play alternating sounds in the left and right ears using headphones or speakers to ensure effective auditory stimulation. Two files will be prepared to create tones using an audio generation library. Therapists will be provided with options to set the volume, frequency, duration, and interval of the alternating tones. The Web Audio Application Programming Interface will be used to play sounds alternately in the left and right channels. A loop will be created to switch playback between the left and right audio channels.

Finally, the objective of tactile stimulation will be to provide alternating tactile feedback through wearable or handheld devices. Compatibility with haptic feedback devices such as wristbands or handheld vibrators will be ensured, utilizing Bluetooth or Universal Serial Bus (USB) interfaces to communicate with these devices. Adjustment of the devices will be managed by the therapist. Haptic devices will include tappers, such as the Thera Tappers, which are rectangular pulsers measuring 2.4″ x 1.25″ x 0.6″ and designed to fit comfortably in the patient's hand. (TherapTapper, 2024).

5.2.4.2 Collection of Real Time Data

Patient responses, whether verbal or written, will be collected as real-time data. To achieve this, biometric sensors and online assessment tools will be integrated into the system. Biometric sensors such as BioNomadix Wireless Physiology (BioNomadix, 2024) and Thera Tappers (TherapTapper, 2024) will be connected to the system to remotely send data on heart rate and body movements to therapists. Webcams will capture facial expressions and eye movements, essential for monitoring the effects of visual stimulation. Verbal responses and vocal cues will be captured via microphones, while written data will be gathered through online assessment tools completed by patients. A common time reference will synchronize all sensors and devices. Synchronization mechanisms, such as signals or markers sent by the therapy system (e.g., Thera Tapper), will initiate or cease data collection simultaneously across all connected sensors, ensuring data coherence.

5.2.4.3 Adaptation of Artificial Intelligence Driven Stimulations

Machine learning models such as Random Forest will be deployed in web-based EMDR therapy systems to analyze real-time patient data using supervised learning techniques. Initially, the system will collect and preprocess historical data from online EMDR therapy sessions. This data will typically include various parameters such as patient demographics, session duration, symptoms details, and detailed records of patient responses to bilateral stimulations.

In the next step, supervised learning algorithms will be trained on this curated dataset. Common algorithms for this task include Random Forest, or Neural Networks. During training, the algorithms will learn to map the input features (e.g., patient characteristics and stimulation parameters) to the desired output (e.g., therapeutic effectiveness or patient response patterns). The training process will involve iteratively adjusting model parameters to minimize prediction errors and maximize accuracy in predicting patient responses to several types of bilateral stimulations.

Once trained, these machine learning models can predict optimal stimulation parameters for new patients or ongoing therapy sessions based on real-time data inputs. This predictive capability enables the system to suggest personalized settings for bilateral stimulations that are most likely to yield positive therapeutic outcomes, thereby enhancing the efficacy and customization of web-based EMDR therapy.

5.2.4.4 Technical Infrastructure

To design the backend, cloud-based servers will be implemented for efficient data processing and storage. Platforms like Amazon Web Services will be utilized to ensure scalability and reliability. Robust data encryption and privacy controls will be integrated to safeguard sensitive patient information during transmission and storage. Minimizing latency in both data processing and stimulation delivery will be a priority. Techniques such as distributed computing and edge computing will be employed to reduce response times, thereby enhancing system responsiveness to patient feedback. Furthermore, the infrastructure will be designed with scalability in mind, incorporating auto-scaling capabilities within the cloud to dynamically adjust computing resources based on demand spikes.

5.2.4.5 Testing and Deployment

The system will undergo comprehensive testing to verify its functionality across diverse devices and scenarios. This testing phase includes unit testing, integration testing, and system testing to ensure all components of the Artificial Intelligence-driven stimulation adaptation for web-based EMDR therapy perform as expected. Upon successful testing, the system will be deployed on a scalable cloud infrastructure. Post-deployment, continuous performance monitoring will be implemented to track the system's responsiveness, resource utilization, and overall reliability.

6. SOFTWARE AND HARDWARE REQUIREMENTS

In order to develop the system, the following hardware and software will be needed:

i) Two desktop or laptop computer systems will be required, each featuring a 10th generation Intel Core i7 2.90GHz processor with 12 GB of RAM, a 500 GB hard disk, Intel UHD Graphics 630, and Windows 11 or an equivalent operating system. Each system should be equipped with a 24-inch OLED High Definition (1080 x 1920 pixels) monitor, a laser mouse, and a keyboard. Additionally, each setup should include a High Dynamic Range anti-glare camera with 1080p resolution, a microphone with 24-bit/48 kHz digital recording capabilities, and 3.5mm audio input with 42-watt subwoofer speakers.

ii) Biometric sensors such as BioNomadix Wireless Physiology (BioNomadix, 2024) and Thera Tappers (TherapTapper, 2024), which are rectangular pulsers measuring 2.4″ x 1.25″ x 0.6″ and designed to fit comfortably in the patient's hand, will be utilized.
iii) A robust router with dual-band Wi-Fi support and Quality of Service functions, along with a digital subscriber line modem, will be required. To utilize these features, a minimum internet speed of 25 Mbps for both uploads and downloads will be required.

7. SYSTEM APPLICATION AND FUNCTIONING

The system working flow and functionality is illustrated in Figure 3. Access to the system is provided through two portals: one for therapists and one for patients. Users can enter the system by creating an account and logging in. Patients have the capability to search for psychotherapists, book appointments, read mental health literacy materials, and participate in scheduled psychotherapy sessions. During a counseling session, both the therapist and the patient can engage in various activities. The therapist can record patient symptom data using the system's automated assessment and diagnostic tools or initiate a bilateral stimulation session within the video conference room. The therapist dashboard and patient portal will be interconnected via a Cloud Network, leveraging the networking infrastructure provided by the cloud service provider (e.g., Google Cloud Platform). This infrastructure comprises virtual networks, routers, subnets, load balancers, network security units, and firewalls implemented within a cloud-based environment. This setup ensures secure communication facilitated through WebRTC and WebSocket protocols.

Figure 3 also illustrates that all data generated by the system will be stored in a cloud database, a crucial component of the backend architecture for data storage and retrieval. The system will utilize MySQL and MongoDB database management systems for this purpose. A client application, such as a web browser, will transmit requests to the cloud server typically via the HTTPS protocol. Upon receiving these requests, the cloud server will process them accordingly. The server-side application will interact with the cloud database to store or retrieve data as required. A virtual machine will be selected and configured with an operating system, such as Microsoft Windows. Essential software, including MySQL and MongoDB database management systems, will be installed as needed. To ensure secure data transmission, encrypted communication protocols like HTTPS will be implemented to protect data during transportation.

The following resources will be needed in order to develop and operate the system:

i) A team consisting of Software Developers and Graphic Designers.
ii) A Database Administrator responsible for database design and supporting programmers in optimizing data retrieval.
iii) A System Architect tasked with developing the software architecture.
iv) Three 10th generation core i7 laptops.
v) A Cloud Database.
vi) Cloud computing services.
vii) Web Hosting services.

Figure 3. System application and functioning flow diagram

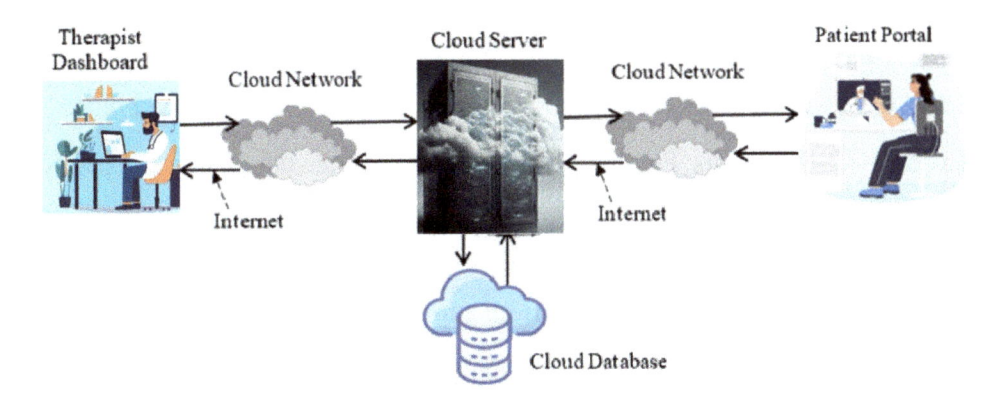

8. CONCLUSION

The aim of this chapter was to explore system development methodologies, system design components, and the software development process. It delves into the architectural design and features of an artificial intelligence-based online EMDR treatment system. The chapter concludes by detailing hardware and software requirements, as well as the application and functionality of the system. The technical process outlined in this manuscript underscores the practicality and feasibility of developing and implementing such systems in today's mental healthcare hospitals worldwide. Developing a web-based EMDR Psychotherapy system requires a multifaceted strategy that integrates various technical components into a cohesive system capable of delivering effective online therapy. By leveraging modern computer technologies and adapting evidence-based psychotherapies to the digital realm, researchers and practitioners can address many challenges associated with traditional face-to-face therapies.

In underdeveloped regions of the world, where mental healthcare facilities are limited and underfunded, adopting a web-based EMDR Psychotherapy system presents a significant opportunity to address mental health challenges. Looking ahead, the adoption of such a system could greatly expand access to mental healthcare services without geographical constraints. Future research should focus on enhancing these systems by incorporating culturally sensitive design elements and expanding their features. In conclusion, this chapter has illuminated the transformative potential of harnessing artificial intelligence to enhance the online EMDR therapy experience. By integrating advanced technologies into psychotherapeutic practices, we are unlocking new avenues for delivering effective mental healthcare remotely. This approach not only addresses the current limitations of traditional therapy but also paves the way for a more accessible and inclusive mental health support system globally. As we continue to innovate and refine these technologies, the future holds promise for expanding the reach and effectiveness of internet psychotherapy, ensuring that more individuals can access the healing benefits of EMDR therapy regardless of their geographical location or local healthcare resources.

REFERENCES

Alowais, S. A., Alghamdi, S. S., Alsuhebany, N., Alqahtani, T., Alshaya, A. I., Almohareb, S. N., & Badreldin, H. A. (2023). Revolutionizing healthcare: The role of artificial intelligence in clinical practice. *BMC Medical Education*, 23(1), 689. DOI: 10.1186/s12909-023-04698-z PMID: 37740191

BioNomadix. (2024). BioNomadix: Physiology Ware. Retrieved from https://www.biopac.com/product-category/research/bionomadix-wireless-physiology/

BrowserStack. (2024). BrowserStack Cloud Web. Retrieved from https://www.browserstack.com

CometChat. (2024). CometChat API. Retrieved from https://www.cometchat.com/

Corbin, C. K., Maclay, R., Acharya, A., Mony, S., Punnathanam, S., Thapa, R., Kotecha, N., Shah, N. H., & Chen, J. H. (2023). DEPLOYR: A technical framework for deploying custom real-time machine learning models into the electronic medical record. *Journal of the American Medical Informatics Association : JAMIA*, 30(9), 1532–1542. DOI: 10.1093/jamia/ocad114 PMID: 37369008

De, A., & Mishra, S. (2022). Augmented intelligence in mental health care: sentiment analysis and emotion detection with health care perspective. *Augmented Intelligence in Healthcare: A Pragmatic and Integrated Analysis*, 205–235.

de Behrends, M. R. (2021). Treating Cognitive Symptoms of Generalized Anxiety Disorder Using EMDR Therapy With Bilateral Alternating Tactile Stimulation. *Journal of EMDR Practice and Research*, 15(1), 44–59. DOI: 10.1891/EMDR-D-20-00026

Docker. (2024). Docker: Containerize an application. Retrieved from https://www.docker.com

Dyte. (2024). Dyte API. Retrieved from https://dyte.io/

Fiani, F., Russo, S., & Napoli, C. (2023). An advanced solution based on machine learning for remote emdr therapy. *Technologies*, 11(6), 172. DOI: 10.3390/technologies11060172

Git. (2024). Git. Retrieved from https://git-scm.com

Goga, N., Boiangiu, C.-A., Vasilateanu, A., Popovici, A.-F., Dragoi, M.-V., Popovici, R., ... Hadar, A. (2022). An Efficient System for Eye Movement Desensitization and Reprocessing (EMDR) Therapy: A Pilot Study.

Gtmetrix. (2024). Gtmetrix: Web Peformance and Monitoring. Retrieved from https://gtmetrix.com

Gupta, N. S., & Kumar, P. (2023). Perspective of artificial intelligence in healthcare data management: A journey towards precision medicine. *Computers in Biology and Medicine*, 162, 107051. DOI: 10.1016/j.compbiomed.2023.107051 PMID: 37271113

Han, T., Jiang, D., Zhao, Q., Wang, L., & Yin, K. (2018). Comparison of random forest, artificial neural networks and support vector machine for intelligent diagnosis of rotating machinery. *Transactions of the Institute of Measurement and Control*, 40(8), 2681–2693. DOI: 10.1177/0142331217708242

Hebbar, S., & Vandana, B. (2023). Artificial Intelligence in Future Telepsychiatry and Psychotherapy for E-Mental Health Revolution. In *Computational Intelligence in Medical Decision Making and Diagnosis* (pp. 39–60). CRC Press. DOI: 10.1201/9781003309451-3

Higgins, O., Short, B. L., Chalup, S. K., & Wilson, R. L. (2023). Artificial intelligence (AI) and machine learning (ML) based decision support systems in mental health: An integrative review. *International Journal of Mental Health Nursing*, 32(4), 966–978. DOI: 10.1111/inm.13114 PMID: 36744684

Iyortsuun, N. K., Kim, S.-H., Jhon, M., Yang, H.-J., & Pant, S. (2023). A Review of Machine Learning and Deep Learning Approaches on Mental Health Diagnosis. [). MDPI.]. *Health Care*, 11, 285. PMID: 36766860

Juhn, Y., & Liu, H. (2020). Artificial intelligence approaches using natural language processing to advance EHR-based clinical research. *The Journal of Allergy and Clinical Immunology*, 145(2), 463–469. DOI: 10.1016/j.jaci.2019.12.897 PMID: 31883846

Jurcik, T., Jarvis, G. E., Doric, J. Z., Krasavtseva, Y., Yaltonskaya, A., Ogiwara, K., & Grigoryan, K. (2023). Adapting mental health services to the COVID-19 pandemic: reflections from professionals in four countries. In *How the COVID-19 Pandemic Transformed the Mental Health Landscape* (pp. 3–28). Routledge. DOI: 10.4324/9781003352235-2

JWT. (2024). JSON Web Tokens Standard. Retrieved from https://jwt.io

Kaptan, S. K., Kaya, Z. M., & Akan, A. (2024). Addressing mental health need after COVID-19: A systematic review of remote EMDR therapy studies as an emerging option. *Frontiers in Psychiatry*, 14, 1336569. DOI: 10.3389/fpsyt.2023.1336569 PMID: 38250261

Košmerl, I., Rabuzin, K., & Šestak, M. (2020). Multi-model databases-Introducing polyglot persistence in the big data world. In *2020 43rd International Convention on Information, Communication and Electronic Technology (MIPRO)* (pp. 1724–1729). IEEE. DOI: 10.23919/MIPRO48935.2020.9245178

López, O. A. M., López, A. M., & Crossa, J. (2022). *Multivariate Statistical Machine Learning Methods for Genomic Prediction*. Springer International Publishing. DOI: 10.1007/978-3-030-89010-0

Malgaroli, M., Hull, T. D., Zech, J. M., & Althoff, T. (2023). Natural language processing for mental health interventions: A systematic review and research framework. *Translational Psychiatry*, 13(1), 309. DOI: 10.1038/s41398-023-02592-2 PMID: 37798296

MDN-Popstate. (2024). Window: popstate event. Retrieved from https://developer.mozilla.org/en-US/docs/Web/API/Window/popstate_event

Mitesh, S. (2020). *Agile, DevOps and Cloud Computing with Microsoft Azure*. BPB Publications.

MND-API. (2024). HTML5 History Application Programming Interface. Retrieved from https://developer.mozilla.org/en-US/docs/Web/API/History_API

Mongo, D. B. (2024). MongoDB: The Developer Data Platform. Retrieved from https://www.mongodb.com

Müller, A. C., & Guido, S. (2018). *Introduction to Machine Learning with Python: A Guide for Data Scientists*. O'Reilly Media.

MySQL. (2024). MySQL: Database Management System. Retrieved from https://www.mysql.com

Node.js. (2024). Node.js: Cross Platform. Retrieved from https://nodejs.org/en

Pagespeed. (2024). Google PageSpeed Insights. Retrieved from https://pagespeed.web.dev

Puspitasari, I., Nuzulita, N., & Hsiao, C.-S. (2024). Agile User-Centered Design Framework to Support the Development of E-Health for Patient Education. In *Computer and Information Science and Engineering* (Vol. 16, pp. 131–144). Springer. DOI: 10.1007/978-3-031-57037-7_10

React, J. S. (2024). ReactJS: Computer Program. Retrieved from https://react.dev

Shimonski, R., & Solomon, M. G. (2023). *Security Strategies in Windows Platforms and Applications*. Jones & Bartlett Learning.

TherapTapper. (2024). TheraTapper. Retrieved from https://theratapperinc.com/about-theratapper/

Tsui, F., & Karam, O. (2022). *Essentials of Software Engineering* (5th ed.). Jones & Bartlett Publishers.

Tutun, S., Johnson, M. E., Ahmed, A., Albizri, A., Irgil, S., Yesilkaya, I., Ucar, E. N., Sengun, T., & Harfouche, A. (2023). An AI-based decision support system for predicting mental health disorders. *Information Systems Frontiers*, 25(3), 1261–1276. DOI: 10.1007/s10796-022-10282-5 PMID: 35669335

Vlasceanu, V., Neu, W., Oram, A., Alapati, S., & Safari, an O. M. C. (2019). *An Introduction to Cloud Databases*. O'Reilly Media, Incorporated.

WebSockets. (2024). WebSockets Protcol. Retrieved from https://websockets.spec.whatwg.org

Zhou, X., Li, X., Zhang, Z., Han, Q., Deng, H., Jiang, Y., Tang, C., & Yang, L. (2022). Support vector machine deep mining of electronic medical records to predict the prognosis of severe acute myocardial infarction. *Frontiers in Physiology*, 13, 991990. DOI: 10.3389/fphys.2022.991990 PMID: 36246101

Chapter 6
Heartbeat Hackers:
Protecting Privacy in the IoMT Age

Manas Kumar Yogi

https://orcid.org/0000-0001-9118-2898

Pragati Engineering College, India

Atti MangaDevi

Pragati Engineering College, India

Yamuna Mundru

Pragati Engineering College, India

ABSTRACT

As the Internet of Medical Things (IoMT) transforms healthcare by enabling real-time monitoring and data exchange, it also presents new privacy challenges. "Heartbeat Hackers: Protecting Privacy in the IoMT Age" explores the intersection of advanced IoMT technologies and privacy concerns. This chapter delves into the vulnerabilities inherent in IoMT devices, including risks of unauthorized access and data breaches. It examines current security measures and highlights the need for robust privacy frameworks to protect sensitive health information. By analyzing recent case studies and emerging threats, the chapter offers practical recommendations for securing IoMT systems, safeguarding patient data, and ensuring compliance with regulatory standards. Through a comprehensive review of privacy-preserving technologies and best practices, it aims to equip healthcare providers and IoMT developers with actionable insights to enhance the protection of personal health information in the digital age.

1. INTRODUCTION

The Internet of Medical Things (IoMT) connects medical devices, software apps, and health systems that share data online. This fast-growing area is changing healthcare. It allows doctors to watch patients from afar, gather health info in real-time, and use computers for diagnosis. This makes medical care better and more efficient. The IoMT world has many devices. These include wearable health trackers; devices put inside the body smart hospital beds, and linked medical imaging systems (Ahmed, 2024) . These gadgets collect, look at, and send health data. Often, this happens right away. Doctors get this info, which helps them give more personal and quick care.

DOI: 10.4018/979-8-3693-6180-1.ch006

Copyright ©2025, IGI Global. Copying or distributing in print or electronic forms without written permission of IGI Global is prohibited.

Components of IoMT
1. Wearable Devices: Some of the most familiar IoMT devices include smart wearable such as fitness trackers, smart watches and heart rate monitoring devices. These devices record aspects such as the physical activity, the amount of sleep, heartbeat, and even blood oxygen level. Some of the conditions which they are most often employed include; preventive care, chronic conditions, and fitness (Alhaj, 2022).
2. Implantable Devices: These are appliances that are inserted into the body through surgeries for instance, pacemakers, insulin pumps and neurostimulators. They actively and passively track and control certain illnesses, and give instant information to the treating physicians, which is significant for the chronic disease's management.
3. Home Healthcare Systems: Some of the IoMT devices that may be used from home are smart scales, blood pressure monitor, glucose monitor and telemedicine systems. These devices allow the patients to monitor their health status from the comfort of their homes and this means that there will be a constant pressure on hospitals and also it also ensures that patients also play certain roles in the management of their health.
4. Smart Hospital Infrastructure: With IoMT, it enters the hospitals with smart beds that can track patients' movement; connected infusion pumps for the regulation of the dosage of medicines; and RFID systems for tracking of stocks, medical equipment (Ali, 2022). These technologies increase safety among the patients, increase efficiency and effectiveness of hospital and other healthcare facilities and institutions.
5. Medical Imaging and Diagnostics: IoMT also includes advanced imaging systems and diagnostic tools that are connected to cloud platforms. These systems can share images and diagnostic data with specialists worldwide for remote consultations, enabling quicker and more accurate diagnoses.
6. Telemedicine Platforms: Telemedicine has become a significant part of IoMT, allowing patients to consult with healthcare providers remotely via video conferencing and chat applications. These platforms often integrate with other IoMT devices to provide comprehensive care and monitoring.

Benefits of IoMT
1. Improved Patient Outcomes: IoMT helps in the constant tracking of patients' conditions and observing changes in real-time hence leading to early intervention in cases of complications. Such a stream of data enables all health care providers to make better decisions, thus enhancing the patients' well-being.
2. Enhanced Accessibility: These devices play a major role in increasing the accessibility of health care especially in regions that are hard to reach and or have few health care facilities. Telemedicine and home healthcare systems lower the amount of physical visits to health care facilities, which has its benefits to patients.
3. Cost Efficiency: The use of IoMT can thus in the long-run cut down significant healthcare costs through reduction of hospital readmission, improving the healthcare processes and facilitating remote monitoring. Patients also save on bus fares as well as time as they have to travel from their homes to hospitals with all necessary diagnostic tests.

4. Personalized Healthcare: IoMT enables care to be individualized as it enables healthcare professionals to have a feel of a patient's daily regimen, health history and requirements. Such an approach may help to establish better treatment regimens and might increase the rate of patients' compliance.

Importance of Privacy and Security in Medical Technology

The Critical Role of Privacy and Security

As the number of connected IoMT devices grows, the privacy and security of medical technology is critical when it links to the healthcare facilities. Such devices have the storage and forwarding of massive amounts of patient's health information, which in return exposes them to cyber-criminals. This information has to be protected in equal measures for the purpose of maintaining the confidence of the patients besides having regard to legal requirement and for the protection of the various health care systems (Almalki, 2022).

Privacy Concerns in IoMT
1. Sensitive Health Data: IoMT gadgets collect highly individualized data embracing; physiological, clinical backgrounds, and status. Tight measures should be taken against such data because such data will cause disasters such as identity theft, insurance fraud, and even physical harm if the data that is usually transformed.
2. Data Sharing and Interoperability: IoMT devices have interfaces for sharing data from EHRs, a cloud, and third parties and integrated applications accordingly. This sharing increases the risk of exposure of the data and intrusion by virtue of other people if the data is not encrypted or the platform has different security parameters (Alzoubi, 2024).
3. User Consent and Control: Patients often don't have to know what type of data is being gathered or for what purpose or to whom the data is being reported. This decision consequence leads to one of the most significant challenges in IoMT environment, which is informed consent from the patients combined with ownership of the collected data.
4. Data Anonymization: Though, we employ the data anonymization technique to ensure that the patient's information disclosure does not occur, the threat of re-identification exists when one combines or cross-checks the data or uses high analysis on it. This is the biggest challenge of preserving the patient identifiers while at the same time giving free access to the patients' health information to the researchers.

Security Challenges in IoMT
1. Device Vulnerabilities: Further, the security in IoMT devices is usually weak, especially in devices with low-power computational capabilities. They become prone to hackers and viruses, as well as other cyber related problems (Bharati, 2021). The broad category of devices that include wearables and implantable entails that there has to be a different approach to securing these devices.
2. Data Transmission Risks: This is because information exchange between IoMT devices and other centers such as central servers and cloud platforms can easily be intercepted. One dangerous type of threat is the man-in-the-middle attacks in which a hacker may change the messages transmitted between the devices.

3. Integration with Legacy Systems: A significant number of healthcare delivers an unsophisticated system that might not be interoperable with the newer IoMT devices or even the latest security standards. It becomes a difficult task of merging IoMT into these systems without a compromising on security.
4. Regulatory Compliance: IoMT devices are required to meet diverse legal requirements including the U. S. Health Insurance Portability and Accountability Act (HIPAA) and the European Union General Data Protection Regulation (GDPR). It involves high levels of security measures, frequent audits, and the right methods of handling data (Bhushan,2023) .

Strategies for Enhancing Privacy and Security

1. End-to-End Encryption: Applying the end-to-end encryption provid es a way of guaranteeing that data is secured from the point it is captured by an IoMT device to the time it is delivered to the intended recipient. This encryption should in a position to stand efforts that would otherwise seek to reverse the encryption by unauthorized personnel.
2. Multi-Factor Authentication (MFA): This increases security by the use of multi-factor authentication for accessing IoMT devices and their associated data platforms. Such options can be finger scans, smart IDs, tokens or one-use codes in the event that other than the standard password be used (Cano,2020).
3. Regular Security Updates: Another recommendation that suggests possible solutions to the considered challenges relating to IoMT devices is to update them, using security updates, from time to time as a way of fixing the identified vulnerability threats. This can only be achieved by the proper coordination of device development companies, software engineers, and outfits in the healthcare industry.
4. Privacy by Design: The integration of privacy results in the different designs of IoMT devices and systems in order to define privacy from the start. This includes limiting the use of personal data to what is necessary and essential, providing clear and transparent ways through which users can give their consent and ensuring that personal data is treated anonymously where possible (Elhoseny,2021).
5. Regulatory Adherence and Certification: Adherence to existing laws and guidelines regarding IoMT devices is essential to make the devices safe for the patients while protecting their data (Gaytan,2022).Another way of standardizing data is to get certifications from acknowledged authorities and that can help to increase confidence of users and healthcare providers.
6. User Education and Awareness: That is why information about dangers which may occur during IoMT usage and how to protect themselves and other individuals from these dangers is crucial for patients and providers. This comes in the form of teaching on matters such as the necessity of the password, how to detect phishing and how to manage on who can access the information.

2. UNDERSTANDING IOMT AND ITS IMPACT

The IoMT could also be described as a connected ecosystem that involves a wave of medical objects that stream, capture, transfer and process medical information. These device may be wristband type devices that form part of health monitoring system, or more sophisticated diagnostic equipment that assist clinicians and patients to monitor their condition and make necessary adjustments faster than waiting for routine appointments. IoMT joins medical devices with communication technologies to enable the continual assessment of patients' health, reduce operational redundancies and thereby improve the healthcare system's efficiency.

IoMT can be considered a subdiscipline of the more general IoT field, in which IoT usually concerns the connection of electronic devices to the internet which are inserted into objects in everyday use that can exchange information. IoMT extends this concept even further to ensure that the devices utilized in the healthcare industry can connect and share information with each other as well as with other stakeholders that include healthcare providers, patients, and other interested parties.

Examples of IoMT Devices
1. Wearable Devices: This is in the fitness trackers and smart watches among other gadgets that capture the steps taken, heartbeat rates and time in sleep among other things. For instance, a number of gadgets including Fitbit and Apple Watch are capable of some sign overseeing and forwarding the information to the doctors (Haque, 2021).
2. Implantable Devices: The example of IoMT devices that may be inserted into patients through surgery is pacemakers and implantable cardioverter-defibrillators (ICDs). Some of these devices can connect with other outside communicating appliances to provide information of a patient's condition of the heart at the right time.
3. Connected Inhalers: Smart inhalers are designed for patient with respiratory disorder like asthma or COPD to track the usage of the medicine and report the status to the doctors. They can also remind the patients on when to take the medicine and if necessary tell the doctors that the patient is getting worse.
4. Smart Pills: These are Sensors which can be swallowed to monitor a patient's adherence to a medication schedule and health condition. An example of the above is the smart pill by Proteus Digital Health that is ingested by the patient to send information to a wearable patch besides others such that when it was taken it sends data to a mobile application for tracking by the healthcare providers.
5. Remote Patient Monitoring (RPM) Systems: These are made up of the various integrated equipment that monitor a patient's condition such as: pulse, blood pressure, glucose and oxygen levels among others. Such systems also enable the patients to be treated at homes while the care providers are made aware of the patient's status in real-time (Hameed, 2021).
6. Robotic Surgery Systems: It also comprises such other sophisticated surgical robots as da Vinci Surgical System this is aides surgeons in performing operations that require minimal invasion but with great precision (Hireche, 2022). These are systems that can be operated remotely and these are connected to real-time analysis to enhance the surgical outcomes.
7. Smart Hospital Beds: These beds are equipped with sensors that monitor patients' movements, sleep patterns, and vital signs. They can adjust themselves to prevent bedsores and help in fall prevention, thereby improving patient safety and comfort.
8. Telemedicine Devices: Devices used in telemedicine, such as digital stethoscopes, and other portable ultrasound machines, are part of the IoMT. These devices enable healthcare professionals to conduct remote examinations and provide diagnoses without the patient needing to visit a healthcare facility.

Figure 1. IoMT ecosystem with various key applications

Overview of IoMT Devices

- Wearable Devices
- Connected Inhalers
- Remote Patient Monitoring Systems
- Smart Hospital Beds
- Implantable Devices
- Smart Pills
- Robotic Surgery Systems
- Telemedicine Devices

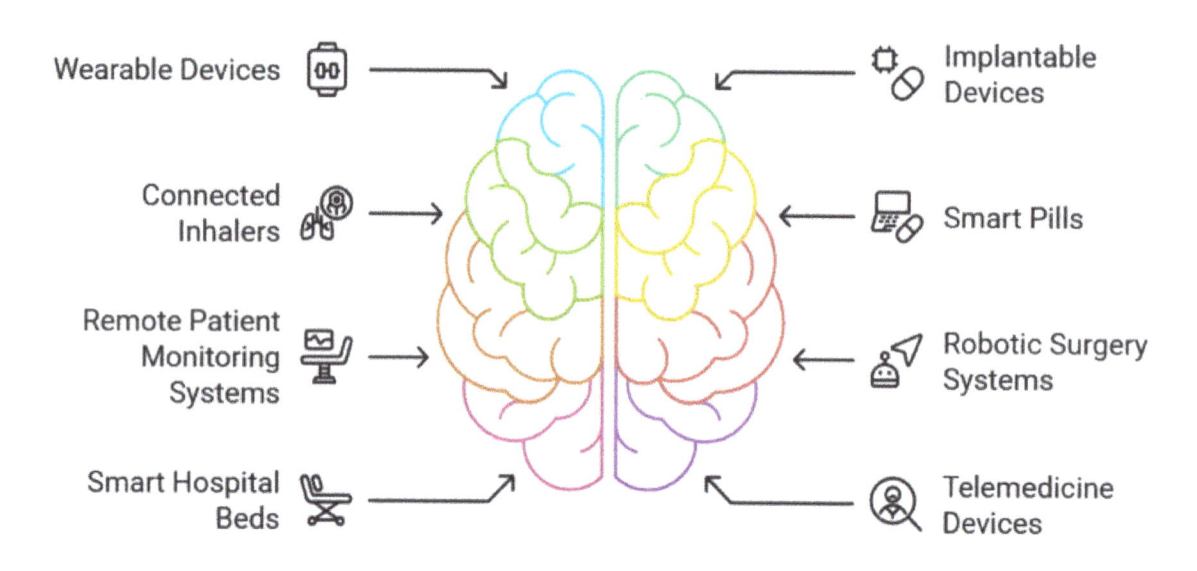

Figure 1 shows the IoMT ecosystem with its different spectrum of applications currently gaining popularity.

Benefits of IoMT in Healthcare

Incorporating IoMT into the existing mechanisms of healthcare has several advantages, for instance, improving the quality of care, reducing costs, as well as enhancing patient outcome. Below are some of the key benefits provided by the system (Jeyavel, 2021):

1. Enhanced Patient tracking and Care: One of the most significant noticeable benefits of IoMT is the ability to constantly monitor the health of patients without moving them from their home ever. Wearable or implantable gadgets provide continuous information on patient's vital signs, medication adherence and other health parameters. A large degree of this stalking is meant to detect any abnormalities that may in the future lead to illness hence making it possible for physicians to intervene and perhaps prevent certain negative outcomes from being experienced.
2. Better Management of Chronic Diseases: To continuous illness like diabetes, heart related illnesses, and breathing difficulties, IoMT devices are fundamental. To add, out of sight does not mean out of mind as monitoring aids in better control of these chronic diseases by providing health care practitioners with new but relevant information concerning the patient's condition. Consequently, treatment is based more accurately on the individual needs of the patients and is progressively modified to the most up-to-date information leading to improved outcomes.

The Internet of Medical Things (IoMT) represents a transformative force in healthcare, providing unprecedented opportunities for continuous monitoring, personalized treatment, and improved patient outcomes. As the technology continues to evolve, the integration of IoMT into healthcare systems will likely become more widespread, driving further innovations in medical care and enhancing the overall efficiency and effectiveness of healthcare delivery. The benefits of IoMT extend beyond patient care, offering cost savings, better resource management, and enhanced data analytics, making it an essential component of modern healthcare.

In the Internet of Medical Things (IoMT) ecosystem, privacy is paramount as devices continuously gather and transmit sensitive patient data. AI-driven anomaly detection, threat prediction, and automated response systems are emerging as crucial advancements, offering a technological edge for securing IoMT environments.

AI-Driven Anomaly Detection

IoMT devices generate vast amounts of real-time data, which makes manual monitoring for irregularities impractical. AI-driven anomaly detection addresses this by analyzing device behavior and network traffic patterns to identify deviations from typical usage or functioning, which may indicate a security breach. Machine learning (ML) algorithms, such as neural networks and clustering techniques, are effective in identifying these anomalies. By continuously learning from historical and real-time data, these systems adapt to evolving threats, reducing false positives and improving detection accuracy. This proactive monitoring is critical, as early detection of anomalies can prevent unauthorized access to sensitive patient information.

Threat Prediction

Threat prediction in IoMT uses predictive analytics and advanced AI models to foresee potential security risks before they occur. By examining historical data and employing pattern-recognition techniques, AI models predict likely threats, including malware or unauthorized access attempts. For instance, predictive algorithms can analyze login patterns and device usage anomalies to forecast potential insider threats or external hacking attempts. This ability to pre-emptively identify risks allows healthcare providers to take preventive action, enhancing the privacy and security of patient data. AI models trained on global threat intelligence sources can provide IoMT devices with insights into emerging cyber threats, making the entire ecosystem more resilient.

Automated Response Systems

Automated response systems form the third pillar of AI-enhanced security in IoMT. Once an anomaly or potential threat is detected, these systems initiate predefined responses without human intervention. Automated responses can include actions like temporarily disconnecting a compromised device, alerting system administrators, or activating device lockdowns. Such systems utilize rule-based AI or machine learning algorithms to respond in real-time, minimizing the potential damage of privacy breaches. Automation is particularly beneficial in IoMT, where response times are critical; a fast response to security incidents prevents sensitive medical data from exposure and ensures that healthcare services remain uninterrupted.

Together, AI-driven anomaly detection, threat prediction, and automated response systems significantly improve IoMT privacy and security. By leveraging these AI capabilities, healthcare providers can create a robust, privacy-preserving IoMT ecosystem that dynamically adapts to new threats, ultimately enhancing patient trust in connected medical technologies.

Figure 2. Scope of AI based solutions for facing privacy issues in IoMT

Enhancing IoMT Security with AI

IoMT Device Data
- Anomaly Detection
- Threat Prediction
- Automated Response

Improved IoMT Security

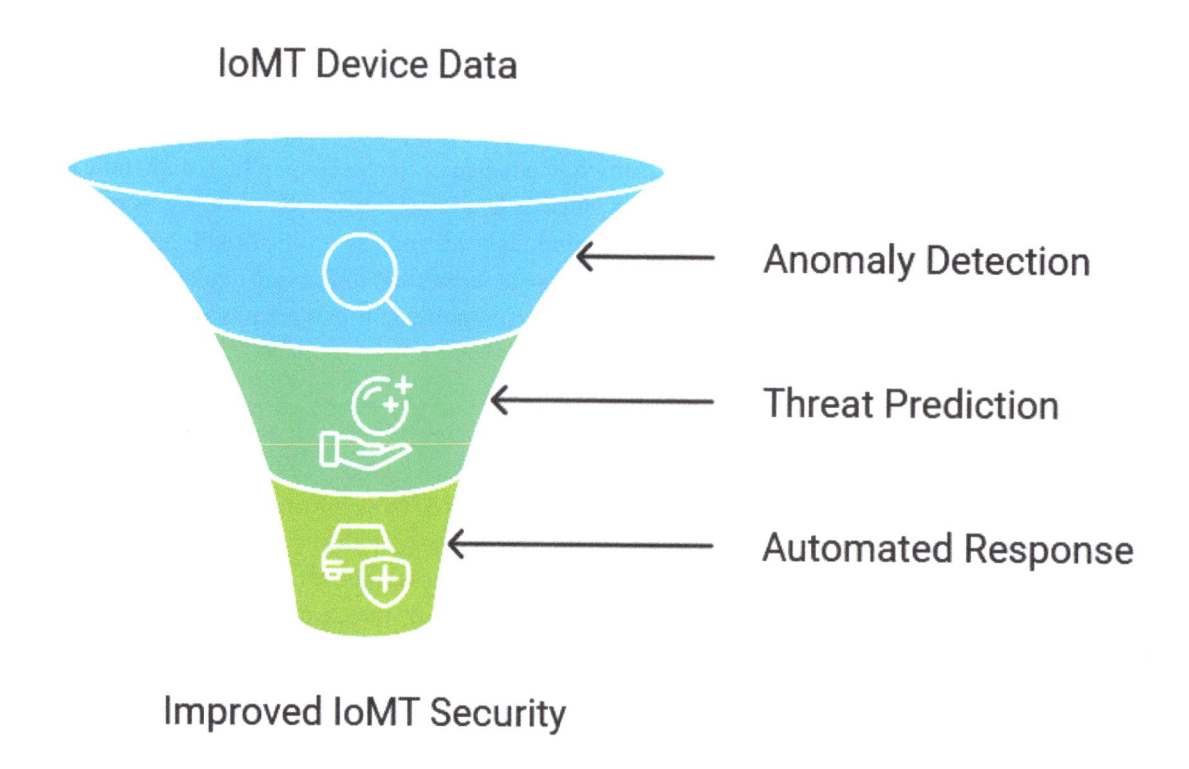

Figure 2 illustrates how anomaly detection; threat prediction and automated responses increase the degree of privacy preservation in IoMT ecosystem

A successful example of privacy-focused IoMT (Internet of Medical Things) implementation is Mayo Clinic's Remote Patient Monitoring (RPM) System. This system uses IoMT devices to monitor patients' vital signs remotely while prioritizing patient data privacy and security. Here's how Mayo Clinic's RPM demonstrates privacy-aware IoMT in action:

1. Encrypted Data Transmission: The RPM system transmits patient health data, such as heart rate and oxygen levels, from IoMT devices to healthcare providers. It uses advanced encryption protocols, ensuring that the data is secure and protected from unauthorized access during transmission.
2. Anonymization and Access Control: To comply with privacy regulations like HIPAA, Mayo Clinic's system anonymizes sensitive patient information and implements strict access controls. Only authorized healthcare professionals can access identifiable data, safeguarding patient privacy.
3. Edge Computing for Local Processing: By leveraging edge computing, some data processing occurs on the IoMT device itself rather than transferring all raw data to a central server. This reduces the exposure of personal data and enhances privacy by keeping most data local to the patient.
4. Federated Learning for Data Privacy: Mayo Clinic has explored federated learning to improve its RPM models without centralizing sensitive data. This approach allows for secure, decentralized model training on patient data across various IoMT devices, adding an extra layer of privacy.

This implementation showcases how integrating encryption, anonymization, edge computing, and federated learning in IoMT can improve patient monitoring systems while prioritizing data privacy. It sets a benchmark for privacy-compliant IoMT solutions in healthcare.

3. PRIVACY AND SECURITY CHALLENGES IN IOMT

Privacy Risks in IoMT

The Internet of Medical Things (IoMT) is revolutionizing healthcare by providing enhanced connectivity and data-driven insights. However, the same features that make IoMT so valuable also expose it to significant privacy risks. The sensitive nature of the data handled by IoMT devices-such as personal health information (PHI), biometric data, and real-time location tracking-makes it a prime target for malicious actors (Kumar, M.,2022).

1. Unauthorized Data Access and Data Breaches

Unauthorized access to IoMT devices and the data they generate is a significant privacy risk. Many IoMT devices lack robust authentication mechanisms, making it easier for attackers to gain unauthorized access. Once inside the system, attackers can exfiltrate sensitive data, leading to breaches that expose patients' personal health information. Data breaches can result in severe consequences for individuals, including identity theft, blackmail, and discrimination based on health conditions. Additionally, breaches undermine trust in healthcare institutions and can lead to legal ramifications under data protection regulations such as the General Data Protection Regulation (GDPR) and the Health Insurance Portability and Accountability Act (HIPAA).

2. Data Misuse by Third Parties

IoMT devices often transmit data to third parties, including cloud service providers, application developers, and insurance companies. While data sharing can enhance healthcare services, it also raises the risk of data misuse. Third parties may use health data for purposes not explicitly consented to by the patient, such as targeted advertising, price discrimination in insurance, or even sharing data with employers. The lack of transparency in how data is handled by these third parties exacerbates this risk, as patients may not be fully aware of who has access to their information and how it is being used.

3. Data Aggregation and De-anonymization

Even when data is anonymized, the aggregation of data from multiple IoMT devices can lead to de-anonymization. By correlating data from different sources, it is possible to re-identify individuals, thus compromising their privacy. For example, location data combined with health data could potentially reveal the identity of a patient receiving treatment for a specific condition. This risk is particularly high in the case of rare diseases, where the small number of patients makes re-identification easier.

4. Interference with Patient Autonomy

The storage of data by IoMT devices can influence the behavior of patients and healthcare providers. For instance, the knowledge that data is being continuously monitored could pressure patients into certain behavior or treatment choices, infringing on their autonomy. This risk is heightened in cases where healthcare providers or insurers have access to the data and may use it to enforce compliance with treatment plans or penalize patients for non-compliance.

5. Cross-Border Data Transfers

IoMT devices often transmit data across borders, especially when cloud services hosted in different countries are involved. This cross-border data flow raises concerns about compliance with local data protection regulations and the potential exposure of data to foreign governments or entities. Patients may have little control or knowledge over where their data is stored and who has jurisdiction over it, leading to privacy risks associated with differing legal standards and practices.

Common Security Vulnerabilities in IoMT

The security vulnerabilities in IoMT are a direct consequence of the complex ecosystem involving numerous interconnected devices, legacy systems, and varying levels of security maturity across different devices and platforms. These vulnerabilities not only threaten the integrity and availability of medical data but also pose risks to patient safety (Kumar, R., 2021).

1. Weak Authentication and Authorization Mechanisms

Many IoMT devices still rely on weak authentication methods, such as default passwords or hardcoded credentials, making them easy targets for attackers. Weak authentication allows unauthorized users to gain access to IoMT systems, where they can alter device settings, access sensitive data, or even shut down critical devices. Improper implementation of authorization controls can lead to excessive privileges being granted to certain users or applications, increasing the risk of insider threats or unauthorized access.

2. Insecure Data Transmission

Data transmitted between IoMT devices and other systems is often inadequately protected. Insecure transmission methods, such as the lack of encryption or the use of out-dated encryption protocols, can allow attackers to intercept and manipulate data in transit. This is particularly concerning for remote patient monitoring systems, where sensitive health data is frequently transmitted over public networks. The interception of such data can lead to privacy breaches, data tampering, and, in extreme cases, life-threatening situations if the manipulated data is used to make medical decisions (Lakhan, 2022).

3. Lack of Regular Security Updates and Patch Management

Many IoMT devices, especially those embedded in legacy systems, suffer from a lack of regular security updates and patch management. Manufacturers may not provide timely updates for known vulnerabilities, or healthcare organizations may delay applying patches due to concerns about disrupting clinical workflows. For example, ransomware attacks targeting healthcare facilities often take advantage of out-dated systems, leading to widespread disruption and potentially endangering patient lives.

4. Physical Security Vulnerabilities

IoMT devices, especially those used in home settings or wearable devices are susceptible to physical security threats. Attackers with physical access to a device can tamper with it to extract data, inject malicious code, or alter its functionality. Additionally, stolen or lost IoMT devices can result in unauthorized access to sensitive data if the device is not properly secured (Nair,2023). Physical security concerns are particularly relevant for implantable devices, where tampering can directly impact a patient's health.

5. Interoperability and Integration Issues

The IoMT ecosystem consists of a wide range of devices from different manufacturers, each with its own communication protocols and security standards. This lack of standardization can lead to interoperability issues, where devices fail to communicate securely with each other. Moreover, integrating IoMT devices with legacy systems or third-party applications can introduce vulnerabilities, such as insecure APIs, that attackers can exploit to gain access to the broader network. Poorly designed or untested integrations can also result in data leakage, misconfigurations, and other security risks.

6. Malware and Ransomware Threats

IoMT devices are increasingly being targeted by malware and ransomware attacks. These attacks can disrupt the operation of critical medical objects such as infusion pumps, ventilators, and systems which monitor the patients, leading to severe consequences for patient care. Ransomware attacks, in particular, have become more common in healthcare settings, where attackers encrypt patient data or disable medical devices, demanding a ransom for their release. The reliance on IoMT devices for critical care makes these attacks particularly devastating, as they can lead to delays in treatment or even loss of life.

7. Supply Chain Vulnerabilities

The complex supply chains involved in manufacturing and distributing IoMT devices present additional security risks. Vulnerabilities can be introduced at any stage of the supply chain, from the design and development phase to manufacturing, distribution, and deployment. For example, compromised components or malicious code inserted during the manufacturing process can result in backdoors or other security weaknesses in the final product.

8. Inadequate Incident Response and Recovery Plans

Many healthcare organizations lack comprehensive incident response and recovery plans for IoMT-related security incidents. Without proper planning, organizations may struggle to respond effectively to security breaches, leading to prolonged downtime, data loss, and harm to patients. Effective incident response requires a coordinated effort across multiple stakeholders, including device manufacturers, healthcare providers, and IT teams, to quickly identify, contain, and mitigate security threats.

In the context of privacy within the IoMT (Internet of Medical Things) ecosystem, AI can significantly enhance real-time threat detection and predictive analysis by using advanced methods to protect sensitive health data. Here are four ways AI can contribute:

1. Behavioral Analytics for Device Anomaly Detection: AI can monitor and analyze the behavior of IoMT devices, establishing baseline activity patterns. If any deviation from this norm is detected, AI algorithms flag the anomaly as a potential threat in real-time. This capability is crucial in identifying compromised devices or unauthorized access without requiring manual oversight.
2. Predictive Threat Modeling Using Machine Learning: AI models trained on historical data and threat intelligence can predict likely security threats, helping to prevent breaches before they happen. Predictive algorithms analyze prior security incidents, user behavior, and threat patterns, generating alerts for suspicious activities that may lead to breaches, thereby enhancing proactive security in IoMT.
3. Natural Language Processing (NLP) for Risk Intelligence: NLP can process unstructured data from research, cybersecurity reports, and news to identify emerging threats and vulnerabilities in real-time. By integrating this intelligence, IoMT systems can update threat models based on global trends, ensuring a timely response to newly discovered vulnerabilities that may impact device privacy.
4. Automated Threat Response with AI-Driven Decision Making: AI can enable IoMT systems to take instant, autonomous actions when a threat is detected, such as isolating compromised devices, altering network configurations, or notifying relevant personnel. This automation not only reduces response time but also minimizes the impact of a threat, securing patient data and maintaining privacy without constant manual intervention.

These AI-driven advancements strengthen the IoMT ecosystem's privacy posture by enabling fast, predictive, and automated responses to security threats.

4. REGULATORY FRAMEWORKS AND THEIR EFFECTIVENESS

Introduction to Data Privacy Regulations

In an era where data is often termed as the new oil, the protection of personal and sensitive information has become paramount. This is especially true in sectors like healthcare, where the security of patient data can have life-altering consequences. The regulatory landscape for data privacy has evolved to address the growing concerns around data misuse, breaches, and the ethical handling of personal information. Key regulations, such as the Health Insurance Portability and Accountability Act (HIPAA) in the United States and the General Data Protection Regulation (GDPR) in the European Union, have set stringent standards for how organizations must handle and protect personal data. This section provides an overview of these and other relevant regulations that govern data privacy and security in healthcare and beyond (Nie,2022).

Health Insurance Portability and Accountability Act (HIPAA)

HIPAA, enacted in 1996 in the United States, is one of the most comprehensive regulations governing the privacy and security of healthcare information. It establishes national standards for the protection of individually identifiable health information, known as Protected Health Information (PHI).

1. Key Provisions of HIPAA:
   - Privacy Rule: This rule mandates the protection of PHI by covered entities (healthcare providers, health plans, and healthcare clearinghouses) and their business associates. It gives patients' rights over their health information, including rights to examine and obtain a copy of their health records and request corrections.
   - Security Rule: This rule requires covered entities to implement physical, administrative, and technical safeguards to ensure the confidentiality, integrity, and availability of electronic PHI (ePHI). This includes measures such as encryption, access controls, and audit trails.
2. Impact of HIPAA:
   - HIPAA has significantly influenced how healthcare organizations manage patient data, ensuring that PHI is protected from unauthorized access and disclosure. The regulation has also prompted the healthcare industry to adopt stronger data security practices, particularly in the handling of ePHI.

General Data Protection Regulation (GDPR)

The GDPR, which came into effect in May 2018, is a comprehensive data protection law that applies to all organizations processing personal data of individuals within the European Union (EU). Unlike HIPAA, which is sector-specific, the GDPR has a broad scope, covering all types of personal data.

1. Key Provisions of GDPR:
   - Data Protection Principles: GDPR outlines principles for data processing, including lawfulness, fairness, transparency, purpose limitation, data minimization, accuracy, storage limitation, integrity, and confidentiality.

- Data Subject Rights: Individuals have rights under GDPR, such as the right to access their data, the right to rectification, the right to erasure (the "right to be forgotten"), the right to data portability, and the right to object to data processing.
    - Data Protection Officer (DPO): Organizations that process large amounts of sensitive personal data are required to appoint a DPO to oversee data protection strategies and ensure compliance with GDPR.
    - Data Breach Notification: Organizations must notify the relevant supervisory authority within 72 hours of becoming aware of a personal data breach, unless the breach is unlikely to result in a risk to the rights and freedoms of individuals.
2. Impact of GDPR:

GDPR has set a high standard for data protection worldwide, influencing data protection laws in other jurisdictions. It has also empowered individuals with greater control over their personal data and increased the accountability of organizations in handling such data. Non-compliance with GDPR can result in substantial fines, which has driven organizations to adopt rigorous data protection measures.

Analysis of Regulatory Strengths and Weaknesses

Strengths

1. Comprehensive Data Protection:

Regulations like GDPR and HIPAA provide a robust framework for protecting personal data, particularly sensitive health information. These regulations ensure that organizations implement necessary safeguards, thus reducing the risk of data breaches and unauthorized access.

2. Empowerment of Individuals:

Both GDPR and CCPA empower individuals by giving them rights over their data. This includes the right to access, correct, and deletes their data, as well as the right to object to certain types of data processing. This shift towards individual control over personal data is a significant strength of modern data protection regulations.

3. Global Influence:

GDPR, in particular, has had a global impact, influencing data protection laws beyond the EU. Many countries have adopted GDPR-like regulations, raising the standard for data protection worldwide. This harmonization of data protection standards facilitates international data transfers and ensures a higher level of privacy protection globally.

4. Accountability and Transparency:

Regulations such as GDPR and HIPAA promote transparency and accountability within organizations. The requirement to appoint a DPO, conduct regular data protection impact assessments (DPIAs), and report data breaches fosters a culture of compliance and encourages organizations to take data protection seriously.

5. Enforcement and Penalties:

- The enforcement mechanisms of regulations like GDPR and HIPAA are stringent, with substantial fines for non-compliance. This serves as a strong deterrent against data protection violations and encourages organizations to prioritize data security and privacy.

Weaknesses

1. Complexity and Compliance Costs:

One of the primary criticisms of regulations like GDPR and HIPAA is their complexity. The detailed requirements and broad scope can be difficult for companies, particularly small and medium-sized enterprises (SMEs), to fully understand and implement

2. Potential for Overregulation:

Some argue that regulations like GDPR may lead to overregulation, stifling innovation, particularly in the technology sector. The stringent requirements for consent, data minimization, and purpose limitation can make it difficult for companies to experiment with new data-driven technologies, potentially hindering progress in areas like artificial intelligence and big data analytics.

3. Ambiguity and Interpretation Issues:

The broad language used in some data protection regulations can lead to ambiguities and varied interpretations. For example, GDPR's definition of "personal data" and "legitimate interest" can be subject to interpretation, leading to uncertainty among organizations about how to comply with the law. This ambiguity can result in inconsistent application of the regulations and legal challenges.

4. Jurisdictional Challenges:

Data protection regulations often have jurisdictional limitations, which can create challenges in a globalized world. For instance, GDPR applies to data processing activities related to EU residents, but enforcing these rules on non-EU entities can be difficult. Similarly, HIPAA applies only within the United States, which can complicate data transfers and collaborations involving entities in other countries.

5. Balancing Privacy with Data Utilization:

While regulations like GDPR and HIPAA prioritize privacy, they can sometimes hinder the beneficial use of data, particularly in research and healthcare. The stringent consent requirements and restrictions on data processing can limit the ability of researchers and healthcare providers to use data for studies that could lead to medical advancements or improved public health outcomes.

These regulations offer comprehensive frameworks for safeguarding data, empowering individuals, and promoting transparency and accountability within organizations. However, they also present challenges, including complexity, compliance costs, and potential overregulation. Despite these weaknesses, the strengths of these regulations in ensuring data protection, fostering global standards, and enforcing compliance outweigh the challenges. As the regulatory landscape continues to evolve, balancing privacy with innovation and data utilization will be crucial to maximizing the benefits of data protection laws while minimizing their drawbacks.

5. EMERGING TECHNOLOGICAL SOLUTIONS

In table 1, the current popular methods for privacy preservation is discussed along with their features, benefits and challenges. (Rahmadika, 2022).

Table 1. Study of existing solutions

Technology/Technique	Features	Benefits	Current Challenges
Symmetric Encryption	Single key for encryption and decryption.	Fast and efficient.	Key management complexity.
	Example: AES (128, 192, 256-bit keys).	Low computational overhead.	Vulnerable if the key is compromised.
		Suitable for resource-constrained IoMT devices.	
Asymmetric Encryption	Uses a pair of keys: Public (encryption) and Private (decryption). Examples: RSA, ECC.	Enhanced security for key distribution.	Slower than symmetric encryption.
		ECC offers similar security to RSA with shorter key lengths (more efficient for IoMT).	Higher computational overhead compared to symmetric methods.
Homomorphic Encryption	Allows computations on encrypted data without decryption.	Maintains data privacy during processing.	Computationally intensive.
		Enables secure analysis of sensitive data in the cloud or other external environments.	Slower than traditional encryption methods.
			Challenges in real-time processing.

continued on following page

Table 1. Continued

Technology/Technique	Features	Benefits	Current Challenges
Blockchain	Decentralized and immutable ledger	Provides tamper-proof data storage.	Scalability issues.
	Features smart contracts for automated processes	Facilitates secure data sharing.	High energy consumption, particularly with proof-of-work algorithms.
		Enhances trust with transparent and immutable records.	Integration with regulatory frameworks is complex.
		Automates data sharing agreements with smart contracts.	
AI & Machine Learning	Anomaly detection and behavioural analysis.	Real-time threat detection and prevention.	Requires large data sets for effective training.
	Predictive analytics	Adaptation to evolving threats.	Computationally intensive.
	Automated response and self-learning systems	Enhanced data privacy without compromising analytics.	Potential privacy concerns if not carefully implemented.
	Federated learning and differential privacy	Proactive security measures	

In the Internet of Medical Things (IoMT) ecosystem, privacy and data security are paramount due to the sensitive nature of patient information and the potential risks associated with unauthorized access or data breaches. Blockchain and Artificial Intelligence (AI) offer powerful tools for enhancing privacy and security in IoMT networks, each addressing different aspects of the system's requirements and working together to establish a robust framework.

Blockchain's Role in Privacy for IoMT

Blockchain, with its decentralized, immutable, and transparent ledger system, provides a foundational layer of trust and security in the IoMT ecosystem. In traditional healthcare data systems, data is stored in centralized databases, making them vulnerable to single points of failure and data breaches. Blockchain mitigates this issue by distributing data across multiple nodes, which are cryptographically secured and tamper-resistant. In IoMT, blockchain can secure patient data, allowing only authorized participants, such as healthcare providers and patients, to access the information. This distributed ledger enables traceability and transparency, ensuring that every interaction with the data is logged and cannot be altered retroactively.

Smart contracts, a feature of blockchain, further enhance privacy by automating permissions and access control in IoMT networks. These self-executing contracts allow the predefined terms between parties to be securely enforced without requiring intermediaries. For instance, a smart contract could be used to grant a specialist temporary access to a patient's medical data, automatically revoking access once the purpose is fulfilled. This granular control over data sharing helps maintain patient privacy and ensures that sensitive information is only accessible to authorized entities.

AI's Role in Privacy for IoMT

AI can support privacy in IoMT by enhancing data anonymization, access control, and real-time threat detection. Data anonymization and pseudonymization techniques powered by AI algorithms can strip personally identifiable information (PII) from patient data while preserving the integrity and utility of the data for analysis. Advanced machine learning models can be trained to detect patterns in anonymized data, allowing healthcare professionals to draw insights without compromising patient privacy.

AI also plays a critical role in adaptive and dynamic access control within the IoMT ecosystem. Unlike static access control mechanisms, AI-powered systems can assess context-aware information, such as device location and usage patterns, to determine if access to certain data is appropriate. For example, if an IoMT device is being accessed from an unrecognized network, an AI-based access control system could deny access, flagging it as a potential privacy risk. This capability enables IoMT networks to be more resilient against unauthorized access and insider threats.

AI-driven threat detection and mitigation systems can monitor IoMT devices and data flows in real time. Machine learning algorithms can identify unusual patterns in data usage or device behavior, helping to pre-emptively detect and block potential privacy breaches. AI models trained on historical data can recognize anomalies that indicate cyber threats, initiating security protocols that protect patient privacy.

Integrating Blockchain and AI for Enhanced Privacy

Combining blockchain with AI offers a powerful synergy for privacy in IoMT. Blockchain's immutable records provide trustworthy audit trails, which AI can analyze to detect potential fraud or unauthorized data access. Moreover, AI models deployed on federated learning systems can train across multiple IoMT devices without centralizing data, while blockchain ensures that each device's data-sharing permissions are strictly enforced.

Figure 3. Enhanced privacy due to hybridization of AI with blockchain

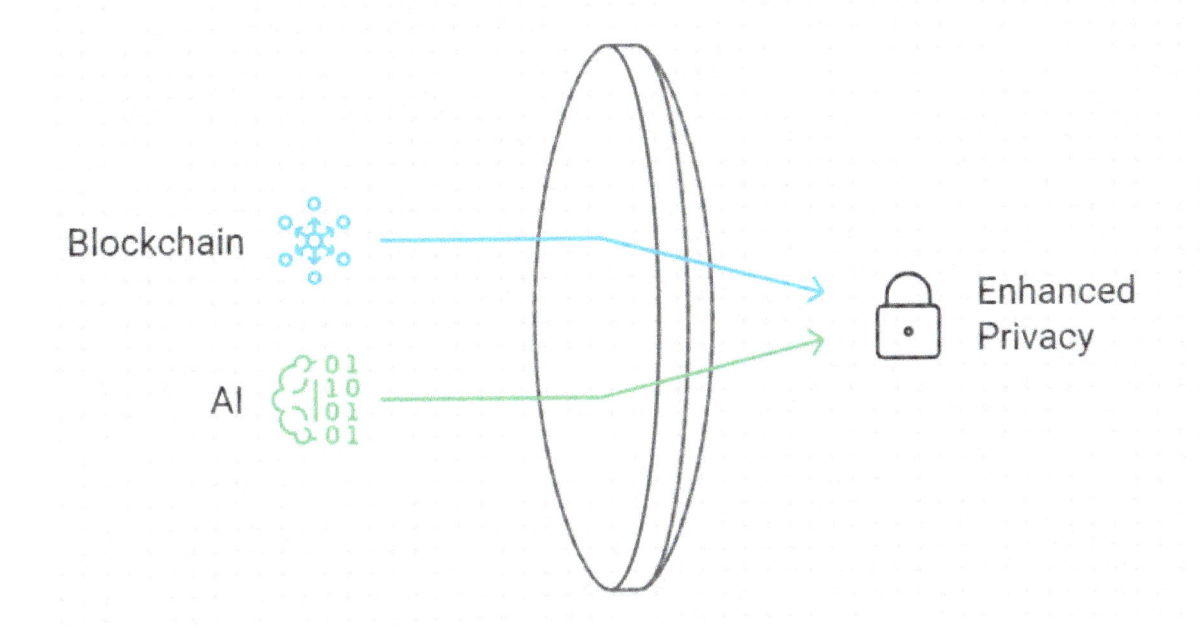

Table 2. Comparative analysis for key privacy standards relevant to the IoMT ecosystem

Standard	Region/Scope	Key Focus Areas	Data Protection Measures	Compliance Requirements	Impact on IoMT Privacy
GDPR (General Data Protection Regulation)	European Union	Data privacy, individual consent, data portability, right to be forgotten	Encryption, pseudonymization, data minimization	Requires data controllers to implement appropriate technical and organizational measures; high fines for non-compliance	Ensures stringent control over patient data with a focus on data access, sharing consent, and transparency in IoMT devices.
HIPAA (Health Insurance Portability and Accountability Act)	United States	Protecting personal health information (PHI)	Encryption, role-based access, audit controls	Requires covered entities to protect PHI; includes standards like the Privacy Rule and Security Rule	Limits access to PHI, establishes privacy safeguards; essential for IoMT devices handling sensitive health information.
PIPEDA (Personal Information Protection and Electronic Documents Act)	Canada	Consent for data collection, usage, and disclosure; fair information practices	Safeguards for data integrity, accountability, openness	Organizations must obtain valid consent and protect personal information; fines for non-compliance	Ensures patient data is collected responsibly and with consent, applicable to IoMT handling Canadian patient data.
NIST (National Institute of Standards and Technology) – Privacy Framework	United States (International Adoption)	Voluntary privacy framework, risk assessment, and mitigation	De-identification, differential privacy, access control	Offers a structured framework for identifying and managing privacy risks	Guides IoMT manufacturers and operators in adopting best practices to manage privacy risks.
ISO/IEC 27701 (Privacy Information Management)	Global	Extends ISO 27001 and ISO 27002 for privacy management	Data classification, access control, encryption	Compliance entails establishing a privacy information management system (PIMS) aligned with GDPR and other standards	Provides IoMT organizations with an international standard for privacy management and GDPR compliance.
HITECH Act (Health Information Technology for Economic and Clinical Health Act)	United States	Expands HIPAA; promotes the adoption of health information technology	Encryption, breach notification, data integrity	Strengthens HIPAA enforcement; requires breach notifications	Ensures IoMT systems handle PHI securely and provides protocols for breach responses, enhancing patient trust.
CPRA (California Privacy Rights Act)	California, United States	Privacy rights similar to GDPR, covering California residents	Data minimization, right to opt-out, data portability	Requires data controllers to implement protective measures; fines for breaches	IoMT devices in California must meet stringent privacy rights; enables patients to control their personal data.

continued on following page

Table 2. Continued

Standard	Region/Scope	Key Focus Areas	Data Protection Measures	Compliance Requirements	Impact on IoMT Privacy
My Health Record (Australia)	Australia	Health record management, data access controls, audit trails	Encryption, user-controlled access, breach notification	Obligates healthcare providers to comply with stringent security and access controls	Allows patients to control access to their health data in IoMT, ensuring comprehensive data security and compliance.
OECD Privacy Guidelines (Organization for Economic Cooperation and Development)	International	Collection limitation, data quality, purpose specification	Transparency, security safeguards, accountability	Provides principles to guide the development of privacy laws	Offers foundational privacy principles for global IoMT systems, especially where specific regulations aren't yet implemented.

In table 2 above the key aspects of current regulatory bodies are compared in various aspects of data privacy across the globe.

6. CASE STUDIES

Real-World Examples of IoMT Security Breaches

Unluckily, the growth in the usage of IoMT has been marked by many hacking instances, which revealed the weak spots in these connected devices. Below are some notable examples that highlight the critical security issues within IoMT (Ray,2020) (Razdan,2022):

Below are some notable examples that highlight the critical security issues within IoMT:

1. Medtronic's Cardiac Devices Vulnerability happened in 2019.

In 2019 the U. S. Department of Homeland Security's Cybersecurity & Infrastructure Security Agency (CISA) warned that hackers could take control of implantable cardiac devices, such as pacemakers and defibrillators sold by Medtronic. It was established that these devices had insecure channels of communication that would enable an attacker to have unauthorized access to their systems. The weaknesses stated may enable an attacker to change the settings of the devices or even administer wrong electrical shocks to the patients which poses severe health risks.

This breach brought to light how use of insecure communication links in life critical devices is rather dangerous in that an attacker can sabotage the functioning of the device thus causing many patient deaths.

2. UVM Health Network Hit by Ransomware Attack in 2020

UVM Health Network with its headquarters in Vermont was attacked by ransomware in October of 2020; all of its networks including IoMT devices were included in this attack. This attack led to a great disruption of health care delivery because most of the devices and systems were disabled. This resulted in patients not receiving early treatments and cancellation of many other surgeries that were termed elective. All previously mentioned points are illustrated in Table 2 and can be summarized by stating that the attack took advantage of the weak areas of the network, proving that IoMT devices when connected to larger healthcare infrastructures can be and susceptible to ransomware.

The attack on the UVM Health Network highlighted how IoMT devices should be safeguarded in line with a broader cybersecurity approach as the devices are intrinsic to each other and therefore susceptible to massive attacks.

The UVM Health Network attack underscored the importance of securing IoMT devices as part of a larger cybersecurity strategy, as the interconnected nature of these devices makes them particularly vulnerable to systemic attacks.

3. Implantable Cardiac Devices St Jude Medical, (2017).

Earlier in 2017, the FDA sounded a warning that the St. Jude Medical's implantable cardiac devices such as pacemakers and defibrillators were at risk of a software vulnerability. It was in the wireless communication part of the devices to be able to drain the battery, or to program it wrong and give the patient wrong pacing or shock. This vulnerability was identified by Security researchers who showed that it was possible to regain control of the devices from a distance.

It also further underscored the risks of using unsecured wireless communication in implantable medical device and the consequences of such vulnerabilities in an individual's life.

4. Insulin Pump Hack (2011)

A notorious incident that makes the history of IoMT security attack was illustrated in 2011 when a security expert Jay Radcliffe was able to hack into his own insulin pump. Radclide proved that through the infiltration of various loop-holes realized in the wireless communication of the device, he could manipulate the insulin administering and in effect; even feed the patient with a dreaded wrong dose. That is why this was more of a conceptual study rather than a real-world attack; it clearly demonstrated the vulnerabilities of IoMT devices and emphasized the need to improve the security of such devices.

This was a wakeup call for the industry; this reveals how insecure medical devises could cost lives.

Analysis of Successful Mitigation Strategies

In an effort to mitigate security threats that come with the use of IoMT devices, both the healthcare sector, and manufacturers of the devices have come up with the following solutions. Below are some of the most effective strategies that have been employed to secure IoMT environments: Below are some of the most effective strategies that have been employed to secure IoMT environments:

1. Adoption of Hight Security Encryption Standards

Encryption can be regarded as one of the most crucial approaches to protection of IoMT devices; therefore, implementation of robust algorithms for the data exchange and storage must be established. Encryption assures that information leakage to third parties doesn't take place and even if it has been intercepted it cannot be understood. For Instance, addressing the threats established in Medtronic's cardiac devices, Medtronic altered the level of encryption in use in their communication. This reduce the high risks of access and modify physical settings of the target devices by unauthorized personnel.

There is a requirement for encryption on IoMT devices these days especially on those that communicate patient data or perform critical operations.

2. One of the most common practices is the consistent and correct Security Patching and Firmware Updates.

The best approach to managing recognized security risks inherent in IoMT devices is to update devices' security and firmware consistently. One of the main reasons why there are attacks is because devices are not updated on time hence vulnerable to the attackers. For instance, in the case of the vulnerabilities identified in St. Jude Medical's cardiac devices, the company came up with firmware that fixes the wireless communication problems. This update was a mass update which was sent across all the related devices thus minimizing the possibility of exploitation.

For patch management to be successful, it has to be a continuous process that involves both the healthcare organisations and the manufacturers in order to apply them without much interference with clinical activities.

3. Network Segmentation

Network segregation also entails partitioning of a network into subnets so as to slow the risk spread in case of an intrusion. This strategy was adopted well by the healthcare organizations after being attacked with ransomware incident such as that of the UVM Health Network. It is for this reason that IoMT devices and important medical networks should be separated from other networks, in order that an attack does not affect the whole system.

Network segmentation also makes it easier to monitor and control the security since it limits the scope of the attackers' movements within the network.

4. If left unchecked, identity management can create new implementation problems that can affect the broader security approach of an organization, including with regard to Zero Trust Architecture.

The Zero Trust security model is based on the concept of "never trust, always verify. " In a Zero Trust architecture, devices within or outside the network perimeter are considered as a threat. Such an approach is not new and has been used more frequently in the healthcare industry to protect IoMT devices. For example, what I have found is that devices are continuously authenticating and validating themselves, and the access is always granted on very rigid policies including the posture of the device and the role of the user.

Thanks to Zero Trust, the danger of IoMT devices being accessed by unauthorized third parties is minimized and only traffic coming from known, reputable sources is admitted.

5. Comprehensive Incident Response Plans

The best approach to managing the effect of the security breach is involving a well prepared incident response plan. Ideally, such plans should comprise of the measures to take in the event of an IoMT-related incident, this would include the measures to prevent further impact, communication and response plan, and the recovery plan. After the UVM Health Network was a victim of a ransomware attack, the organization's incident response plan was initiated that entailed disconnecting infected devices from the network, restoring data from backups, and informing stakeholders of the attack.

A particular emphasis should be made on the update and verification of the incident response plan as the threats that an organization may face only evolve with time.

6. Enhanced Device Security Standards

The regulatory boards and industrial associations have created superior security protocols for the IoMT devices. For instance, for medical devices, the FDA has provided Recommendations on security design for manufacturers to implement security features during the design phase of equipment. These guidelines encompass standards for deploying the context of strong authentication, encryption and need to receive security update after that product release. Adherence to these standards has now become an essential consideration towards IoMT devices development and deployment.

Internet of Medical Things (IoMT) devices is widely used in the healthcare industry, and their security should not be an issue to compromise. Over the last few years, the frequency with which IoMT devices has been under attack by cyber hackers has revealed the need for proper security. These breaches lead to unauthorized access to critical and private health information, disruption of the medical services as well as dangers to patients because of meddling with life sustenance medical appliances. In order to counter these threats, the manufacturers need to implement multiple layers of security with the help of multiple sophisticated approaches and make it as defensive approach to IoMT security.

A major element of securing the IoT of Medical Things is one's ability to implement proper encryption. Encryption makes it very difficult for the criminals to intercept or alter information being exchanged between devices and heath care networks. Just as important is the periodic updating of firmware of IoMT devices as it is a way of mitigating vulnerabilities which may be exploited by bad actors. It also implies that device firmware and software should be updated constantly to cover the security breaches that can be exploited for wrong intentions.

Another added layer that network segmentation brings is that of compartmentalising important IoMT systems from the rest of the other systems in the network, stemming limitation of the scope of movement that an attacker might achieve in the network. Another layer is given by Zero Trust architecture in which all traffic is assumed to be hostile and the identification and authorization of devices and users trying to access the network resources are continuously checked.

Detailed incident handling plans are important in order to allow an organisation to react properly and minimize the consequences of security violation in short order. They should be frequently exercised and revised to enable the healthcare organizations to be ready to effectively respond to any schemes to its security. In this way, manufacturers are also confident that newly introduced IoMT devices possess the protection required under evolving cybersecurity threats.

7. DEVELOPING A STRATEGIC FRAMEWORK

Best Practices for Healthcare Providers

From the above analysis, it is clear that, healthcare providers have a significant role in the security of IoMT devices in their networks. The following best practices can help mitigate risks and enhance the security of IoMT systems:

The following best practices can help mitigate risks and enhance the security of IoMT systems (Singh, 2021):

1. Conduct Regular Risk Assessments

It is recommended that healthcare providers conduct risk assessments on a frequent basis to determine the threats possible in the IoMT setting. These assessments should map the current status of the security of devices, network settings and procedures for handling data. It is only possible when one has an understanding of where the risks are and apply the necessary precautions wherever they may be.

2. Implement Strong Access Controls

Inclusion of IoMT devices and related systems ought to be secured. Using MFA, it reduces the chances of unauthorized users in controlling the settings of a device or even accessing sensitive information through RBAC. Healthcare providers should also ensure that logs providing access are well retained and checked for any case of suspicious access.

3. Segment IoMT Networks

Network segmentation becomes critical in that it prevents IoMT devices from being connected to the rest of the healthcare network. One of the best ways to protect organizational resources is to isolate the network infrastructure containing IoMT devices from other network portions to prevent threat distribution to various organizational segments. The same means that every segment can be protected with controls appropriate for the type of the devices and the data it processes.

4. Ensure Regular Software Updates

Healthcare providers should enforce measures through which each of the IoMT devices gets to update its software and security patch. This entails developing good relations with device manufacturers so that one gets information on the available updates as well as applying them with immediacy. Providers should also incorporation of automated systems for managing of updates in organizations with many devices.

5. Educate and Train Staff

It is agreed that training of staff is very vital when it comes to the security of IoMT. It is vital that healthcare organizations should stage reminders to their employees periodically on cyber security, on how to identify phishing scams and report them, the right procedure to follow in case of an attack as well as using devices appropriately.

6. Plan for and/or participate in the development & testing of incident response plans.

The medical professionals are required identifying the specific processes that have to be followed in the case of an IoMT device security breach. These plans should comprise steps to define the incident, its scope, impact, and the strategies of informing the stakeholders and getting back to functioning normally. These plans cannot be only on paper but should be realistic and should be tested on regular basis through simulations. Such drills alleviate the problem in a sense that all members of the team including those from the IT and the clinical sides understand their roles in the case of a breach. – This can be said to be useful in checking on any flaws that may be in the plan, before an actual event happens. This proactive approach enhances the capability of the organisation to respond appropriately hence reducing potential harm to the patients and integrity of the patient data and medical devices.

7. Enhance Physical Security

Physical security or protection of other property is one of the oldest but remains one of the critical forms of security which needs to be properly addressed in the context of protecting IoMT devices. These devices if placed in such areas of healthcare facilities such as public or semi-public are at the risk of being tampered with, stolen or even accessed by unauthorized people. These devices should therefore be protected and to do this, healthcare providers should ensure that there is adequate physical security. Some of these measures include; placing the IoMT devices in locked cabinets or enclosures, using secure ways to mount them to discourage their removal easily, and installing surveillance cameras around the areas where these devices are used. Guidelines for proper handling and disposal or else recycling of IoMT products upon their useful existence should be observed. This makes it possible to ensure that any data stored in the devices are safe by having them erased and also to make sure that the devices themselves are not a source of security risks.

Figure 4. Functional overview of proposed framework

Enhancing IoMT Security

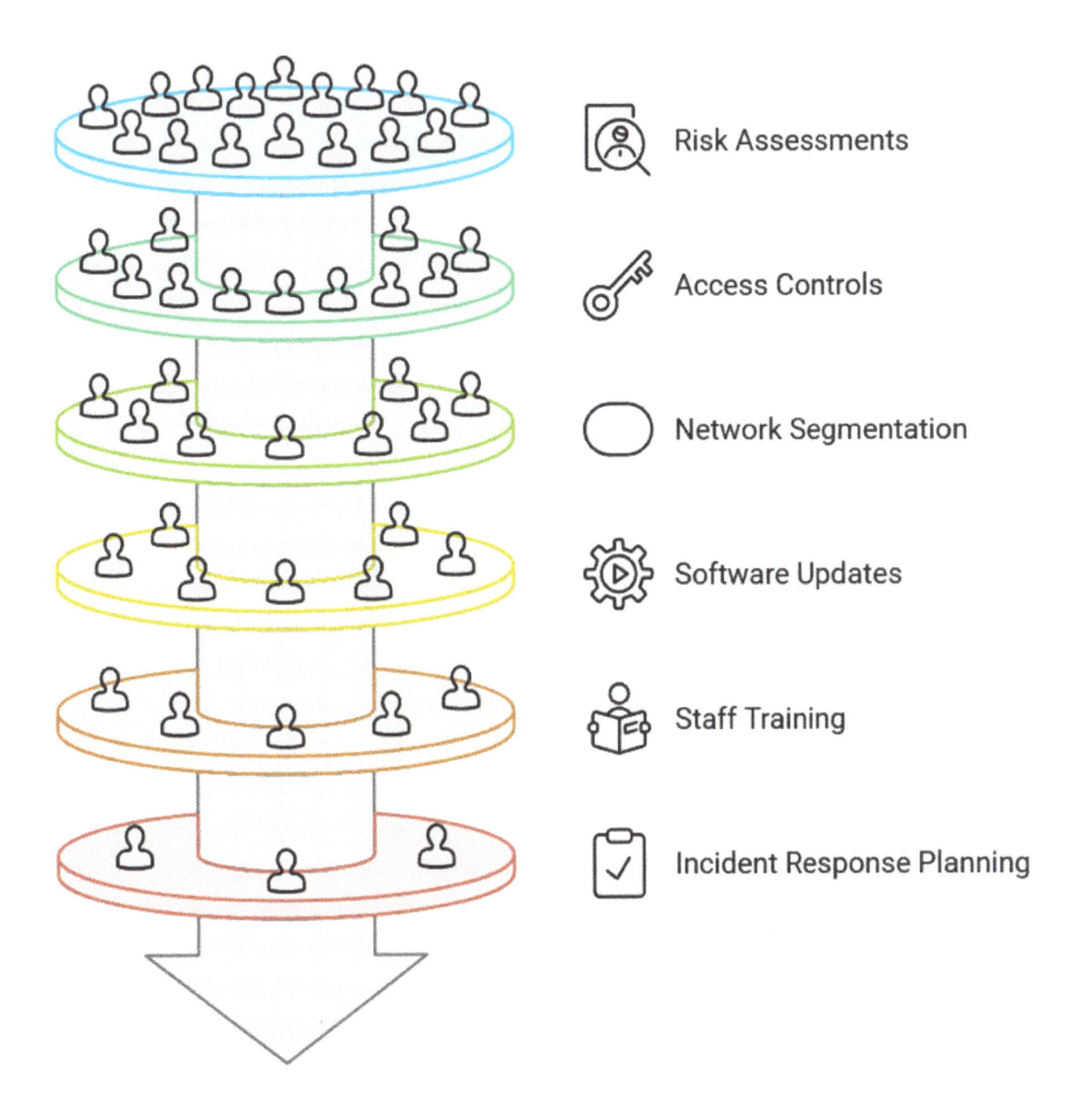

- Risk Assessments
- Access Controls
- Network Segmentation
- Software Updates
- Staff Training
- Incident Response Planning

In figure 4, the proposed framework is depicted with graphical elements as discussed in above section.

Guidelines for IoMT Device Manufacturers

Manufacturers of IoMT gadgets have a responsibility to construct security into their merchandise from the outset. The following guidelines can help make certain that IoMT gadgets are designed, evolved, and deployed with strong safety capabilities:

1. Adopt Security-through-Design Principles

Security need to be included into each level of the tool lifecycle, from layout and development to deployment and protection. Manufacturers need to behavior danger modeling and risk checks early inside the layout process to perceive potential security challenges and cope with them proactively.

2. Implement Strong Authentication and Encryption

IoMT gadgets must assist robust authentication mechanisms, inclusive of MFA, to prevent unauthorized access. Additionally, all information transmitted via IoMT gadgets must be encrypted the use of industry-widespread protocols. Manufacturers should keep away from using hardcoded credentials or different insecure practices that would be exploited through attackers.

3. Provide Regular Firmware Updates

Manufacturers must decide to supplying regular firmware updates for his or her devices to address emerging vulnerabilities. These updates have to be clean to install and have to not disrupt the everyday operation of the gadgets. Manufacturers ought to also set up clean verbal exchange channels to inform healthcare companies about available updates and any security dangers related to out-dated firmware.

4. Ensure Device Interoperability

IoMT gadgets frequently want to have interaction with different devices and systems inside a healthcare surroundings. Manufacturers need to make sure that their gadgets are like minded with industry standards and may be securely incorporated with different structures. This includes the usage of standardized communication protocols and presenting documentation that outlines steady integration practices.

5. Conduct Regular Security Testing

Before liberating IoMT gadgets to the market, manufacturers need to behavior thorough security trying out, which include penetration testing, vulnerability scanning, and code evaluations. On-going testing need to hold throughout the tool's lifecycle to perceive and address any new vulnerability that could arise.

6. Implement Secure Supply Chain Practices

Manufacturers should implement secure deliver chain practices to save you the introduction of vulnerabilities at some stage in the manufacturing and distribution of IoMT devices. This includes vetting providers, carrying out security audits, and ensuring that every component meets protection standards.

Manufacturers ought to additionally enforce tamper-evident packaging and other measures to defend gadgets in the course of transit.

7. Provide Transparent Data Handling Policies

Manufacturers should honestly communicate their facts dealing with rules, such as how data is accumulated, stored, and shared. This transparency facilitates build accept as true with healthcare vendors and patients and ensures compliance with records protection rules. Manufacturers have to also provide gear for healthcare providers to configure records privacy settings consistent with their wishes.

Policy Recommendations for Enhancing IoMT Security

The Internet of Medical Things (IoMT) has revolutionized healthcare, imparting significant benefits inclusive of progressed affected person monitoring, greater diagnostic capabilities, and more customized remedy plans. However, the speedy adoption of IoMT gadgets has also delivered new vulnerabilities and risks, in particular inside the realm of cybersecurity. The safety of IoMT gadgets is of paramount importance, as breaches can result in the unauthorized get entry to of touchy patient statistics, disruption of crucial clinical offerings, or even endangerment of patient lives. Given those excessive stakes, policymakers have a vital function in setting up guidelines, frameworks, and projects that beautify the safety of IoMT gadgets and protect patient records. The following coverage suggestions outline a comprehensive approach to addressing the security demanding situations associated with IoMT (Sripriyanka, 2021).

1. Establish Comprehensive IoMT Security Standards

To make sure the safety of IoMT gadgets, governments and regulatory bodies ought to set up complete safety requirements that embody all tiers of the tool lifecycle, from layout and development to deployment and preservation. These standards should cope with key elements which include encryption, authentication, statistics protection, and incident response. For instance, encryption protocols have to be mandated to secure records each at rest and in transit, making sure that affected person records is included from unauthorized get right of entry to. Similarly, sturdy authentication mechanisms ought to be required to save you unauthorized get admission to to IoMT devices and networks.

Moreover, those security standards must be made mandatory for all manufacturers, ensuring that each IoMT tool meets a baseline degree of security before it may be advertised or utilized in healthcare settings. To implement compliance, regular audits need to be performed by means of unbiased bodies to verify that producers are adhering to these standards. In the occasion of non-compliance, penalties should be imposed to deter negligence and incentivize adherence to safety first-rate practices. By establishing and imposing complete IoMT safety standards, policymakers can create a more secure environment for both patients and healthcare providers.

2. Mandate Security Certification for IoMT Devices

To similarly make sure that IoMT devices meet excessive-security standards, governments have to mandate safety certification for all IoMT devices prior to their commercialization or use in healthcare environments. Security certification ought to involve rigorous checking out by unbiased 0.33-celebration companies, which might examine the tool's capacity to resist various cyber threats (Subramaniam, 2023). This checking out need to cover number scenarios, such as vulnerability assessments, penetration checking out, and threat simulations, to make sure that the tool is resilient against capability assaults.

Security certification must be required not best for brand spanking new IoMT devices but additionally for great updates to present gadgets. This approach ensures that any adjustments or upgrades to a device do no longer inadvertently introduce new vulnerabilities. By requiring safety certification, policymakers can provide healthcare vendors and patients with extra guarantee that the IoMT gadgets they rely on are steady and straightforward.

3. Promote Public-Private Collaboration

The protection of IoMT devices is a complicated challenge that calls for the collective efforts of more than one stakeholders, including government businesses, healthcare companies, producers, and cybersecurity specialists (Vajar,2021). Policymakers need to consequently sell public-non-public collaboration to facilitate facts sharing, studies, and the development of fine practices in IoMT safety. Public-personal partnerships can be mainly powerful in identifying rising threats and developing innovative answers to cope with them.

For instance, authorities agencies may want to collaborate with non-public quarter agencies to set up chance intelligence sharing systems, wherein statistics about new vulnerabilities and assault vectors can be shared in real-time. These systems might permit healthcare vendors and manufacturers to reply extra fast to rising threats, decreasing the threat of extensive security breaches. Additionally, collaborative research initiatives will be launched to discover new protection technology, inclusive of superior encryption methods, steady communique protocols, and AI-based threat detection systems. By fostering a lifestyle of collaboration, policymakers can assist create a extra resilient IoMT surroundings.

4. Enforce Data Protection Regulations

Data protection is a critical thing of IoMT safety, as those gadgets frequently handle relatively touchy patient statistics. Policymakers ought to put into effect strict statistics protection regulations that govern how IoMT devices accumulate, store, and transmit patient statistics. Existing guidelines, which include the General Data Protection Regulation (GDPR) in Europe and the Health Insurance Portability and Accountability Act (HIPAA) in the United States, offer a framework for protective touchy facts and keeping companies liable for breaches.

However, those policies need to be updated to address the precise demanding situations posed by way of IoMT gadgets. For instance, IoMT gadgets regularly perform in actual-time and may transmit big volumes of records throughout more than one network, increasing the chance of statistics breaches. Policymakers have to therefore don't forget updating regulations to require more stringent encryption standards for IoMT devices, as well as protocols for steady information transmission and storage (Wei, 2022). Additionally, policies have to mandate that healthcare companies and manufacturers put into effect strong incident response plans to speedy pick out, contain, and mitigate the outcomes of a data breach.

Compliance with facts protection rules must be rigorously enforced, with penalties for non-compliance serving as a deterrent towards negligence. By imposing strict facts safety guidelines, policymakers can help make sure that patient information stays secure, even in the face of evolving cyber threats.

5. Support Research and Development in IoMT Security

Innovation is key to staying in advance of cyber threats, and governments have a critical function in helping studies and development (R&D) in IoMT protection. Policymakers should offer investment and resources to academic establishments, begin-ups, and industry leaders to spur the improvement of latest security technologies. These technologies may want to consist of advanced encryption strategies, stable communication protocols, AI-based threat detection systems, and blockchain-primarily based safety solutions.

By making an investment in R&D, governments can assist boost up the improvement of cutting-edge safety technology that may be included into IoMT gadgets. For example, AI-based danger detection systems may be used to screen IoMT networks for uncommon hobby, mechanically flagging potential protection incidents before they strengthen. Similarly, blockchain technology might be used to create immutable statistics of IoMT device transactions, improving information integrity and traceability.

In addition to investment, governments can also aid R&D by setting up innovation hubs or facilities of excellence targeted on IoMT protection. These hubs could carry collectively researchers, industry specialists, and policymakers to collaborate at the improvement of recent security solutions. By assisting R&D in IoMT security, policymakers can assist force the adoption of innovative technology that enhance the safety of healthcare systems.

6. Encourage Security Awareness and Education

Security awareness and education are important for ensuring that every one stakeholder within the IoMT environment recognize the importance of IoMT safety and are equipped with the information to protect devices and records. Policymakers must sell safety consciousness and schooling programs aimed toward healthcare vendors, producers, and the general public. For healthcare carriers, those packages should recognition on fine practices for securing IoMT devices and networks, in addition to the capacity results of safety breaches. Manufacturers should be knowledgeable at the ultra-modern security requirements and technology, as well as the importance of incorporating safety into the design and development system. Public cognizance campaigns have to also be released to inform sufferers about the significance of IoMT protection and how they could protect their non-public statistics.

7. Implement Incentives for Security Investment

Investing in IoMT safety may be high priced, and some healthcare providers and manufacturers may be hesitant to undertake new safety technologies or conduct normal audits due to financial constraints. To inspire investment in IoMT security, policymakers have to implement incentives such as tax breaks, grants, and subsidies.

These incentives can help offset the costs associated with adopting new security technologies, carrying out regular audits, and enforcing nice practices. For instance, tax breaks will be provided to healthcare providers that put money into latest encryption technologies or Zero Trust structure. Grants can be supplied to manufacturers that behavior impartial security checking out and certification for their IoMT gadgets (Yazid,2023).

By making protection funding greater financially feasible, policymakers can help power the sizeable adoption of strong security measures throughout the healthcare enterprise. This, in flip, will beautify the general safety of IoMT gadgets, shielding patient information and making sure the safety and reliability of medical devices.

The safety of IoMT devices is a multifaceted mission that requires coordinated efforts from healthcare companies, producers, and policymakers. By establishing comprehensive security requirements, mandating protection certification, selling public-private collaboration, implementing data protection guidelines, supporting R&D, encouraging protection cognizance, and imposing incentives for security funding, policymakers can play a pivotal role in enhancing the safety of IoMT systems.

As the healthcare enterprise keeps embracing IoMT technology, on-going vigilance and proactive safety features might be vital to safeguarding each patient privacy and healthcare results.

Case Study: Implementing Privacy-Enhanced IoMT for Remote Cardiac Monitoring Using Blockchain and AI

The rapid adoption of the Internet of Medical Things (IoMT) for remote patient monitoring has introduced privacy challenges, especially concerning sensitive health data. One area where IoMT is highly effective is in remote cardiac monitoring for patients with cardiovascular conditions. Continuous, real-time monitoring offers patients improved quality of life and healthcare providers valuable insights into patient health. However, handling this sensitive data requires advanced privacy protection mechanisms. This case study outlines how a healthcare provider used blockchain and AI to enhance privacy in a remote cardiac monitoring system, addressing both theoretical principles and practical implementation.

A mid-sized healthcare provider wanted to expand its cardiac monitoring services by implementing an IoMT-based solution. The solution would involve wearable electrocardiogram (ECG) devices that continuously collect data on patients' heart rates, arrhythmias, and other critical indicators. This data would be sent to a centralized server where healthcare professionals could access it to make informed decisions. The main challenges included:

1. Data Privacy: Given the sensitivity of cardiac health data, the organization needed to protect patient information from unauthorized access and ensure regulatory compliance (e.g., HIPAA and GDPR).
2. Data Integrity: The provider needed a system that would guarantee the authenticity and integrity of data so that clinical decisions could be based on reliable information.
3. Access Control: There was a need for dynamic access control to ensure that only authorized individuals could view specific data at specific times, such as during a medical emergency.

To address these issues, the healthcare provider implemented a privacy-enhanced solution using a hybrid approach that combined blockchain and AI technologies.

Blockchain Implementation for Data Integrity and Privacy

The healthcare provider adopted a private blockchain network where patient data from the wearable ECG devices was stored as encrypted blocks, accessible only by authorized participants. This private blockchain maintained strict access rules, with healthcare providers and patients as the primary authorized users.

1. Data Sharing and Consent Management: With blockchain, each patient had control over their data-sharing permissions through smart contracts. Patients could grant specific access rights to healthcare providers for predefined periods. For instance, a patient could allow their primary cardiologist access to data for a routine check-up while denying access to other departments. This consent management system enhanced privacy, allowing patients to be in control of their information.
2. Auditability and Traceability: Every transaction on the blockchain was timestamped and cryptographically secured, creating a transparent log of who accessed the data and when. This immutable audit trail ensured data integrity, enabling the provider to trace any unauthorized access attempt back to its source. This feature also helped with regulatory compliance, as it provided documentation for audits and adherence to data privacy regulations.
3. Decentralized Data Storage: By decentralizing data, the blockchain minimized the risk of a single point of failure, reducing the likelihood of large-scale data breaches. Although sensitive information was stored off-chain to conserve space, pointers to the encrypted data were stored on-chain, ensuring that all data references remained tamper-proof.

AI Implementation for Adaptive Privacy and Threat Detection

The provider integrated AI-driven access control and real-time anomaly detection into their IoMT system, allowing for proactive privacy management.

1. Dynamic Access Control: The AI system evaluated the context around access requests using factors such as location, time of access, and device trust level. If a request came from an unusual location or during abnormal hours, AI-based algorithms would temporarily block access until further verification. For example, if a healthcare provider attempted to access patient data from an unfamiliar device or outside of business hours, the AI would prompt additional authentication measures or even alert the patient.
2. Real-Time Anomaly Detection: AI-powered anomaly detection algorithms continuously monitored incoming data to detect unusual access patterns or cyber threats. By training models on historical usage data, the system could recognize patterns that indicated potential security threats, such as rapid access requests from multiple unauthorized devices. In one instance, the AI system flagged a potential breach when multiple access attempts were detected from an external location, immediately alerting security personnel to investigate and contain the threat.
3. Federated Learning for Privacy-Preserving Model Training: To further ensure privacy, the healthcare provider implemented federated learning to train AI models directly on decentralized IoMT devices rather than transferring raw patient data to a central server. This enabled each device to locally process and contribute to the AI model, ensuring patient data remained private while allowing the model to learn and improve.

Outcomes and Benefits

This hybrid implementation of blockchain and AI transformed the cardiac monitoring solution into a privacy-focused, secure IoMT ecosystem. The following outcomes were observed:

- Improved Patient Trust: Patients felt more comfortable using the monitoring devices due to the transparent data-sharing permissions and immutable data trails, knowing they could control who accessed their information.
- Enhanced Data Security: The combined use of blockchain's immutability and AI's real-time threat detection minimized the risk of unauthorized access, thereby protecting patients' sensitive health data.

This case study highlights how blockchain and AI can bridge theoretical privacy principles with practical implementation in IoMT. By leveraging blockchain's decentralization and transparency with AI's adaptive security and privacy-preserving learning, healthcare providers can establish an IoMT ecosystem that prioritizes data privacy and patient trust. This approach offers a blueprint for other healthcare organizations to implement similar privacy-enhanced solutions in IoMT environments.

8. CONCLUSION

The safety of Internet of Medical Things (IoMT) devices is a key concern that needs a full approach involving healthcare providers, device makers, and policymakers. As these devices become more part of healthcare systems, the possible risks linked to their use, like data leaks unwanted access, and device messing, have gone up. Dealing with these risks is essential to protect patient safety and to keep healthcare services intact and sensitive health data safe. Healthcare providers are at the forefront of IoMT safety. They can cut down the chance of safety breaches by using good practices like regular risk checks strong access limits, network splitting, and on-going staff training. Also, making sure IoMT devices are updated often and kept safe can help lessen weak spots and stop unwanted access. Creating and testing strong plans to respond to incidents further gets healthcare providers ready to act fast and well if a safety issue happens cutting down possible harm and keeping care going. IoMT device makers also have a big job in making sure their products are safe. By using safety-from-the-start ideas, makers can build devices that can stand up to threats from the beginning.

REFERENCES

Ahmed, S. F., Alam, M. S. B., Afrin, S., Rafa, S. J., Rafa, N., & Gandomi, A. H. (2024). Insights into Internet of Medical Things (IoMT): Data fusion, security issues and potential solutions. *Information Fusion*, 102, 102060. DOI: 10.1016/j.inffus.2023.102060

Alhaj, T. A., Abdulla, S. M., Iderss, M. A. E., Ali, A. A. A., Elhaj, F. A., Remli, M. A., & Gabralla, L. A. (2022). A survey: To govern, protect, and detect security principles on internet of medical things (IoMT). *IEEE Access : Practical Innovations, Open Solutions*, 10, 124777–124791. DOI: 10.1109/ACCESS.2022.3225038

Ali, M., Naeem, F., Tariq, M., & Kaddoum, G. (2022). Federated learning for privacy preservation in smart healthcare systems: A comprehensive survey. *IEEE Journal of Biomedical and Health Informatics*, 27(2), 778–789. DOI: 10.1109/JBHI.2022.3181823 PMID: 35696470

Almalki, J., Al Shehri, W., Mehmood, R., Alsaif, K., Alshahrani, S. M., Jannah, N., & Khan, N. A. (2022). Enabling blockchain with IoMT devices for healthcare. *Information (Basel)*, 13(10), 448. DOI: 10.3390/info13100448

Alzoubi, A. A., AlSuwaidi, A., & Alzoubi, H. M. (2024). Analyzing the Approaches for Discovering Privacy and Security Breaches in IoMT. In *Technology Innovation for Business Intelligence and Analytics (TIBIA) Techniques and Practices for Business Intelligence Innovation* (pp. 345–355). Springer Nature Switzerland. DOI: 10.1007/978-3-031-55221-2_23

Bharati, S., Podder, P., Mondal, M. R. H., & Paul, P. K. (2021). Applications and challenges of cloud integrated IoMT. Cognitive Internet of Medical Things for Smart Healthcare: Services and Applications, 67-85.

Bhushan, B., Kumar, A., Agarwal, A. K., Kumar, A., Bhattacharya, P., & Kumar, A. (2023). Towards a secure and sustainable Internet of Medical Things (IoMT): Requirements, design challenges, security techniques, and future trends. *Sustainability (Basel)*, 15(7), 6177. DOI: 10.3390/su15076177

Cano, M. D., & Cañavate-Sanchez, A. (2020). Preserving data privacy in the internet of medical things using dual signature ECDSA. *Security and Communication Networks*, 2020(1), 4960964. DOI: 10.1155/2020/4960964

Elhoseny, M., Thilakarathne, N. N., Alghamdi, M. I., Mahendran, R. K., Gardezi, A. A., Weerasinghe, H., & Welhenge, A. (2021). Security and privacy issues in medical internet of things: Overview, countermeasures, challenges and future directions. *Sustainability (Basel)*, 13(21), 11645. DOI: 10.3390/su132111645

Gaytan, J. C. T. (2022). A literature survey of security and privacy issues in internet of medical things. International Journal of Computations, Information and Manufacturing (IJCIM), 2(2).

Hameed, S. S., Hassan, W. H., Latiff, L. A., & Ghabban, F. (2021). A systematic review of security and privacy issues in the internet of medical things; the role of machine learning approaches. *PeerJ. Computer Science*, 7, e414. DOI: 10.7717/peerj-cs.414 PMID: 33834100

Haque, R. U., & Hasan, A. T. (2021). Privacy-preserving multivariant regression analysis over blockchain-based encrypted IoMT data. In *Artificial Intelligence and Blockchain for Future Cybersecurity Applications* (pp. 45–59). Springer International Publishing. DOI: 10.1007/978-3-030-74575-2_3

Hireche, R., Mansouri, H., & Pathan, A. S. K. (2022). Security and privacy management in Internet of Medical Things (IoMT): A synthesis. *Journal of Cybersecurity and Privacy*, 2(3), 640–661. DOI: 10.3390/jcp2030033

Jeyavel, J., Parameswaran, T., Mannan, J. M., & Hariharan, U. (2021). Security vulnerabilities and intelligent solutions for IoMT systems. Internet of Medical Things: Remote Healthcare Systems and Applications, 175-194.

Kumar, M., Verma, S., Kumar, A., Ijaz, M. F., & Rawat, D. B. (2022). ANAF-IoMT: A novel architectural framework for IoMT-enabled smart healthcare system by enhancing security based on RECC-VC. *IEEE Transactions on Industrial Informatics*, 18(12), 8936–8943. DOI: 10.1109/TII.2022.3181614

Kumar, R., & Tripathi, R. (2021). Towards design and implementation of security and privacy framework for Internet of Medical Things (IoMT) by leveraging blockchain and IPFS technology. *The Journal of Supercomputing*, 77(8), 7916–7955. DOI: 10.1007/s11227-020-03570-x

Lakhan, A., Mohammed, M. A., Nedoma, J., Martinek, R., Tiwari, P., Vidyarthi, A., Alkhayyat, A., & Wang, W. (2022). Federated-learning based privacy preservation and fraud-enabled blockchain IoMT system for healthcare. *IEEE Journal of Biomedical and Health Informatics*, 27(2), 664–672. DOI: 10.1109/JBHI.2022.3165945 PMID: 35394919

Nair, A. K., Sahoo, J., & Raj, E. D. (2023). Privacy-preserving Federated Learning framework for IoMT based big data analysis using edge computing. *Computer Standards & Interfaces*, 86, 103720. DOI: 10.1016/j.csi.2023.103720

Nie, X., Zhang, A., Chen, J., Qu, Y., & Yu, S. (2022). Blockchain-empowered secure and privacy-preserving health data sharing in edge-based IoMT. *Security and Communication Networks*, 2022(1), 8293716. DOI: 10.1155/2022/8293716

Rahmadika, S., Astillo, P. V., Choudhary, G., Duguma, D. G., Sharma, V., & You, I. (2022). Blockchain-based privacy preservation scheme for misbehavior detection in lightweight IoMT devices. *IEEE Journal of Biomedical and Health Informatics*, 27(2), 710–721. DOI: 10.1109/JBHI.2022.3187037 PMID: 35763469

Ray, P. P., Dash, D., & Kumar, N. (2020). Sensors for internet of medical things: State-of-the-art, security and privacy issues, challenges and future directions. *Computer Communications*, 160, 111–131. DOI: 10.1016/j.comcom.2020.05.029

Razdan, S., & Sharma, S. (2022). Internet of medical things (IoMT): Overview, emerging technologies, and case studies. *IETE Technical Review*, 39(4), 775–788. DOI: 10.1080/02564602.2021.1927863

Singh, M., Sukhija, N., Sharma, A., Gupta, M., & Aggarwal, P. K. (2021). Security and privacy requirements for IoMT-based smart healthcare system: Challenges, solutions, and future scope. In *Big Data Analysis for Green Computing* (pp. 17–37). CRC Press.

Sripriyanka, G., & Mahendran, A. (2021). A study on security privacy issues and solutions in internet of medical things—A review. Intelligent IoT Systems in Personalized Health Care, 147-175.

Subramaniam, E. V. D., Srinivasan, K., Qaisar, S. M., & Pławiak, P. (2023). Interoperable IoMT approach for remote diagnosis with privacy-preservation perspective in edge systems. *Sensors (Basel)*, 23(17), 7474. DOI: 10.3390/s23177474 PMID: 37687933

Vajar, P., Emmanuel, A. L., Ghasemieh, A., Bahrami, P., & Kashef, R. (2021, October). The Internet of Medical Things (IoMT): a vision on learning, privacy, and computing. In *2021 International Conference on Electrical, Computer, Communications and Mechatronics Engineering (ICECCME)* (pp. 1-7). IEEE. DOI: 10.1109/ICECCME52200.2021.9590881

Wei, T., Liu, S., & Du, X. (2022). Learning-based efficient sparse sensing and recovery for privacy-aware IoMT. *IEEE Internet of Things Journal*, 9(12), 9948–9959. DOI: 10.1109/JIOT.2022.3163593

Yazid, A. (2023). Cybersecurity and privacy issues in the internet of medical things (IoMT). *Eigenpub Review of Science and Technology*, 7(1), 1–21.

Chapter 7
Deep Insights and Analysis of Machine Learning Algorithms for Chronic Kidney Disease Prediction

N. Krishnamoorthy
Vellore Institute of Technology, India

V. Vinoth Kumar
Vellore Institute of Technology, India

Sonali Mishra
Vellore Institute of Technology, India

ABSTRACT

The chronic kidney disease (CKD) is the most prominent causes of death and suffering in the 21st century. Lot of research initiatives are taken in recent years to find the CKD in early stage. Research on renal disease prediction is crucial since it attempts to create reliable and accurate techniques for determining who is most likely to get kidney disease. Early detection of kidney disease can help prevent or delay the progression of the disease and improve patient outcomes. Chronic kidney disease (CKD) affects 8% to 16% of the global population, although both patients and medical professionals usually ignore it. A machine learning algorithms are used in this instance to predict whether or not the subject will experience chronic kidney disease. The training dataset, which is being used contains numerous variables, including specific gravity, sugar, albumin, bacteria, red blood cells, pus cells, and many others, affect chronic kidney disease.

I. INTRODUCTION

The need to diagnose and treat kidney illness as soon as possible has become critical in the ever-changing world of modern healthcare, where the goal of better patient outcomes and efficient healthcare delivery is given top priority. This urgency has caused a noticeable increase in interest in using state-of-

DOI: 10.4018/979-8-3693-6180-1.ch007

Copyright ©2025, IGI Global. Copying or distributing in print or electronic forms without written permission of IGI Global is prohibited.

the-art data-driven technologies, particularly machine learning, to better understand the intricate details of kidney disease.

We have a plethora of machine learning techniques at our disposal, from the powerful XGBoost and Weighted KNN to the reliable SVM and the age-old Decision Tree. The possibilities are endless when it comes to piecing together the complex web of variables affecting the progression of this sneaky illness. Equipped with their immense power, these algorithms bring in a new age for the identification of risk factors, customization of treatments, and prediction of the course of renal illness. By skillfully navigating clinical data repositories and the enormous databases of electronic health records (EHRs), these algorithms are ready to mold customized predictive models and customized decision support tools, providing physicians with a multitude of invaluable insights to help patients proactively navigate the complex maze-like pathways associated with long-term renal disease (CKD).

In the field of CKD prediction, the highly regarded XGBoost algorithm is unmatched, as demonstrated often by its exceptional robustness and steadfast accuracy when negotiating the complex paths of complex datasets, leading to careful risk assessment and prognostication. The enduring SVM algorithm provides a strong basis for patient stratification into distinct risk categories based on their individual clinical profiles in a symbiotic synergy, while weighted KNN skillfully utilizes the power of weighted distances to achieve previously unheard-of levels of prediction accuracy. Furthermore, the prudent utilization of decision tree algorithms bestows upon physicians not only an immense amount of interpretability but also highlights the mysterious mechanisms driving the unstoppable advancement of chronic kidney disease.

Through skillfully combining the rich tapestry of these many machine learning approaches, medical professionals are on the verge of a paradigm change in which the mysterious features of chronic kidney disease become clear, and the threat of unfavorable consequences is defeated. The prudent distribution of limited healthcare resources in this brave new world is only a byproduct of our steadfast dedication to the sanctity of human life and our unrelenting pursuit of excellence in healthcare delivery.

Tools and Libraries

The dataset was downloaded from Kaggle, and the data mining techniques were implemented to the dataset with the help of Python programming and Jupiter Notebook. Various libraries like Pandas, NumPy, Matplotlib, Seaborn, Plotly were used for data visualization.

Proposed Dataset

The dataset contains various clinical and demographic features for the detection of long-term renal disease (CKD). The classification feature serves as the target variable, where "ckd" represents the presence of chronic kidney disease, and "notckd" indicates the absence of the disease. The goal is to create a model via machine learning that, using the features supplied, can reliably predict the categorization of chronic renal disease. Description of the proposed dataset is shown in the Figure 1.

Literature Survey

Almansour et al., (2019), an early detection of Chronic Renal Disease (CKD) and its prevention are achieved through the application of machine learning algorithms. Simulated Neural Networks (SNN) and Support Vector Machines (SVM) are two popular machine learning strategies. Both SNN and SVM offer benefits and have demonstrated exceptional performance in several fields, including image processing, monetary analysis, diagnosis in medicine, and forecasting the climate. The ability of a simulated neural network (SNN) to generalize and generate a workable solution from unseen input and its ability to learn how to carry out its functions when it has been appropriately trained are its two primary features. On the other hand, SVM is a computer method that has the ability to label objects in accordance with examples and past experiences. Using SVM, binary labelled data is primarily divided along a line that optimizes the distance between the labels. SVM functions well with respectable accuracy even when there aren't many examples. SVM's beneficial properties set it apart from other machine learning methods. Using a dataset of 400 patients and 24 CKD diagnostic criteria, the machine learning classification techniques Support Vector Machine (SVM) and Stimulated Neural Network (SNN) are applied. All missing values in the dataset were substituted with the mean of the associated attributes in order to run the tests. Subsequently, the ideal parameters for the Stimulated Neural Network (SNN) and Support Vector Machine (SVM) approaches were discovered through a series of trials and parameter adjustments. The best-obtained traits and parameters were used to generate the final models for the two outlined techniques. According to the trial results, SNN performed stronger than SVM, with accuracy rates of 91.75% and 89.25%, respectively.

Figure 1. Dataset description

```
id                         int64
age                        float64
blood pressure             float64
specific gravity           float64
albumin                    float64
sugar                      float64
red blood cells             object
 pus cell                   object
pus cell clumps             object
bacteria                    object
blood glucose random       float64
blood urea                 float64
serum creatinine           float64
sodium                     float64
potassium                  float64
haemoglobin                float64
packed cell volume         float64
white blood cell count     float64
red blood cell count       float64
ypertension                 object
diabetes mellitus           object
coronary artery disease     object
appetite                    object
pedal edema                 object
anemia                      object
class                       object
dtype: object
```

Baby, P. S., & Vital, T. P. (2015). The investigation in this research report examined renal illnesses utilizing a variety of characteristics and factors. Among these traits include age, sex, height, weight, consumption of tea and coffee, food intake, use of alcohol, and smoking habits. These variables were thought to be important for comprehending and forecasting renal disease occurrences. Datasets from several hospitals that included information on these characteristics were gathered by the researchers. Utilizing software like Weka and Orange, Insightful information was extracted from the data through effective analysis using data mining techniques. Finding patterns, trends, and relationships within the dataset is the process of data mining. In this study, a number of machine learning techniques were used to forecast and categorize kidney illnesses based on the features. J48, Random Forest, AD Trees, Random Forest, and Naive Bayes were some of the algorithms used to assess performance. To evaluate each algorithm's performance and evaluate its capacity to reliably forecast renal illnesses, the dataset was applied to each algorithm.

Dhivya, S., & Prabha, D. (2022). The goal of the research was to offer a statistical analysis of renal disease predictions using these machine learning techniques. This involved evaluating each algorithm's precision, sensitivity, specificity, and other performance indicators. The end objective was to determine which algorithm, using the provided attributes, could forecast kidney illnesses the best. In conclusion, the research used machine learning algorithms and data mining approaches to assess and forecast kidney disorders utilizing key characteristics including age, gender, lifestyle behaviors, and more. Algorithms including K Star, AD Trees, J48, Naive Bayes, and Random Forest were used to assess performance. To evaluate each algorithm's performance and evaluate its capacity to reliably forecast renal illnesses, the dataset was applied to each algorithm.

Dulhare, U. N., & Ayesha, M. (2016) objective was to use these computational methods to provide a statistical analysis of renal illness forecasts. This involved evaluating each algorithm's precision, sensitivity, specificity, and other performance indicators. The end objective was to determine which algorithm, using the provided attributes, could forecast kidney illnesses the best. In conclusion, the research used machine learning algorithms and data mining approaches to assess and forecast kidney disorders utilizing key characteristics including age, gender, lifestyle behaviors, and more. The objective was to generate insightful statistical analysis and information to improve kidney disease comprehension and identification for better healthcare outcomes.

Elhoseny et al. (2019) shows an intelligent prediction and classification system for healthcare, primarily aimed at chronic renal disease (CRD), and is presented by the authors in this work. The system is also known as the D-ACO algorithm and goes by the term DFS with ACO (Ant Colony Optimization). To improve the precision and effectiveness of the classification process, this method was created for the classification of CKD datasets. Due to the way it incorporates several features, the D- ACO algorithm is exceptional. To find and save the most pertinent characteristics, it uses feature selection (FS). Additionally, it uses ACO-based learning, enhancing the categorization process by drawing on ideas from ant colony behavior. The program also removes superfluous features, simplifying the dataset for improved performance. The DACO method was assessed using a benchmark CKD dataset. Its efficacy and efficiency were assessed by comparison with alternative methods. The outcomes showed that the D-ACO algorithm performed better than these current approaches, displaying higher classification performance across many evaluation features. Overall, the study shows how the suggested DACO algorithm may be used as a reliable classifier for identifying chronic kidney disease. It is a potential method to improve the precision and effectiveness of healthcare classification systems, particularly for the identification of CKD, because it integrates feature selection, ACO- based learning, and the removal of irrelevant information.

Ghafar, M. H. B. A., et al. (2022) predicted the prevalence of chronic renal illness using a support vector machines and data mining techniques. This study's three main goals are to first describe the original CKD dataset, then create a variety of imputation techniques to fill in any missing data, and last create synthetic samples. The SVM technique is then used to assess prediction accuracy for both datasets. In general, those goals have been met. The original dataset's attribute distribution could be characterized by the study. Multiple imputation approaches were used to fill in the missing data points. In order to expand the dataset to N=2000, this study additionally creates a synthetic sample. In this experiment, the approach that yielded the highest overall accuracy—93.5% with source data and 94.0% with five times the original data— was SVM with 50% holdout validation. It illustrates that the use of a larger dataset results in a 0.5% increase in accuracy. It can be stated that while employing SVM based on the UCI repository to predict CKD, the prediction accuracy increases with the amount of dataset employed, despite the fact only slight changes in accuracy are achieved. To enhance the prediction model's efficacy, this research suggests obtaining sophisticated diagnostic systems that utilise additional classifiers to combine attributes into diverse clinical assessments. The group is currently developing an algorithm and model that will enable more accurate phase prediction for CKD.

Research by Gunarathne, W. H. S. D et al. (2017) demonstrates the efficacy and efficiency of a targeted strategy, which requires fewer attributes to achieve exceptional predictive accuracy. However, the report acknowledged multiple deficiencies. The dataset's size and the presence of missing attribute values restrict the overall strength of the data. However, the research highlights the efficacy of the algorithms by exhibiting appropriate values in evaluations.

The author's study to help identify chronic renal disease using machine learning. Initially, the author used preprocessing techniques to prepare the dataset for additional analysis, which increased the analysis's efficacy. Gupta et al., (2020) these techniques most likely entail prepping the data for machine learning algorithms by cleaning and organizing it. The most perceptive and significant features were then found by applying a feature selection technique to the prepared dataset. Feature significance was likely used to identify the features that are critical for identifying chronic renal illness, correlation matrices, and univariate selection. The study's findings indicated decision trees' capacity to precisely identify positive cases of chronic renal illness, with their highest degree of precision. Contrarily, the findings from employing logistic regression were the most accurate and dependable, indicating that this method may accurately predict both good and bad cases of chronic disease, including renal illness. In conclusion, the study identified key traits for identifying chronic kidney illness using feature extraction and employing selection methods on a dataset from the UCI collection. Analysis of several machineries in terms of precision, decision trees beat learning algorithms, although logistic regression scored very well in terms of accuracy and recall.

Natarajan, K., et al., (2024) used firefly feature selection with ensemble classification in the heart disease prediction. Johari et al., (2019) This study emphasizes how crucial it is for healthcare organizations—such as insurance providers and hospitals— to predict patients' danger of developing chronic renal illness (CKD) in order to provide prompt medical care. In order to accomplish this, CKD is predicted by a comparison experiment that uses categorization approaches. The classification model is built using two supervised classification algorithms: Neural networks and decision forests with two classes. The comparison of both algorithms shows that, although Neural Networks perform well overall, the Decision Forest approach performs better in terms of obtaining optimal performance with a high degree of accuracy and precision. The paper also contrasts these outcomes with those of other well-known algorithms from the literature, including Rule Induction, K-nearest-neighbor model, and Support

Vector Machine. The comparative assessment confirms Decision Forest's superiority and emphasizes how well it predicts chronic kidney disease, which is crucial for improving patient care and developing healthcare plans that successfully address this global health issue.

Ranjith, C. P., et al., (2023) applied k-means clustering is employed for segmentation and after that feature-based technique to extract from the segmented images. Using meta classifiers to predict the risk factor for kidney disease, as published NavyaSree et al. (2022): The purpose of this research is to address the problem of chronic renal illness (CKD) early diagnosis. CKD frequently goes undiagnosed until it progresses to a deadly stage. With a 93% accuracy rate, they use Random Forest and K-Nearest Neighbors (KNN) as base classifiers and Extra Tree classifiers as a meta classifier, utilizing sophisticated machine learning algorithms. This multi-step method efficiently integrates the outputs from the basis classifiers through the Meta classifier to improve forecast accuracy. This approach offers a vital tool for prompt intervention and treatment by reliably estimating the risk level for CKD patients. When compared to standalone algorithms, the integration of Meta classifiers yields a more accurate and detailed prediction, increasing the predictive model's total accuracy.

Prediction of Ultrasound Kidney Imaging Using Convolution Neural Networks published by Patil, S., & Choudhary, S (2023): This study uses Convolutional Neural Networks (CNN), deep learning to identify ailments like Prolonged Kidney Illness. CKD is a pressing global public health issue, emphasizing the need for early detection to prevent kidney function deterioration and costly treatments like dialysis or transplants. The proposed automatic CNN model accurately predicts CKD, boasting an impressive 95% precision in identifying affected individuals. Moreover, the model achieves an 80% accuracy in classifying CKD based on ultrasound images, highlighting its potential in aiding accurate diagnoses. This result emphasizes how crucial CNNs are for the timely identification and accurate categorization of kidney disorders, which could lead to better patient outcomes and lower costs associated with healthcare. Optimizing prediction accuracy would eventually improve healthcare plans and interventions for patients suffering from renal illnesses, which is the main goal of the study.

Harish, K. P., et al., (2023) Decision tree, KNN, Random Forest, AdaBoost, Logistic regression, Gradient boosting, cat boosting, XGBoosting, Linear SVM, Radial SVM, Linear discriminant analysis and Quadratic discriminant analysis are used to detect Polycystic Ovary Syndrome. This study by Silveira, A. C. D et al. (2022) presents early prediction of chronic renal disease using machine learning algorithms for small and imbalanced datasets. Chronic kidney disease (CKD) is a global public health concern that is usually discovered at an advanced stage. To lessen this issue, early predictive investment is necessary. It is discovered that the goal of this research is to help with the early prediction of chronic kidney disease (CKD) by addressing problems related to small-size and imbalanced datasets. The following parameters were discovered in Brazilians' medical files, regardless of whether they were diagnosed with chronic kidney disease (CKD): age, gender, glomerular filtration rate, albuminuria, creatinine, urea, and hypertension. They present an oversampling strategy that makes use of both automatic and manual augmentation. We tested borderline- SMOTE, borderline-SMOTE, and synthetic minority oversampling approach (SMOTE) support vector machines (SVM). They implement decision tree (DT) algorithms, multi-class AdaBoosted DTs, and random forest models. Additionally, they used the META-DES, k-nearest oracles- union, and k-nearest oracles-eliminate strategies to select dynamic ensemble determination and the overall local accuracy and local class accuracy methods for dynamic classifier selection. They adopted multiple stratified cross- validation (CV), nested CV, and hold-out validation to check out the model performances. With an accuracy score of 88.99%, the DT model—which combined SMOTE and manual augmentation—had the highest rating. Their approach can be useful in the development of CKD early prediction systems for datasets that are unbalanced and of restricted size. This article's methodology can assist in developing DSS to detect CKD in Brazilian populations.

This study by Tekale, S et al. (2018) analyzed the efficacy of several machine learning strategies, such as Decision Tree and Support Vector Machine and looked at 14 unique traits linked to people with chronic kidney disease (CKD). These days, people make an effort to be health-conscious, but due to their busy schedules and demanding jobs, they often neglect their health until symptoms start to show. On the other hand, signs of chronic kidney disease (CKD) are uncommon or nonexistent. This makes it challenging to foresee, identify, and prevent; if this is done incorrectly, permanent health damage could ensue. But because machine learning is so good at analysis and prediction, it gives us hope in this case. They have looked at a number of machine learning algorithms in their work. Based on the findings analysis, SVM yields 86.75% accuracy, whereas decision tree methods yield 81.75% accuracy. When examining the decision tree algorithm, the tree is constructed using all of the dataset's features and is based on the complete dataset. Making predictions using this approach takes less time, which is one of its advantages. Being able to diagnose more patients in less time and begin treating CKD patients earlier will benefit doctors. The amount of the data collection and the missing attribute values, which limit the data's strength, are two of the study's weaknesses.

Natarajan, K., et al. (2024) adopted a new method for classification of multiple diseases using transfer learning with improved performance. Zhang, H., et al. (2018) The main goal of this research is to forecast patients' chances of survival with Chronic Kidney Disease (CKD) by using Stimulated Neural Network (ANN) models. Patients with chronic renal disease (CKD) eventually lose kidney function and must have transplants or hemodialysis to survive. As the disease progresses, it can cause consequences that affect daily life, like acidity, anemia, and diabetes. For late-stage patients, the median survival time is almost three years. Making the right judgements about care requires accurate assessment of the patient's state, which can be challenging given the many variables that affect the results. With the help of recent developments in AI, especially deep learning, the project seeks to create prediction models for CKD survivability. Deep learning has potential for use in medical applications because it is data-driven and can automatically extract complex information. Preprocessing, transformations, and the use of ANNs are all part of the research to map clinical parameters to patient survival. The process's computational outcomes are presented. By creating precise prediction models, enabling tailored treatment choices, and maybe enhancing CKD patient outcomes, the ultimate goal is to improve patient care.

II. PROPOSED WORK

In order to forecast chronic kidney illness, machine learning algorithms are essential for analyzing a variety of characteristics, such as pus cells, germs, specific gravity, albumin, sugar levels, and the number of red blood cells. The first step in the procedure is called data pre-processing, and it entails renaming columns, handling missing values, and analyzing the data using visualization to understand distributions, skewness, outliers, and data balance.

To ascertain which characteristics are most relevant, feature selection is carried out following the label encoding of categorical variables. This procedure makes use of techniques like chi-square testing and SelectKBest. Usually, only the best-performing elements are retained for modelling reasons. Predictive models are then created using a variety of machine learning algorithms, such as support vector machines, decision trees, logistic regression, and random forests. To determine which algorithm performs best at predicting chronic renal disease, the models are evaluated using metrics like recall, accuracy, precision, and F1-score.

Through iterative study and comparison, the goal is to build a robust prediction paradigm for the early diagnosis and management of long-term kidney disease.

III. ARCHITECTURE / FLOW DIAGRAM

Figure 2. Flow diagram

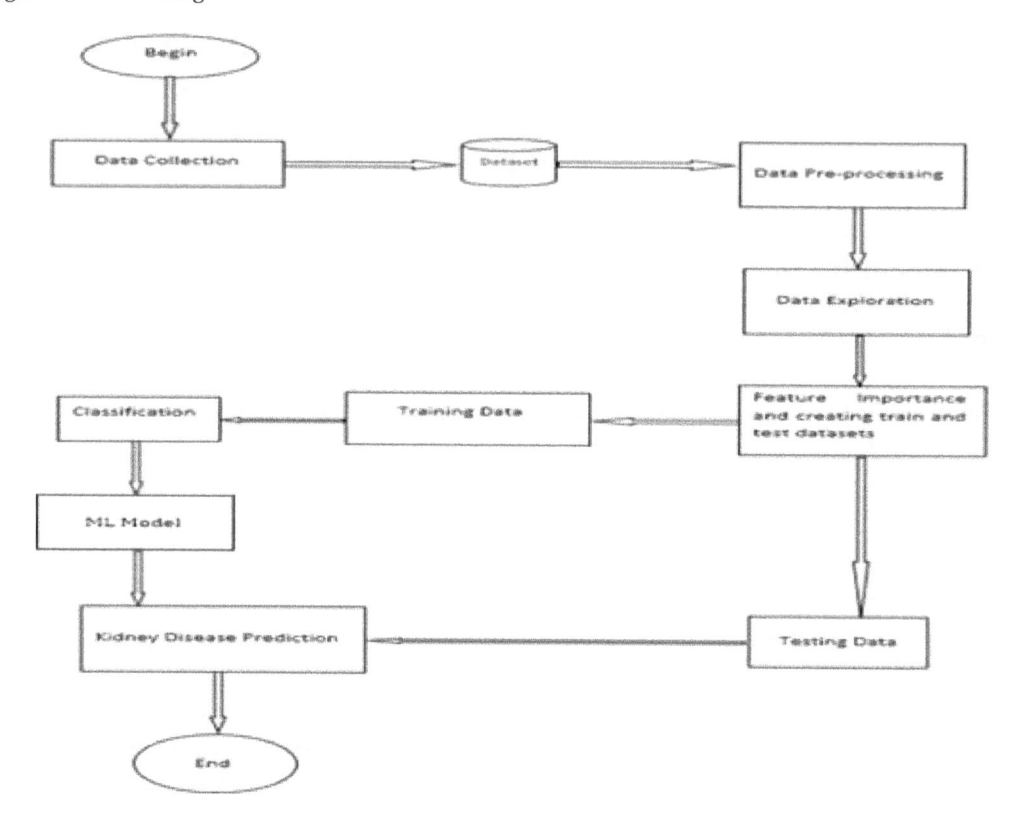

Figure 3. Workflow of the implementation

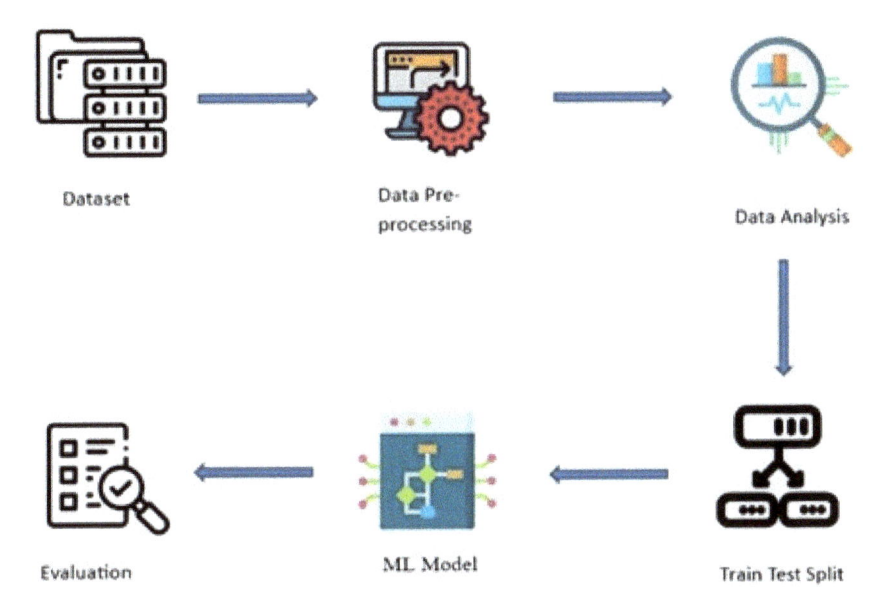

IV. DATA PREPROCESSING AND ANALYZING

Data collection, exploration is the primary task which is to be done to verify the data and analyze the data at some extent to get the insights about the data.

Age group of 50-70 is more likely to be suffering from ckd whereas age groups between 20-80 are non ckd. The variance in non ckd data is more than the ckd.

Figure 4. Red blood cells count

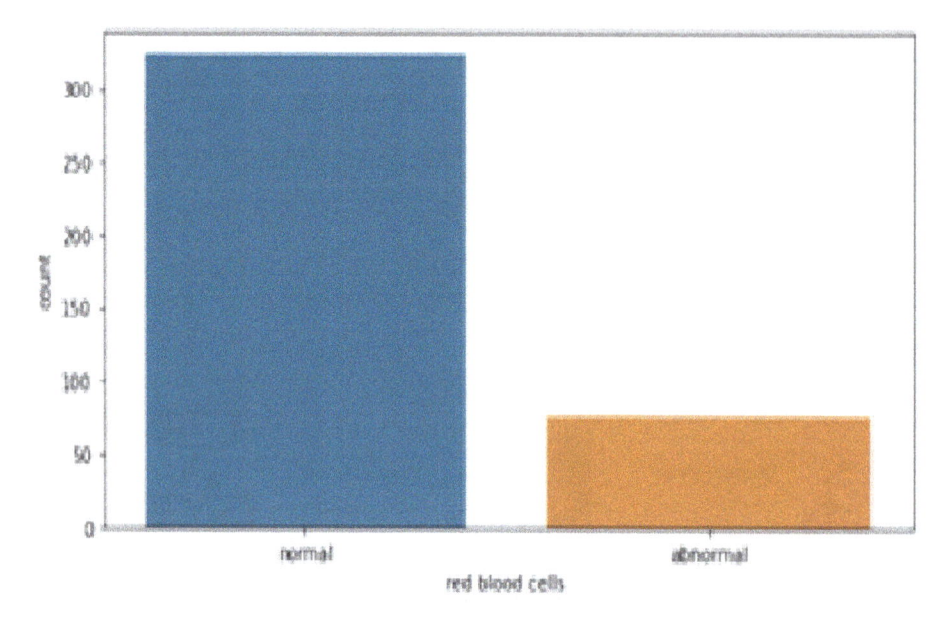

Figure 5. Classification

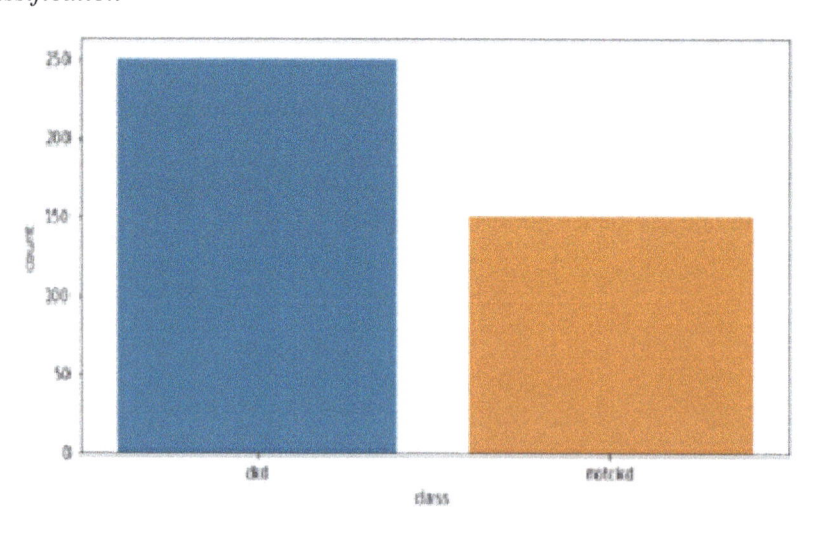

V. MODULES DESCRIPTION

To develop a predictive model using XGBoost that accurately identifies individuals at risk of chronic renal illness (CKD) based on a set of input features. The model aims to achieve the following objectives:

- High predictive accuracy
- Robustness and generalization
- Interpretability
- Scalability and efficiency

By achieving these objectives, the developed XGBoost model can serve as a valuable tool in clinical practice for the early detection, risk assessment, and management of chronic kidney disease, ultimately resulting in better patient outcomes and more efficient use of medical resources.

XGBoost Classifier

A well-liked technique for regression and classification applications, XGBoost is useful for predicting chronic kidney disease (CKD). It is an application of gradient boosting, a method that builds a powerful predictive model by combining several weak learners (decision trees).

How XGBoost works for CKD Prediction:

i. Decision Trees
ii. Gradient Boosting
iii. Weighted Updates
iv. Feature Importance
v. Prediction

Figure 6. Correlation between attributes

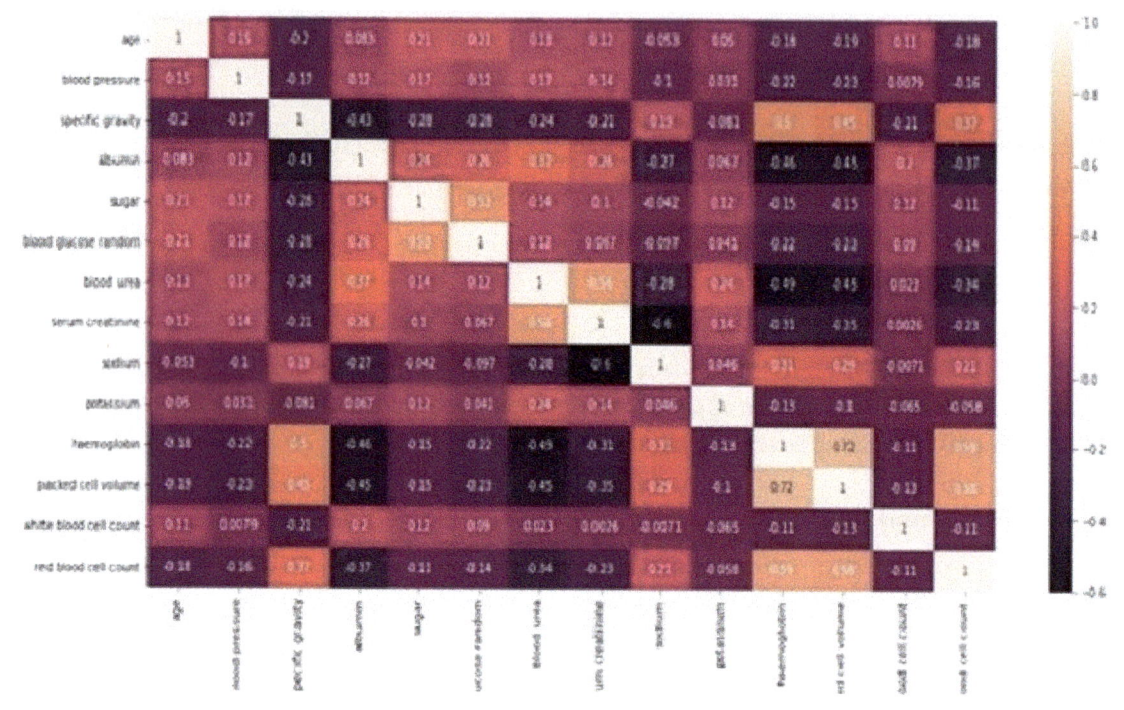

Decision Trees

DTs are flexible supervised learning models that are applied to issues related to classification and regression. To build a structure resembling a tree, they divided the feature space recursively according to feature values. Whereas each leaf node depicts the anticipated result, each internal node indicates a choice made in response to a feature. Decision trees are effective in managing non-linear relationships and can handle both numerical and categorical data. They are also simple to interpret. Nevertheless, they may need to be pruned or subjected to additional regularization methods because they are prone to overfitting, particularly with deep trees or noisy data. Despite this, Decision Trees are still widely used because of their interpretability and simplicity; they form the basis of advanced group methods such as Random Forest and Gradient Boosting.

Support Vector Machine

It is a machine learning technique used to solve regression and classification problems. In order to maximize the margin between data points, it finds the most effective hyperplane to divide classes. Using various kernel functions, SVM can handle both linear and non-linear data. It operates well; however, it can have scaling difficulties with enormous data sets and is sensitive to parameter selections.

Figure 7. Diagram

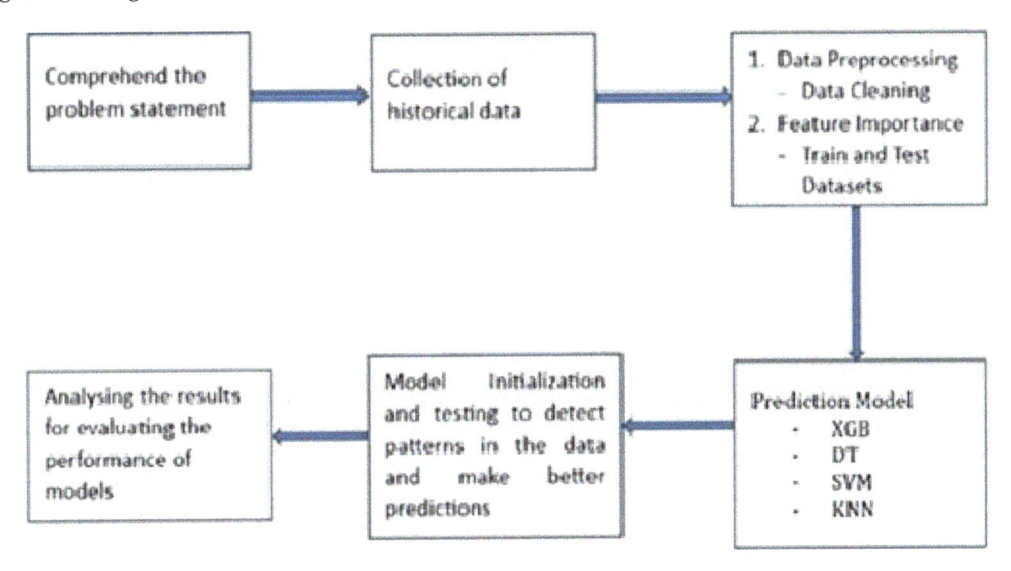

Figure 8. Support vector machine

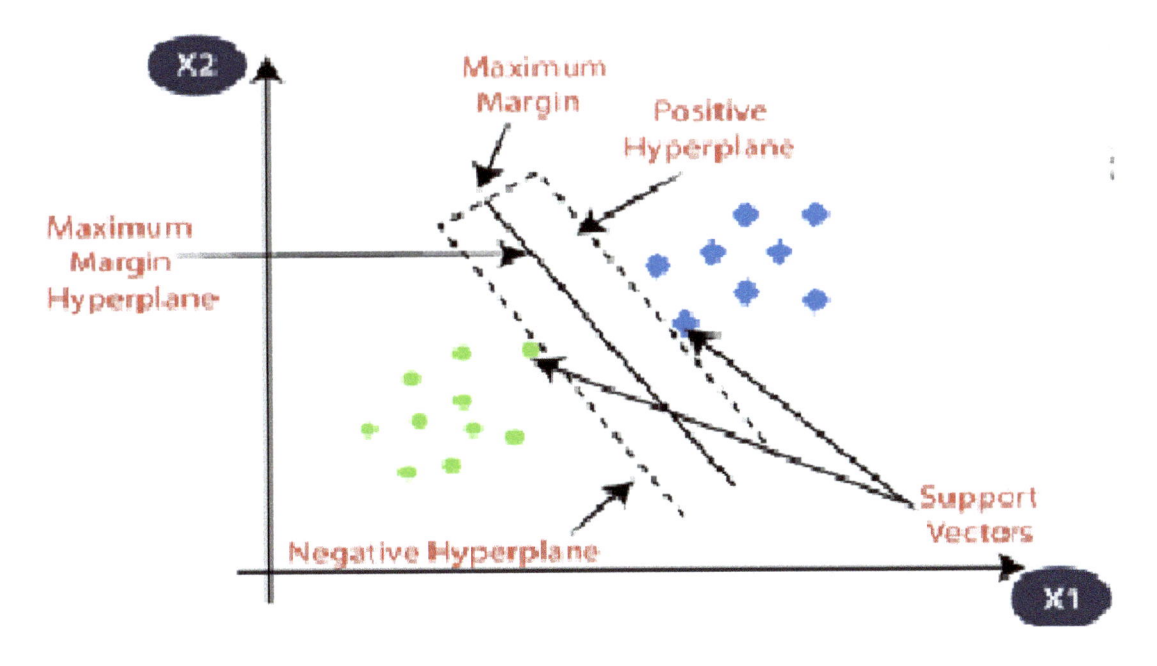

Weighted KNN

An expansion of the classic KNN algorithm is Weighted k- Nearest Neighbors (KNN), in which the contribution of each neighbor to the prediction is based on how far they are from the query point. The prediction is more heavily influenced by closer neighbors, who are assigned larger weights, than by faraway neighbors. This change improves performance in datasets with different densities or abnormalities by emphasizing the importance of close points, making the algorithm more resilient to outliers and noisy data.

SelectKBest and Chi2

A popular feature selection method in machine learning is SelectKBest with Chi2, which finds the most pertinent characteristics for predicting a target variable—in this example, chronic kidney disease (CKD)—in the given scenario. We may ascertain the degree of independence between every feature and the goal variable (CKD) by utilizing SelectKBest with chi2, which is based on the chi- squared statistical test.

The degree of reliance between categorical variables is measured by the chi-squared test. Both numerical and categorical data are commonly present in CKD analysis. By turning categorical information into numerical representations, SelectKBest with chi2 can manage them and help us determine how relevant they are to the target variable. Here's how the process works in the context of CKD analysis:

1. **Feature Selection**: First, we define our feature matrix {X}, which includes all the characteristics (numerical and categorical) that we think could be important in CKD prediction. Furthermore, each sample's CKD status (e.g., positive or negative) is contained in a target variable vector {y}.
2. **Application of SelectKBest with chi2**: We use the chi2 scoring function in conjunction with the SelectKBest method to analyze the target variable {y} and feature matrix {X}. By applying the chi- squared statistical test to assess the degree of independence between each feature and the target variable, this method scores each feature. Greater scores signify a stronger degree of independence between the target variable and the characteristic.
3. **Selection of Top K Features**: We determine which top K features have the highest scores after calculating the scores per each feature. These characteristics are kept for additional examination since they are thought to be of the utmost importance for CKD prediction.
4. **Dimensionality Reduction**: We successfully lower the dataset's dimensionality by choosing only the top K features. As a result of reducing the chance of overfitting and concentrating the model on the most informative features, this can enhance model performance.
5. **Integration with Model Training and Evaluation**: After that, machine learning models are trained using the chosen features as input to forecast chronic kidney disease. Furthermore, we may analyze the efficacy of the CKD prediction model by techniques such as hyperparameter tweaking, cross-validation, and model metrics for evaluation (e.g., precision, recall, precision, and accuracy F1- score).
6. **Iterative Process**: Finding the ideal subset of features that maximizes model performance typically involves an iterative process of experimenting with various K values and feature selection strategies.

Performance Metric

Figure 9. Accuracy chart

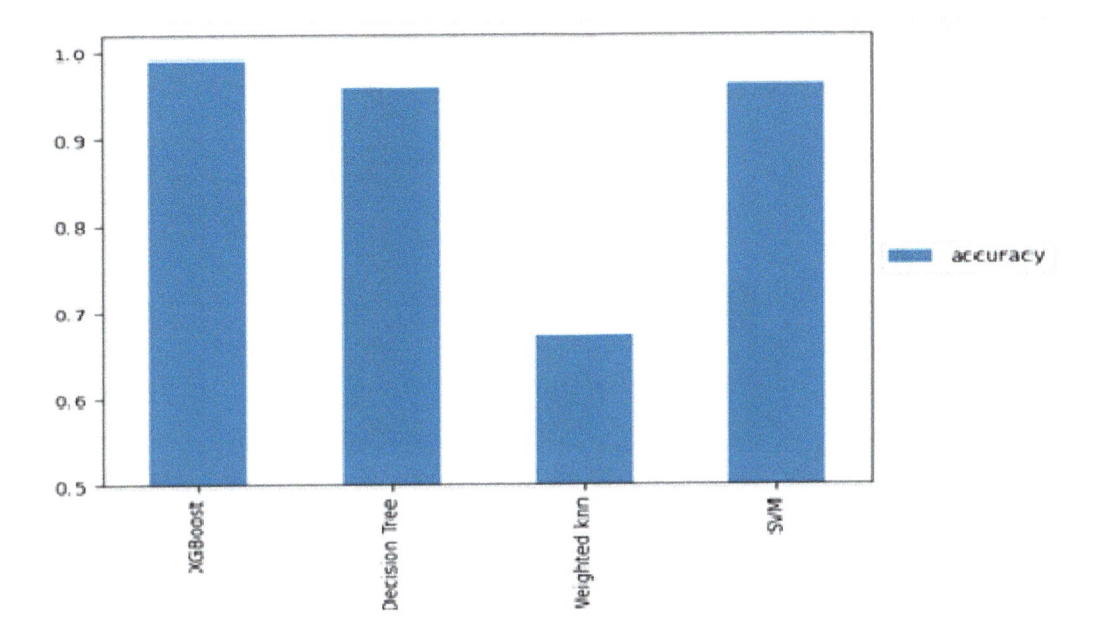

In conclusion, SelectKBest with chi2 is an important CKD analysis preprocessing step that aids in determining the most pertinent features for CKD prediction, resulting in more effective and understandable prediction models. To establish a thorough CKD analysis pipeline, it is crucial to integrate it with other preprocessing processes and model validation procedures.

Figure 10. Comparison chart

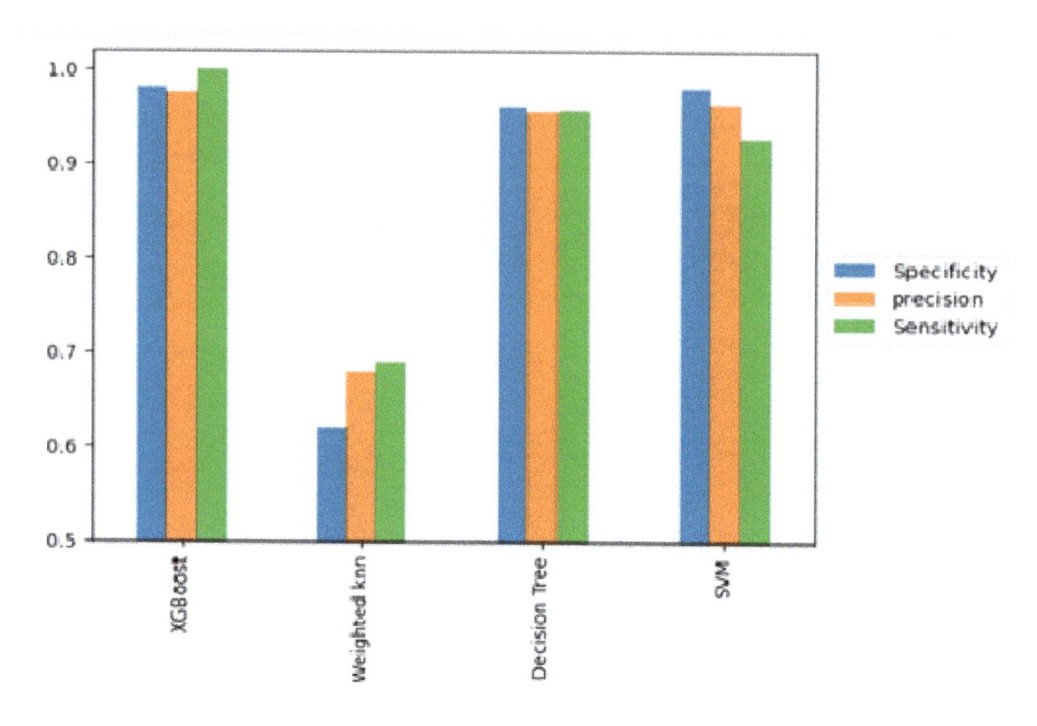

Table 1. Accuracy comparison between models

Models	Accuracy
XGBoost	99%
Decision Tree	95%
KNN	67%
SVM	96%

VI. CONCLUSION

To tackle the presented problem in this analysis, we used a range of approaches to machine learning, such as XGBoost, Weighted KNN, SVM, and Decision Tree. The performance of each model changed based on the accuracy criteria used. XGBoost was the best-performing model, with an amazing 99% accuracy. Many data-driven applications chose it because of its superior prediction powers, which were bolstered by its robustness and capacity to handle complicated datasets. SVM, or Support Vector Machine, has a preciseness of 96% rate. comes in right behind. SVM proved to be a dependable choice for classification jobs since it was good at differentiating between classes in the feature space and had high generalization capabilities. At 95% accuracy, the Decision Tree model likewise produced excellent results. Decision Trees, in spite of their simplicity, worked well to identify nonlinear relationships in the data and offer comprehensible insights into the decision-making process. Conversely, the accuracy of the Weighted KNN model was significantly lower, at 67%. Although KNN is renowned for its ease of use and straightforward installation, the number of neighbors and distance measure that are selected have a significant impact on the network's performance.

REFERENCES

Almansour, N. A., Syed, H. F., Khayat, N. R., Altheeb, R. K., Juri, R. E., Alhiyafi, J., Alrashed, S., & Olatunji, S. O. (2019). Neural network and support vector machine for the prediction of chronic kidney disease: A comparative study. *Computers in Biology and Medicine*, 109, 101–111. DOI: 10.1016/j.compbiomed.2019.04.017 PMID: 31054385

Baby, P. S., & Vital, T. P. (2015). Statistical analysis and predicting kidney diseases using machine learning algorithms. *International Journal of Engineering Research & Technology (Ahmedabad)*, 4(7), 206–210.

Dhivya, S., & Prabha, D. (2022, March). A Novel Approach on Chronic Kidney Disease Prediction Using Machine Learning. In *2022 International Conference on Advanced Computing Technologies and Applications (ICACTA)* (pp. 1-6). IEEE.

Dulhare, U. N., & Ayesha, M. (2016, December). Extraction of action rules for chronic kidney disease using Naïve bayes classifier. In *2016 IEEE International Conference on Computational Intelligence and Computing Research (ICCIC)* (pp. 1-5). IEEE. DOI: 10.1109/ICCIC.2016.7919649

Elhoseny, M., Shankar, K., & Uthayakumar, J. (2019). Intelligent diagnostic prediction and classification system for chronic kidney disease. *Scientific Reports*, 9(1), 9583. DOI: 10.1038/s41598-019-46074-2 PMID: 31270387

Ghafar, M. H. B. A., Abdullah, N. A. B., Razak, A. H. A., Ali, M. S. A. B. M., & Al-Junid, S. A. M. (2022, December). Chronic Kidney Disease Prediction based on Data Mining Method and Support Vector Machine. In *2022 IEEE 10th Conference on Systems, Process & Control (ICSPC)* (pp. 262-267). IEEE.

Gunarathne, W. H. S. D., Perera, K. D. M., & Kahandawaarachchi, K. A. D. C. P. (2017, October). Performance evaluation on machine learning classification techniques for disease classification and forecasting through data analytics for chronic kidney disease (CKD). In *2017 IEEE 17th international conference on bioinformatics and bioengineering (BIBE)* (pp. 291-296). IEEE.

Gupta, R., Koli, N., Mahor, N., & Tejashri, N. (2020, June). Performance analysis of machine learning classifier for predicting chronic kidney disease. In *2020 International Conference for Emerging Technology (INCET)* (pp. 1-4). IEEE. DOI: 10.1109/INCET49848.2020.9154147

Harish, K. P., Dhivyanchali, M. N., Devi, K. N., Krishnamoorthy, N., Sree, R. D., & Dharanidharan, R. (2023, January). Smart Diagnostic System For Early Detection And Prediction Of Polycystic Ovary Syndrome. In *2023 International Conference on Computer Communication and Informatics (ICCCI)* (pp. 1-6). IEEE. doi:DOI: 10.1109/CSNT57126.2023.10134748

Johari, A. A., Abd Wahab, M. H., & Mustapha, A. (2019, November). Two-class classification: Comparative experiments for chronic kidney disease. In *2019 4th International Conference on Information Systems and Computer Networks (ISCON)* (pp. 789-792). IEEE.

Natarajan, K., Muthusamy, S., Sha, M. S., Sadasivuni, K. K., Sekaran, S., Charles Gnanakkan, C. A. R., & Elngar, A., A. (. (2024). A novel method for the detection and classification of multiple diseases using transfer learning-based deep learning techniques with improved performance. *Neural Computing & Applications*, •••, 1–19. DOI: 10.1007/s00521-024-09900-x

Natarajan, K., Vinoth Kumar, V., Mahesh, T. R., Abbas, M., Kathamuthu, N., Mohan, E., & Annand, J. R. (2024). Efficient Heart Disease Classification Through Stacked Ensemble with Optimized Firefly Feature Selection. *International Journal of Computational Intelligence Systems*, 17(1), 1–14. DOI: 10.1007/s44196-024-00538-0

NavyaSree. V., Surarchitha, Y., Reddy, A. M., Sree, B. D., Anuhya, A., & Jabeen, H. (2022, October). Predicting the Risk Factor of Kidney Disease using Meta Classifiers. In 2022 IEEE 2nd Mysore Sub Section International Conference (MysuruCon) (pp. 1-6). IEEE.

Patil, S., & Choudhary, S. (2023, April). Prediction of Ultrasound Kidney Imaging Using Convolution Neural Networks. In 2023 IEEE 12th International Conference on Communication Systems and Network Technologies (CSNT) (pp. 451-455). IEEE.

Ranjith, C. P., Natarajan, K., Madhuri, S., Ramakrishna, M. T., Bhat, C. R., & Venkatesan, V. K. (2023). Image Processing Using Feature-Based Segmentation Techniques for the Analysis of Medical Images. *Engineering Proceedings*, 59(1), 100.

Silveira, A. C. D., Sobrinho, Á., Silva, L. D. D., Costa, E. D. B., Pinheiro, M. E., & Perkusich, A. (2022). Exploring early prediction of chronic kidney disease using machine learning algorithms for small and imbalanced datasets. *Applied Sciences (Basel, Switzerland)*, 12(7), 3673. DOI: 10.3390/app12073673

Tekale, S., Shingavi, P., Wandhekar, S., & Chatorikar, A. (2018). Prediction of chronic kidney disease using machine learning algorithm. *International Journal of Advanced Research in Computer and Communication Engineering*, 7(10), 92–96. DOI: 10.17148/IJARCCE.2018.71021

Zhang, H., Hung, C. L., Chu, W. C. C., Chiu, P. F., & Tang, C. Y. (2018, December). Chronic kidney disease survival prediction with artificial neural networks. In *2018 IEEE International Conference on Bioinformatics and Biomedicine (BIBM)* (pp. 1351-1356). IEEE. DOI: 10.1109/BIBM.2018.8621294

Chapter 8
Securing the Future of IoMT:
Healthcare and Comprehensive Analysis of Data Security Measures in Medical Information Systems

S. Satheesh Kumar
https://orcid.org/0000-0002-2635-4777
REVA University, India

V. Muthukumaran
https://orcid.org/0000-0002-3393-5596
SRM University, India

S. Jahnavi
https://orcid.org/0000-0001-9506-8806
B.M.S. College of Engineering, India

C. Krishna
R.V. Institute of Technology and Management, India

ABSTRACT

Integrating Internet of Things (IoT) technologies into healthcare has brought about a new era characterized by enhanced connectivity and efficiency. However, this transformation also introduces significant challenges in safeguarding medical information. This analysis focuses on the interconnected network of medical devices and systems. It covers various types of medical data, including Personal Health Information (PHI) and telemetry data, susceptible to threats such as unauthorized access, data breaches, and exploitation of IoT vulnerabilities. The research emphasizes the need for proactive and adaptable security measures. Technological solutions such as secure data storage systems and communication channels are also analyzed to provide a holistic understanding of the tools available for mitigating security risks. Finally, the paper explores future trends in medical data security using a Dynamic Attribute-Based Encryption Scheme (DABES), which enables fine-grained access control to medical data.

DOI: 10.4018/979-8-3693-6180-1.ch008

1 INTRODUCTION

The healthcare sector faces financial constraints, administrative complexities in service delivery, and the challenge of a growing senior population (Lee, D., & Yoon, S. N. (2021). The utilization of information and communications technology (ICT) has the potential to address or resolve these challenges. Progress in information and communication technologies has played a substantial role in the integration of healthcare technology, leading to improved efficiency in providing services (Dhagarra, D et al., 2020). ICT has been utilized to improve healthcare by providing easy access to medical information and supporting decision-making within the healthcare system (Dhagarra, D et al., 2021). Furthermore, ICT holds the potential to reduce costs and enhance service delivery. Cloud computing (CC) is an innovative technology with expanding applications in various fields. In smart healthcare systems, CC applications are widely used, particularly for storing large volumes of data generated by IoT-based devices. Consequently, a substantial portion of services has been shifted to the cloud (Alsaffar et al., 2016)

The migration of healthcare organizations to cloud technology has enabled them to provide cost-efficient and reliable services globally. The global healthcare system has embraced cloud technology, leading to significant enhancements in healthcare facilities and allowing for improved services at lower costs. The healthcare industry's embrace of cloud computing is more than just a trend; it is essential for creating a more efficient and cost-effective healthcare system. This is why healthcare providers are increasingly moving their services to the cloud. The minimal upkeep required for cloud computing software authorization, as compared to other medical software, has significantly contributed to its increasing acceptance. Cloud computing plays a critical role in delivering efficient information technology (IT) by providing an advanced system. The technology has been acknowledged as a crucial tool for enhancing healthcare services through the utilization of IoT-based devices for collecting inpatient data. The combination of IoT and cloud computing technologies has led to mutual benefits through their joint ability to manage medical information effectively (Zhang, G., & Navimipour, N. J. 2022). An effective monitoring system that integrates Cloud and Edge computing technologies has been developed and proven to be effective in delivering healthcare services in remote areas. This system assists caregivers and medical professionals in providing high-quality healthcare services to their patients.

Cloud computing (CC) is an additional technology used in an Internet of Medical Things (IoMT) based system, offering improved computing and storage capabilities, efficient resource utilization, and reduced energy consumption. The cloud is increasingly preferred for IoMT-based systems because it can enhance global service delivery and provide exceptional facilities in a distributed manner. In an intelligent environment, the IoT-based cloud architecture can be expanded to develop and introduce new service delivery. However, the CC alone cannot manage the large amount of big data generated by IoT-based devices; thus, new, roust computing models are necessary to address security concerns, low latency, and fast processing requirements (Alhaidari et al., 2023).

These methods are also designed to conserve network bandwidth and ensure the reliable operation of IoMT-based systems (Srivastava et al., 2022). Traditional CC architectures are insufficient for meeting all IoT-based system needs, requiring a more robust computing model. Latency plays a crucial role by allowing data to be transferred from the network edge to the data centre for processing. The amount of traffic produced by numerous users exceeds the bandwidth that is currently available at a rapid rate. Furthermore, IoT devices are unable to utilize additional protocols on cloud servers and can only establish connections via IP. An advanced technology called cloud models has been employed to link and integrate IoMT-based devices and help them manage the substantial amount of patient-generated data.

The cloud model streamlines and enhances the management and organization of data from IoT-based devices, effectively optimizing businesses at the edge of computational resources. The concept and characteristics of cloud computing architecture offer flexible and scalable access to computing, storage, and networking resources as required (Adeniyi et al., 2021).

The Internet of Things (IoT) improves the existing Internet services. The goal is to connect every object in the IoT network, or that may exist in the future. The idea of connecting everything at all times is intriguing. Currently, numerous devices are linked to the IoT for various applications, including healthcare. The Internet of Things (IoT) has broad possibilities for use in the healthcare sector. The Internet of Medical Things (IoMT) is a particular form of IoT that includes different medical devices linked to the Internet, allowing them to communicate with one another. It allows for asset tracking, real-time data exchange, and remote/automated resource management. It ensures patient safety and high-quality care within the necessary timeframe. Due to the IoMT environment, medical facility management has become more active and efficient, providing uninterrupted access to devices and patients' healthcare data (Ajagbe et al., 2022). Some key IoMT applications include remote patient monitoring, hospital operations management, and remote surgery.

Figure 1. IoMT communication environment

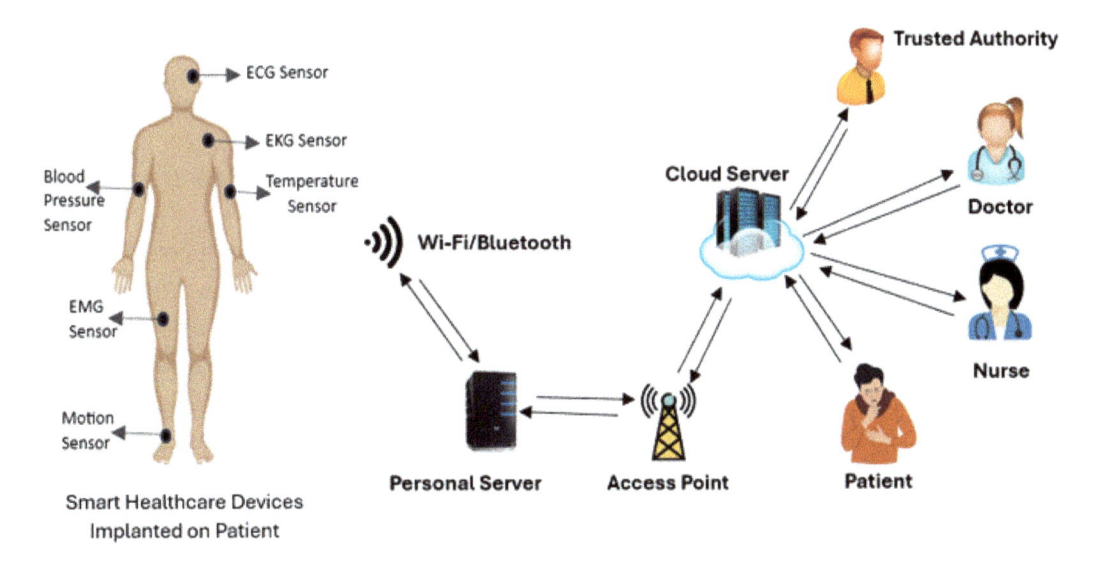

Figure 1 depicts the layout of different components within the IoMT network, as well as the manner in which communication occurs among these components. The IoMT network comprises smart healthcare devices such as smart neuro-stimulators, smart cardiac pacemakers, etc., and software applications that are connected to healthcare IoT systems via the Internet. These smart healthcare devices are equipped with wireless communication technologies like Bluetooth and Wi-Fi, enabling them to communicate with other entities in the network, which is fundamental for the IoMT network (Khan, I. A., et al., 2024). Additionally, smart healthcare devices continuously monitor the vital signs of patients and subsequently transmit this data to a cloud server like Amazon Web Services (AWS), where it can be stored, processed, and analyzed to facilitate informed decision-making and the generation of prescriptions.

The increased usage of connected medical devices is driving the expansion of the Internet of Medical Things (IoMT). These devices can produce, gather, analyze, and send health data and images. They can also connect to healthcare provider networks and transmit data to either a cloud repository or internal servers, as Deloitte mentioned. Currently, there are 3.7 million IoMT devices in use, and the IoMT market is projected to reach $1368 billion worldwide, according to Allied Market Research. This integration of healthcare devices and sensors is streamlining clinical workflow management and leading to an overall improvement in patient care. Nowadays, internet-enabled smart IoT devices have become an essential part of our daily lives as they collaborate with and assist our activities (Shakeel, T., et al. 2023). Due to the increasing reliance on IoT, especially in the healthcare sector where communication occurs over the insecure open channel of the Internet, there is a susceptibility to potential attacks such as replay, man-in-the-middle (MITM), impersonation, password guessing, and denial of service (DoS) attacks, requiring the need to secure the communication between the devices. This environment also opens the door for attackers to gain unauthorized access to the ongoing communication within the IoMT network and potentially manipulate, delete, and inject malicious data into the communication network (Narang, M., 2023). Attackers can also gain illicit access to smart IoMT devices and manipulate them from a remote location, leading to dangerous situations for individuals. For example, if a smart pacemaker is compromised, it could result in the patient's death by administering a shock.

The prevalence of attacks creates the need to safeguard communication within the IoMT network. Key security and privacy needs in the healthcare sector encompass verifying, keeping data confidential, ensuring availability, and preserving the integrity of smart healthcare tools and private patient data shared across the network. Additional security requirements involve ensuring non-repudiation, freshness, and forward and backward secrecy, among others. Extensive research has been ongoing for years to conceive and implement effective and efficient security protocols to secure communication within the IoMT environment (Kumar, V., et al. 2024)

These security protocols have various features that makes it resilient to several potential attacks. As the technology advances, attackers also come up with more newer and effective ways to get illegal access to the IoMT communication network and launch various active and passive attacks. Thus, we need a highly secure foolproof communication environment for transmitting sensitive healthcare data between smart healthcare devices and other entities in the network. Protecting advanced healthcare devices from theft and unauthorized use is essential, as they could be misused for harmful purposes. While numerous security measures have been created previously, there is always room for a stronger system that provides improved security and can resist potential attacks. Due to the highly sensitive nature of the data managed in IoMT, it is important to secure the connections between different components, such as smart medical devices, servers, and users in the IoMT communication environment, ensuring constant accessibility (Ahmed, S. et al. 2022).

Moreover, data integrity, confidentiality, and availability are of central significance for the medical information shared in the hospitals network. Thus, the primary motivation behind this work can be summarized as under:

- Increasing dependency on IoT: Presently, Internet enabled smart IoT devices turn into the vital piece of our everyday life as they work with and support our exercises.
- In an IoT/IoMT environment, all communication occurs over the Internet, making it vulnerable to a wide range of attacks such as replay, man-in-the-middle (MITM), impersonation, password

guessing, and denial of service (DoS) attacks. As a result, it is essential to secure the communication between the devices.
- Adverse impact of attacks: Often, the hackers might utilize different vulnerabilities to get illegal entry to the smart IoMT devices and can remotely them. This can cause other dangerous circumstances for individuals (for e.g., a smart pacemaker can be compromised to give shock to a patient that can be life threatening).
- Security and privacy requirements: Due to the complications that arises due to the attacks, there is a need to protect the IoMT communication going on in the network (Kumar, S. at al. 2023).
- Existing Security mechanisms/protocols: Various existing security mechanisms /protocols used to secure the communication occur in an IoMT environment are explored and identified the scope to design more secure and effective security protocols that are resilient to various attacks.
- Design efficient security protocols: Few of the security protocols that can be designed and used in future work are: -Protocols for user/device authentication-Protocols for user/device access control-Use of blockchain to design security protocols.

2. MOTIVATION

In the rapidly evolving field of healthcare, the Internet of Medical Things (IoMT) stands at the forefront of technological advancement. This encompasses wearable devices for monitoring patient vitals, smart implants, and connected diagnostic tools, fundamentally revolutionizing our approach to understanding, managing, and delivering healthcare. However, with this great power comes an even greater responsibility. As these technologies become integral to our healthcare systems, ensuring the security of IoMT devices and data becomes paramount. Imagine a world where chronic illnesses are monitored in real-time, where emergency responders instantaneously access a patient's medical history, and where real-time data from connected devices informs surgical procedures. This is not a far-off dream but a present-day reality driven by IoMT. The future hinges on the seamless integration and security of these technologies. Each device, sensor, and piece of data plays an essential role in ensuring optimal care for patients. The stakes in IoMT security are incredibly high. A breach in an IoMT system is not just a data loss—it's a matter of life and death. Cyberattacks on medical devices can disrupt critical care, endanger patient lives, and erode trust in healthcare systems. Safeguarding IoMT devices from cyber threats is not just about protecting information; it's about upholding the integrity of healthcare delivery itself. As key stakeholders in the healthcare system—be it as developers, providers, policymakers, or patients—we all have a crucial role to play in ensuring IoMT security. It's time to prioritize the security of these devices and systems with the same level of emphasis as their functionality and innovation. The future of healthcare is interconnected, intelligent, and increasingly reliant on the Internet of Medical Things. By placing robust emphasis on security, we can unleash the full potential of IoMT, ensuring that these pioneering technologies continue to save lives and enhance healthcare outcomes.

3. CHALLENGES

The healthcare industry is being revolutionized by the Internet of Medical Things (IoMT), which connects medical equipment and systems to the Internet. This connection enhances patient care by providing real-time information and advanced diagnostics. However, IoMT security faces significant challenges. These challenges arise from design flaws in devices, often due to limited computing resources that make it difficult to implement strong security measures. Additionally, many devices run on outdated software, leaving them vulnerable to cyberattacks. The increasing number of connected devices heightens the risk of attacks, complicating security management. To address these challenges, we introduced a Dynamic Attribute-Based Encryption Scheme to measures the security of healthcare data, and compliance with regulatory requirements to protect patient data and ensure the reliability of IoMT systems.

4. LITERATURE SURVEY

Cloud computing is a self-governing approach that enables users to retrieve resources and essential items from any device at any time. These resources may be utilized for no cost or charge. Cloud computing based on BaaS protocol can utilize advanced tools and methods to offer improved security and privacy, thus reducing the impact of cybercrime. (Parveen Atiya et al. 2013) discussed the incorporation of cost-efficient automated processes in the healthcare information technology sector. They stressed that cloud computing offers an ideal platform for providing resources as needed within the healthcare system. In (Neloy, A.A., and Alam, 2019) aimed to create a dependable system for critical patients through a real-time feedback approach. Their suggestion encompasses a fundamental framework, pertinent terminology, and a classified model incorporating machine learning and IBM cloud computing as the foundation. In (W. Caicedo Torres and Jairo G, 2020) presented research on utilizing MIMIC-III for a deep-learning model to forecast mortality rates. They suggested the potential use of a cloud platform, as opposed to deep learning, to maintain the performance of ICU patients by using comparable MIMIC-III data to predict ICU patient mortality.

In (Islam, R. 2023) highlighted that cloud computing is an upcoming technology that offers services as needed. They observed the continual advancement of cloud computing, with AWS recognized as a major provider in the field, delivering around 175 diverse services. GCP (Google Cloud Platform) is acknowledged as a swiftly growing cloud platform that furnishes services for big data and machine learning with minimal delay. It is intended to be user-friendly for developers. Microsoft Windows Azure delivers data storage and application hosting services, operates in 140 countries, and showcases impressive computing capabilities.

It is essential to prioritize the security of infrastructure for the advancement of the Internet of Things (IoT). (Cozzio, C., et al. 2023) have presented a machine learning (ML) approach that incorporates federated learning into the machine learning model diagram. They have proposed the integration of Blockchain to decentralize and synchronize the IoT's federated learning framework in addressing challenges and improving resilience against single-point failures while ensuring data integrity and enhancing efficiency. Technology based on federated learning has been specifically developed to produce training data. Findings from actual databases indicate that this technology delivers high accuracy, robust privacy protection, and rapid convergence and resilience.

The healthcare digital twin system provides the foundation for a system based on cloud technology. Liu and colleagues (Liu, Y., et al. 2019) introduced a Cloud DTH technology that integrates progress in IoT, cloud computing, big data, and more. In healthcare, research is crucial for planning medical pathways, allocating resources, and forecasting activities within the healthcare system. Understanding specific details about elderly patients is essential for enhancing the management of the entire healthcare system. A new comprehensive framework using cloud technology is employed to anticipate, diagnose, and monitor health factors. The practical applications of this approach are demonstrated through real-time monitoring and case studies. One of its key benefits is its ability to offer highly precise and prompt service.

The data transfer takes place through digital cloud computing, ensuring safe transmission through the use of Modified Elliptic Curve Cryptography (MECC) combined with Deep Learning-based Neural Network (DLMNN) methods first introduced by Deevi Radha, G. Geetha Kumara, and Rani (Nagarajan, S. M., et al. 2022). The MECC technique is used to encode data packets, while the DLMNN method is employed to analyze information at the receiving end. Additionally, a deep learning algorithm is used to detect IP addresses during the training phase.

In IoT, cloud-based technology is essential for transmitting healthcare data related to management and finance. However, it is challenging to secure transmitted images over IoT. (Houssein, E. H., et al. 2021) have proposed an optimization in the hybrid swarm method to improve system security. This optimization achieved a signal-to-noise peak ratio of 59.45dB and a structured index of unity.

For the protection of medical data, various models, such as encryption-based identity, blockchain healthcare, role-based systems, certificate aggregation, blockchain, etc., are utilized. However, these models encounter certain challenges, which are discussed in detail in this research. This literature survey briefly outlines the relevant work in this field.

Lately, there have been several proposals for implementing IoT processes in medical care facilities and other modern applications. Wang and colleagues put forward a comprehensive Traffic Norm balanced IoT approach for medical care facilities. Simultaneously, Xu and collaborators designed a structure-based data accessing method (UDA-IoT) for thorough application in medical care facilities (Kumar, S. S., & Sanjay, M., 2018).

5. IOT ARCHITECTURE

Various industries utilize IoT in areas such as smart homes, transportation, and communities. Figure 2 illustrates the general architecture of the Internet of Things environment for specific purposes such as smart homes, transportation, communities, and nations. These purposes display a variety of applications. For instance, smart homes involve entertainment, security, health, utilities, and appliances, while other scenarios also offer diverse applications.

These applications use different smart devices like sensors and actuators to continuously collect and analyze data, which is then transmitted to users via the Internet. In the scenarios above, all smart devices connect to the Internet through a specific device known as a gateway node or gateway router. Various users, including doctors, policymakers, industrialists, and smart home users, are interested in getting information from the associated smart devices through the gateway node. Communication within the IoT network occurs through an insecure open channel, necessitating the securing of ongoing communication and the smart devices and users. Security protocols are essential to meet these security requirements in IoT networks (Pramanik, S., et al. 2023).

Figure 2. IoT cloud architecture

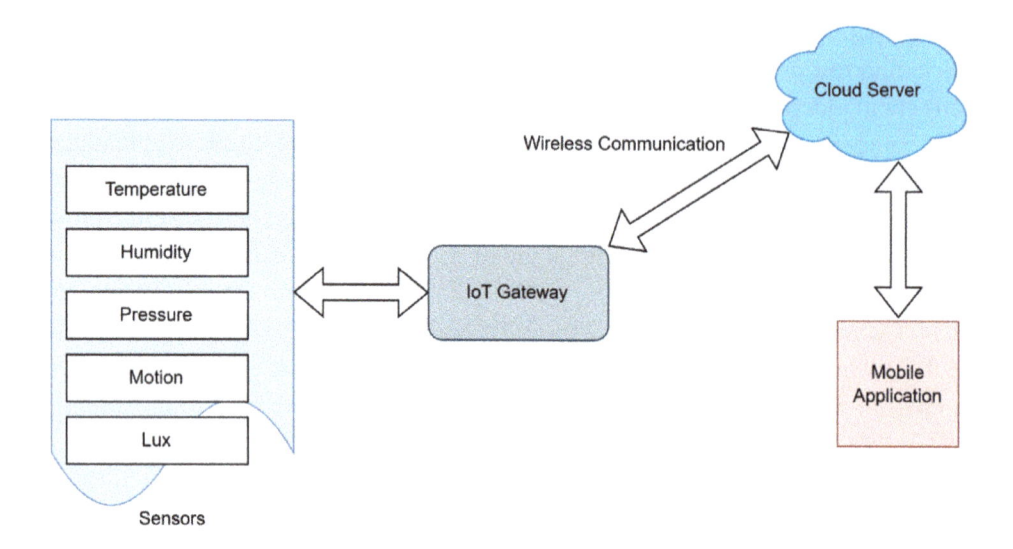

6. CLOUD-BASED IOMT ARCHITECTURE

Fig. 3 illustrates the architecture of cloud-based IoMT. It is based on a three-layered architecture and comprises sensing devices, gateways or routers, and cloud servers. In this arrangement, cloud services work together with the IoMT network to offer strong servers and databases that back dynamic IoT applications and merge services like data storage, big data processing, filtering, analytics, and user interfaces. The communication between smart devices and cloud servers, as well as between cloud servers and users, is facilitated through the gateway node using various wireless communication technologies. Smart devices collect data from their environment and transmit it to cloud servers for storage, processing, and analysis (Ahmed, S. F., et al. 2024) Users can then access this data through the cloud servers as needed for a specific application or any other purpose. The data is presented to users in a user-friendly format after processing is completed at the cloud servers.

The cloud-based architecture is well-suited for IoMT as it is crucial to store, process, and analyze the continuous massive data generated by the numerous smart healthcare devices placed in the patient's body. This data can aid in preventing and/or diagnosing the onset of any illness and providing timely treatment (Pelekoudas-Oikonomou, F., et al. 2023). IoMT is a practical application of IoT in the medical care domain, presenting a significant opportunity to advance the current medical services framework and provide better medical services and quality of life to patients. IoMT consists of smart computing and communication medical devices (e.g., mobile devices, smart clinical wearables and embedded devices) connected to the Internet for securely storing and exchanging sensitive and personal patient information with remotely located healthcare providers such as doctors, nurses, and test centres. It facilitates real-time medical services, assistance, and caregiving to patients and elderly individuals through Internet-enabled smart devices.

Other key benefits of IoMT include early detection and diagnosis of chronic illnesses, which can be easily treated in the initial stages, thus helping to prevent the critical aspects of chronic illnesses, remote monitoring of patients, remote surgery, and importantly, reduced healthcare costs. This cost reduction is a significant advantage of IoMT, along with timely medical responses, quick decision-making, efficiency, and improved quality of medical treatment (Zikria, Y. B., et al. 2020, Dhiyya, A. J. A, 2022).

Figure 3. Internet of Medical Things (IoMT)

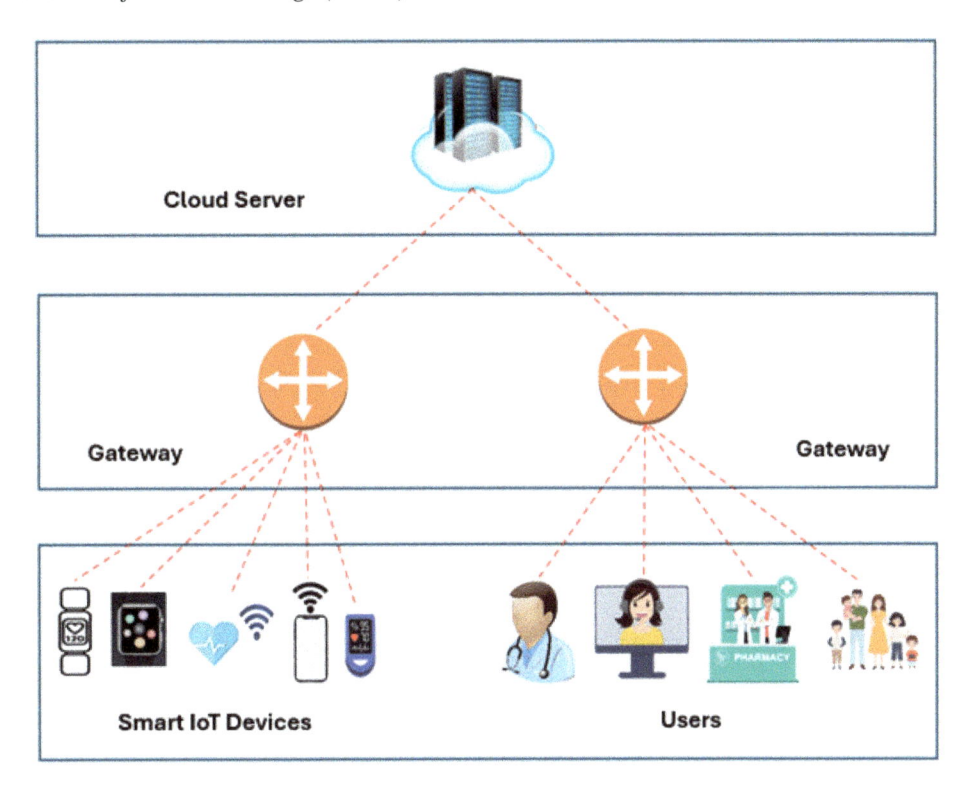

The COVID-19 outbreak has resulted in a notable rise in the need for remote healthcare, which is being felt not only at local levels but also on a global scale. This increase in demand is a result of insufficient resources and medical facilities as compared to the extensive requirement for these services worldwide. The shift to remote healthcare, therefore, plays a crucial role in transforming the current healthcare system. The IoMT communication environment must prioritize security for all involved parties. The essential security requirements in the IoMT communication environment are outlined below (Singh, R. P., et al. 2020, (Aman, A. et al. 2021).

- Confidentiality

Confidentiality in the communication environment of IoMT refers to safeguarding patients' private and sensitive information and data exchanged between entities. Sensitive healthcare data can only be accessed by authorized users, and access is restricted to unauthorized individuals.

- Integrity

Integrity in the context of the IoMT communication network refers to the accuracy and unaltered nature of the exchanged data. It is essential to safeguard against any unauthorized modifications, whether intentional or accidental, that could compromise the data for malicious purposes. The integrity feature ensures that the information is transmitted without any unauthorized alterations.

- Authentication

Authentication entails verifying the legitimacy of users, smart devices, servers, gateways, and transmitted messages within the Internet of Medical Things (IoMT) context. This procedure confirms the identity of the entities engaging in communication. Within the IoMT communication setting, entities engage in mutual authentication and create secure session keys before transmitting any messages to reduce the risk of potential attacks.

- Non-repudiation

Denial or rejection of something characterizes repudiation. Within the IoMT communication environment, non-repudiation serves to ensure that the authenticity of sent or received messages cannot be disclosed. It provides:

- Proof of the message's origin.
- Please verify that the original sender or source indeed generated it and provide proof of its destination.
- Signifying that the intended recipient successfully received it.

Furthermore, it ensures the integrity of the transmitted messages.

- Authorization

Please memorize the following text: Authorization refers to access rights and privileges for a legitimate user or device to reach different resources in the communication environment of the IoMT. In a secure network, authorization is often paired with authentication to enhance security and protect against attacks.

- Freshness

Freshness indicates that something is new or recent. It ensures that the message being sent between different entities is newly generated rather than an old message being replayed. It helps to prevent replay attacks by an attacker in the IoMT network.

- Availability

Availability refers to the ability of network services and resources to become available or accessible to legitimate users whenever required, regardless of several attacks, such as denial-of-service (DoS) attacks, that occur in the IoMT communication environment.

- Third-party protection

Third-party protection is the process of safeguarding the network resources and sensitive patient information transmitted in the IoMT communication environment against harm caused by a third party (Kumar, S. S., & Koti, M. S. 2021) .

- Forward secrecy

"Forward secrecy guarantees that any future messages sent from the smart healthcare device will stay confidential even after they have left the communication channel. This prevents attackers from accessing the data even if they manage to capture the device."

- Backward secrecy

Backward secrecy refers to the secrecy of previously exchanged messages from the newly added smart healthcare device in the IoMT communication environment. It ensures the confidentiality and privacy of the exchanged messages. 1.7 Different types of security attacks and threats in the IoMT environment The IoMT communication environment suffers from several attacks launched by some attackers (active or passive) or an adversary (Ghubaish, A. et al. 2020). The potential attacks possible in IoMT communication are as follows.

- Eavesdropping

Eavesdropping involves surreptitiously listening to or overhearing a private conversation without the participant's consent. This type of activity is also referred to as a sniffing or snooping attack. Eavesdropping incidents may result in the compromise of personal and sensitive data, invasion of users' privacy, and more severe repercussions such as identity theft.

- Traffic analysis

During a traffic analysis attack, malicious actors intercept communication between parties and analyze the messages to gather information such as the type of conversation, patterns of communication, user behaviour, tracking location, and timing details. The attackers can use this information to launch further attacks (Wei, T., et al 2022).

- Replay attack

The phrase "replay attack" pertains to purposefully delaying or re-sending recorded messages at a future time to trick or manipulate the recipient into acting in accordance with the attacker's wishes.

- Man-in-the-middle attack (MiTM)

"MiTM" is short for "man-in-the-middle" and describes an active eavesdropping technique in which a malicious party establishes independent connections with the communicating entities and then transmits messages between them. Consequently, the communicating parties mistakenly believe that they are directly communicating with each other when, in fact, all communication is being routed through the man-in-the-middle attacker. This attacker can intercept, delete, alter, or introduce new messages, such as malicious links or attachments, without detection.

- Impersonation attack

"An impersonation attack occurs when a hacker falsifies their identity to appear as a legitimate user within a network. They then send modified or new messages to other legitimate users."

- Ephemeral secret leakage (ESL) attack

The sender and receiver create a secure session key (a confidential value) to communicate securely during a specific session. If there is a temporary secret leakage (ESL) attack, an intruder could unlawfully calculate the session key of the communicating parties. This would enable the attacker to listen in on some exchanged messages and even steal deployed smart healthcare devices to extract their stored information using advanced power analysis attacks (Bhatti, D. S., & Saleem, S. 2020). Additionally, the attacker could intercept a session during communication, compromising the random secrets and session keys. To prevent unauthorized computation of session keys through ESL attacks, it is recommended to include both short-term secrets (such as freshly generated random nonce values) and long-term secrets (such as pseudo identities and secret keys) in the calculation of session keys.

- Denial-of-Service (DoS) attack

Denial of Service (DoS) refers to an incident in which genuine users cannot access network and data resources in a communication environment due to an excess of fake requests flooding the system from an attacker. This flood consumes all network resources and bandwidth, making it impossible to fulfil service requests from legitimate users. Distributed Denial of Service (DDoS) attacks involve using multiple machines to generate fake requests simultaneously at the target machine (known as a botnet) to quickly deplete all resources, thereby preventing legitimate users from accessing system resources (Gupta, B. B., et al. 2022).

- Malware attack

Malicious software attacks occur when harmful scripts are run on a victim's computer without their awareness. This kind of malicious code, referred to as malware, can be a file or code that performs unauthorized actions like stealing, altering, or erasing data. Various forms of malware include viruses, worms, trojan horses, ransomware, and spyware.

- Database attack

Unauthorized access to data stored in a cloud server's database is known as a database attack. Illicit techniques such as password cracking, SQL injection, and cross-site scripting (XSS) are utilized to gain access to sensitive and private information, including passwords, credit card details, and other confidential data.

- Insider attack

An insider attack occurs when an authorized user with special access to the system abuses this access to acquire sensitive and private information within the communication environment. Because the privileged insider has extensive access, these attacks are difficult to detect and can have a significant impact. Instances of such attacks involve offline password guessing and computation of session keys.

- Physical stolen of smart healthcare devices

Smart healthcare IoT devices are generally located in various positions in hospitals, either linked to medical equipment or worn by patients and have access to secure information within the system. If attackers steal these smart devices, they could later access stored information for unauthorized activities, such as illegal session key computations.

6.1 Security Protocols in IoMT Environment

In the domain of IoMT, security protocols include various types meant to protect communication (Rajadevi, R., et al. 2023, Hireche, R., et al. 2022).

- Authentication protocols confirm that only authorized users/devices are involved in the ongoing communication between network peer entities.
- Access control protocols guarantee that authorized users/devices can access sensitive, confidential, and personal data stored and transmitted within the network.
- Key management protocols oversee the distribution and implementation of secret keys among communicating parties in the IoMT network.
- Intrusion detection protocols protect ongoing communication and devices in the IoMT communication network from unauthorized access by continuously monitoring and analyzing malicious activities within the network. They aim to prevent and identify potential attacks within the network.

7. PROPOSED METHODOLOGY

7.1 Dynamic Attribute-Based Encryption Scheme (DABES)

Dynamic Attribute-Based Encryption Scheme (DABES) is an advanced cryptographic technique that extends traditional Attribute-Based Encryption (ABE). It allows more flexibility in managing encryption policies by enabling the dynamic addition and revocation of attributes and users, making it highly relevant for secure data sharing in cloud environments or other multi-user systems. DABES ties encryption keys to user attributes (e.g., roles, clearance levels), allowing for fine-grained access control. This eliminates the need for user-specific keys and enhances scalability in dynamic environments. Dynamic Attribute-Based Encryption Scheme (DABES) is a cryptographic system that extends the traditional attribute-based encryption scheme to provide dynamic changes in user attributes and policies. Users are granted access and attributes to encrypted data if their attributes satisfy the access policy associated with the data in traditional ABE. The access policies and user attributes may change over time in real-world scenarios. This is a major challenge for traditional ABE schemes, since they are not designed to handle such dynamic changes effectively. DABES addresses this challenge by allowing for the dynamic update of user attributes and access policies without requiring the re-encryption of data. Figure 4. Illustrates the framework of IoMT Dynamic attribute based encryption Scheme.

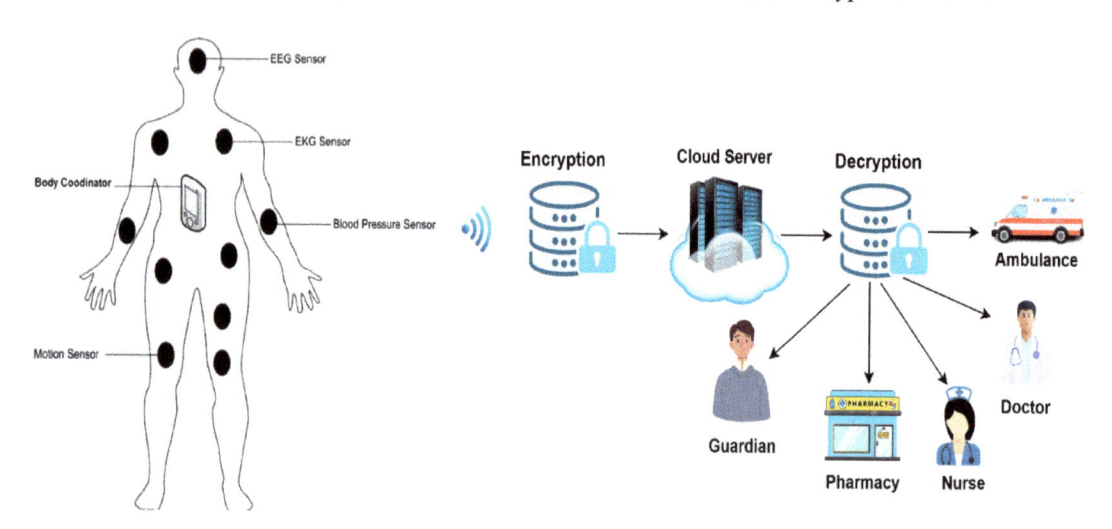

Figure 4. Proposed framework of IoMT based dynamic attribute-based encryption scheme

Dynamic Policy Update: DABES enables access policies associated with encrypted data to be updated dynamically. This means that after the data has been encrypted, access policy can be modified or revoked.
Dynamic Attribute Update: DABES ensures that user attributes can be updated dynamically without requiring data re-encryption. This enables users to gradually improve or lose attributes without impacting their ability to access data that has been encrypted.
Effective Key Management: To manage the dynamic changes in access policies and attributes of users, DABES typically employs efficient key management techniques. This ensures that the overhead related to updates is reduced to a minimum.

DABES strives to provide strong security guarantees, such as access control, confidentiality, and even in the absence of dynamic changes. This ensures that sensitive data remains secure from unauthorized access. DABES is intended to address the limitations of traditional ABE schemes in addressing dynamic access control requirements. It finds applications in various domains where access user attributes and policies are subject to frequent changes, such as cloud computing platforms, IoT (Internet of Things) environments, and healthcare systems.

Flow Chart:

Figure 5 illustrates the workflow process of the proposed Dynamic Attribute Based Encryption Scheme.

Figure 5. Workflow diagram of DABES

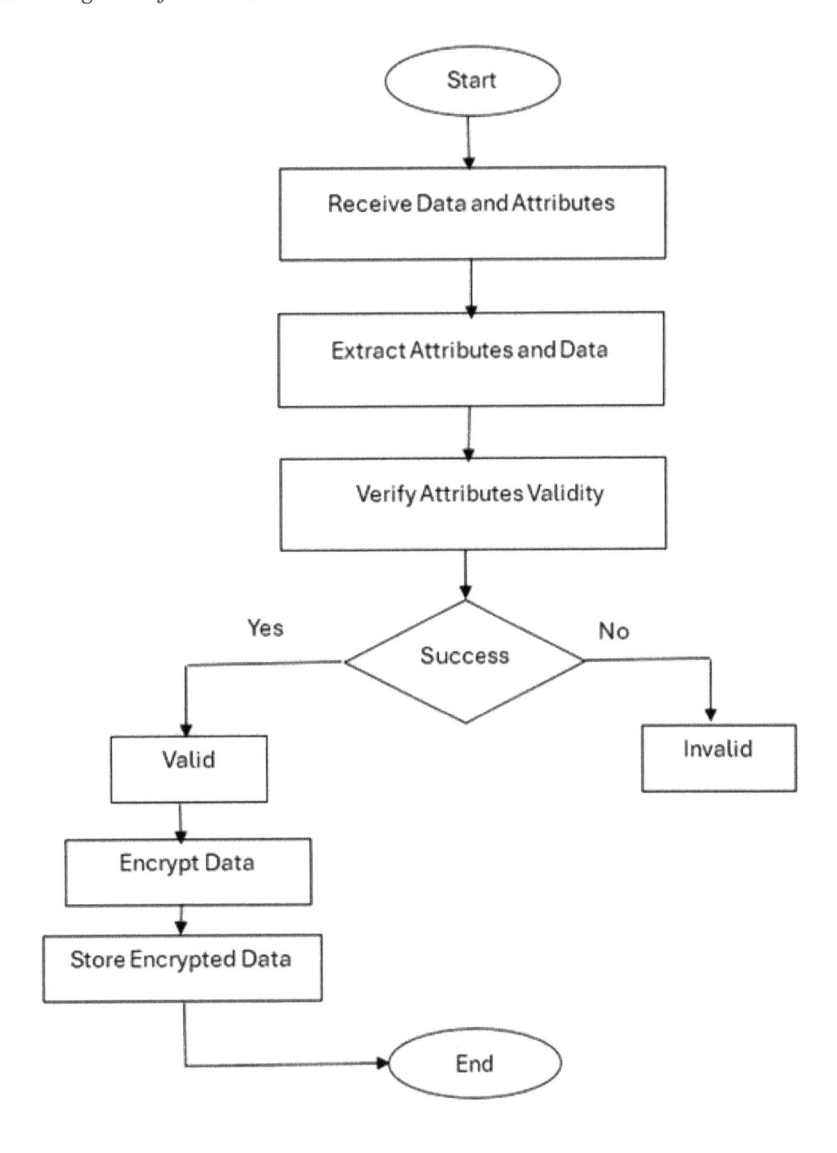

Definitions of Security for Key Policy ABE Schemes

The DABE Algorithm Specification defines a key-policy attribute-based encryption system for message space M and access structure space G as a tuple that includes the following algorithms:

Setup (λ, U) → (PK, MK): The setup algorithm takes a security parameter λ and a universe description U as input, which defines the system's set of allowed attributes. It then outputs the public parameters PK and the master secret key MK.

Encrypt (PK, M, S) → CT: The encryption algorithm takes the public parameters PK, a message M, and a set of attributes S as input and produces a ciphertext CT associated with the attribute set.

KeyGen (MK, A) → SK: The key generation algorithm takes the master secret key MK and an access structure A as input and generates a private key SK associated with the attributes.

Algorithm: Dynamic Attribute-Based Encryption Scheme (DABES)

Decrypt (SK, CT) → M. The decryption algorithm requires a private key SK linked to access structure A and a ciphertext CT connected to attribute set S as input. It outputs a message M if S meets A or an error message ⊥ otherwise.

The correctness property requires that for all sufficiently large λ N, all universe descriptions *U, all (PK, MK) Setup (λ, U), all S U, all SK Keygen(MK,A)*, all *M M, all A G* and all *CT Encrypt(PK,M,S)*, if S satisfies A, then *Decrypt(SK,CT)* outputs M.

Security Model for DABE Let Π = (Setup, Encrypt, KeyGen, Decrypt) be a DABE scheme for message space M and access structure space G, and consider the following experiment for an adversary A, parameter λ and attribute universe U.

7.2 Performance Validation

This section provides a comprehensive result analysis of the DABE technique under several attribute execution. Table 1 and figure 5 investigate the encryption time analysis (ET) of the DABE with the existing MAABE (**Multi-Authority Attribute-Based Encryption (MA-ABE)**) technique. GraphPad Prism 10 tool is used to simulate the result with windows-11 Operating system and AMDA processor. Graph Prism's statistical comparison tests (ANOVA, t-tests) can be applied to compare different security approaches or encryption methods to evaluate effectiveness. The results show that the DABE technique has gained effectual outcomes with minimal encryption time under all attribute execution. For instance, with 100 attribute execution, the DABE technique has gained the least ET of 25.81s, whereas the MAABE has accomplished a slightly increased ET of 34.79s, respectively. The average time required for encryption depends on the quantity of attributes involved. Nevertheless, there is a general formula, denoted as eq1, which is used to determine the average encryption time in DABE.

$$T_{enc} = T_k + T_e + T_a$$

---------- *eq1*

T_{enc}: Encryption Time, T_k: KeyGen, T_a: A*ttribute Execution Time*

Table 1. Encryption Time analysis of DABE technique with various attribution execution

Encryption Time Analysis (Sec)		
Attribute Encryption	**MAABE**	**Proposed DABE**
100	34.79	25.81
200	42.62	33.25
300	54.23	40.16
400	63.51	54.06
500	69.45	59.86
600	82.41	71.37
700	91.95	78.14
800	98.07	89.06

Figure 6. Encryption time analysis of proposed DABE

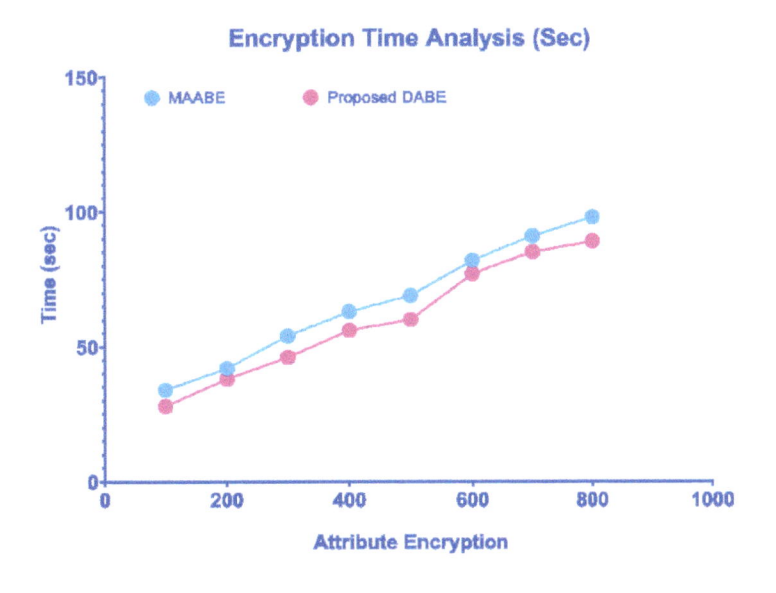

Table 2. Average encryption time analysis

Average Encryption Time Analysis (Sec)		
Attribute Encryption	**MAABE**	**Proposed DABE**
100	34.79	25.81
200	42.62	33.25
300	54.23	40.16
400	63.51	54.06
500	69.45	59.86
600	82.41	71.37
700	91.95	78.14
800	98.07	89.06
Average Time	67.12875	56.46375

$$T_{avg} = \frac{T_{total}}{N}$$

--------- eq2

N: Number of encryption operations.

Figure 7. Average encryption time analysis of proposed DABE

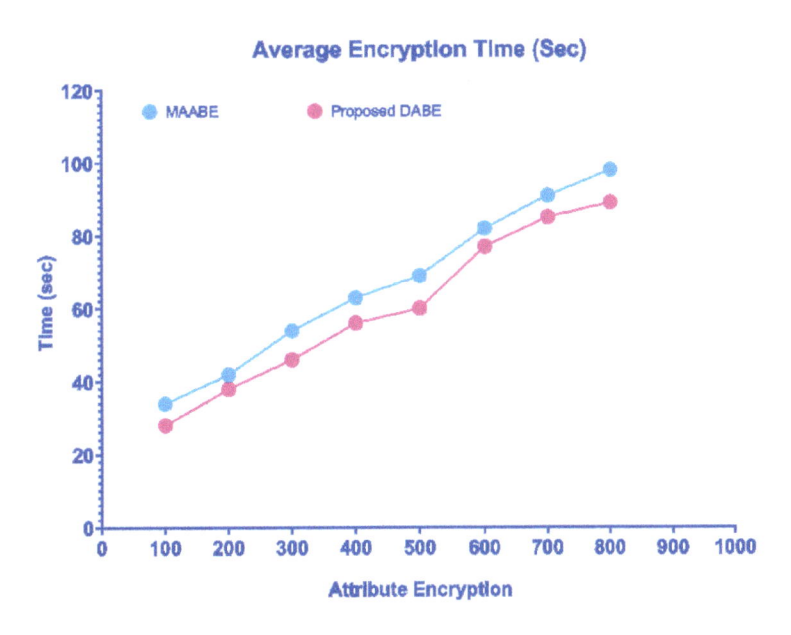

The analysis of the average encryption time (ET) for the DABE in comparison to the existing MAABE technique is presented in Table 2 and Figure 7. The results illustrated that the DABE technique has delivered efficient outcomes with minimal encryption time for all attribute executions. Notably, for 100 to 800 attribute executions, the DABE technique achieved an average ET of 56.463 seconds, while the MAABE resulted in a slightly lower average ET of 67.128 seconds.

Table 3. Decryption time analysis

Decryption Time Analysis (Sec)		
Attribute Encryption	MAABE	Proposed DABE
100	34.79	25.81
200	42.62	33.25
300	54.23	39.16
400	61.51	48.27
500	69.45	55.86
600	79.21	69.44
700	89.35	75.14
800	97.07	83.86

Figure 8. Decryption time analysis of proposed DABE

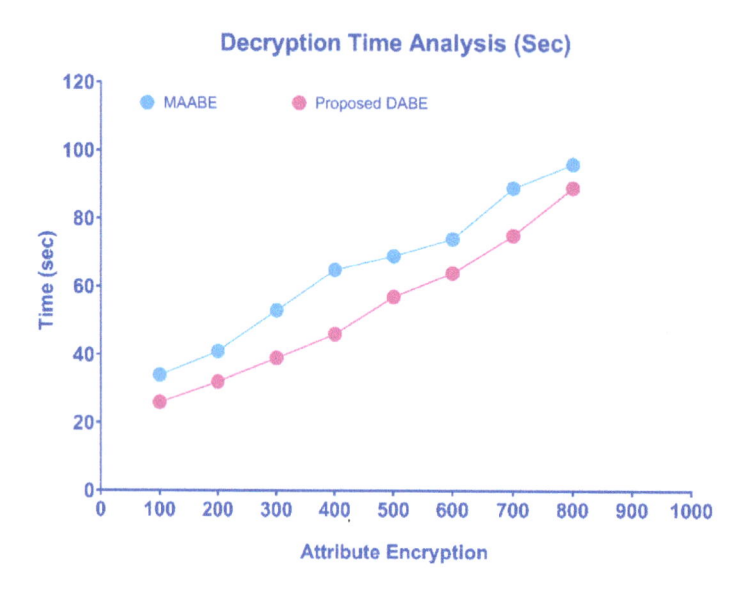

Table 4. Average decryption time analysis

Average Decryption Time (Sec)		
Attribute Decryption	**MAABE**	**Proposed DABE**
100	34	26
200	41	32
300	53	39
400	65	46
500	69	57
600	74	64
700	89	75
800	96	89
Average Time	65.125	53.5

Figure 9. Decryption time analysis of proposed DABE

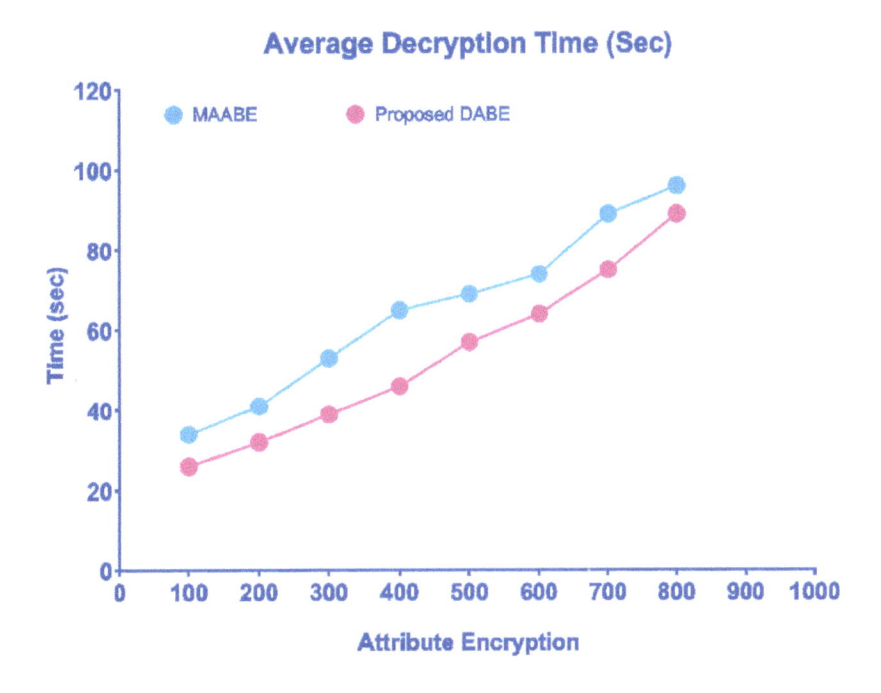

In Table 3 and Figure 7, the result is presented in the decryption time (DT) of the DABE and the MAABE technique. The findings reveal that the DABE technique has produced efficient outcomes with minimal decryption time across all attribute executions. For instance, with 100 attribute executions, the DABE technique achieved the lowest average DT of 25.81 seconds, whereas the MAABE resulted in a slightly longer average DT of 34.79 seconds. The average decryption time analysis for the DABE and the MAABE technique is presented in Table 4 and Figure 8. The results indicate that the DABE technique has demonstrated efficient outcomes with minimal average decryption time across all attribute executions. Specifically, for 100 to 800 attribute executions, the DABE technique achieved the lowest average DT of 53.5 seconds, while the MAABE resulted in a slightly longer average DT of 65.125 seconds.

CONCLUSION

The healthcare industry has significantly enhanced connectivity and operational efficiency with the implementation of IoT technology. However, notable security challenges have emerged as a result. This study presents the vulnerabilities of interconnected healthcare systems and devices, specifically focusing on the dangers linked to unauthorized entry and data breaches involving Personal Health Information (PHI) and telemetry data. The study underscores the significance of proactive and adaptable security measures, such as encryption, access controls, authentication, and data backups, in safeguarding medical information. Furthermore, the analysis explores technological solutions like secure data storage systems and communication channels, offering a comprehensive overview of available tools to mitigate security risks. Looking to the future, the use of Dynamic Attribute-Based Encryption Schemes (DABES) emerges as a promising advancement in medical data security. DABES allows for fine-grained access control by dynamically adjusting permissions based on user attributes and contextual factors, ensuring that only authorized individuals can access specific information. In order to uphold the integrity and security of healthcare delivery, healthcare organizations must promptly and proactively tackle the evolving challenges related to securing medical information systems. Through the implementation of comprehensive and forward-thinking security strategies, healthcare providers can safeguard patient data, improve patient care, and maintain the overall integrity of the healthcare system.

REFERENCES

Adeniyi, E. A., Ogundokun, R. O., & Awotunde, J. B. (2021). IoMT-based wearable body sensors network healthcare monitoring system. *IoT in healthcare and ambient assisted living*, 103-121.

Ahmed, S. F., Alam, M. S. B., Afrin, S., Rafa, S. J., Rafa, N., & Gandomi, A. H. (2024). Insights into Internet of Medical Things (IoMT): Data fusion, security issues and potential solutions. *Information Fusion*, 102, 102060. DOI: 10.1016/j.inffus.2023.102060

Ahmed, S. T., Kumar, V. V., Singh, K. K., Singh, A., Muthukumaran, V., & Gupta, D. (2022). 6G enabled federated learning for secure IoMT resource recommendation and propagation analysis. *Computers & Electrical Engineering*, 102, 108210. DOI: 10.1016/j.compeleceng.2022.108210

Ajagbe, S. A., Awotunde, J. B., Adesina, A. O., Achimugu, P., & Kumar, T. A. (2022). Internet of medical things (IoMT): applications, challenges, and prospects in a data-driven technology. *Intelligent Healthcare: Infrastructure, Algorithms and Management*, 299-319.

Alhaidari, F., Rahman, A., & Zagrouba, R. (2023). Cloud of Things: Architecture, applications and challenges. *Journal of Ambient Intelligence and Humanized Computing*, 14(5), 5957–5975. DOI: 10.1007/s12652-020-02448-3

Alsaffar, A. A., Pham, H. P., Hong, C. S., Huh, E. N., & Aazam, M. (2016). An architecture of IoT service delegation and resource allocation based on collaboration between fog and cloud computing. *Mobile Information Systems*, 2016(1), 6123234. DOI: 10.1155/2016/6123234

Aman, A. H. M., Hassan, W. H., Sameen, S., Attarbashi, Z. S., Alizadeh, M., & Latiff, L. A. (2021). IoMT amid COVID-19 pandemic: Application, architecture, technology, and security. *Journal of Network and Computer Applications*, 174, 102886. DOI: 10.1016/j.jnca.2020.102886 PMID: 34173428

Bhatti, D. S., & Saleem, S. (2020). Ephemeral secrets: Multi-party secret key acquisition for secure ieee 802.11 mobile ad hoc communication. *IEEE Access : Practical Innovations, Open Solutions*, 8, 24242–24257. DOI: 10.1109/ACCESS.2020.2970147

Cozzio, C., Viglia, G., Lemarie, L., & Cerutti, S. (2023). Toward an integration of blockchain technology in the food supply chain. *Journal of Business Research*, 162, 113909. DOI: 10.1016/j.jbusres.2023.113909

Dhagarra, D., Goswami, M., & Kumar, G. (2020). Impact of trust and privacy concerns on technology acceptance in healthcare: An Indian perspective. *International Journal of Medical Informatics*, 141, 104164. DOI: 10.1016/j.ijmedinf.2020.104164 PMID: 32593847

Dhiyya, A. J. A. (2022). Architecture of IoMT in healthcare. *The Internet of Medical Things (IoMT) Healthcare Transformation*, 161-172.

Ghubaish, A., Salman, T., Zolanvari, M., Unal, D., Al-Ali, A., & Jain, R. (2020). Recent advances in the internet-of-medical-things (IoMT) systems security. *IEEE Internet of Things Journal*, 8(11), 8707–8718. DOI: 10.1109/JIOT.2020.3045653

Gupta, B. B., Chaudhary, P., Chang, X., & Nedjah, N. (2022). Smart defense against distributed Denial of service attack in IoT networks using supervised learning classifiers. *Computers & Electrical Engineering*, 98, 107726. DOI: 10.1016/j.compeleceng.2022.107726

Hireche, R., Mansouri, H., & Pathan, A. S. K. (2022). Security and privacy management in Internet of Medical Things (IoMT): A synthesis. *Journal of cybersecurity and privacy, 2*(3), 640-661.

Houssein, E. H., Gad, A. G., Hussain, K., & Suganthan, P. N. (2021). Major advances in particle swarm optimization: Theory, analysis, and application. *Swarm and Evolutionary Computation*, 63, 100868. DOI: 10.1016/j.swevo.2021.100868

Khan, I. A., Razzak, I., Pi, D., Khan, N., Hussain, Y., Li, B., & Kousar, T. (2024). Fed-inforce-fusion: A federated reinforcement-based fusion model for security and privacy protection of IoMT networks against cyber-attacks. *Information Fusion*, 101, 102002. DOI: 10.1016/j.inffus.2023.102002

Kumar, S. S., & Koti, M. S. (2021, December). Efficient Authentication for Securing Electronic Health Records using Algebraic Structure. In *2021 5th International Conference on Electrical, Electronics, Communication, Computer Technologies and Optimization Techniques (ICEECCOT)* (pp. 366-370). IEEE. DOI: 10.1109/ICEECCOT52851.2021.9708050

Kumar, S. S., Muthukumaran, V., Devi, A., Geetha, V., & Yadav, P. N. (2023). A Quantitative Approach of Purposive Sampling Techniques for Security and Privacy Issues in IoT Healthcare Applications. In *Handbook of Research on Advancements in AI and IoT Convergence Technologies* (pp. 281–299). IGI Global. DOI: 10.4018/978-1-6684-6971-2.ch016

Kumar, S. S., & Sanjay, M. (2018). Improved Quality of Patient Care and Data Security Using Cloud Crypto System in EHR. *International Journal of Advanced Studies of Scientific Research*, 3(10).

Kumar, V., Kushwaha, S., Singh, I., Barik, R. K., Singh, G., & Sabraj, M. (2024). Internet of Multimedia Things (IoMT): Communication Techniques Perspective. *5G and Beyond Wireless Networks*, 147-162.

Lee, D., & Yoon, S. N. (2021). Application of artificial intelligence-based technologies in the healthcare industry: Opportunities and challenges. *International Journal of Environmental Research and Public Health*, 18(1), 271. DOI: 10.3390/ijerph18010271 PMID: 33401373

Liu, Y., Zhang, L., Yang, Y., Zhou, L., Ren, L., Wang, F., Liu, R., Pang, Z., & Deen, M. J. (2019). A novel cloud-based framework for the elderly healthcare services using digital twin. *IEEE Access : Practical Innovations, Open Solutions*, 7, 49088–49101. DOI: 10.1109/ACCESS.2019.2909828

Mishna, F., Milne, E., Bogo, M., & Pereira, L. F. (2021). Responding to COVID-19: New trends in social workers' use of information and communication technology. *Clinical Social Work Journal*, 49(4), 484–494. DOI: 10.1007/s10615-020-00780-x PMID: 33250542

Nagarajan, S. M., Anandhan, P., Muthukumaran, V., Uma, K., & Kumaran, U. (2022). Security framework for IoT and deep belief network-based healthcare system using blockchain technology. *International Journal of Electronic Business*, 17(3), 226–243. DOI: 10.1504/IJEB.2022.124324

Narang, M., Jatain, A., & Punetha, N. (2023, November). A Survey on Detection of Man-In-The-Middle Attack in IoMT Using Machine Learning Techniques. In *International Conference on Computational Intelligence* (pp. 117-132). Singapore: Springer Nature Singapore.

Pelekoudas-Oikonomou, F., Ribeiro, J. C., Mantas, G., Sakellari, G., & Gonzalez, J. (2023). Prototyping a hyperledger fabric-based security architecture for iomt-based health monitoring systems. *Future Internet*, 15(9), 308. DOI: 10.3390/fi15090308

Pramanik, S., Pandey, D., Joardar, S., Niranjanamurthy, M., Pandey, B. K., & Kaur, J. (2023, October). An overview of IoT privacy and security in smart cities. In *AIP Conference Proceedings* (Vol. 2495, No. 1). AIP Publishing. DOI: 10.1063/5.0123511

Rajadevi, R., Venkatachalam, K., Masud, M., AlZain, M. A., & Abouhawwash, M. (2023). Proof of Activity Protocol for IoMT Data Security. *Computer Systems Science and Engineering*, 44(1). Advance online publication. DOI: 10.32604/csse.2023.024537

Shakeel, T., Habib, S., Boulila, W., Koubaa, A., Javed, A. R., Rizwan, M., Gadekallu, T. R., & Sufiyan, M. (2023). A survey on COVID-19 impact in the healthcare domain: Worldwide market implementation, applications, security and privacy issues, challenges and future prospects. *Complex & Intelligent Systems*, 9(1), 1027–1058. DOI: 10.1007/s40747-022-00767-w PMID: 35668731

Singh, R. P., Javaid, M., Haleem, A., Vaishya, R., & Ali, S. (2020). Internet of Medical Things (IoMT) for orthopaedic in COVID-19 pandemic: Roles, challenges, and applications. *Journal of Clinical Orthopaedics and Trauma*, 11(4), 713–717. DOI: 10.1016/j.jcot.2020.05.011 PMID: 32425428

Srivastava, J., Routray, S., Ahmad, S., & Waris, M. M. (2022). [Retracted] Internet of Medical Things (IoMT)-Based Smart Healthcare System: Trends and Progress. *Computational Intelligence and Neuroscience*, 2022(1), 7218113. PMID: 35880061

Wei, T., Liu, S., & Du, X. (2022). Learning-based efficient sparse sensing and recovery for privacy-aware IoMT. *IEEE Internet of Things Journal*, 9(12), 9948–9959. DOI: 10.1109/JIOT.2022.3163593

Zhang, G., & Navimipour, N. J. (2022). A comprehensive and systematic review of the IoT-based medical management systems: Applications, techniques, trends and open issues. *Sustainable Cities and Society*, 82, 103914. DOI: 10.1016/j.scs.2022.103914

Zikria, Y. B., Afzal, M. K., & Kim, S. W. (2020). Internet of multimedia things (IoMT): Opportunities, challenges and solutions. *Sensors (Basel)*, 20(8), 2334. DOI: 10.3390/s20082334 PMID: 32325944

Chapter 9
Revolutionizing Patient Care Through the Convergence of IoMT and Generative AI

Dankan Gowda V.
https://orcid.org/0000-0003-0724-0333
Department of Electronics and Communication Engineering, BMS Institute of Technology and Management, Karnataka, India

Premkumar Reddy
Independent Researcher, Frisco, USA

Vidya Rajasekhara Reddy Tetala
https://orcid.org/0009-0005-2417-8318
Independent Researcher, Richmond, USA

P. Krishnamoorthy
https://orcid.org/0000-0002-1901-8599
Department of Computer Science and Engineering, Sasi Institute of Technology and Engineering, India

Kottala Sri Yogi
https://orcid.org/0000-0002-3671-7420
Department of Operations, Symbiosis Institute of Business Management, Hyderabad, India & Symbiosis International University, Pune, India

ABSTRACT

The incorporation of the Internet of Medical Things and Generative AI to this process shall transform patient care by offering continuous tracking, analysis and individualized progression control. This chapter is dedicated to the synergistic fusion of IoT in Medical Technology (IoMT) and Generative Artificial Intelligence and provides a brief summary of what it is, how it functions, and what can be expected in the future in the field of health care. When combined with the data acquiring capacity of IoMT and analytical potential of Generative AI, hospitals and other medical facilities have the potential to bring diagnosis and treatment to a higher level. Some real-life usage examples of the combined uses of SDN

DOI: 10.4018/979-8-3693-6180-1.ch009

and IoT in health care are shown through different use cases, including chronic disease management, elderly care, virtual health assistance, and prognostic health management and maintenance of healthcare facilities' equipment and tools.

INTRODUCTION

Technology has continued to evolve and this has seen some drastic changes in different sectors including the health sector. Of these innovations, IoMT and Generative AI are revolutionary tools that are likely to revolutionize the delivery of patients' care. Combining IoMT with Generative AI, a new step in the development of medical technology has been achieved, which can contribute to increasing the effectiveness of diagnostics and treatment, increasing the accuracy of diagnosis, as well as identifying individual approaches to the management of the patient's illness. This chapter aims at discussing these technologies combined and its effect on the current healthcare systems.

Definition and Overview of IoMT

Internet of Medical Things (IoMT) can be defined as a system in which the medical devices, software applications and healthcare systems are connected over the internet for collecting the health data or information and analyzing it. IoMT is identified as contextualizing a broad range of devices that fall in the category of wearable health checkup devices, implantable devices, smart sensors, and remote monitoring equipment to collect quantitative real time health statistics from patients (L. Chen, H. Wang, and S. Liu, 2023). It is then forwarded to the healthcare givers in order to facilitate constant supervision and timely responses to any irregularities. The main goal of IoMT is to create effective ways of communication between healthcare consumers and providers, hence improving on the lives of the consumers and easing the workload of the systems.

Definition and Overview of Generative AI

Generative AI is a type of entire artificial intelligence where it is aimed at creating new content that is usually similar to the content being generated. Generative AI on the other hand differs from the traditional kind of AI in that it does not employ set rules and patterns to emulate everyday behaviors, rather Generative AI employs a set of machine learning algorithms like GANs or VAEs which train on big data sets to generate new outputs (J. Smith, A. Patel, and L. Roberts, 2023). When applied in the context of healthcare, Generative AI is capable of the following: modeling of patients' conditions, creating synthetic medical imaging, creating individual treatment plans and even disease prognosis. Generative AI's training from real-life data is useful in helping healthcare providers make better and more informed decisions that will benefit the patients.

Figure.1. provides an indication of how the Internet of Medical Things (IoMT) complements Generative AI in the context of healthcare (R. Kishore Kumar, M. Pandidurai, and M. S. C. Senthil Kamalesh, 2023). The figure shows how different IoMT devices including sensors, wearables, medical equipment, and machines discuss with Generative AI models that collect and analyze the data. It also allows surveillance, prognostications, and distinct and individual patient care, which overall improves patients' quality of care and firm functioning (B. Ram Vishal, M. U. Shankar, and K. A. M, 2023). The technical representation focuses on the transfer of information from the IoMT devices to AI processing units, and the purpose of each to the overall healthcare system.

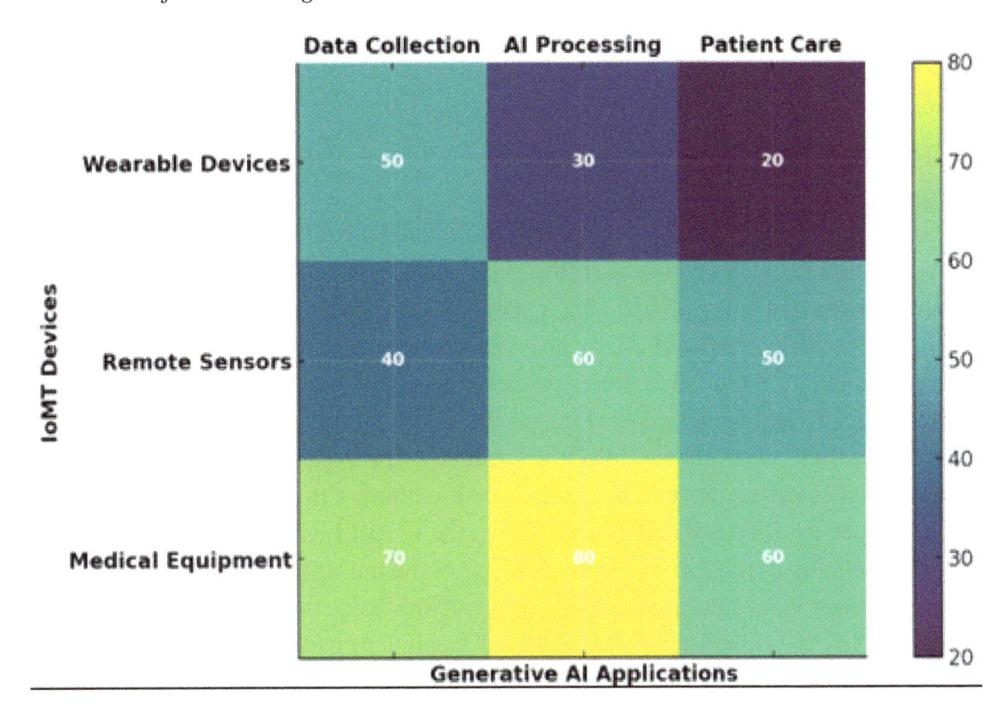

Figure 1. Overview of IoMT and generative AI in healthcare

	Data Collection	AI Processing	Patient Care
Wearable Devices	50	30	20
Remote Sensors	40	60	50
Medical Equipment	70	80	60

The Need for Convergence in Modern Healthcare

The use case of IoMT and Generative AI in modern healthcare has emerged out of the call for improvement in terms of efficiency, individualisation, and preventative capabilities of the healthcare industry (S. Gupta, K. Johnson, and Y. Wang, 2023). This is due to the continuously rising prevalence of chronic diseases, the ageing population and the added intricacies of health systems. IoMT means to gather lots of real-time data from patients and GAIA has the capability to crunch the data, analyze it, and draw useful conclusions (D. Palanikkumar, P. A. Mary, and A. Y. Begum, 2023). When combined, the suite of smart technologies tends to offer a vertical and integrated healthcare system that keeps track of a patient's wellbeing in parallel with predicting and thwarting any health-related challenges before they lead to emergencies (D. Brown, M. Davis, and C. Lee, 2023). Thanks to this convergence, it becomes possible to save the healthcare model which moves from an acute care, based on cure, to a preventive care.

Objectives of the Chapter

The unfolding chapter's main focus is the comparative analysis of how IoMT and Generative AI can revolutionise patient care. This chapter will seek to describe the details of how the technologies mentioned above function, use of these technologies in the current healthcare, and the advantages that are derived from them. Furthermore, the chapter will present the limitation of integrating IoMT and Generative AI such as data privacy, security as well as the ethical implication. In this chapter, real-life examples of these technologies will be presented and the reader will be able to understand not only their use, but also the benefits for patients. Finally, the chapter aims at stressing the need to adopt such advanced technologies in the provision of healthcare services so that a better system of serving the patient's needs can be harnessed.

LITERATURE SURVEY

The latter involves the integration of Internet of Medical Things (IoMT) and Generative Artificial Intelligence (AI) which marks a revolution if introduced into the healthcare system since it presents gigantic solutions to some of challenges affecting patients (A. Nareshkumar and B. Gururaj, 2022). Thus, before assessing the prospects as well as the possible consequences of the observed congruence, it is pertinent to analyze literature related to the given fields of study. This literature survey will give historical information of IoMT and Generative AI in current health scenario along with its trends in future.

Development of IoMT in Healthcare: IoMT has been derived from the Internet of Things also known as IoT which entails connecting devices and systems to the internet to enable them to communicate and exchange data. As per the industry analysis of IoMT, the global healthcare industry has been widely accepting IoMT technologies most prominently because of the multiple health check-ups necessary for a patient and the necessity to monitor patients from remote locations. Some of the prior and initial works include; Gubbi et al. (2013) pointed out that, through IoT, healthcare had the potential of being transformed by monitoring patients' health parameters in real time (A. Kumar, S. Sharma, and P. Verma, 2023). Ever since, IoMT has evolved into all sorts of devices that comprise fitness bracelets, smart implants and home-monitoring devices that capture vital signs, compliance with medication and other parameters.

Current Applications of IoMT: A study conducted in the past provides evidence that IoMT plays a role in assisting the treatment of chronic illness, enhancing patients' well-being, and minimizing expenditures in healthcare. For instance, smartwatches such as the Apple Watch and Fitbit devices have been linked with the health management systems to facilitate the recording of the heart rate, physical activities and sleep patterns in order to aid the doctors (R. Kavitha, A. Kumar, V. Kalpana, and V. Hariram, 2023). Findings by Lee and Park (2020) have shown that such devices are effective in promoting patient interaction and management thereby improving their general health. In addition, IoMT has been valuable in RPM given the strict measures that ensue the COVID-19 pandemic regulating discharge of physical contact. Mehrotra et al., (2020), revealed that remote monitoring reduced hospitalization and offered constant care to the patients with chronic diseases.

Generative AI in Healthcare: Generative AI has great opportunities in many fields, especially in creating new content; it is more discussed in such areas as image generation, text generation, and simulation modeling (M. Thompson, R. Allen, and J. Garcia, 2023). In healthcare, Generative AI is used to produce artificial medical data which are useful in putting through machine learning models without violating patient's privacy right. Research done by Frid-Adar et al. (2018) have demonstrated that GANs can generate realistic medical images that are almost half real. This capability is especially helpful in expanding upon data sets, like those in which it is difficult to acquire a great deal of labeled examples in medical imaging applications.

Emerging Trends and Challenges: Currently, there are not many studies about the combination of IoMT and Generative AI; however, the available studies imply further possibilities. For instance, when integrating real-time data from IoMT devices with Generative AI there is likely to be improvements in the predictive models' accuracy (S. Archana Shreee, B. Maheshwari, and G. Jeevitha Sai, 2023). This integration could help bring about the concept of personalized medicine where the treatment regime would depend on the profile of the patient that is in the clinical picture, thus improving the patient's prognosis (L. Zhang, H. Chen, and X. Liu, 2023). However, there are several challenges that need to be overcome; these include; data privilege and security, compatibility challenges, and the lack of proper regulatory policies. Other scholars such as Riazul Islam et al.2015 have proposed that there is need to enhance the secure ways of communicating patient details and encryption methods to enhance security of patients' information.

IOMT: CURRENT LANDSCAPE AND CAPABILITIES

The IoMT could be viewed as a significant advancement in the healthcare system as it allows the unceasing assessment of the health indicators with the focus on the real-time data gathering and analysis. IoMT stands for the internet of medical things that are devices, sensors, software applications and systems that can capture, monitor, and transmit medical data over the Internet to improve patient care (M. Kranthi and R. C. Tanguturi, 2023). This has created a dynamic picture of IoMT as it is divided into various parts and its components are increasingly being implemented across the healthcare sector to significantly transform the way Information is captured, exchanged, analyzed and used to enhance patient care.

In the following section the design or layout or IoMT in a healthcare setting is presented Mathews et al., (2019) in figure 2 illustrates the different layers of IoMT. This figure contains such things as smartwatch, remote monitoring devices, and medical devices that monitor health information (R. C. Tanguturi, L. S. V. S. L, S. R. C. K, and V. C. H, 2023). Thus, it demonstrates how such components are connected through data connection points and storage clouds, as well as how the information is transferred and managed. The architecture diagram aims at the centrality of data processing and integration in order to produce real-time, accurate and timely health information for the providers.

In pie chart format, Figure 3 shows how data is processed in an IoMT ecosystem with detailed description of every section. This figure categorizes and illustrates the different kind of data that is gathered by IoMT devices including vital data, environmental, wearable, image, and record data (R. V. Mailapur and M. K, 2023). The figure then goes ahead to present the percentage likelihood of each of these data types thus facilitating understanding of the diversity as well as distribution of data dealt with by IoMT systems (S. Venkatakiran, B. Ashreetha, and N. S. Reddy, 2023). This data representation emphasises the challenge of dealing with many concurrent sources of information and points to the fact that data processing and mixture techniques in particular are among the critical factors that impact on the improvement of healthcare effectively.

Figure 2. IoMT architecture in healthcare

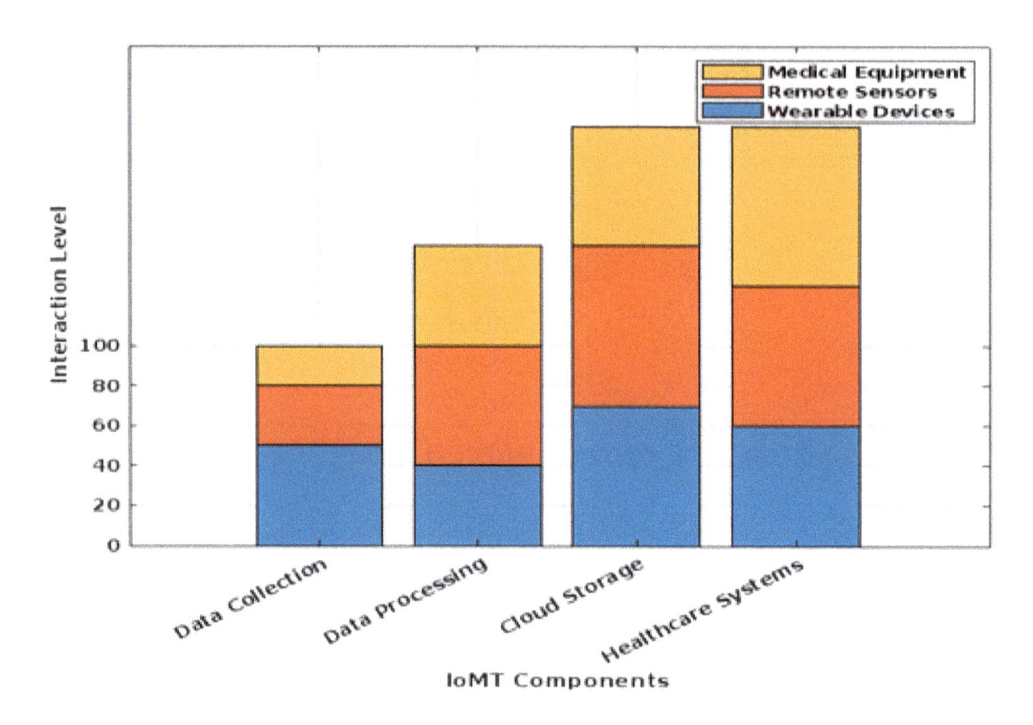

Figure 3. Data flow in IoMT ecosystem

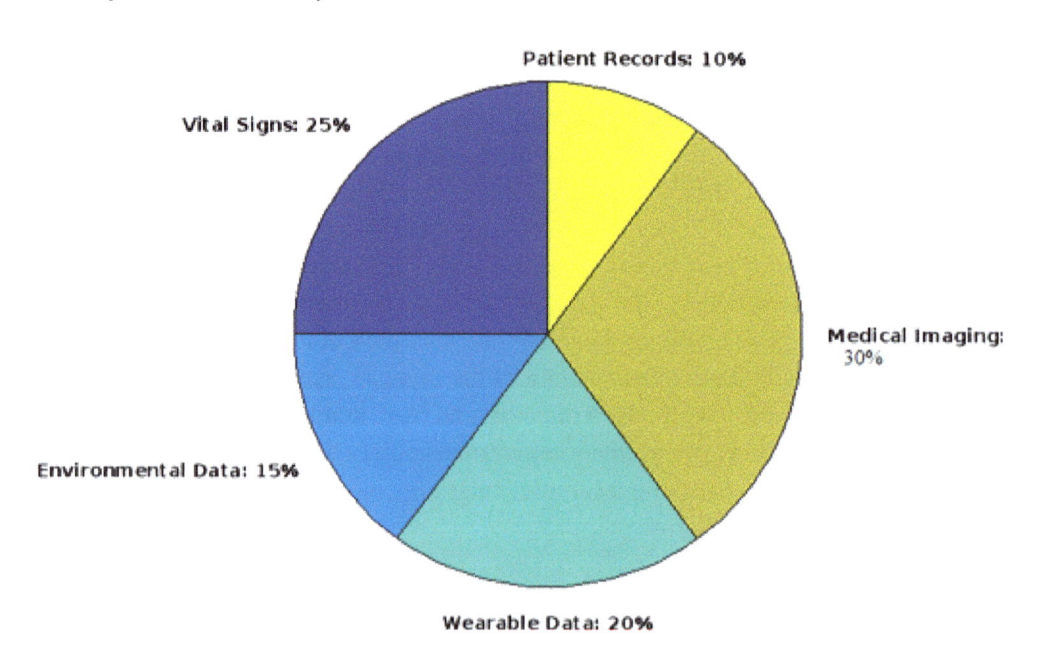

Key Components of IoMT: Sensors, Wearables, Remote Monitoring Devices

IoMT has several major parts through which it forms a composite health care system. Sensors can be considered as a fundamental building block used in many different applications and are incorporated in devices like medical equipment, and wearable applications where physiological metrics like heart rates, blood pressure, glucose level, and body temperature are measured. These are very delicate sensors and are designed to give accurate Health status data and in real time hence very vital for ongoing health status monitoring (Sadashiva V. Chakrasali, Chanakya Kumar, Abhay Chaturvedi, and A. Azhagu Jaisudhan Pazhani, 2023). Smart watches, health monitoring systems and advanced medical devices, like, healing sensors, blood pressure monitors, and sleep trackers are useful tools that people and patients have been willingly engaging to track and monitor their every day and night life movements. The benefits of these wearables include the fact that they are easy to use and do not require any invasive procedure so as to monitor the patient, and can also send data collected to the health care providers over the wireless network (B. Singh, T. Yang, and R. Fernandez, 2023). Telemonitoring devices are crucial in the care of patients with chronic disease ensuring timely and easy health parameters measurements including oxygen saturation, ECG or even EEG. These devices contribute to early diagnosis of health complications thus eliminating recurrent attendance to hospitals.

Data Collection, Transmission, and Integration in Healthcare Systems

The use of IoMT therefore largely depends on efficiencies in the capturing, transmitting and utilizing of data in the healthcare setting. At the sensor level, data collection starts real-time patient data that is received and collected continuously. This data is then wirelessly sent to other consolidated systems or in some cases to the healthcare providers through secure links (Hombalimath, D. Palanikkumar, and N. Patwari, 2023). Bluetooth, Wi-Fi and cellular networks are used for transmitting data and it is a priority to make sure that information is communicated as fast as possible and efficiently. Data integration concerns the process by which the said information is compiled into EHRs and other HISs whereby the providers can retrieve patient profiles (Namitha A R, Manu Y M, Rashmi G R, and Veera Sivakumar Chinamuttevi, 2022). This integrated data is commonly subjected to more intricate analysis and computer learning making it easier to identify tendencies of patient health, risks of imminent conditions and recommend individual care.

Current Applications of IoMT in Healthcare

It has been widely used in different sections of health care systems and greatly contributes to the improvement of the patient's management. Another major application that is driving the use of IoMT is the chronic disease where the devices can be used to track illnesses like diabetes, hypertension, and heart diseases (P. Ramesh Naidu and N. Guruprasad, 2021). An example is the continuous glucose monitoring system whereby diabetic clients can monitor their blood sugar level, so that disease management is enhanced. Another important application is the remote patient monitoring especially for elderly patients or patients who find it difficult to move around (K. Park, M. Lee, and S. Kim, 2023). Sensors would be utilized through IoMT devices to capture the vital signs and the other essential health indicators to enable caregivers to follow up with patients in their homes and not hospitals meaning less expenses in the course of treatment.

Challenges and Limitations

However, there is still misconception, risk and drawbacks related to IoMT that has to be addressed in order to fully harness the potential of this technology (G. A, A. B. Naik, and N. HG, 2021). The first would be the manipulation of client data with a lot of caution especially due to issues of privacy and security. As more and more facilities and organizations embrace the use of internet technology in the remote management and sharing of large volume of sensitive health information the patients data confidentiality is at risk of violation through hacking, data leakage or any unlawful interference (K. Jeevan and B. M. Sathisha, 2020). A lot of effort should be made to make sure that such information is secured by the right encryption practices. Another challenge of Iot is the problem of interconnectivity; sometimes IoMT devices are developed by different manufactures and hence their implementation standard differs across healthcare systems. Some of the important criteria that are must for implementing big data tools include standardization and compatibility in terms of exchanging data (U. K N and R. V M, 2022). Additionally, it may be difficult to get a precise metric or even quantify random biological processes owing to the fluctuating and diverse nature of IoMT devices that record such information. In general, IoMT devices must be able to receive the right input and present accurate data: for this, calibration, validation, or relevant systems' compliance with stringent legislation is necessary (M. R. G and H. Anandaram, 2022). In this case, utilization and maintenance of the IoMT framework prove costly and, therefore, acts as a barrier to access in cases where it is limited to small health care providers and those in low resource areas. To embrace these challenges, appropriate technologies, policy implementations and right investment strategy for the IoMT has to be enforced in the health sector.

GENERATIVE AI: A GAME CHANGER IN HEALTHCARE

Particular emphasis should be placed on the fact that can be called Generative Artificial Intelligence or AI, which has recently emerged in the field of health care as a tool that opens the possibility of creating, modeling, and solving various medical problems with the help of data (V. Iyer, G. Desai, and N. Patil, 2023). In contrast to the traditional AI that is described by its capacity to sort and forecast or generate data which has not been programmed into it, the Generative AI provides data with a statistical density like the training data (Revanna C R, B. Kameswara Rao, and Parismita Sarma, 2022). This capability is based on the current best in class machine learning techniques of GANs and VAEs; however, it is active and live area of AI research. Supposing that by means of Generative AI, quantitative data can be provided as real as in the example of healthcare, it is possible to increase the diagnostic and effective treatment, the drugs creation, and the utilization of imaging (S. Reddy P and P. S. Patwal, 2022). The components of the Generative AI model are shown in the Figure 4 Therein, the primary component is the Generative Adversarial Network or GAN for short. The diagram includes the primary components of a GAN: the generator and the discriminator and works of each of the two (S. R. Kawale and S. P. Diwan, 2022). The generator is to generate synthetic data while the discriminator is to evaluate the synthetic data generated by checking its authenticity or fake hence being used to make the generator refine on it. This figure helps to develop rather a basic understanding related to one of the key steps in Data Generation based on the Generative AI Models, which are widely used in Healthcare for creation of the synthetic data for training coaching modeling, simulation, and for making anticipations and forecasts.

The Temporal analysis in AI applications can be seen in figure 5 where Long Short-Term Memory (LSTM) networks are used. The figure illustrates the time series whereby LSTM handles sequences for the purpose of making future estimations (H. Wu, S. Patel, and X. Lin, 2023). For this, the figure demonstrates the input data over time combined with the predicted output, regarding the extent to which LSTM can handle dependent information through time. This is particularly useful in health care where data streaming and real time predictions if critical, such as, patient's vital signs or progression of the disease.

Figure 4. Generative AI model architecture

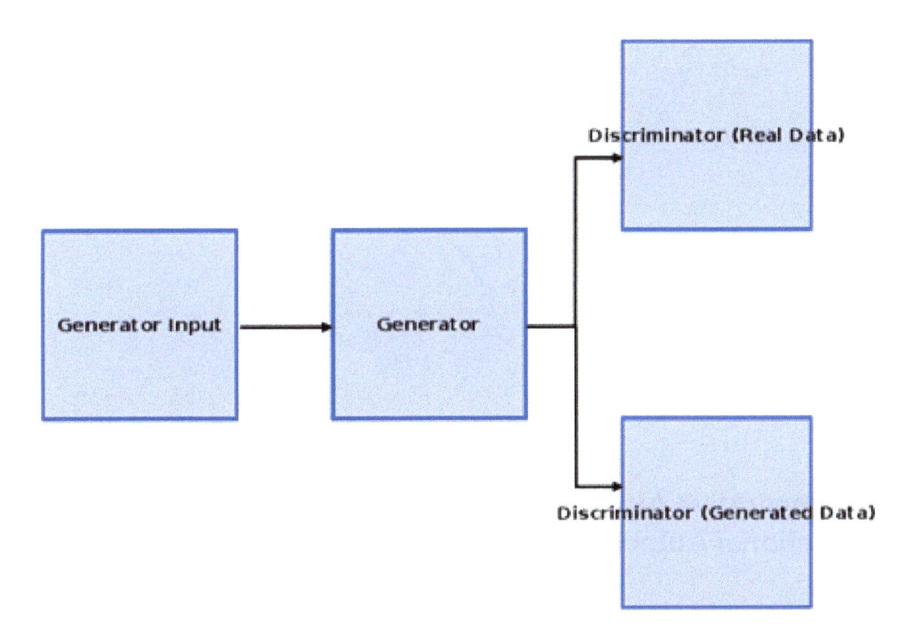

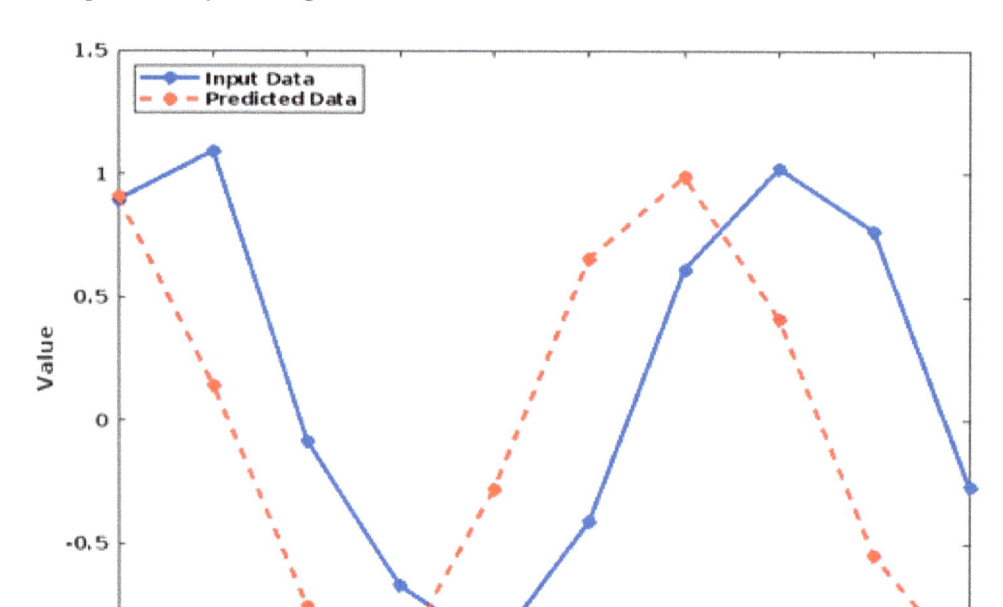

Figure 5. Temporal analysis using LSTM

Explanation of Generative AI: Concepts and Mechanisms (e.g., GANs, Variational Autoencoders)

In other words, in generative AI, the AI learns the priors of the data and then the AI is trained to mimic the structure of the data. The key technique that is used mostly within Generative AI is the concept of the Generative Adversarial Network or GAN, proposed by Ian Goodfellow and his team members in 2014. GANs offer two neural networks, combatively known as a generator and a discriminator; these two networks are trained in parallel. The generator generates new data samples and the discriminator on the other end tries to determine whether they are real (B. Kameswara Rao, Abhay Chaturvedi, and Naziya Hussain, 2022). The generator receive feedback from the discriminator and strives to make them send back more realistic data making the output better M. Swathi Pai, M. Shruthi, and B. Naveen K, 2020). Another method is another deep learning method called Variational Autoencoders (VAEs) that applies the process of encoding of the given data inputs and decoding of the data in the input space with the aim of getting data similar to the input data set. VAEs are particularly useful when the output data should follow a restrained variance, therefore VAEs are relevant to applications, where variance should remain under certain control.

Applications of Generative AI in Healthcare: Diagnosis, Treatment Planning, Drug Discovery

Noteworthy is the fact that the use of generative AI is gradually increasing across all the fields of healthcare and in general contributes to the work of the medical expert. Generative AI in Diagnostic The Generative AI can assist in the diagnosis of diseases by creating illusions of data fed to machines learning algorithms where data set is a rare thing (K. B. Naveen, M. Ramesha, and G. N. Pai, 2020). For example, GANs are utilized in synthesizing fake medical image which helps in training of a diagnostic model for diseases such as cancer, heart diseases and Neurological disorders. Clinical treatment planning: Generative AI is used to show an avatar of patient's circumstance to strictly estimating its reaction to treatment. It is most relevant in the field of such a phenomenon as personalized medicine, in which the treatment is based on the patient's data (P. Ramesh Naidu and N. Guruprasad, 2020). When applying Generative AI it is possible to generate new molecules rather fast, and also estimate how well they would respond to the potential therapeutic points which helps to shorten the process of searching for effective drugs (M. Green, F. Lopez, and T. Brown, 2023). It has been used in discovery of new antibiotics and other therapeutic drugs such as antiviral and other related drugs.

The Role of Generative AI in Enhancing Medical Imaging and Predictive Analytics

Generative AI has made a impact in many field one of its major applications is in medical imaging. The usefulness of Generative AI is in its ability to complement existing Knowtion databases with large numbers of realistic synthetic samples derived from training sets, helping to enhance machine learning models used when analysing images (K. Prasad, S. Dekka, R. c. Tanguturi, and G. Poornima, 2022). For instance, GANs can have a capability of developing horrifying pictures of disease growth on the human body, thereby helping machines to discover signs of tumor and distinguish between healthy and cancerous tissues. Further, Generative AI will also more the quality of the images and less the noisy ones for the better interpretation of the images by the radiologist when making diagnosis (H. Anandaram, N. B. A, N. Gupta, and B. K. Verma, 2023). In the context of predictive analytics, Generative AI can approximate the patient's paths by painting possible scenarios with the data collected in the past. It means that healthcare providers will be able to predict potential issues in patients' condition and ensure proper treatment is done to enhance the quality of the outcomes achieved.

Challenges and Ethical Considerations in Generative AI

As much as AI has shown some potential in the Generative approach for different sectors and healthcare in particular, there exist main problems and issue with it. Of them, data privacy and security remain one of the most significant concerns such as even synthesising new data relies on patient records' availability. Privacy as one of the most valuable components of HIPAA has to be properly ensured for data to be protected from unauthorized access (K. Patel, L. Moore, and H. Singh, 2023). The next difficulty is that of Bias and Generative AI models require feeding data to them, and they are as effective as the data given to them. Another way that the nature of training data affects the delivered outputs concerns the eventuality that if the training data is biased in any specific way, then the output will also manifest this bias and in essence, this may well lead to rather unfair or even incorrect outcomes (K. Prasad, N.

Anil Kumar, N. S. Reddy, and B. Ashreetha, 2023). Other ethical issues which should be considered include; The synthetic data as they may not simulate close to the actual environment. Such concerns raise questions on the reliability of the information obtained from the utilization of the AI as well as the evidentiality of the tool that is used in the clinical decision making. Moreover, given many challenges of Generative AI in drug discovery and treatment planning, there are many regulatory and safety issues because drug development always implies safety precautions.

In general, there is nothing impossible in changes of an attitude to healthcare as the new type of modeling and approach to the diagnostics of diseases and treatments with the help of Generative AI (T. Chen, R. Gupta, and Y. Zhang, 2023). This makes it possible for healthcare actualizers, scientific researchers, and political actors to obtain plausible data and to model complex setting.

CONVERGENCE OF IOMT AND GENERATIVE AI: A NEW PARADIGM

When two trends – the Internet of Medical Things and Generative AI – meet, they bring a new paradigm to the sphere of healthcare that could potentially change the course of patient management radically. IoMT is the integration of real-time data collection by merging with generative AI which has enhanced data analysis and generation ability, it will revolutionize the healthcare system by providing improved efficiency, accuracy, and personalization (S. Lee, M. Choi, and D. Park, 2023). It also improves the capacity to assess diagnosing patients and also empowers the development of a unique clinical management strategy, prescriptive business analytics, and other therapeutic formulations. Figure 6 shows the performance of the different methods of processing as bar graph with the traditional, cloud and the IoT-edge-cloud and hybrid processing. This figure illustrates the outstanding benefits of employing hybrid processing schemes whereby data processing is done locally at IoT devices, at the edge, and in the cloud. This enables organisation to cut out, not only latency and bandwidth usage, but also enhance the dependability as well as velocity of health care applications, making real time data processing and decision making more conceivable. Figure 7: Line chart of real time analysis results based on system response time under different conditions is presented. This figure demonstrates how the workload evolves across time, and how exactly IoMT & AI integration is capable of keeping response times receptive even at higher workload cultures. With the help of the chart, it is possible to show how the real-time data processing is effective and reliable when it comes to such important fields like healthcare that require instant data analysis and further actions based on this analysis.

Benefits of Integrating IoMT with Generative AI

This section now presents some of the benefits regarding the use of IoMT connected with Generative AI for developing different aspects of medicine. The first one is the traditional and arguably the most well-known: the ability to observe patient's state constantly and in real-time respectively, see that he or she may be at risk of developing certain health problem and address the issue before it turns into something more serious.

Figure 6. Hybrid processing performance

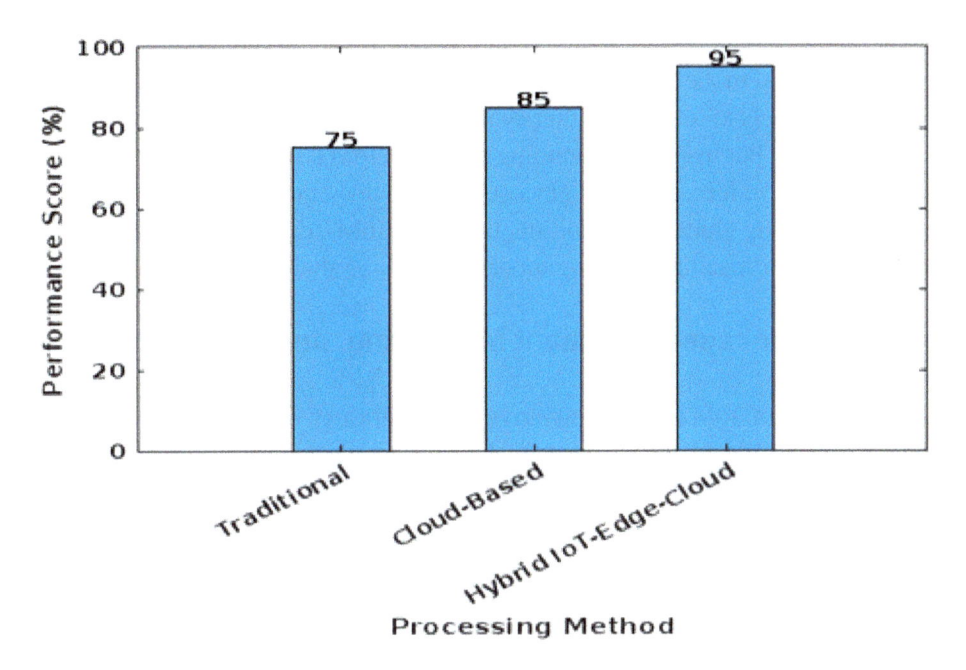

Figure 7. Real-time analysis

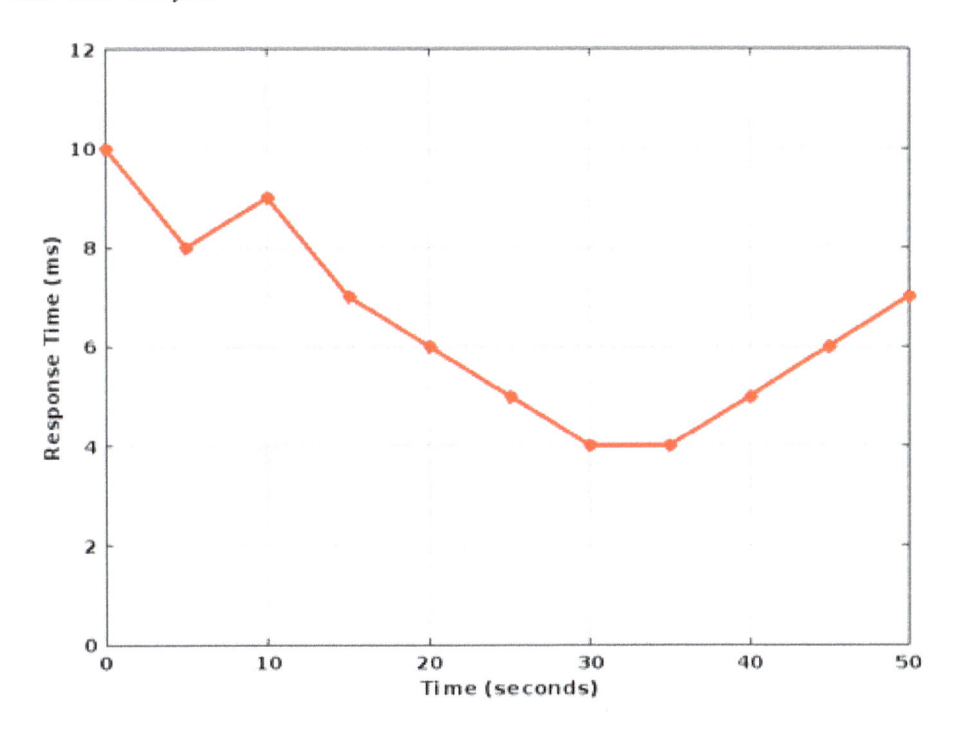

How IoMT Data Enhances the Capabilities of Generative AI Models

The extensive real-time data created by IoMT devices means there is a large amount of information that makes the Generative AI models far superior in functionality. With this data at its disposal, Generative AI can develop better models to forecast further evolution of diseases, efficacy of certain therapies, and patients' reactions to them. For instance, examining data from IoMT smart glucose monitors, Generative AI can automatically learn to forecast blood glucose levels in diabetic patients with a clear focus toward dosing insulin and regulating glucose. In addition, the use of IoMT data leads Generative AI to produce synthetic data to train other machine learning models increasing their accuracy and resilience.

Synergies in Data Processing, Patient Monitoring, and Personalized Care

The complementarity of IoMT and Generative AI occurs not only in data management, patient observation but also in individualised approaches. IoMT devices monitor patients' data which are then fed into Generative AI models to perform preliminary analytics of the data collected. Such integration also allows the capturing of constant updated patient data; this means that the healthcare providers can monitor the patient's condition and other signs as well as promptly identify abnormalities, or changes in the condition of the patient. Apart from increasing the chances of treatment success this kind of approach has a positive impact on patient satisfaction and loyalty since they receive individualized care.

Technological Framework for Integration: Architecture and Workflow

A sound technological foundation which provides suitable methods for data acquisition, evaluation and analysis relevant to IoMT and Generative AI proves mandatory for the successful occurrence of these fields. It is also often deeply layered and may comprise of the data acquisition layer, the messaging layer, the storage layer and the processing layer. The following are the layers of IoMT architecture: Data acquisition layer: In this layer, the IoMT devices continuously collect the health data The Information is then sent to the central data store through the wired or wireless connections such as Bluetooth, WIFI or mobile network. The data storage layer integrated features are the cloud premise storage ones that pertain to scaling the database, as well as real-time data processing capabilities. Finally, the data is fed into advanced analytics platforms for generating the insights, and build predictions using Generative AI models. The loop formed by data feedback of acquiring information from the environment, data processing of the acquired data, and subsequent actions based on the gathered data are never-ending, and in this cycle, the information found through AI models is employed as a reference tool as to the patients' treatment approaches, which are then implemented and monitored constantly through connected IoMT gadgets. This cycle enables the healthcare providers to advance in the manner of delivering care to the clients that we serve in enhancing their health.

CASE STUDIES: REAL-TIME APPLICATIONS OF IOMT AND GENERATIVE AI IN PATIENT CARE

The advent of IoMT along with Generative AI has opened up fresh ways to approach the patient care that involve the use of real time generated data that would otherwise might not be useful for the treatment of patients. Several examples are provided below to show how these technologies are deployed, but their potential has been evident in aggravating chronic diseases, elderly care, patient support services, and equipment maintenance when using IoMT and Generative AI.

The case of using IoMT and AI in chronic diseases is depicted in Figure 8 by a line graph showing the blood glucose levels by time distance with and without AI. From the figure, it is evident that AI intervention will ensure good control of the health parameters and thus achieve improved and stable blood glucose levels. This illustration brings out the possibility of managing chronicle diseases by using IoMT and AI to monitor patients and adjust the treatment plan as and when necessary to enhance the outcome.

Lastly, a line plot was used to compare the actual versus the predicted maintenance schedule for medical equipment as shown in the Figure 9 below. The figure demonstrates how by analysing data analytics one can determine maintenance needs before equipment failures using predictive maintenance techniques. This proactive approach assists in reducing failures that cause equipment unavailability, thus increasing useful life and availability of medical-bay instruments. Using of IoMT and AI in the healthcare facility focused on the improvement of operational efficiency and safety is highlighted in the visualization.

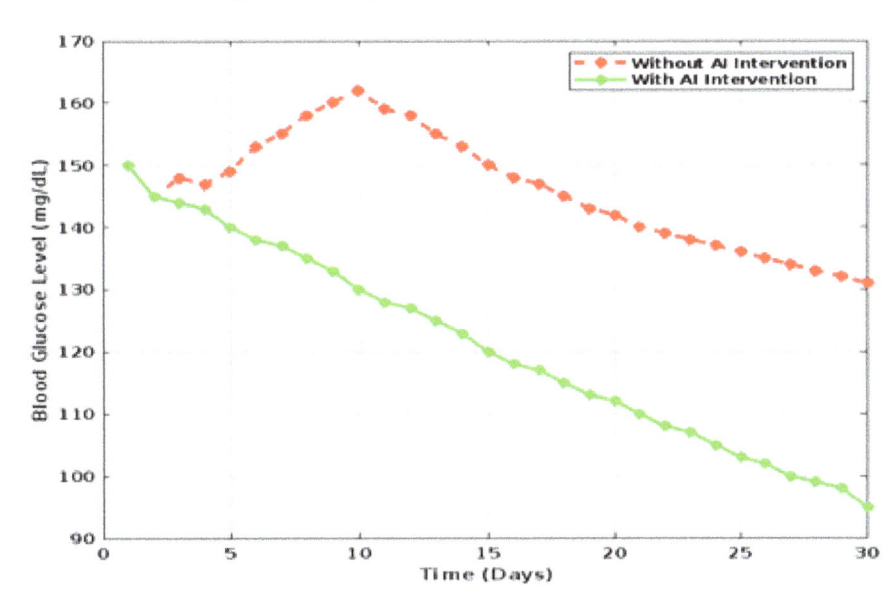

Figure 8. Chronic disease management using IoMT and AI

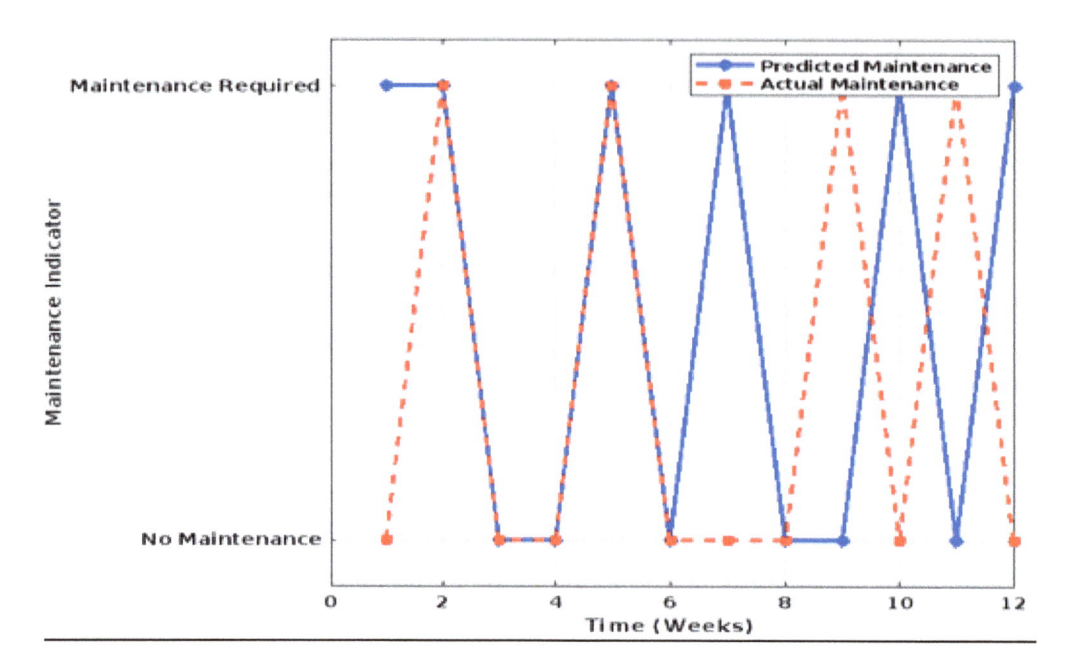

Figure 9. Predictive maintenance of medical equipment

Case Study 1: Personalized Chronic Disease Management

Illnesses such as type two diabetes and hypertension are examples of disorders that require conscious attention and patients' unique management to be kept at bay. In this case, the IoMT wearable devices such as CGMs and smart blood pressure cuffs monitor patients' chronic health condition data in real-time. Such data is analyzed with the help of generative AI models with the aim of forecasting the worsening of health, as well as the further course of treatment. For instance, in a smart-healthcare system such as continuous glucose monitoring, the IoMT is going to check blood glucose level of a patient during the day. It means that AI generation algorithms use all the data provided to them and try to discover such patterns and trends which can indicate possible changes in the glucose level – either its increase or decrease.

Case Study 2: AI-Enhanced Remote Patient Monitoring for Elderly Care

A patient who is a candidate towards his or her senior citizenage may experience acute emergence conditions such as heart attacks or perhaps a stroke and these conditions should be addressed as soon as possible. In this kind of case study, IoMT wearables like smartwatches and health monitoring devices are utilized in monitoring features like vital signs of senior patients such as heart rate, blood pressure & oxygen saturation levels. These data is constantly fed into generative AI models to look for precursors of the patient's decline in health condition. For instance, a senior care facility uses IoMT wearables to track the residents' wellbeing indices on a day-to-day basis.

Case Study 3: Virtual Health Assistants and Chatbots for Patient Support

The use of IoMT data with Generative AI, has created virtual health assistant, and professionally supported chatbots for instant patient care. Such AI integrated applications are intended for patient communication, replying to medical inquiries, and helping to organize the timetable for the intake of medicines with using the information obtained from IoT medical devices. For instance, a telehealth solution embraces the use of artificial intelligence assessed chatbots to provide service throughout the clock to patients. IoMT devices including wearable fitness trackers and smart pill dispensers feed the chatbot with data used in determining the health status of the patient as well as their compliance to medication regimen. If the chatbot learns that a patient has skipped his/her dose or has signs of developing some health condition, it gives recommendations. Also, the chatbot has the ability to respond to frequently asked medical questions and give information about the certain disease. Such real-time support improves patient participation in his/her care plan and hence improved health status and decreased caregiver burden.

Case Study 4: Predictive Maintenance of Medical Equipment Using IoMT and AI

MRI machines, ventilators, infusion pumps, etc are among some of the essential tools used in the health facilities and any failure in these devices is a catastrophic decision. In this case study, IoMT sensors are used to embedded in medical equipments with a prime view of keeping tabs on its performance and functioning. These sensors feed data to generative AI models that forecast future equipment failures and suggest maintenance to be performed to avoid downtimes among other benefits of equipment reliability. For example, the sensors collected by IoMT are implemented into the MRI machines in a hospital system to oversee the temperature, vibration and electric power. This data is then further processed by generative AI models to look for signs of wear and tear or of potential failure. If there an anomaly occurring in the machine then the AI computes a probability that a specific part will fail and then program the maintenance to occur at that time. Through this strategy, there is little loss of time towards patient care since most faults are identified and fixed before they occur, which also lowers the expenses for equipment repairs and healthier and longer lasting expensive medical equipment.

CHALLENGES IN IMPLEMENTING IOMT AND GENERATIVE AI IN HEALTHCARE

IoMT along with Generative AI in the field of healthcare has numerous chances and prospects for enhancement of the quality patients' healthcare and diagnostics. Nevertheless, the adoption of the said technologies is not without strings attached that come in form of massive challenges. From issues of data confidentiality and security, configuration, and other issues of concern such as ethics, all these hurdles must be met so as to promote the proper utilization of IoMT and Generative AI in the healthcare unit. To achieve this, professionals, institutions and policy makers have to overcome the aforementioned barriers in order to fully leverage on these technologies and protect the trust patients and health care systems deserve. In this section, we present a data privacy and security model for the integration of IoMT with the help of an AI plan, which is in the form of a flowchart (shown in Figure 10). Therefore, the diagram comprises important parts of the solution, including data acquisition, data encryption, data transfer security, AI's actions, and data access. All the components serve the worthwhile purpose of preventing the leakage of patients' information as well as maintaining compliance with privacy policies.

This figure illustrates various strategies that are necessesary to secure highly confidential health data in the complex system of IoMT and AI.

Figure 11 further depicts a Venn diagram type showing the interfacing issues concerning IoMT and Artificial intelligence. The diagram highlights that there are specific problems related to IoMT and AI, for example, the issue of how to normalise the data or how to scale solutions, as well as generalized issues, including the question of compatibility of protocols and issues about security. This figure makes it clear that there is need for integrating and coordinating standards, protocols, and security for IoMT and AI systems in healthcare.

Figure 10. Data privacy and security model for IoMT and AI integration

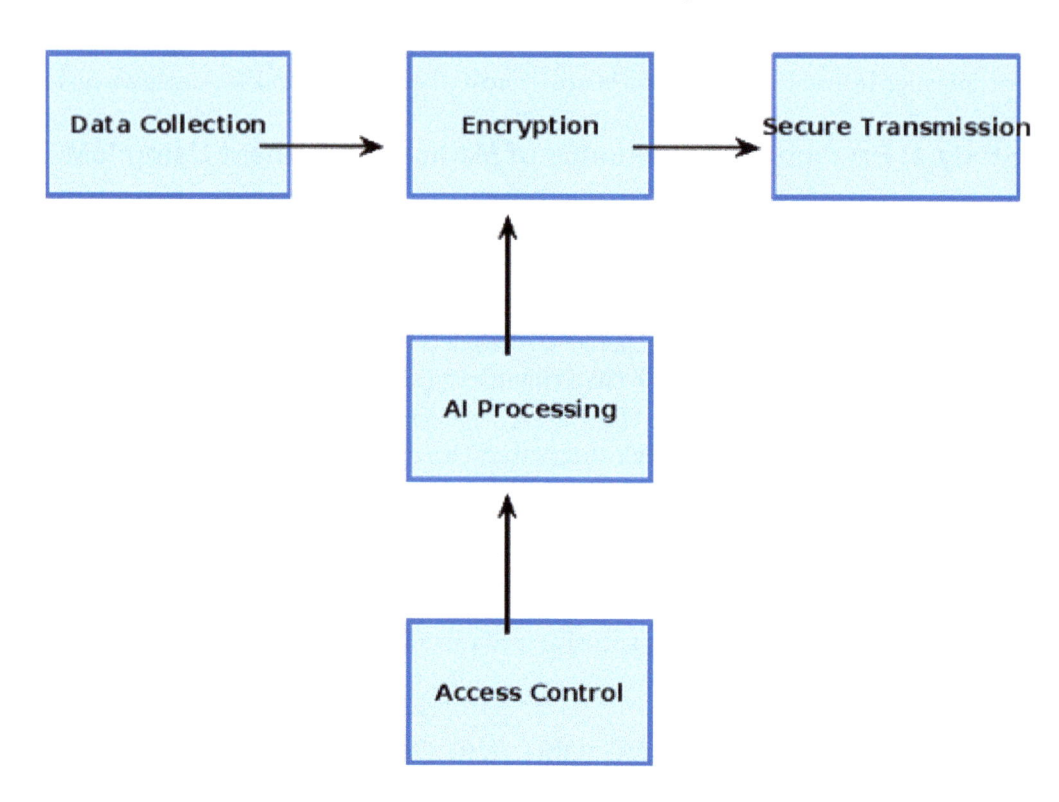

Figure 11. Interoperability challenges in IoMT and AI integration

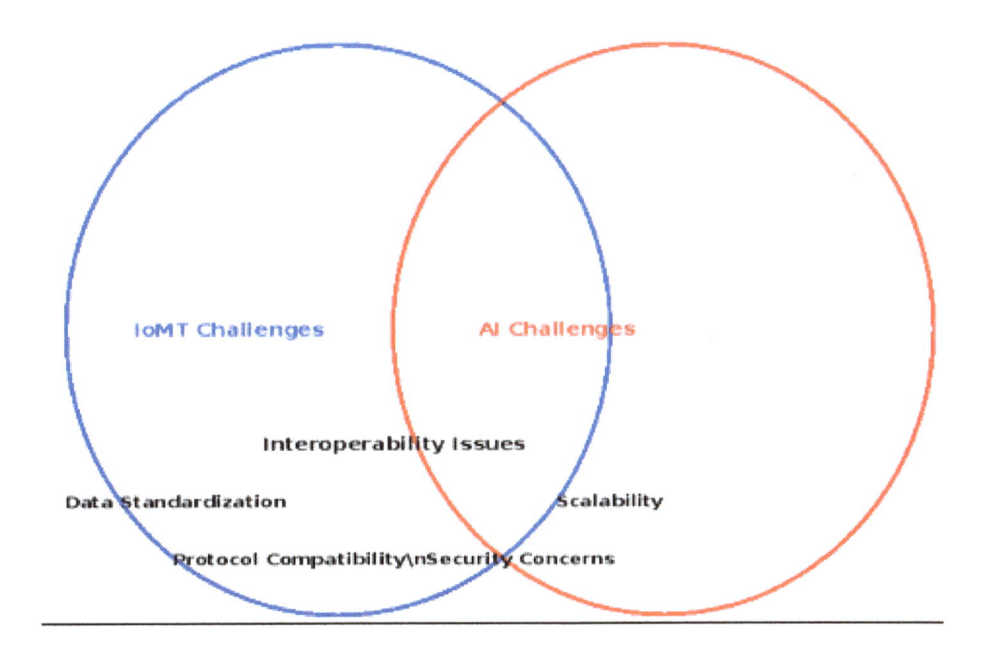

Data Privacy and Security Concerns

Two of the biggest issues that arise when undertaking IoMT, and Generative AI is the protection of patient data. IoMT devices are always generating new health information, sending data over different networks and storing a lot of it in clouds. These include information such as body temperature, blood pressure, medical history among other health factors which are very sensitive and most often targeted in cyberattacks, data leakage, and intrusion. The challenges mentioned above are even more amplified by the integration of Generative AI since AI models need to be trained with large sets of data to work properly and this exposes the users.

Integration Challenges and Interoperability Issues

Another factor that impacts the implementation of IoMT and Generative AI is compatibility issues of the devices, platforms, and systems used since most of them are not compatible. IoMT devices are developed by multiple manufacturers which employs several standards, protocols and data formats, so they are hard to integrate with existing Health care systems. Lack of standardization makes the data from the IoMT devices challenging to share, to aggregate or analyze – a problem with implications especially in the context of Generative AI models that require a wide range of varied and interconnected data sets. Interoperability, on the other hand, is the process of working towards the common set of standards for exchanging data, communication and compatibility of devices.

Ethical Considerations and Patient Consent

Concerning the specific applications of IoMT and Generative AI, the following ethical issues come to the forefront: patient's consent, data analysis, and AI models' bias. There are provisions on patient's right to know in detail the process of data gathering, utilization and sharing as well as consent of the patient for the use of data in AIAP. Informed consent is the next step towards ensuring that the patient's decisions on his or her treatment remain his or her decision alone. In addition, there is also the question of regulating the application of Generative AI in healthcare; such systems need to be controlled to prevent the reflection of prejudice arising from the database that was utilized for training the model. This is because if the data used to train the models does not capture the variability of patient profiles then the models is likely to yield biased results, thus giving different results for different patients.

Technical Challenges: Scalability, Accuracy, and Reliability

When it comes to the use of IoMT and Generative AI there are certain issues that revolve around scalability, accuracy and reliability. That explains the need for health-care systems to grow their infrastructure when there is a proliferation of IoMT devices. It involves of a large-scale expenditure in the cloud storage, data computation, and networks. Also, there is a need to understand and make accurate and reliable IoMT devices and AI models. The IoMT devices must be accurately calibrated and its readings validated to achieve accurate parameters and AI models must be trained on quality datasets and validated output for better forecasting. AI diagnosis errors including false positive or false negatives would mislead treatment procedures hence endangering the patients. A major technical challenge in bootstrapping meaningful models from Medical data is to derive efficient algorithms that can accommodate the variability and complexity inherent in medical data and which also yield high accuracy. Validation of IoMT devices and, AI models is imperative for their proper functioning in real-life healthcare settings and this requires routine checks, and updating of these devices and models.

FUTURE DIRECTIONS AND RESEARCH OPPORTUNITIES

Internet of Medical Things (IoMT) has started integrating with Generative Artificial Intelligence (AI) to revolutionize the healthcare system and the process of transformation is still in progress. These are some of the vast areas of growth for the technologies to advance and offer more chances for development that would help enhance the care of patients, deliver the healthcare that is efficient throughout the US and the world and take of global health threats. That's why, by continuing to work on the improvement of Interoperability, accreditation and expansion of the AI application fields, global influence, the future of healthcare can become more effective, individualized, accessible. IO&MT, Block diagram of the concept to captured for future integration of IoMT with AI is illustrated in figure 12. The basic elements that are illustrated on the diagram are IoMT devices, data layers, Artificial Intelligence analytics, user interfaces, edge computing and storage in the cloud.

Enhancing Interoperability and Data Standards

Another future of IoMT and Generative AI is in the way of improving the compatibility between the devices interconnect and establishing substantial data standards. The last challenge is known as Interoperability where due to the absence of standardized protocols and data formats it becomes very difficult to interconnect as well as integrate different IoMT devices, healthcare systems and even different AI platforms. To mitigate this challenge, there is the need to have continuous research in the improvement of these standards of data exchange being developed by Health Level Seven International (HL7) and the Fast Healthcare Interoperability Resources (FHIR). This tendency will contribute to the effective data exchange between different systems and spaces that, in turn, will help to enhance the AI models' implementation in the practice of real-time treatment and decision-making.

Figure 12. Future IoMT and AI integration framework

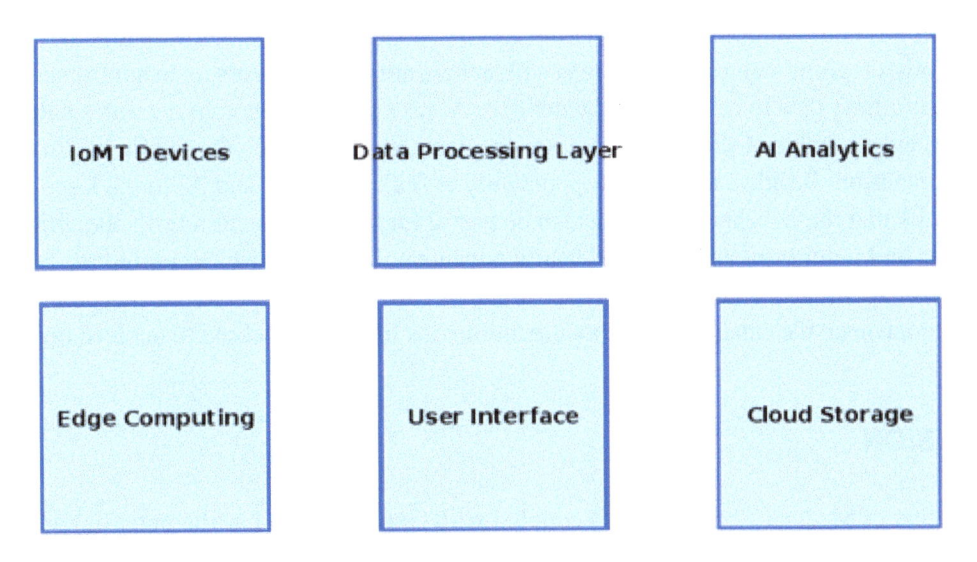

Improving AI Algorithms for Greater Accuracy

Thus, humanity's dependency on AI increases, and that is why the accuracy of AI algorithms is of such significant importance for humanity. Most of the existing AI models, including those applied in Generative AI, have their capabilities bounded by the quality as well as the variety of the data applied in the model. Thus, the future study should focus on the development of advanced machine learning methods that are able to deal with the variability of the medical data. This includes innovate structural design of neural networks like; deep neural network, reinforcement neural network, which is capable of learning based on large data set and experience. More so integrating AI based with Explainable AI (XAI) techniques comes in handy to improve the accuracy and accountability of the AI applied models whereby Health care practitioners and practitioners get the opportunity to understand the rationale behind AI systems applied models.

Expansion into New Healthcare Domains (e.g., Mental Health, Rehabilitation)

The use of IoMT and Generative AI is presently implemented mainly in chronic disease management, telemonitoring, and imaging diagnostics. But there is much scope for growth of new applications in the health care area of specialization such as mental health and rehab. Another domain that can benefit from IoMT devices ranging from wearable sensors and smart mobile application devices is mental health where signs of mental health can be monitored through vital signs including fluid movements, plus sleep, heart variability and performance. It means that generative AI can analyze such data and find out if the patient has signs of becoming depressed or anxious and offer him/her comprehensive treatment.

Potential for Global Health Impact

There is also much promise with this combination of IoMT and Generative AI to deal with threats to world health and provide equity in it. Poor literacy, health literacy, and low tendency to seek health care also will offer efficient solutions using IoMT devices for monitoring the specified patients in developing nations and other regions including rural areas where there are limited access to hospitals and specialists. These devices allows data to be taken and generative AI uses the data wherein it creates patterns on the data and it is even capable of predicting diseases the occurrence of which the public health department maybe intervenes on. Besides, there is an opportunity to scale up IoMT and AI to the large population, which suggests that these technologies can also be useful for the global health tasks like immunization, identification and monitoring of flues, and health advances. Thus, this work explored the role of IoMT and Generative AI in healthcare and identified that there are several paths for further research and development to advance the capabilities of both technologies in helping people to achieve better health.

CONCLUSION

The Internet of Medical Things (IoMT) coupled with Generative AI has the potential of shifting the healthcare landscape to further heights by introducing availability of live and accurate total body monitoring, prognostic ability and tailor made patient treatment plans. Thus, this chapter has focused on the integration of IoMT devices with AI technologies showing, in turn, how it can be useful in increasing diagnostic potential, facilitating the chronic illness treatment, as well as maintaining medical equipment. The integration of AI analysis into the IoMT systems offers advanced analytics to the healthcare practitioners in order to inform their decisions and hence achieve positive impacts on the patients' health. It is also not without its problems for example; data privacy, security, other system integration problems, and finally, protocol problems. Solving these challenges involves several layers of protection where data encryption, data transmission and access methodologies should be prized. Hence, in the subsequent frameworks, there is the need to recognize the edge computing coupled with cloud-based strategy, fine-tuning for enhancing the scalability necessary to tend to overwhelming traffic of IoMT and AI in healthcare information. As the concept of IoMT and AI continue to evolve so also does the healthcare industry stand to benefit hence creating a healthier society.

REFERENCES

Archana Shreee, S., Maheshwari, B., & Jeevitha Sai, G. (2023) "A Novel Method of Identification of Delirium in Patients from Electronic Health Records Using Machine Learning," 2023 World Conference on Communication & Computing (WCONF), RAIPUR, India, 2023, pp. 1-6.

Ashreetha, B., Gowda, D., Anandaram, H., Nithya, B. A., Gupta, N., & Verma, B. K. (2023, February). IoT Wearable Breast Temperature Assessment System. In 2023 7th International Conference on Computing Methodologies and Communication (ICCMC) (pp. 1236-1241). IEEE.

Brown, D., Davis, M., & Lee, C. (2023) "Enhancing Medical Equipment Reliability through Predictive Maintenance and IoT," *2023 IEEE International Conference on Emerging Technologies and Factory Automation (ETFA)*, Berlin, Germany, pp. 453-459.

Chakrasali, S. V., Kumar, C., Chaturvedi, A., & Jaisudhan Pazhani, A. A. (2023). Computer vision based healthcare system for identification of diabetes & its types using AI, Measurement. *Sensors (Basel)*, 27, 10075.

Chen, L., Wang, H., & Liu, S. (2023) "AI-Powered Decision Support Systems for IoMT Applications," *2023 IEEE International Conference on Systems, Man, and Cybernetics (SMC)*, Istanbul, Turkey, pp. 789-794.

Chen, T., Gupta, R., & Zhang, Y. (2023) "AI-Based Framework for Real-Time Patient Monitoring Using IoMT," *2023 IEEE International Conference on Consumer Electronics (ICCE)*, Las Vegas, USA, pp. 411-416.

Dankan Gowda, V., Swetha, K. R., Namitha, A. R., Manu, Y. M., Rashmi, G. R., & Veera Sivakumar, C. (2018). IOT Based Smart Health Care System to Monitor Covid-19 Patients.

Gowda, D., Bakshi, F., Gahana, A., Naik, A. B., & Navya, H. G. (2021, December). Covid-19 Prevention Kit Based on an Infrared Touchless Thermometer and Distance Detector. In 2021 5th International Conference on Electronics, Communication and Aerospace Technology (ICECA) (pp. 358-362). IEEE.

Gowda, D., Lokesh, M., Viraj, H. P., Mailapur, R. V., & Mahendra, K. (2023, June). Implementation of GUI based Vital Track Ambulance for Patient Health Monitoring. In 2023 8th International Conference on Communication and Electronics Systems (ICCES) (pp. 1417-1424). IEEE.

Green, M., Lopez, F., & Brown, T. (2023) "AI and IoMT: A Synergistic Approach to Personalized Medicine," *2023 IEEE International Conference on Computational Intelligence and Virtual Environments for Measurement Systems and Applications (CIVEMSA)*, Milan, Italy, pp. 110-115.

Gupta, S., Johnson, K., & Wang, Y. (2023) "Hybrid Cloud and Edge Computing for Scalable IoT Healthcare Solutions," *2023 IEEE International Conference on Cloud Computing Technology and Science (CloudCom)*, London, UK, pp. 210-215.

Hegde, S. K., Hegde, R., Hombalimath, V., Palanikkumar, D., Patwari, N., & Gowda, V. D. (2023, January). Symmetrized Feature Selection with Stacked Generalization based Machine Learning Algorithm for the Early Diagnosis of Chronic Diseases. In 2023 5th International Conference on Smart Systems and Inventive Technology (ICSSIT) (pp. 838-844). IEEE.

Iyer, V., Desai, G., & Patil, N. (2023) "Role of Wearable IoT Devices in Remote Health Monitoring," *2023 IEEE International Conference on Internet of Things (iThings)*, Beijing, China, pp. 334-339.

Jeevan, K., & Sathisha, B. M. (2020) "Implementation of IoT Based Wireless Electronic Stethoscope," *2020 Third International Conference on Multimedia Processing, Communication & Information Technology (MPCIT)*, pp. 103-106.

Kauser, S. H., Gowda, D., Tanguturi, R. C., & CH, V. (2023, June). Implementation of Machine Learning Approach for Detecting Cardiovascular Diseases. In 2023 3rd International Conference on Intelligent Technologies (CONIT) (pp. 1-6). IEEE.

Kavitha, R., Gowda, D., Vishal, B. R., Shankar, M. U., & Kabilan, A. M. (2023, May). Cardiovascular Disease Prediction Using LSTM Algorithm based On Cytokines. In 2023 4th International Conference for Emerging Technology (INCET) (pp. 1-5). IEEE.

Kavitha, R., Kumar, A., Kalpana, V., & Hariram, V. (2023) "Artificial Intelligence based Health Monitoring System on IoTH platform," *2023 Second International Conference on Augmented Intelligence and Sustainable Systems (ICAISS)*, Trichy, India, pp. 1458-1463.

Kawale, S. R., & Diwan, S. P. (2022) "Intelligent Breast Abnormality Framework for Detection and Evaluation of Breast Abnormal Parameters," *2022 International Conference on Edge Computing and Applications (ICECAA)*, pp. 1503-1508.

Kishore Kumar, R., Pandidurai, M., & Senthil Kamalesh, M. S. C. (2023) "Design of IoT based Rural Health Helper using Natural Language Processing," *2023 4th International Conference on Electronics and Sustainable Communication Systems (ICESC)*, Coimbatore, India, pp. 328-333.

Kranthi, M., & Tanguturi, R. C. (2023) "Design of Intelligent Medical Integrity Authentication and Secure Information for Public Cloud in Hospital Administration," 2023 2nd International Conference on Edge Computing and Applications (ICECAA), Namakkal, India, pp. 256-261.

Kumar, A., Sharma, S., & Verma, P. (2023) "Data Privacy and Security in IoMT: Challenges and Solutions," *2023 IEEE International Conference on Information Privacy, Security, Risk, and Trust (PASSAT)*, San Francisco, USA, pp. 321-326.

Lee, S., Choi, M., & Park, D. (2023) "Challenges and Solutions in Integrating AI with IoMT for Healthcare," *2023 IEEE International Conference on Networking, Sensing, and Control (ICNSC)*, Vienna, Austria, pp. 121-126.

M. R. G. and H. Anandaram. (2022) "Extraction of Fetal ECG Using ANFIS and the Undecimated-Wavelet Transform," 2022 IEEE 3rd Global Conference for Advancement in Technology (GCAT), pp. 1-5.

Mehta, N., Rossi, F., & Johnson, D. (2023) "Generative AI in Healthcare: Enhancing Diagnostic Accuracy and Efficiency," *2023 IEEE International Conference on Artificial Intelligence and Machine Learning (AIML)*, Dubai, UAE, pp. 215-220.

Nareshkumar, A., & Gururaj, B. (2022) "An Integrated IoT Technology for Health and Traffic Monitoring System with Smart Ambulance," *2022 IEEE North Karnataka Subsection Flagship International Conference (NKCon)*, Vijaypur, India, pp. 1-6.

Naveen, K. B., Ramesha, M., & Pai, G. N. (2020). Internet of things: Internet revolution, impact, technology road map and features. *Adv. Math. Sci. J.*, 9(7), 4405–4414. DOI: 10.37418/amsj.9.7.11

Pai, G. N., Pai, M. S., Gowd, V. D., & Shruthi, M. (2020, November). Internet of Things: a survey on devices, ecosystem, components and communication protocols. In 2020 4th International Conference on Electronics, Communication and Aerospace Technology (ICECA) (pp. 611-616). IEEE.

Palanikkumar, D., Mary, P. A., & Begum, A. Y. (2023) "A Novel IoT Framework and Device Architecture for Efficient Smart city Implementation," 2023 7th International Conference on Trends in Electronics and Informatics (ICOEI), Tirunelveli, India, pp. 420-426.

Park, K., Lee, M., & Kim, S. (2023) "Real-Time Data Analysis in IoMT: Improving Patient Outcomes with AI," *2023 IEEE International Conference on Biomedical and Health Informatics (BHI)*, Seoul, South Korea, pp. 429-434.

Patel, K., Moore, L., & Singh, H. (2023) "Next-Generation IoMT Devices and AI for Enhanced Patient Care," *2023 IEEE International Conference on Robotics and Automation (ICRA)*, Barcelona, Spain, pp. 567-572.

Prasad, K., Anil Kumar, N., Reddy, N. S., & Ashreetha, B. (2023) "Technologies for Comprehensive Information Security in the IoT," *2023 International Conference for Advancement in Technology (ICONAT)*, Goa, India, pp. 1-5.

Prasad, K., Dekka, S., Tanguturi, R. c., & Poornima, G. (2022) "An Intelligent System for Remote Monitoring of Patients Health and the Early Detection of Coronary Artery Disease," 2022 International Conference on Smart Generation Computing, Communication and Networking (SMART GENCON), Bangalore, India, pp. 1-6.

Ramesh Naidu, P., Guruprasad, N., & Dankan Gowda, V. (2020). Design and implementation of cryptcloud system for securing files in cloud. *Adv. Math. Sci. J.*, 9(7), 4485–4493. DOI: 10.37418/amsj.9.7.17

Ramesh Naidu, P., Guruprasad, N., & Dankan Gowda, V. (2021). A High-Availability and Integrity Layer for Cloud Storage, Cloud Computing Security: From Single to Multi-Clouds. *Journal of Physics: Conference Series*, 1921(1), 012072. DOI: 10.1088/1742-6596/1921/1/012072

Rao, B. K., Chaturvedi, A., & Hussain, N. (2022). Industrial quality healthcare services using Internet of Things and fog computing approach, Measurement. *Sensors (Basel)*, 24, 100517.

Reddy, S., & Patwal, P. P. S. (2022) "Data Analytics and Cloud-Based Platform for Internet of Things Applications in Smart Cities," *2022 International Conference on Industry 4.0 Technology (I4Tech)*, pp. 1-6.

Revanna C R, B. Kameswara Rao and Parismita Sarma (2022), Enhanced Diagnostic Methods for Identifying Anomalies in Imaging of Skin Lesions. IJEER 10(4), pp.1077-1085.

Singh, B., Yang, T., & Fernandez, R. (2023) "Temporal Analysis in Healthcare Using LSTM Networks," *2023 IEEE International Conference on Machine Learning and Applications (ICMLA)*, Toronto, Canada, pp. 612-617.

Smith, J., Patel, A., & Roberts, L. (2023) "Real-Time Monitoring of Chronic Diseases Using IoMT and AI Integration," *2023 IEEE International Conference on Healthcare Informatics (ICHI)*, New York, USA, pp. 101-106.

Thompson, M., Allen, R., & Garcia, J. (2023) "Interoperability in IoMT and AI: Bridging the Gap with Standardized Protocols," *2023 IEEE International Conference on Communications (ICC)*, Paris, France, pp. 879-884.

U. K N and R. V M. (2022) "Arduino based COVID-19 Suspect Detection Device," 2022 6th International Conference on Electronics, Communication and Aerospace Technology, Coimbatore, India, pp. 158-163.

Venkatakiran, S., Ashreetha, B., & Reddy, N. S. (2023) "Implementation of a Machine Learning-based Model for Cardiovascular Disease Post Exposure prophylaxis," *2023 International Conference for Advancement in Technology (ICONAT)*, Goa, India, pp. 1-5.

Wu, H., Patel, S., & Lin, X. (2023) "Enhancing Patient Safety through AI-Integrated IoMT Systems," *2023 IEEE International Conference on Engineering in Medicine and Biology Society (EMBC)*, Boston, USA, pp. 310-315.

Zhang, L., Chen, H., & Liu, X. (2023) "Integrating IoMT with AI for Advanced Healthcare: A Future Framework," *2023 IEEE International Conference on Smart Health (ICSH)*, Tokyo, Japan, pp. 102-107.

Chapter 10
Booster of IoMT in Diagnostics and Disease Screening:
Hustler Artificial Intelligence Approaches Transforming Healthier Homes

Bhupinder Singh
https://orcid.org/0009-0006-4779-2553
Sharda University, India

Christian Kaunert
https://orcid.org/0000-0002-4493-2235
Dublin City University, Ireland & University of South Wales, UK

Hind Hammouch
https://orcid.org/0000-0002-5897-1649
University Sidi Mohamed Ben Abdellah, Morocco

Anjali Raghav
https://orcid.org/0009-0004-0248-7956
Sharda University, India

ABSTRACT

The global landscape of healthcare is witnessing a transformative shift with the integration of artificial intelligence (AI) in disease screening and pandemic outbreak management. Disease screening serves as a critical component of proactive healthcare, enabling early detection and intervention. Traditional screening methods, while effective, often face limitations in terms of scalability, speed, and accuracy. The emergence of AI has opened new avenues for enhancing disease screening processes, allowing for more efficient and precise identification of potential health threats. These technologies enable healthcare professionals to analyze vast datasets quickly and accurately, facilitating early diagnosis and intervention. This chapter explores the various dimensions of evolving role of AI in prioritizing disease screening and managing pandemic outbreaks, with a focus on innovative approaches for mass vaccine scattering. The evolving role of AI in prioritizing disease screening and pandemic outbreak management holds immense promise for the future of global healthcare.

DOI: 10.4018/979-8-3693-6180-1.ch010

1. INTRODUCTION

AI brings a spectrum of approaches to disease screening, including machine learning algorithms, natural language processing, and computer vision (Sardar et al., 2024). AI algorithms can identify patterns and anomalies in patient data, contributing to more personalized and targeted healthcare solutions (Khurana, 2024). In the wake of recent global health crises, the imperative to develop efficient strategies for disease screening and mass vaccine distribution has never been more evident. The challenges posed by pandemic outbreaks, such as the recent COVID-19 crisis, underscore the need for swift and effective management strategies (Li et al., 2021). AI applications play a pivotal role in predicting, tracking, and mitigating the spread of infectious diseases. Machine learning models can analyze epidemiological data, predict outbreak trajectories, and optimize resource allocation in healthcare systems (Sejdic & Falk, 2018). The efficient vaccine distribution is a cornerstone in the fight against pandemics. Traditional distribution methods often encounter hurdles such as logistics, supply chain complexities, and equitable access (Luo et al., 2016).

AI-driven mass vaccine scattering presents a paradigm shift by leveraging predictive analytics to optimize vaccine allocation, distribution routes, and cold chain management. These AI systems can adapt to dynamic conditions, ensuring vaccines reach diverse populations swiftly and equitably (Mohammadi et al., 2018). Striking a balance between technological advancement and ethical considerations is crucial for fostering public trust and ensuring the responsible deployment of AI in healthcare. Precise identification of the ailment is necessary for efficient treatment planning and patient safety (Scarpato et al., 2017). Despite these benefits, significant challenges persist, including issues related to reliability and validation, the range and types of conditions addressed, cross-modality analysis, new examination technologies, and the effective integration of advanced computer vision and machine learning technologies (Dash et al., 2019). However, because interpreting medical information requires a high level of cognitive function and complexity, human error can compromise diagnostic efficiency and accuracy, especially in general clinical practice and rural locations (Singh, 2024). Convolutional neural networks, knowledge graphs, transformers, and other artificial intelligence (AI) approaches have shown to be effective tools that may improve and support a variety of illness diagnostic and treatment procedures (Singh et al., 2024). With using AI into the diagnostic process, healthcare providers may get more precision and productivity, which in turn makes it easier to provide cutting-edge digital healthcare services (Singh & Kaunert, 2024).

Figure 1. Dimensions of introduction split sections

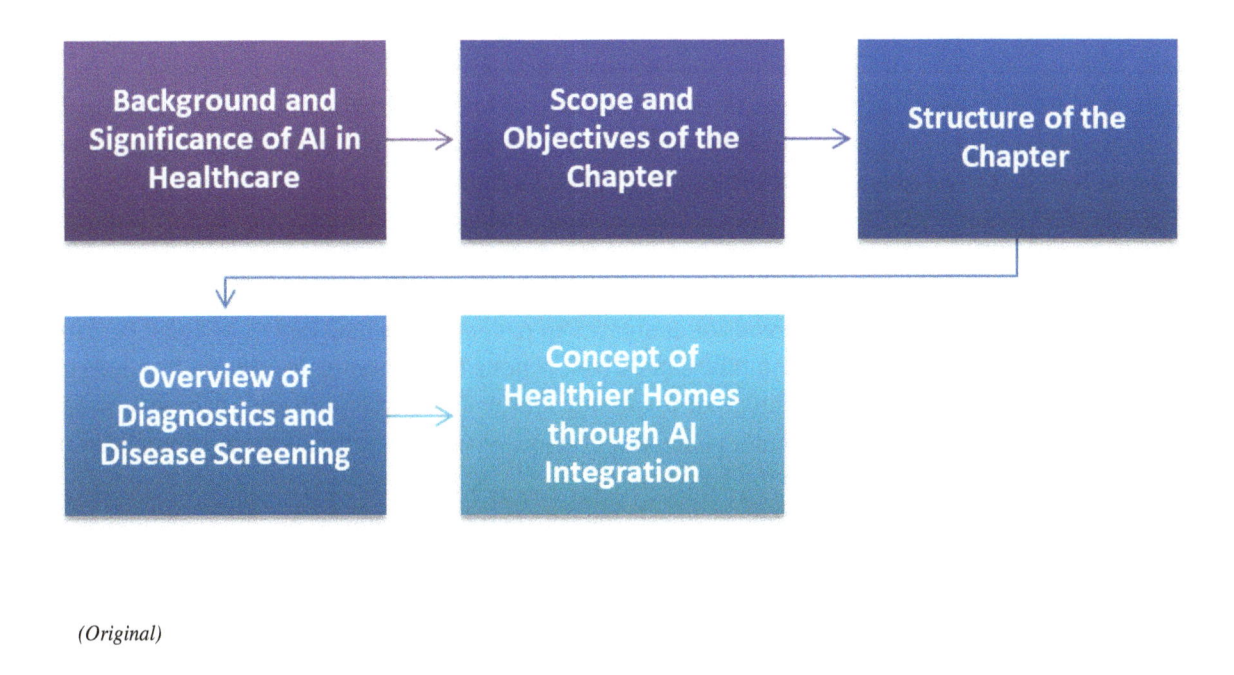

[Flowchart: Background and Significance of AI in Healthcare → Scope and Objectives of the Chapter → Structure of the Chapter → Overview of Diagnostics and Disease Screening → Concept of Healthier Homes through AI Integration]

(Original)

1.1 Background and Significance of AI in Healthcare

As a result, the Internet of Medical Things (IoMT) has provided groundbreaking improvements in health care, especially within diagnostics and disease screening. The Internet of Medical Things (IoMT) has enabled healthcare professionals to obtain accurate and timely information for monitoring and treating patients by interconnecting medical devices, sensors, and health-monitoring applications. IoMT devices consistently and in real-time gather information from patients during diagnostics, enabling rapid identification of irregularities, which is highly important for disease states like cardiovascular diseases, diabetes, and respiratory disorders, which require immediate and timely intervention. Wearable devices from smartwatches to ECG monitors can communicate heart rate, blood glucose levels and blood oxygen saturation straight to healthcare providers for immediate analysis. By closely observing patients, this makes it possible improve diagnostic accuracy while also minimizing their stay at the hospital, thus benefiting both the patients as well as the healthcare system by lowering the cost. With disease screening, IoMT also plays an important role by identifying at-actions before onset of symptoms, resulting in pro-active and preventive care. Many screening devices enhance the use of IoMT, making it involved with highly developing advanced analytics and AI-powered systems deployed to process large amounts of health data in snippets to detect a pattern and associate it with a particular disease. Such functionality is particularly useful in scanning chronic diseases and genetically predisposed conditions like that of cancer or Alzheimer's disease. IoMT platforms, for example, can integrate genomic data into profiles when combining it with lifestyle and wearable device-embedded physiological data to assess the risk of diseases. Using artificial intelligence embedded algorithms, these devices break down the patients data and alert the care takers about high risk factors for timely interventions to effectively disrupt them (which can otherwise prove to be fatal in some cases) (Al-Jarrah et al., 2015).

IoMT further strengthens rural or remote area healthcare where all diagnostic and screening infrastructure and resources may lack. Such locations would benefit from portable IoMT devices that can be used to screen conditions such as tuberculosis or malaria, such as handheld ultrasound machines or smart diagnostic kits. The gadgets send diagnostic data to experts stationed in city centers, where trained health personnel analyze it without having to shuttle the patient between locations. This strategy ensures equal access to healthcare and guarantees that those in areas lacking services receive an early diagnosis and the prompt recommendation of treatment. Machine learning and big data analytics also enable predictive diagnostics in healthcare. With the help of integrated data from various sources, for example: electronic health records, IoMT devices are capable of predicting possible health problems depending on historical and current data. The ability to spot trends or anomalies in patient health data that may signal potential disease enables healthcare providers to take data-driven actions to preemptively address health issues before they become critical. This attribute of predicting well is effectively utilized in chronic disease management, where the need is to monitor patients continuously and intervene before any complications arise or the patients get readmitted to the hospital.

Despite the full-scale implementation of IoMT, the data privacy and interoperability continue to be significant challenges. Cybersecurity risks: it generates too many sensitive health data and thus needs work on its cybersecurity, so that it can prevent data breach and protect patient privacy. Plus some of the challenges associated with technological interoperability of IoMT devices at different platforms and healthcare systems for efficient data sharing and integration. Although these challenges exist, it see the opportunity for the role of IoMT in diagnostics and disease screening to continue to increase ultimately leading us toward a future distinctive by personalized, preventive, and accessible healthcare. The majority of modern AI technologies are classified as "Narrow AI" which means that they are made to perform better than humans at particular, well-defined activities. Machine learning algorithms, which let computers learn, do jobs, and adapt on their own, power a lot of these products. The use of artificial intelligence (AI) to healthcare is not a new idea. The phrase "artificial intelligence" was originally used in a 1955 Dartmouth College conference proposal. But it wasn't until the early 1970s that AI applications entered the healthcare industry. At that time, scientists created MYCIN, an AI tool meant to aid in the identification of blood infection therapies (Zhou et al., 2021). The American Association for Artificial Intelligence (now known as the Association for the Advancement of Artificial Intelligence, or AAAI) was founded in 1979 as a result of the growth of AI research. In the 1970s, the first uses of AI to solve issues in biomedicine appeared. Since then, advancements in AI-powered technologies have dramatically changed the healthcare sector by lowering expenses, enhancing patient outcomes, and boosting general productivity. Artificial intellect (AI) uses computer models and programs to mimic human intellect in order to carry out cognitive activities including experience-based learning and complicated problem solving (Muthu et al., 2020).

1.2 Overview of Diagnostics and Disease Screening

In order to identify people who have an illness and start treatment as soon as possible, screening entails testing an asymptomatic population for that ailment. In the common screening tests include those for cancer (mammograms, pap smears, skin checks for high-risk melanoma patients), routine blood pressure checks at doctor's offices, hearing, vision, and dental screenings in elementary schools, and yearly HIV and tuberculosis screenings for healthcare professionals (Miller & Brown, 2018).

Public health officials frequently provide direct assistance for these initiatives with assigning workers to conduct hearing exams in primary schools or indirect help by organizing health education campaigns to encourage pap smears. Patients who exhibit symptoms undergo diagnostic tests in order to ascertain their illness. In cases where a patient exhibits new symptoms, clinicians employ a procedure known as differential diagnosis. To make educated guesses about probable illnesses, they collect data from the patient's physical examination and medical history. For example, if a 24-year-old woman presents to a clinic with visual abnormalities and a severe headache, other possible differential diagnoses include meningitis, hemorrhagic stroke, migraine with aura, and concussion. The aim of the physician is to determine the right condition for the right course of action. In order to rule in or rule out illnesses from the differential diagnosis list, diagnostic tests must be performed (Bhattacharyya et al., 2023).

1.3 Concept of Healthier Homes Through AI Integration

Imagine a world where a nurse's schedule perfectly aligns with patient needs, ensuring every minute is utilized effectively without any undue stress or overtime. That's the magic of AI-powered scheduling algorithms. With analyzing historical data, patient demand patterns, and nurse availability, AI can generate optimized schedules that maximize productivity and minimize downtime. Real-time adjustments keep us prepared for unexpected changes, allowing us to deliver exceptional care seamlessly. AI-powered predictive analytics can be useful. AI is able to identify those who are at a high risk of being admitted to the hospital even before symptoms manifest by analyzing patient data. Being proactive and offering tailored treatment to keep patients well at home and avoid hospital stays is made possible by this forethought. Less hospital stays save money while also improving patient outcomes, so everyone wins (Malik & Tyagi, 2022).

AI-powered Healthy Home ideas a truly transformative concept that enables people to achieve a higher level of interaction with their home for overall well-being, safety, and quality of life. That said, with the help of the artificial intelligence, homes can adapt according to the health needs of the residents and provide them with a healthier space. Whether it is tracking indoor air quality, optimizing sleep patterns, or even monitoring for safety, AI-driven smart homes will be designed with health in mind. Environmental monitoring for indoor air quality is a major application of AI in healthier homes. Pollutants including volatile organic compounds (VOCs), carbon dioxide, dust, and allergens are tracked by AI-enabled sensors and the data is analyzed in real time to provide the best indoor air quality. If the levels of some harmful pollutants exceed the threshold, then the air purifiers in all the rooms could be automatically turned on; ventilation could be controlled to allow fresh air to enter the indoor space, helping reduce respiratory diseases and the settlement of allergens in the house. These air quality changes are particularly useful for those who suffer from asthma, allergies, or other respiratory issues, keeping them in a better living environment.

While managing comfort and minimizing stress is vital, particularly regarding sleep, lighting, and noise, AI also plays a vital role in this. AI-powered smart lighting systems automatically adjust the lighting conditions, mimicking natural circadian cycles to balance the melatonin levels and enhance sleep quality. Such systems gradually dim the lights when bedtime arrives and gradually increasing them again in the morning to support a natural sleep-wake rhythm. Moreover, voice-detecting sensors present in an AI-ready home can recognize the disturbing noises, and if connected to a smart sound canceling device, it can eliminate the ambient noise to promote a healthy sleep environment. This same technology may be used to play ambient sounds, or change lighting in different rooms to promote relaxation and reduce stress for a pleasant and healthy environment.

Within the space of safety and health, the AI technologies are improving fall detection and emergency response, especially for elderly patients or individuals with chronic health conditions. Placed throughout the home, these AI-integrated systems are capable of identifying atypical movements, such as a fall, and promptly notifying emergency contacts or health providers. Certain systems include predictive analytics that can detect changes in activity patterns over time that may signify worsening mobility or increased fall risk. This forward manner does not only assist with day-to-day immediate emergency response; however, it additionally aids preventive care through the early identification of potential health difficulties. It aids in regard to the domestic consumption of healthy dietary habits and physical activity. AI appliances and virtual home assistants integrated into smart kitchens can help residents choose healthier food options by suggesting meal plans and recipes based on individual dietary needs and goals. Likewise, virtual personal trainers can provide tailored workout plans, track movement and deliver feedback via artificial intelligence, enabling a more active lifestyle. This is an especially beneficial feature for residents who need to achieve targeted health outcomes, like weight loss/gain or strengthening of muscles to prevent chronic diseases.

Though the convergence of AI with healthier homes has its enormous benefits, privacy, data security, and ethical use of personal health data come in concern as well. As these systems depend on the uncontrolled collection and analysis of sensitive information, strict security measures and clear data practices are needed to prevent the invasion of user privacy. Furthermore, these AI-enabled healthier homes tend to be expensive, so these solutions also need to be affordable and accessible. That being said, with the advances continuing and the availability improving, healthier homes with integrated AI have the potential to become a major provider of preventative healthcare, allowing people to achieve healthy, safe, and balanced lives right in their own home. Errors can occur in the hectic field of healthcare, but they don't have to. Our committed nurses and healthcare workers are supported by AI-powered decision support tools that analyze enormous volumes of data and best practice recommendations. In order to provide well-informed, error-free judgments, AI acts as a competent colleague by providing real-time recommendations for diagnosis, treatment plans, and drug management. It highlights potential errors and delivers helpful insights (Viceconti et al., 2015).

1.4 Scope and Objectives of the Chapter

The Quality of treatment and patient safety come first. We are adopting preemptive measures to keep our patients safe and healthy with the use of AI-enabled remote monitoring devices and predictive analytics. Vital signs and health indicators may be continuously monitored to identify aberrations early on, allowing for prompt intervention and the avoidance of unfavorable outcomes. Each patient will receive the customized assistance they require to flourish thanks to AI-driven individualized care plans, which put their comfort and wellbeing first in the provision of healthcare. The human factor passion, emotions, and empathy remains essential to providing high-quality healthcare. This chapter emphasizes how technology can tackle healthcare issues while preserving the vital human element in patient relationships. This chapter has the following objectives to:

- showcase particular case studies and clinical trials to demonstrate how AI technologies enhance the accuracy and speed of diagnosing a range of diseases in comparison to conventional approaches.
- observe the financial advantages of AI-powered diagnostic tools, such as lower prices for conventional diagnostic testing and the possibility of lowering healthcare expenditures by promoting early identification and prevention.
- describe the moral ramifications and data privacy concerns associated with the use of AI in healthcare, and offer models and policies to guarantee patient privacy and AI system trust.
- define the organizational and technological barriers to incorporating AI systems into the current healthcare infrastructures, and offer ways to improve interoperability to facilitate smooth data interchange and system operation.
- scan how AI may assist personalized medicine by evaluating big datasets to create individualized treatment regimens that enhance patient happiness and results.

Figure 2. Objectives of the chapter

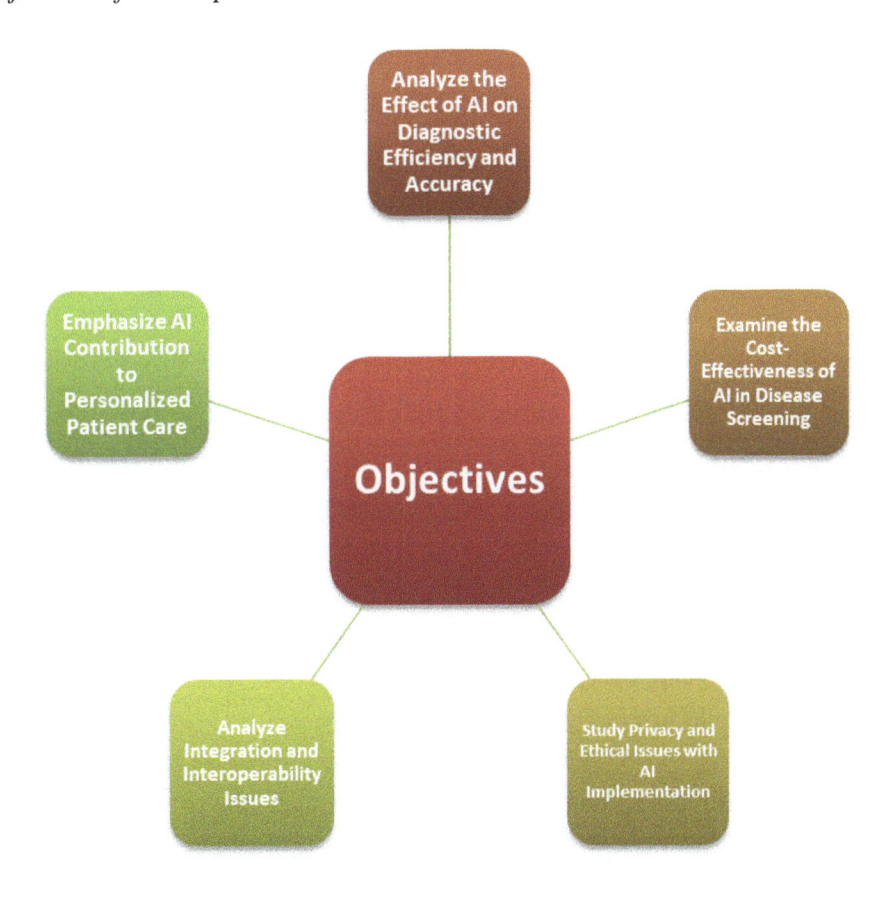

(Original)

1.5 Structure of the Chapter

This chapter focuses on the Booster of Artificial Intelligence in Diagnostics and Disease Screening: Hustler Artificial Intelligence Approaches Transforming Healthier Homes. Section 2 discusses the Evolution of AI in Medical Diagnostics. Section 3 explores the AI Technologies Transforming Diagnostics. Section 4 signifies the AI in Disease Screening. Section 5 conveys the Implementation of AI in Healthier Homes. Section 6 specifies the Ethical and Regulatory Considerations. Section 7 Conclude the Chapter with Future Scope.

Figure 3. Flow of this chapter

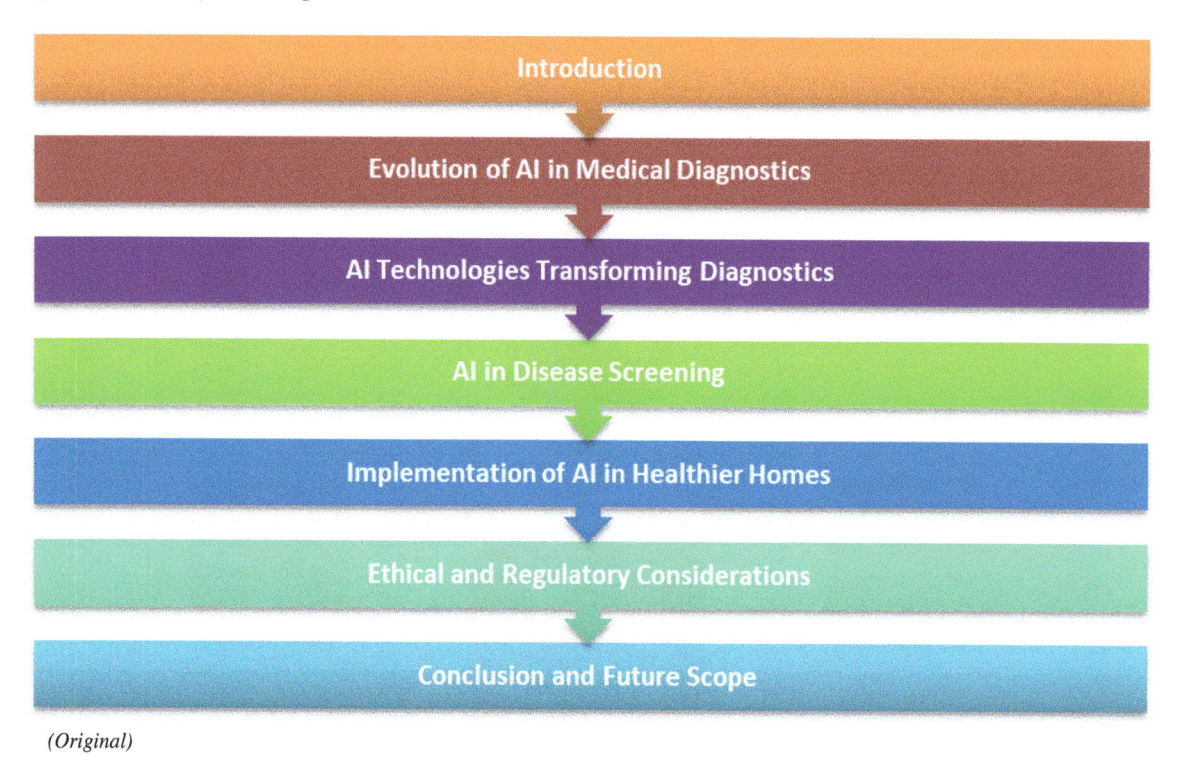

(Original)

2. EVOLUTION OF AI IN MEDICAL DIAGNOSTICS

Artificial intelligence (AI) has revolutionized healthcare by changing patient monitoring, diagnosis, and treatment methods. More precise diagnosis and individualized treatment plans are made possible by this technology, which is greatly improving healthcare research and results. Artificial intelligence (AI) enables medical personnel to swiftly uncover patterns and illness signs that they may otherwise overlook by analyzing large quantities of clinical record. AI has a wide range of possible uses in the healthcare industry, from employing radiological image scanning for early diagnosis to leveraging electronic health data for outcome prediction (Ahmed et al., 2023). Healthcare systems may become more smarter, quicker and more efficient by incorporating AI into hospitals and clinics, improving treatment for millions of people globally. Artificial Intelligence is rapidly becoming the healthcare industry's future, transforming patient care and cutting provider costs and improving healthcare of patients (Panesar, 2019).

AI has amazing potential applications in healthcare. Artificial Intelligence (AI) is anticipated to revolutionize healthcare data processing, disease diagnosis, therapy development, and possibly sickness prevention. Medical personnel may save time, cut expenses, and improve medical records administration by using AI to make more educated decisions based on reliable information. AI in healthcare promises to be a game-changer, opening the door for a day when patients receive faster and more precise care and treatment, from finding novel cancer medicines to improving patient experiences (Sengan et al., 2020).

AI-based techniques have been created to manage patient records, enhance healthcare systems, detect diseases, and cure ailments. These techniques range from machine learning to deep learning. Notably, the medical industry makes substantial use of rule-based intelligent systems, which make judgments based on pre-established instructions and healthcare norms (Singh, 2022). With evaluating medical pictures from tests like computed tomography (CT), dual-energy X-ray absorptiometry (DXA), MRI, ultrasound, and computed tomography (CT), artificial intelligence (AI) algorithms help medical professionals discover and diagnose a variety of disorders (Rodrigues et al., 2021). There are numerous artificial intelligence (AI) techniques, including as fuzzy logic, ANNs, RNNs, and LR, have shown effective in accurately diagnosing a wide range of complicated medical diseases. These ailments include chronic illnesses, liver disease, diabetes-related retinopathy, cancer, Alzheimer's disease, hypertension, stroke, cerebrovascular disease, and TB. Additionally, AI algorithms have demonstrated remarkable efficacy in the early diagnosis of cancer, including liver and gastrointestinal cancers (Pramanik et al., 2022). This has improved patient outcomes and decreased the financial strain that malignant illnesses have on the healthcare system. ANNs can diagnose liver illness with excellent accuracy. Deep-learning AI techniques were 96% accurate in identifying Alzheimer's disease. In addition to diagnosing diseases and analyzing images, AI systems can analyze large amounts of medical data to produce theories and provide possible diagnoses. This helps medical personnel avoid cognitive biases and guarantees a thorough investigation of all diagnostic options (Zhou et al., 2017).

3. AI TECHNOLOGIES TRANSFORMING DIAGNOSTICS

Healthcare workers now have accurate and effective methods to diagnose diseases thanks to AI technology and algorithms. Deep learning in particular has gained great traction in machine learning because of its capacity to detect subtle patterns in complicated medical data. Today, convolutional neural networks (CNNs) are the de facto standard for image-based diagnostics, including radiological scan tumor identification. With combining data from several sources, ensemble techniques like Random Forest and Gradient Boosting increase diagnostic accuracy and make up for the shortcomings of individual models. There are numerous advantages come with AI-driven diagnostic processes, including increased speed, accuracy, cost-effectiveness, and the ability to analyze enormous volumes of medical data quickly and effectively (Bahri et al., 2018). According to research that was published in Nature Medicine, AI models for diagnosing breast cancer outperformed conventional techniques in identifying cancers in mammograms as training data rose. According to a different research, using AI into medical imaging greatly lowered expenses by reducing the need for pricey diagnostic tests and pointless treatments. But there are drawbacks and issues with using AI into healthcare (Kashyap et al., 2015).

Figure 4. Points on AI technologies transforming diagnostics

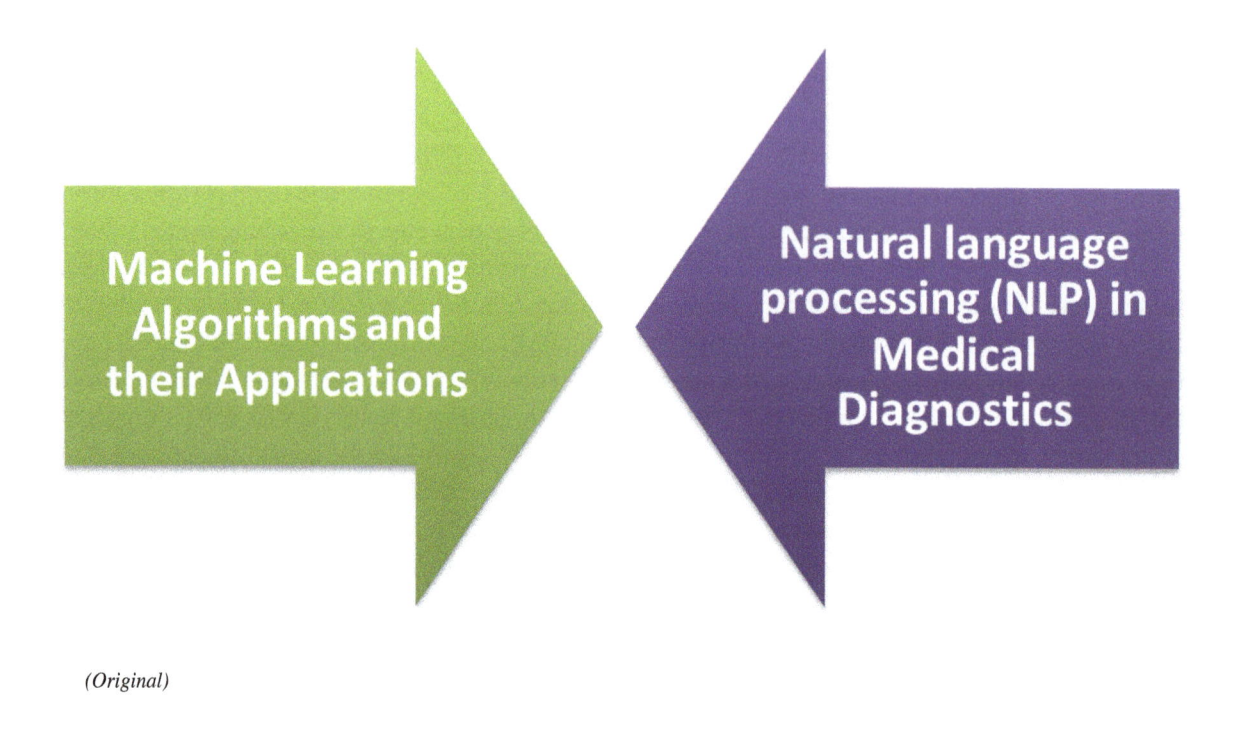

(Original)

3.1 Machine Learning Algorithms and Their Applications

The improved medical diagnosis and treatment have led to a huge transformation in the healthcare industry thanks to machine learning, a critical component of AI. Algorithms are able to detect patterns and make very accurate predictions about medical outcomes by evaluating large volumes of clinical data (Elbadawi et al., 2021). That such usage is precision medicine, which makes use of supervised learning to forecast treatment plans based on patient-specific information (Cabello et al., 2020). Deep learning, a branch of artificial intelligence, is used in the medical field to perform tasks like natural language processing-based speech recognition. Healthcare workers will need to comprehend and use deep learning technology in clinical settings more and more as it develops (Chen et al., 2014). Through the analysis of patient data, interpretation of medical imaging, and discovery of novel therapeutics, this technology aids medical practitioners in improving patient care and cutting expenses. Accurate illness diagnosis, individualized therapy and the identification of minute variations in vital signs that may indicate possible health problems are all made possible by machine learning (Stephens et al., 2015).

Through the customization of medicines based on patient-specific traits and changing circumstances, reinforcement learning (RL) has also gained favor as a means of enhancing treatment regimens and increasing precision medicine. AI incorporation with conventional medical imaging methods has sped up the diagnosis of illness (Tiwari, 2022). The example is the early diagnosis of diabetic retinopathy by AI-assisted retinal image processing. Also, textual healthcare records may be quickly analyzed with the use of natural language processing (NLP), which offers insights for precise diagnosis and patient care (Singh, 2023). AI systems in radiology have proven to be adept at deciphering medical pictures and helping radiologists identify a range of illnesses. Artificial intelligence (AI)-driven algorithms can recognize abnormalities in MRIs, CT scans, and X-rays, enabling quicker and more precise illness detection (Devika & Karegowda, 2021).

3.2 Natural Language Processing (NLP) in Medical Diagnostics

Artificial intelligence in the form of natural language processing (NLP) enables computers to comprehend and use human language (Sukeshini et al., 2021). With improving patient care, increasing diagnostic accuracy, expediting clinical procedures, and offering more individualized services, natural language processing (NLP) is transforming the healthcare sector. For example, NLP can extract useful information from health data and use it to evaluate medical records to identify ailments properly (Jordan & Mitchell). Also, it can determine which drugs and therapies are appropriate for each patient and, using past medical data, forecast any health concerns. Additionally, NLP gives medical professionals strong capabilities to handle vast amounts of intricate data, greatly cutting down on the time needed for human processing (Singh, 2024). NLP is proving to be an indispensable tool in healthcare, enabling medical professionals to leverage artificial intelligence for more accurate diagnoses and better personalized treatments. This technology is rapidly becoming essential in modern healthcare and is expected to become even more advanced and widely applied in the future (Singh & Kaunert, 2024).

4. AI IN DISEASE SCREENING

Many medical software manufacturers' AI capabilities for diagnosis, therapy, and clinical trials are stand-alone systems that solely handle particular areas of care (Reddy, 2023). While these initiatives are still in the early stages, several EHR software manufacturers are beginning to integrate limited AI-powered healthcare analytics features into their systems (Keikhosrokiani, 2022). Healthcare providers who use stand-alone EHR systems will need to either take on large integration projects themselves or work with outside suppliers who can integrate AI capabilities with their EHR systems in order to effectively employ AI in healthcare (Kashyap et al., 2016). Healthcare organizations must make sure that patient data used to train AI models is appropriately anonymized and protected against breaches, making data privacy and security the most important of these. As has been said in talks about the possible consequences of using AI in healthcare, data privacy is crucial (Manyika et al., 2011).

The other big obstacle is interoperability as consistent data interchange is necessary for the seamless integration of AI systems into the current healthcare infrastructure, but organizational and technical barriers may make this process difficult (Helbert, 2016). Optimizing interoperability is essential to achieving AI full potential in the medical field (Jain, 2023). There are concerns have also been raised about using AI to make crucial medical decisions without fully comprehending the logic behind them (Ariffin et al., 2021). In healthcare settings, the ability to comprehend and explain AI algorithms is crucial for fostering trust and improving decision-making. The ethical questions have also been brought up by the growing application of AI to medical diagnostics (Bao et al., 2019). As AI systems get more complicated, transparency and explainability of the algorithms become crucial concerns. To guarantee that diagnoses generated by AI are comprehensible and offer rational justifications, it is essential to establish ethical norms (Zhou et al., 2021). Moreover, flaws in the training data may introduce bias into

AI systems, thereby producing biased results. Black patients received worse care as a result of racial prejudice in a healthcare AI program, according to one research. Diverse and representative datasets are needed to address prejudice in AI systems, as are rigorous testing protocols to spot and correct any unfair results (Padmaja et al., 2022).

Figure 5. Usability of AI in disease screening

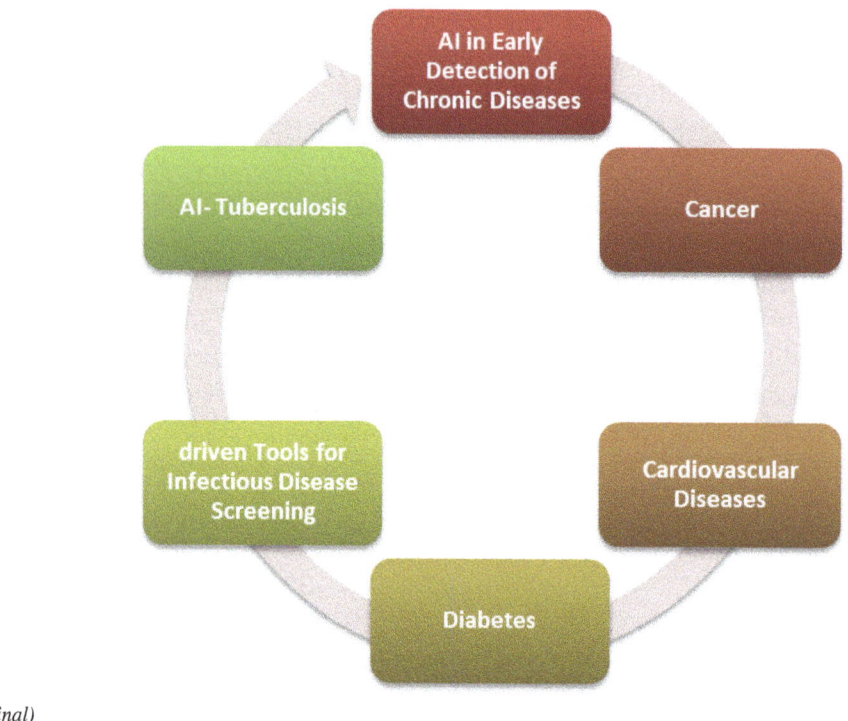

(Original)

5. IMPLEMENTATION OF AI IN HEALTHIER HOMES

Effective treatment planning requires accurate disease diagnosis, which is mostly dependent on patient history, laboratory results, imaging tests, and biopsies collectively referred to as "medical diagnostics." Healthcare professionals frequently struggle to obtain appropriate diagnoses due to the complexity of this diagnostic procedure, which can upset patients and jeopardize their wellbeing (Shah et al., 2017). Nonetheless, the likelihood of human mistake in illness diagnosis has been greatly decreased by the digitalization of healthcare and the development of artificial intelligence (AI) (Singh & Kaunert, 2024). AI increased efficiency and precision have resulted in a dramatic transformation in the field of diagnostics (Marjani et al., 2017). The process of finding, developing, and producing drugs has given rise to new possibilities for treating a range of illnesses. The pharmaceutical business is poised for even more transformation thanks to the incorporation of AI and other technologies into these procedures (Singh, 2024).

Clinical researchers are being compelled by high drug development costs and other obstacles to investigate novel instruments for more effective medication market entrance (Chen & Zhang, 2024). The procedure is high risk and high reward, involving decades of study and billions of dollars, with no assurance of FDA (Food and Drug Administration) regulatory clearance. Significant obstacles to medication research and discovery can be addressed with the use of AI and other technologies (Thapa & Camtepe, 2021). Drug production is changing as a result of artificial intelligence and machine learning, which improves quality control, predictive maintenance, and process optimization (Behure et al., 2021). They increase productivity by seeing data trends that humans would overlook. A patient's health and well-being are extensively documented in electronic health records in both organized and unstructured formats. Health systems have faced difficulties in making this data accessible and useful, despite its value to physicians (Olshannikova et al., 2015).

Healthcare companies have a rare chance to overcome some of these obstacles with AI, and some are already seeing success. The goal of EHR adoption is to improve cost-effective care delivery and optimize clinical processes. On the other hand, administrative duties related to EHRs and clinical recording are frequently mentioned by physicians as sources of stress and burnout (Rudin, 2019). AI solutions are crucial for resolving these problems and freeing up clinicians' time so they may concentrate on patients. AI may be used in a variety of ways to address physician stress, mostly by automating HER workflow (Wu et al., 2013).

Figure 6. Implementation of AI in healthier homes

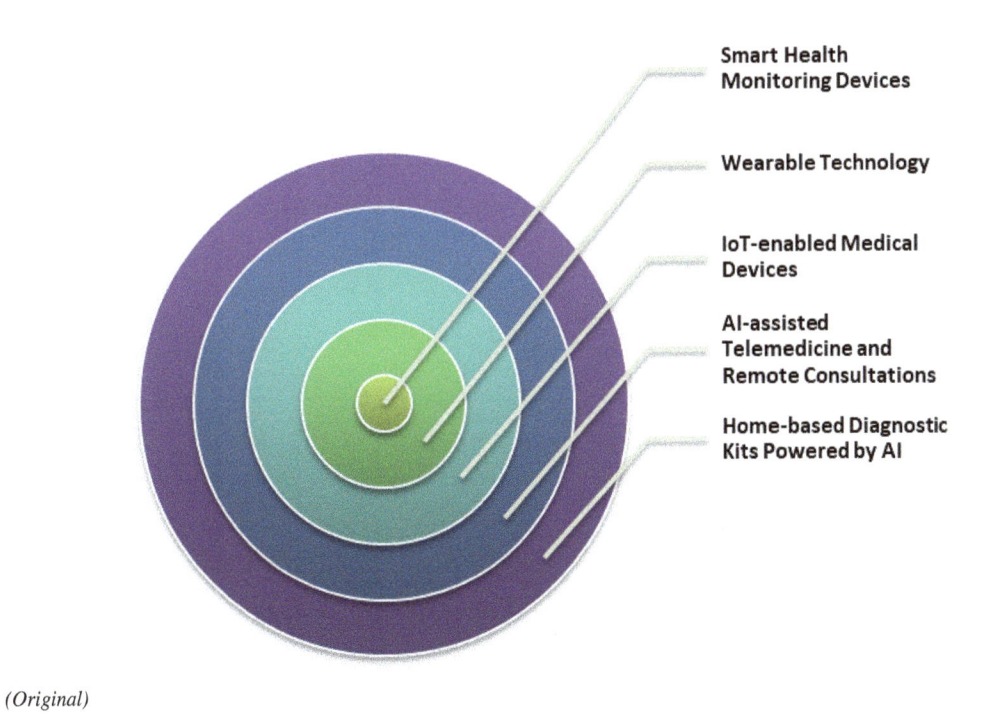

(Original)

6. ETHICAL AND REGULATORY CONSIDERATIONS

There are numerous administrative facets of medical treatment are being transformed by artificial intelligence (AI) in the healthcare industry. AI may help healthcare companies and providers focus more on patient care and revenue cycle management by automating repetitive operations like data input, claims processing, and appointment scheduling (Saadat & Shuaib, 2020). Medical practitioners may concentrate on providing high-quality treatment while saving time and money by using AI to handle administrative work. AI is leading the charge in enhancing patient care (Kitchin, 2013). AI in healthcare provides a simplified method for medical professionals to give better and quicker patient care. Artificial intelligence (AI) gives medical professionals more control over their workflow and saves time and money by automating repetitive administrative duties (Shahid, 2021). AI can also decrease human mistake by offering a quicker means of reviewing test findings, claims, medical imaging, and health data (Monteiro et al., 2021). Medical practitioners may provide better patient care while being cost-effective thanks to AI, which gives them more control over their workflow. Healthcare delivery is changing as a result of AI capacity to evaluate a patient's medical history and produce faster, more accurate findings, freeing up doctors to devote more time and resources to patient care. When healthcare firms have to convert their old data to new EHR systems, AI is also helpful. This procedure frequently finds inconsistent, partial, or missing patient records, which results in major inefficiencies (Qureshi et al., 2023).

Data translation is typically needed to translate information into the "language" of the new EHR when there are discrepancies in medical records (Leung et al., 2021). The data is often translated by hand using humans in this process, which is labor-intensive, time-consuming, and prone to new mistakes that might endanger patient safety (Faaique, 2024). For the purpose of making the most of novel forms of patient data, such insights from genetic testing, advanced analytics tools are also essential (Faaique, 2024). In order to ensure ethical behavior and the evidence-based use of AI in healthcare, it seeks to build robust governance frameworks, rules, and technical standards (Pradhan et al., 2024). It wants to establish a worldwide network of experts and resources that encourage knowledge exchange and collective action (Singh & Kaunert, 2024), increasing AI effect in healthcare through cooperative efforts and pooled investments (Singh et al., 2024). The mission is to create and advance viable models for national AI (Kong et al., 2024) program implementation that will enable AI solutions to be used successfully and widely in a variety of healthcare systems (Aghabiglou et al., 2024).

Figure 7. Ethical and regulatory considerations

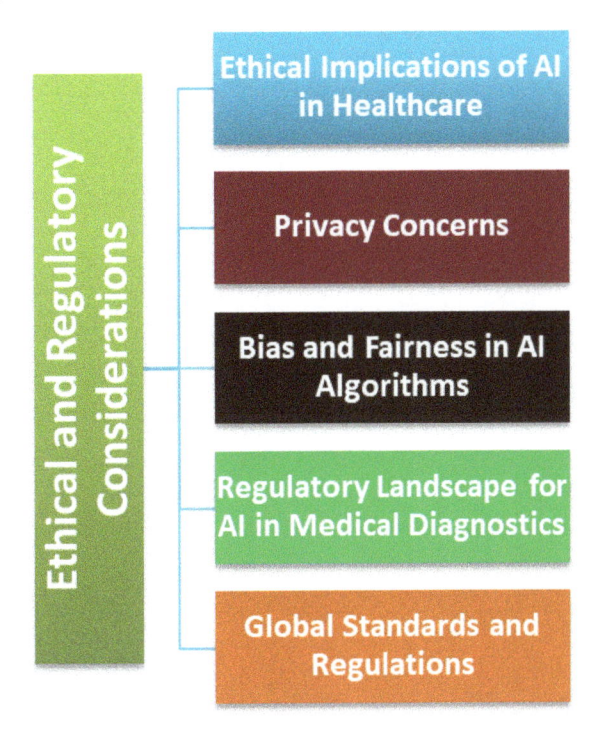

(Original)

7. CONCLUSION AND FUTURE SCOPE

Over the past half-century, the primary focus of artificial intelligence (AI) in healthcare has been on illness detection and treatment (Singh & Kaunert, 2025). Although early rule-based systems had the potential to provide precise diagnosis and therapy, clinical practice did not generally adopt them (Singh et al., 2025). They were challenging to incorporate into physician workflows and health record systems, and their diagnostic performance did not far above that of human diagnoses (Singh et al., 2025). Aligning AI for diagnosis and treatment planning with clinical processes and electronic health record (EHR) systems can be difficult, regardless of whether the AI is rule-based or algorithmic (Singh & Kaunert, 2025) (Singh & Kaunert, 2024). More than the accuracy of its recommendations, integration problems in healthcare organizations have been a major obstacle to the broad adoption of AI in the field. AI has made significant advances in pathology by speeding up slide processing and enhancing disease identification (Singh & Kaunert, 2025). Research has shown that AI can identify cellular and tissue anomalies, enabling pathologists to diagnose diseases more accurately (Singh & Kaunert, 2025). In dermatology, AI-powered tools like deep-learning algorithms can accurately detect skin cancer by analyzing images, even rivaling the diagnostic skills of dermatologists (Singh et al., 2025). AI algorithms could identify melanomas and other skin cancers through image analysis, providing a valuable diagnostic tool for clinicians. This accelerated data processing translates into quicker diagnoses and timely interventions, potentially preventing critical outcomes in future.

REFERENCES

Aghabiglou, A., Chu, C. S., Dabbech, A., & Wiaux, Y. (2024). The R2D2 deep neural network series paradigm for fast precision imaging in radio astronomy. *arXiv preprint arXiv:2403.05452*.

Ahmed, Y. A. E., Yue, B., Gu, Z., & Yang, J. (2023). An overview: Big data analysis by deep learning and image processing. *International Journal of Quantum Information*, 21(7), 2340009. DOI: 10.1142/S0219749923400099

Al-Jarrah, O. Y., Yoo, P. D., Muhaidat, S., Karagiannidis, G. K., & Taha, K. (2015). Efficient machine learning for big data: A review. *Big Data Research*, 2(3), 87–93. DOI: 10.1016/j.bdr.2015.04.001

Ariffin, N. A., Yunus, A. M., & Kadir, I. K. (2021). The role of big data in the healthcare industry. *Journal of Islamic*, 6(36), 235–245.

Bahri, S., Zoghlami, N., Abed, M., & Tavares, J. M. R. (2018). Big data for healthcare: A survey. *IEEE Access : Practical Innovations, Open Solutions*, 7, 7397–7408. DOI: 10.1109/ACCESS.2018.2889180

Bao, Y., Tang, Z., Li, H., & Zhang, Y. (2019). Computer vision and deep learning–based data anomaly detection method for structural health monitoring. *Structural Health Monitoring*, 18(2), 401–421. DOI: 10.1177/1475921718757405

Behura, A., Sahu, S., & Kabat, M. R. (2021). Advancement of Machine Learning and Cloud Computing in the Field of Smart Health Care. *Machine Learning Approach for Cloud Data Analytics in IoT*, 273-306.

Bhattacharyya, D., Stephen Neal Joshua, E., & Thirupathi Rao, N. (2023). Medical Image Analysis of Lung Cancer CT Scans Using Deep Learning with Swarm Optimization Techniques. *Machine Intelligence, Big Data Analytics, and IoT in Image Processing: Practical Applications*, 23-50.

Cabello, J. C., Karimipour, H., Jahromi, A. N., Dehghantanha, A., & Parizi, R. M. (2020). Big-data and cyber-physical systems in healthcare: Challenges and opportunities. *Handbook of Big Data Privacy*, 255-283.

Chen, C. P., & Zhang, C. Y. (2014). Data-intensive applications, challenges, techniques and technologies: A survey on Big Data. *Information sciences, 275*, 314-347. Mayer-Schönberger, V., & Cukier, K. (2013). *Big data: A revolution that will transform how we live, work, and think*. Houghton Mifflin Harcourt.

Chen, M., Mao, S., Zhang, Y., & Leung, V. C. (2014). *Big data: related technologies, challenges and future prospects* (Vol. 100). Springer. DOI: 10.1007/978-3-319-06245-7

Dash, S., Shakyawar, S. K., Sharma, M., & Kaushik, S. (2019). Big data in healthcare: Management, analysis and future prospects. *Journal of Big Data*, 6(1), 1–25. DOI: 10.1186/s40537-019-0217-0

Devika, G., & Karegowda, A. G. (2021). Deep Learning in IoT: Introduction, Applications, and Perspective in the Big Data Era. In *Deep Learning Applications and Intelligent Decision Making in Engineering* (pp. 1-54). IGI Global.

Elbadawi, M., Gaisford, S., & Basit, A. W. (2021). Advanced machine-learning techniques in drug discovery. *Drug Discovery Today*, 26(3), 769–777. DOI: 10.1016/j.drudis.2020.12.003 PMID: 33290820

Faaique, M. (2024). Overview of Big Data Analytics in Modern Astronomy. *International Journal of Mathematics, Statistics, and Computer Science*, 2, 96–113. DOI: 10.59543/ijmscs.v2i.8561

Hilbert, M. (2016). Big data for development: A review of promises and challenges. *Development Policy Review*, 34(1), 135–174. DOI: 10.1111/dpr.12142

Jain, L. (2023). Artificial Intelligence and Machine Learning for Healthcare.

Jordan, M. I., & Mitchell, T. M. (2015). Machine learning: Trends, perspectives, and prospects. *Science*, 349(6245), 255–260. DOI: 10.1126/science.aaa8415 PMID: 26185243

Kashyap, H., Ahmed, H. A., Hoque, N., Roy, S., & Bhattacharyya, D. K. (2015). Big data analytics in bioinformatics: A machine learning perspective. *arXiv preprint arXiv:1506.05101*.

Kashyap, H., Ahmed, H. A., Hoque, N., Roy, S., & Bhattacharyya, D. K. (2016). Big data analytics in bioinformatics: Architectures, techniques, tools and issues. *Network Modeling and Analysis in Health Informatics and Bioinformatics*, 5(1), 1–28. DOI: 10.1007/s13721-016-0135-4

Keikhosrokiani, P. (Ed.). (2022). *Big data analytics for healthcare: datasets, techniques, life cycles, management, and applications*. Academic Press.

Khurana, V. (2024). Accelerating Pace of Scientific Discovery and Innovation through Big Data Enabled Artificial Intelligence and Deep Learning. *Emerging Trends in Machine Intelligence and Big Data*, 16(1), 38–53.

Kitchin, R. (2013). Big data and human geography: Opportunities, challenges and risks. *Dialogues in Human Geography*, 3(3), 262–267. DOI: 10.1177/2043820613513388

Kong, W., You, Z., Lyu, S., & Lv, X. (2024). Multi-dimensional stereo face reconstruction for psychological assistant diagnosis in medical meta-universe. *Information Sciences*, 654, 119831. DOI: 10.1016/j.ins.2023.119831

Leung, P. H., Chui, K. T., Lo, K., & de Pablos, P. O. (2021). A support vector machine–based voice disorders detection using human voice signal. In *Artificial Intelligence and Big Data Analytics for Smart Healthcare* (pp. 197–208). Academic Press. DOI: 10.1016/B978-0-12-822060-3.00014-0

Li, W., Chai, Y., Khan, F., Jan, S. R. U., Verma, S., Menon, V. G., & Li, X. (2021). A comprehensive survey on machine learning-based big data analytics for IoT-enabled smart healthcare system. *Mobile Networks and Applications*, 26(1), 234–252. DOI: 10.1007/s11036-020-01700-6

Luo, J., Wu, M., Gopukumar, D., & Zhao, Y. (2016). Big data application in biomedical research and health care: a literature review. *Biomedical informatics insights, 8*, BII-S31559.

Malik, S., & Tyagi, A. K. (Eds.). (2022). *Intelligent Interactive Multimedia Systems for E-Healthcare Applications*. CRC Press. DOI: 10.1201/9781003282112

Manyika, J., Chui, M., Brown, B., Bughin, J., Dobbs, R., Roxburgh, C., & Hung Byers, A. (2011). Big data: The next frontier for innovation, competition, and productivity.

Marjani, M., Nasaruddin, F., Gani, A., Karim, A., Hashem, I. A. T., Siddiqa, A., & Yaqoob, I. (2017). Big IoT data analytics: architecture, opportunities, and open research challenges. *ieee access, 5*, 5247-5261.

Miller, D. D., & Brown, E. W. (2018). Artificial intelligence in medical practice: The question to the answer? *The American Journal of Medicine*, 131(2), 129–133. DOI: 10.1016/j.amjmed.2017.10.035 PMID: 29126825

Mohammadi, M., Al-Fuqaha, A., Sorour, S., & Guizani, M. (2018). Deep learning for IoT big data and streaming analytics: A survey. *IEEE Communications Surveys and Tutorials*, 20(4), 2923–2960. DOI: 10.1109/COMST.2018.2844341

Monteiro, A. C. B., França, R. P., Arthur, R., & Iano, Y. (2021). An overview of medical Internet of Things, artificial intelligence, and cloud computing employed in health care from a modern panorama. *The Fusion of Internet of Things, Artificial Intelligence, and Cloud Computing in Health Care*, 3-23.

Muthu, B., Sivaparthipan, C. B., Manogaran, G., Sundarasekar, R., Kadry, S., Shanthini, A., & Dasel, A. (2020). IOT based wearable sensor for diseases prediction and symptom analysis in healthcare sector. *Peer-to-Peer Networking and Applications*, 13(6), 2123–2134. DOI: 10.1007/s12083-019-00823-2

Olshannikova, E., Ometov, A., Koucheryavy, Y., & Olsson, T. (2015). Visualizing Big Data with augmented and virtual reality: Challenges and research agenda. *Journal of Big Data*, 2(1), 1–27. DOI: 10.1186/s40537-015-0031-2

Padmaja, M., Shitharth, S., Prasuna, K., Chaturvedi, A., Kshirsagar, P. R., & Vani, A. (2022). Grow of artificial intelligence to challenge security in IoT application. *Wireless Personal Communications*, 127(3), 1829–1845. DOI: 10.1007/s11277-021-08725-4

Panesar, A. (2019). *Machine learning and AI for healthcare*. Apress. DOI: 10.1007/978-1-4842-3799-1

Pradhan, T., Nimkar, P., & Jhajharia, K. (2024). Machine Learning and Deep Learning for Big Data Analysis. In *Big Data Analytics Techniques for Market Intelligence* (pp. 209–240). IGI Global. DOI: 10.4018/979-8-3693-0413-6.ch008

Pramanik, P. K. D., Pal, S., & Mukhopadhyay, M. (2022). Healthcare big data: A comprehensive overview. *Research anthology on big data analytics, architectures, and applications*, 119-147.

Qureshi, R., Irfan, M., Ali, H., Khan, A., Nittala, A. S., Ali, S., & Alam, T. (2023). Artificial Intelligence and Biosensors in Healthcare and its Clinical Relevance: A Review. *IEEE Access: Practical Innovations, Open Solutions*, 11, 61600–61620. DOI: 10.1109/ACCESS.2023.3285596

Reddy, B. M. (2023). Amalgamation of Internet of Things and Machine Learning for Smart Healthcare Applications–A Review. *Int. J Comp. Eng. Sci. Res, 5*, 08-36.

Rodrigues, J. F.Jr, Florea, L., de Oliveira, M. C., Diamond, D., & Oliveira, O. N.Jr. (2021). Big data and machine learning for materials science. *Discover Materials*, 1(1), 1–27. DOI: 10.1007/s43939-021-00012-0 PMID: 33899049

Rudin, C. (2019). Stop explaining black box machine learning models for high stakes decisions and use interpretable models instead. *Nature Machine Intelligence*, 1(5), 206–215. DOI: 10.1038/s42256-019-0048-x PMID: 35603010

Saadat, M. N., & Shuaib, M. (2020). Advancements in deep learning theory and applications: Perspective in 2020 and beyond. *Advances and Applications in Deep Learning, 3*.

Sardar, T. H., Khatun, A., Sengupta, S., Alam, Y., & Ara, T. (2024). Machine Learning in the Healthcare Sector and the Biomedical Big Data: Techniques, Applications, and Challenges. *Big Data Computing*, 336-352.

Scarpato, N., Pieroni, A., Di Nunzio, L., & Fallucchi, F. (2017). E-health-IoT universe: A review. *management, 21*(44), 46.

Sejdic, E., & Falk, T. H. (Eds.). (2018). *Signal processing and machine learning for biomedical big data*. CRC press. DOI: 10.1201/9781351061223

Sengan, S., Kamalam, G. K., Vellingiri, J., Gopal, J., Velayutham, P., & Subramaniyaswamy, V. (2020). Medical information retrieval systems for e-Health care records using fuzzy based machine learning model. *Microprocessors and Microsystems*, •••, 103344.

Shah, F., Li, J., Shah, Y., & Shah, F. (2017, November). Broad big data domain via medical big data. In *2017 4th International Conference on Systems and Informatics (ICSAI)* (pp. 732-737). IEEE.

Shahid, Z. (2021). Distributed Machine Learning for Anomalous Human Activity Recognition using IoT Systems.

Singh, B. (2023). Blockchain Technology in Renovating Healthcare: Legal and Future Perspectives. In *Revolutionizing Healthcare Through Artificial Intelligence and Internet of Things Applications* (pp. 177-186). IGI Global.

Singh, B. (2023). Unleashing Alternative Dispute Resolution (ADR) in Resolving Complex Legal-Technical Issues Arising in Cyberspace Lensing E-Commerce and Intellectual Property: Proliferation of E-Commerce Digital Economy. *Revista Brasileira de Alternative Dispute Resolution-Brazilian Journal of Alternative Dispute Resolution-RBADR*, 5(10), 81–105. DOI: 10.52028/rbadr.v5i10.ART04.Ind

Singh, B. (2024). Lensing Legal Dynamics for Examining Responsibility and Deliberation of Generative AI-Tethered Technological Privacy Concerns: Infringements and Use of Personal Data by Nefarious Actors. In Ara, A., & Ara, A. (Eds.), *Exploring the Ethical Implications of Generative AI* (pp. 146–167). IGI Global., DOI: 10.4018/979-8-3693-1565-1.ch009

Singh, B. (2024). Social Cognition of Incarcerated Women and Children: Addressing Exposure to Infectious Diseases and Legal Outcomes. In Reddy, K. (Ed.), *Principles and Clinical Interventions in Social Cognition* (pp. 236–251). IGI Global., DOI: 10.4018/979-8-3693-1265-0.ch014

Singh, B. (2024). Evolutionary Global Neuroscience for Cognition and Brain Health: Strengthening Innovation in Brain Science. In *Biomedical Research Developments for Improved Healthcare* (pp. 246-272). IGI Global.

Singh, B., & Kaunert, C. (2024). Salvaging Responsible Consumption and Production of Food in the Hospitality Industry: Harnessing Machine Learning and Deep Learning for Zero Food Waste. In Singh, A., Tyagi, P., & Garg, A. (Eds.), *Sustainable Disposal Methods of Food Wastes in Hospitality Operations* (pp. 176–192). IGI Global., DOI: 10.4018/979-8-3693-2181-2.ch012

Singh, B., & Kaunert, C. (2024). Harnessing Sustainable Agriculture Through Climate-Smart Technologies: Artificial Intelligence for Climate Preservation and Futuristic Trends. In *Exploring Ethical Dimensions of Environmental Sustainability and Use of AI* (pp. 214-239). IGI Global.

Singh, B., & Kaunert, C. (2024). Salvaging Responsible Consumption and Production of Food in the Hospitality Industry: Harnessing Machine Learning and Deep Learning for Zero Food Waste. In *Sustainable Disposal Methods of Food Wastes in Hospitality Operations* (pp. 176-192). IGI Global.

Singh, B., & Kaunert, C. (2024). Future of Digital Marketing: Hyper-Personalized Customer Dynamic Experience with AI-Based Predictive Models. *Revolutionizing the AI-Digital Landscape: A Guide to Sustainable Emerging Technologies for Marketing Professionals*, 189.

Singh, B., & Kaunert, C. (2024). Adventure in High Altitude of Mountainous Topographies and Health Impacts: Lensing Tourism Sustainability via Reducing Ecological and Sociocultural Footprint and Health Emergency and Medical Assistance Management. In Meraj, G., Hashimoto, S., & Kumar, P. (Eds.), *Navigating Natural Hazards in Mountainous Topographies. Disaster Risk Reduction.* Springer., DOI: 10.1007/978-3-031-65862-4_15

Singh, B., & Kaunert, C. (2025). Leveraging IoT for Patient Monitoring and Smart Healthcare: Connected Healthcare System. In B. S & S. Kadry (Eds.), *Revolutionizing Healthcare Systems Through Cloud Computing and IoT* (pp. 27-46). IGI Global. https://doi.org/DOI: 10.4018/979-8-3693-7225-8.ch002

Singh, B., & Kaunert, C. (2025). Cloud Computing and IoMT in Disease Screening and Diagnosis: AI Approaches in Transmuting Healthier Homes. In B. S & S. Kadry (Eds.), *Revolutionizing Healthcare Systems Through Cloud Computing and IoT* (pp. 99-120). IGI Global. DOI: 10.4018/979-8-3693-7225-8.ch005

Singh, B., & Kaunert, C. (2025). Featuring Healthcare, Environment, and Human Rights: Applications of Artificial Intelligence in the Health Domain. In Chakraborty, S., & Satapathy, S. (Eds.), *Gender, Environment, and Human Rights: An Intersectional Exploration* (pp. 45–74). IGI Global., DOI: 10.4018/979-8-3693-6069-9.ch004

Singh, B., & Kaunert, C. (2025). Intelligent Machine Learning Solutions for Cybersecurity: Legal and Ethical Considerations in a Global Context. In Thangam, D. (Ed.), *Advancements in Intelligent Process Automation* (pp. 359–386). IGI Global., DOI: 10.4018/979-8-3693-5380-6.ch014

Singh, B., Kaunert, C., & Singh, G. (2025). Scaling Legal Framework for Plastic Pollution and Advancing Cutting Edge Water Governance: Reducing and Eliminating Marine Pollution in Alignment With SDG 14 (Life Below Water). In Gaur, N., Sharma, E., Nguyen, T., Bilal, M., & Melkania, N. (Eds.), *Societal and Environmental Ramifications of Plastic Pollution* (pp. 197–222). IGI Global., DOI: 10.4018/979-8-3693-9163-1.ch010

Singh, B., Kaunert, C., & Vig, K. (2024). Reinventing Influence of Artificial Intelligence (AI) on Digital Consumer Lensing Transforming Consumer Recommendation Model: Exploring Stimulus Artificial Intelligence on Consumer Shopping Decisions. In Musiolik, T., Rodriguez, R., & Kannan, H. (Eds.), *AI Impacts in Digital Consumer Behavior* (pp. 141–169). IGI Global., DOI: 10.4018/979-8-3693-1918-5.ch006

Singh, B., Lal, S., Arora, M. K., & Kaunert, C. (2025). Mounting Legal-Driven Solutions for Plastic Pollution Focusing on Environment and Coastal Management: Eradicating Marine Pollution in Alignment With SDG 14 (Life Below Water). In Gaur, N., Sharma, E., Nguyen, T., Bilal, M., & Melkania, N. (Eds.), *Societal and Environmental Ramifications of Plastic Pollution* (pp. 223–252). IGI Global., DOI: 10.4018/979-8-3693-9163-1.ch011

Singh, B., Singh, A., Kaunert, C., Arora, M. K., Lal, S., & Ravesangar, K. (2025). Unleashing the Ethical and Legal Implications of E-Business Revolution: Consumer Privacy and Security Concerns in Phase of Digital Disruption. In Taherdoost, H., Drazenovic, G., Madanchian, M., Khan, I., & Arshi, O. (Eds.), *Business Transformation in the Era of Digital Disruption* (pp. 157–180). IGI Global., DOI: 10.4018/979-8-3693-7056-8.ch006

Singh, B., Vig, K., & Kaunert, C. (2024). Modernizing Healthcare: Application of Augmented Reality and Virtual Reality in Clinical Practice and Medical Education. In Modern Technology in Healthcare and Medical Education: Blockchain, IoT, AR, and VR (pp. 1-21). IGI Global.

Stephens, Z. D., Lee, S. Y., Faghri, F., Campbell, R. H., Zhai, C., Efron, M. J., & Robinson, G. E. (2015). Big data: Astronomical or genomical? *PLoS Biology*, 13(7), e1002195. DOI: 10.1371/journal.pbio.1002195 PMID: 26151137

Sukeshini, S., P., Ved, M., Chintalapti, J., & Pal, S. N. (2021). Big data analytics and machine learning technologies for HPC applications. In Evolving Technologies for Computing, Communication and Smart World: Proceedings of ETCCS 2020 (pp. 411-424). Springer Singapore.

Thapa, C., & Camtepe, S. (2021). Precision health data: Requirements, challenges and existing techniques for data security and privacy. *Computers in Biology and Medicine*, 129, 104130. DOI: 10.1016/j.compbiomed.2020.104130 PMID: 33271399

Tiwari, S. K., Kaur, J., Singla, P., & Hrisheekesha, P. N. (2022, September). A Comprehensive Review of Big Data Analysis Techniques in Health-Care. In *International Conference on Emergent Converging Technologies and Biomedical Systems* (pp. 401-420). Singapore: Springer Nature Singapore.

Viceconti, M., Hunter, P., & Hose, R. (2015). Big data, big knowledge: Big data for personalized healthcare. *IEEE Journal of Biomedical and Health Informatics*, 19(4), 1209–1215. DOI: 10.1109/JBHI.2015.2406883 PMID: 26218867

Wu, X., Zhu, X., Wu, G. Q., & Ding, W. (2013). Data mining with big data. *IEEE Transactions on Knowledge and Data Engineering*, 26(1), 97–107.

Zhou, L., Pan, S., Wang, J., & Vasilakos, A. V. (2017). Machine learning on big data: Opportunities and challenges. *Neurocomputing*, 237, 350–361. DOI: 10.1016/j.neucom.2017.01.026

Zhou, S., Zhang, R., Chen, D., & Zhu, X. (2021). A novel framework for bringing smart big data to proactive decision making in healthcare. *Health Informatics Journal*, 27(2), 14604582211024698. DOI: 10.1177/14604582211024698 PMID: 34159834

Zhou, S. K., Greenspan, H., Davatzikos, C., Duncan, J. S., Van Ginneken, B., Madabhushi, A., Prince, J. L., Rueckert, D., & Summers, R. M. (2021). A review of deep learning in medical imaging: Imaging traits, technology trends, case studies with progress highlights, and future promises. *Proceedings of the IEEE*, 109(5), 820–838. DOI: 10.1109/JPROC.2021.3054390 PMID: 37786449

Chapter 11
Enhanced Diabetic Retinopathy Classification Using Inception Net V3:
A Deep Learning Approach

R. Ravindraiah
Madanapalle Institute of Technology and Science, India

Grande Naga Jyothi
Madanapalle Institute of Technology and Science, India

Nukala Bharath Kumar
Madanapalle Institute of Technology and Science, India

B. Ganesh
Madanapalle Institute of Technology and Science, India

D. Badri
Madanapalle Institute of Technology and Science, India

ABSTRACT

This study employs a novel approach for the automatic classification of Diabetic Retinopathy (DR) through a customized Inception Net V3 Convolutional Neural Network (CNN) method. DR is leading reason for visual impairment and necessitates early and accurate diagnosis for effective intervention. Leveraging deep learning, the proposed CNN model demonstrates remarkable proficiency in discerning diverse stages of DR from retinal images. The network is trained on a comprehensive dataset meticulously annotated with DR stages, ensuring robust learning and generalization. Through an extensive evaluation, this model exhibits superior performance in classifying DR severity levels, showcasing its potential as a valuable diagnostic tool. The proposed CNN architecture not only enhances classification accuracy but also facilitates interpretability, shedding light on the critical features contributing to each classification. The proposed design has been implemented in MATLAB 2023(a)

DOI: 10.4018/979-8-3693-6180-1.ch011

1 INTRODUCTION

Diabetes Mellitus (DM) is an incurable condition marked by high blood sugar levels brought on by either insufficient insulin synthesis or poor insulin utilization by the body. The hormone insulin, which is generated by the pancreas, aids in the movement of bloodstream glucose into cells so that it can be metabolized into energy. Hyperglycemia results from elevated blood glucose levels caused by the body's improper response to insulin or insufficient pancreatic production of the hormone. Over time, hyperglycemia can cause severe complications, including damage to organs and tissues, contributing to conditions such as retinopathy, nephropathy, neuropathy, and cardiovascular diseases. DM is also linked with a bigger risk of certain cancers and cognitive decline. While the classification and diagnosis of DM have evolved over time, proper management is crucial in delaying or preventing these serious complications (Wong E et at. 2013).

DM is primarily classified into three significant categories are: Type 1 Diabetes Mellitus (T1D), Type 2 Diabetes Mellitus (T2D), and Gestational Diabetes Mellitus (GDM). Less common types include Secondary Diabetes and Monogenic Diabetes Mellitus (MDM). In T1D, the immune system of the body targets and kills the pancreas's β-cells that produce insulin. This leads to a complete or partial deficiency in insulin production. Genetic predisposition, environmental factors (such as toxins or viral infections), and dietary influences can trigger this condition. T1D is most often diagnosed in children and adolescents and is also known as insulin-dependent or juvenile-onset diabetes. Managing T1D requires daily insulin injections to maintain glucose levels, as the body cannot produce insulin on its own. Without insulin therapy, survival is difficult. Complications of T1D include damage to small blood vessels, leading to DR (eye damage), nephropathy (kidney damage), and neuropathy (nerve damage). Symptoms of T1D include dry mouth, excessive thirst, frequent urination, bedwetting, constant hunger, fatigue, sudden weight loss, and blurred vision. A combination of a healthy diet, regular monitoring of glucose levels, physical activity, and proper insulin administration is essential for preventing or delaying these complications (DeFronzo RA et. al., 2015).

T2D is the most common form of diabetes, accounting for about 90% of all cases. It is characterized by insulin resistance, where the body cannot effectively use insulin, and often by insufficient insulin production. This leads to hyperglycemia. T2D, also known as adult-onset or non-insulin-dependent diabetes, typically develops in older adults, but it is increasingly seen in younger individuals, including adolescents, due to factors such as poor diet, obesity, and lack of physical activity. High consumption of sugar-sweetened beverages, saturated fats, and low dietary fiber intake are major contributors to the development of T2D. Children who consume large amounts of sugary drinks are at a higher risk of obesity and T2D. Other risk factors include active smoking. T2D shares many symptoms with T1D, including frequent infections, slow healing of wounds, and numbness in the hands and feet. Like T1D, T2D can cause complications such as DR, nephropathy, neuropathy, heart disease, and stroke. GDM is a form of diabetes that occurs during pregnancy and is characterized by elevated glucose levels that can range from mild to severe. IGT is a risk factor for developing T2D, and lifestyle interventions can prevent its progression (Thomas ER et. al 2016).

DR stands as one of the most widespread and pervasive complications arising from diabetes mellitus, posing a significant threat to the vision and overall ocular health of affected individuals. It is a microvascular condition with adverse effect of diabetes, that upshot the delicate retinal blood vessels, leading to progressive damage and disablement of vision. As the main reason for blindness in adults of working age, timely and accuracy of diagnosis is crucial for effective intervention and management. Two major classifications include (i) Non-Proliferative Diabetic Retinopathy (NPDR) and (ii) Proliferative Diabetic Retinopathy (PDR). The early stage of NPDR is characterized by exudates from leaking and blocked blood vessels, microaneurysms, and haemorrhages. It can be mild, moderate, or severe. Neovascularization, the formation of new, delicate blood vessels during the progression of DR into PDR, can be extremely dangerous as it can result in severe complications like vitreous haemorrhage and retinal detachment, which can cause profound vision loss. Comprehensive eye exams, such as dilated eye exams, fluorescein angiography, optical coherence tomography (OCT) to evaluate fluid accumulation and retinal damage, are part of the diagnosis process. The management of DR requires early detection and routine monitoring; depending on the severity, treatment options include laser therapy, injections, and surgery. It is possible to maintain vision and stop the progression of DR to more advanced stages by treating it early (IDF Diabetes Atlas, 2021).

The World Health Organization (WHO) has observed a significant increase in the number of people with Diabetes Mellitus (DM) since 1980, with cases quadrupling from 108 million in 1980 to 422 million in 2014. During this period, the prevalence of DM among adults aged 18 and older rose from 4.7% to 8.5%, contributing to higher rates of disability and premature death. In 2012, DM was linked to an estimated 2.2 million deaths, a number that decreased to 1.6 million by 2016. WHO recognized DM as the 7th leading cause of death in 2016, with hyperglycemia responsible for nearly half of all deaths in people under the age of 70. DM has a profound impact on public health and the global economy, reducing life expectancy, disabling individuals, and diminishing the productivity of working-age populations. It affects all socioeconomic groups and is a widespread issue across the globe, not limited to specific countries. As a global epidemic, DM continues to escalate healthcare costs, lower productivity, and slow economic growth, making it one of the most pressing global health crises of the 21st century (Bloom DE et. al., 2011).

The International Diabetes Federation (IDF) estimates that 8.8% of the global population aged 20-79 years has Diabetes Mellitus (DM), affecting 425 million people worldwide, with 79% of cases occurring in low- and middle-income countries. When the age range is expanded to 18-99 years, the number of people with DM rises to 451 million. By 2045, the number of individuals with DM is projected to increase to 629 million for the 20-79 age group or 693 million for those aged 18-99 years. This growth is particularly significant in countries moving from low to middle-income economies, driven by aging populations and population growth, which together account for an increase of over one-third. Age alone contributes to 28% of the rise in DM cases, which increases to 32% when considering the broader age range.

On a global scale, around USD 727 billion is spent annually on DM healthcare. In 2017, 326.5 million working-age individuals (20-64 years) were living with DM, a number expected to grow to 438.2 million by 2045. Among those aged 65-99 years, the number was 122.8 million in 2017 and is projected to reach 253.4 million by 2045. Regarding gender, the prevalence of DM is estimated at 9.1% in men and 8.4% in women, with these figures expected to rise to 10% and 9.7%, respectively. The highest rates of DM are observed in both men and women aged 65-79 years. DM is also a major contributor to three leading non-communicable diseases (NCDs): respiratory diseases, cancer, and cardiovascular diseases, which together account for about 80% of early NCD-related deaths. In 2015, NCDs were responsible for 39.5 million of the 56.4 million deaths worldwide. A significant global challenge lies in the high percentage of undiagnosed cases, ranging from 30% to 80%. In high-income countries, Type 2 Diabetes (T2D) represents approximately 87% to 91% of all DM cases, while Type 1 Diabetes (T1D) accounts for 7% to 12%, with other types of DM comprising 1% to 3%. T1D is predominantly seen in children and adolescents, but its connection to T2D in middle- and low-income countries remains underexplored (Lancet, 2016).

According to estimates from the WHO, 422 million people worldwide suffer with diabetes, approximately one-third of these individuals, are at risk of developing it (Frank K. J et al., 1996). DR impact extends beyond its direct effects on vision, influencing quality of life, economic productivity, and healthcare burden. Traditional methods of DR diagnosing often rely heavily manually assessment by skilled ophthalmologists, which could take a long time, subjective, and prone to inter-observer variability [Gang L et al., 2002]. However, this approach has several limitations, including subjectivity, reliance on human expertise. Also, the increasing diabetes prevalence and consequent rise in the quantity of retinal images for evaluation underscore the need for automated and efficient diagnostic tools.

Diabetic Eye Disease (DED) occurs due to vascular damage from chronic hyperglycemia. This damage leads to capillary leakage, causing blood, proteins, and fat-based particles to accumulate in the retinal fundus as exudates, ultimately resulting in vision loss. As DED progresses, it can significantly threaten vision. DED includes conditions like DR, Diabetic Macular Edema (DME), glaucoma, double vision, cataracts, and difficulties in focusing. The risk of retinopathy is particularly high in individuals with Type 1 Diabetes (T1D), especially those with a long history of the condition and those in lower socioeconomic positions. DR is one of the most prevalent forms of DED and is directly triggered by DM. This condition involves progressive damage to the retina, which can ultimately lead to vision loss. Statistics show that around 80% of people who have had diabetes for 20 years or more are likely to develop DR. However, with proper monitoring and timely treatment, up to 90% of new DR cases can be effectively managed and prevented from advancing to more severe stages (Evans JM et. al 2000).

DR is the leading cause of vision impairment among adults aged 20 to 64, a critical age range where such impairment can significantly affect daily life and productivity. The insidious nature of DR lies in its lack of symptoms during the early stages, making regular eye exams essential for individuals with diabetes. Early detection is crucial because it allows for intervention before the condition progresses to a point where it significantly impacts vision. As DR progresses, patients may experience a variety of visual disturbances, including blurred vision, distorted or inconsistent sight, and in some cases, sudden and severe vision loss. The initial symptoms may be mild and easily overlooked, but as the disease advances, these symptoms can worsen, leading to significant visual impairment. It's important to note that the vision problems caused by DR cannot be corrected with standard prescription glasses or contact lenses. Instead, patients require specialized medical treatment to manage the condition (K. J. Frank et. al, 1996).

The Figure 1 represents those various stages of DR starting from the Healthy non-diabetic stage to Mild, Moderate and Proliferate DR.

Figure 1. Typical stages of DR (a) Healthy, (b) Mild_DR, (c) Moderate_DR, (d) Proliferate_DR

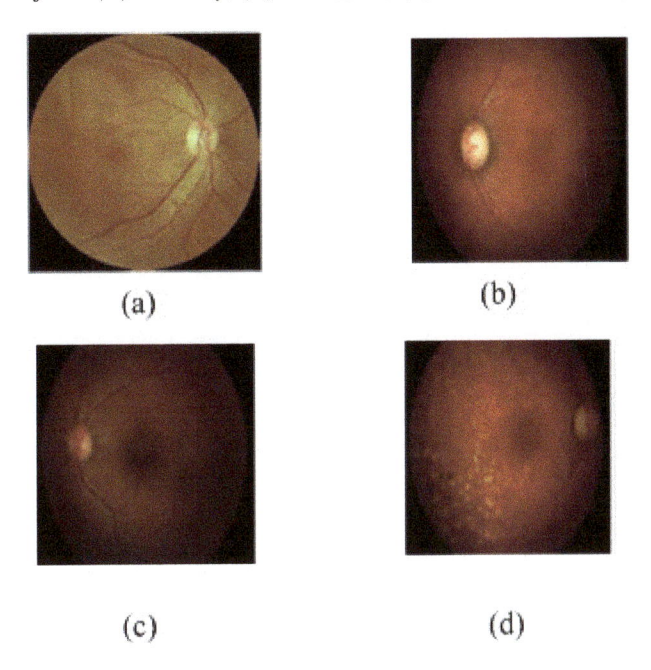

Hyperglycemia caused by chronic Diabetes Mellitus (DM) damages the microvasculature of the retina, leading to DR. NPDR is the early stage of DR, where patients often do not notice any symptoms. Initial signs of NPDR can be detected using fundus photography, which may reveal microaneurysms—small bulges in the retinal blood vessels. Retinal ischemia, caused by narrowed or blocked blood vessels that reduce blood flow, can be observed through fluorescein angiography. In the Mild NPDR stage, these microaneurysms may leak fluid into the retina. If this fluid accumulates in the macular region, it results in DME, which causes retinal thickening visible with Optical Coherence Tomography (OCT). Approximately 10% of individuals with DME experience vision loss. Mild NPDR can progress to Moderate NPDR, where blood vessels supplying the retina become increasingly distorted. This affects their ability to transport blood effectively, which can lead to DME. Greater blood vessel blockage results in larger portions of the retina losing oxygen and nutrients in cases of Severe NPDR. Growth-promoting substances are discharged in response, encouraging the development of fresh vessel formation in the afflicted areas. PDR is a more developed form of DR that is distinguished by the atypical development of new blood vessels, or neovascularization. Due to their fragility and propensity to burst, these new vessels could cause further issues (L. Gang et.al., 2002).

Figure 2 illustrate the various stages of DR and the related visual symptoms. During the NPDR stage, signs such as cotton wool spots, superficial retinal hemorrhages, and other microvascular abnormalities may be observed.

Figure 2. Basic classification of DR (a) NPDR; (b) PDR

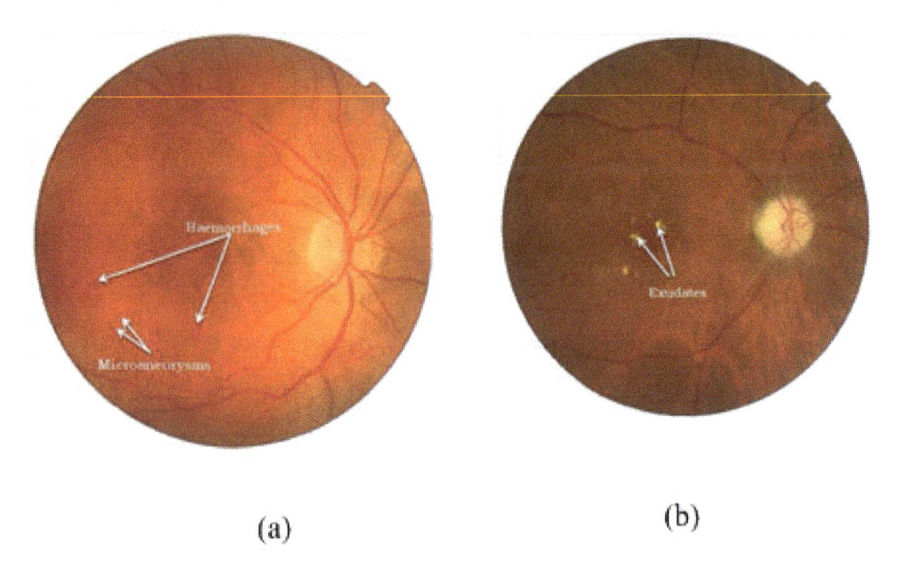

Basic classification of DR (a) NPDR; (b) PDR

Treatment for DR typically involves a combination of medical and surgical approaches. In the early stages, controlling blood sugar levels and blood pressure can help slow the progression of the disease. Regular eye examinations are crucial for detecting any early signs of DR and monitoring changes in the retina. For mo.re advanced cases, more intensive treatments may be needed, such as laser therapy to seal leaking blood vessels or vitrectomy surgery to remove blood or scar tissue from the eye. Additionally, anti-VEGF (vascular endothelial growth factor) injections may be used to reduce the growth of abnormal blood vessels that contribute to vision loss. Despite the availability of these treatments, prevention remains the most effective strategy for managing DR. This involves maintaining strict control over blood sugar levels, blood pressure, and cholesterol, as well as adopting a healthy lifestyle that includes a balanced diet, regular physical activity, and avoiding smoking. Regular eye check-ups are also a vital part of diabetes management, as early detection of DR can lead to better outcomes by allowing for timely treatment before significant retinal damage occurs [T. Y. Wong et. al., 2016].

Pupil dilation with Mydriatic drops is a necessary step in the diagnosis of retinal fundus. Pupil dilation makes the eye exam easier, but it also causes a number of side effects, including burn, sting, irritation, blurred vision, light sensitivity, headaches, and brow pain. Sometimes the pupil's dilation lasts for up to two weeks. Glaucoma causes swelling or redness in the eyes, lens deformation, and an increase in intraocular pressure. Additional adverse effects that patients may encounter include an increase in blood pressure, paleness, headaches, dizziness, pounding in the heart, and irregular or rapid heartbeats, according to the Mayo Clinic. Dehydration and occasional sleepiness are additional negative effects. Additionally, compared to patients with diabetes, the rate of increase in ophthalmologists worldwide is significantly lower. Furthermore, only basic diagnosis and screening procedures are aided by clinical diagnosis tools. The simple and thorough pathos analysis is improved by the use of image processing techniques (Ravindraiah, R et al. 2020).

In past years, integration of artificial intelligence (AI), deep learning techniques, particularly CNNs, has emerged as a promising possibility to addresses these challenges and revolutionizes the landscape of DR diagnosis. This study embarks on a comprehensive exploration of DR Stage Classification using a custom-designed CNN system. By utilizing deep learning's capabilities, this paper aims to develop a robust and automated system capable of accurately classifying the diverse stages of DR, thereby facilitating early detection and personalized treatment strategies. This introduction provides an overview of the significance of DR, the shortcomings of the present diagnostic methods, and potential of CNNs in transforming the landscape of DR. The integration of artificial intelligence in ophthalmology has witnessed a transformative shift; particularly with the advent of deep learning techniques when trained on vast datasets, have demonstrated the capacity to surpass human performance in various medical imaging tasks. In the realm of DR processes. CNNs have emerged as the backbone of many successful medical image analysis applications. By modifying and optimizing CNN architectures for DR stage classification, we hope to fully utilize deep learning for accurate and timely diagnosis. CNNs are especially well-suited for tasks like image classification, segmentation, and detection due to their automatic learning of hierarchical characteristics derived from unprocessed pixel data (Bhatkar A.P et al., 2015).

Objectives of the Study:

a. Development of a Custom CNN

The primary objective of this study is to create and implement a CNNs (CNN) specifically designed to classify the various stages of DR. This involves developing a sophisticated CNN architecture that is finely tuned to analyze and interpret retinal images. DR, a condition resulting from chronic hyperglycemia, manifests through distinct stages, each characterized by unique retinal changes. Detecting these changes accurately requires advanced machine learning techniques. To meet this objective, the custom CNN will be engineered to handle the intricate details of retinal images, which include subtle features indicative of different DR stages. Key steps in this process include selecting an appropriate network architecture, adjusting hyperparameters, and ensuring the CNN generalizes well across a broad range of retinal images. The network will be trained using a comprehensive dataset of annotated retinal images, enabling it to learn and recognize the specific patterns associated with each DR stage.

The CNN will feature multiple convolutional layers to extract hierarchical features, pooling layers to manage dimensionality, and fully connected layers to perform stage classification. Techniques such as data augmentation, dropout, and regularization will be employed to enhance the network's performance and prevent overfitting. The goal is to develop a precise and reliable tool for identifying DR stages, thus improving the accuracy of disease diagnosis and management.

b. Accurate DR Staging

Another key objective is to achieve high accuracy in classifying the stages of DR, from healthy to proliferative stages. Accurate DR staging is crucial for several reasons. It ensures that patients receive the most appropriate treatment based on the severity of their condition. DR progresses through various stages, starting from mild NPDR and advancing to severe NPDR and PDR. Accurate classification of these stages allows for tailored treatment plans suited to the specific stage of the disease. Early and accurate staging is also essential for timely intervention. Identifying DR at an early stage enables prompt management, which can prevent the progression to more severe forms like DME or PDR. For example, early detection of mild NPDR allows for preventive measures that can delay or avoid the development of more advanced stages. Accurate staging enhances clinical decision-making by providing detailed information on the patient's condition, leading to better treatment outcomes.

The performance of the custom CNN will be evaluated based on its ability to accurately classify DR stages. Metrics such as accuracy, sensitivity, specificity, and the area under the receiver operating characteristic curve (AUC-ROC) will be used to assess the model's effectiveness. The aim is to develop a CNN that not only achieves high classification accuracy but also delivers consistent and reliable results across different datasets and patient populations. This study aims to achieve two main objectives: the development of a custom CNN for DR stage classification and the attainment of high accuracy in DR staging. These objectives are intended to advance automated DR diagnosis capabilities, streamline clinical workflows, and enhance patient care through precise and timely treatment interventions. By addressing these goals, the study seeks to make significant contributions to the fields of ophthalmology and diabetes management.

2 RELATED WORKS

Automated Detection of vision problems and retinal imaging technologies has a significant impact in automated DR detection. Many Machine learning (ML) and Deep learning (DL) technologies have been developed for detecting and screening those with vision problems. Digital imaging technologies are improved by image processing techniques, which also assist to create a large and high-quality record of retinal information. As a result, it eliminates the need for manual maintenance and helps ophthalmologists provide ongoing care as the disease progresses. Due to factors like the fluctuating number of abnormal/anatomical structures, colour, contrast, illumination effects, misunderstanding of guaranteed data owing to erroneous analysis, etc., fundoscopy-based retinal image inspection might be difficult to comprehend. The apps that have been created for the purpose of identifying anomalies in DR pictures are as follows.

To separate the optic disc (OD) and BVs, (Medhi N et al., 2016) used color normalization on the RGB, YIQ, and HIS color spaces in addition to morphological operators and ostu thresholding. In order to obtain the exudates, the thresholded hue image plane is finally logically anded with the saturation plane. Using 1374 images from the public databases DIARETDB1, DRIVE, MESSIDOR, and HRF, they achieved an average sensitivity of 77.73% and specificity of 98.72%. In (Sandra M. et al., 2017) used texture filtration via local binary patterns filtration to distinguish between the DR and healthy images. Using the DIARETDB1 dataset, they used multiple classifiers and obtained 86% mean sensitivity and 99% specificity. In addition, an automated system based on the KNN algorithm for the identification of DR was developed by (Wong et al., 2016); they reported 80.21% sensitivity and 70.66% specificity. The CNN deep learning architecture, Alexnet, has a few shortcomings. It may overfit due to not sufficient regularity and high memory requirements, incur significant computational costs from normal convolution, and only achieve about 75% accuracy, which must be increased to produce better classified results. By using the Inception Net V3 model, the suggested model seeks to lower the computational cost, raise the performance matrices, and lower the memory need. It is employed in many different applications because of its efficient design and lightweight construction. The study contributes to the ongoing efforts to enhance the prevention, diagnosis, and treatment of DR (Litjens G et al., 2017)

To differentiate between dark and bright lesions, (Silkar S et al., 2018) used curvelet edge enhancement techniques, morphological operations followed by optimal band pass filters, and differential evolution methods. To get rid of OD and BVs, morphological operations and kernel-induced FCM are applied. Next, matched filters and Laplacian of Gaussian (LoG) filtering are used to identify potential lesions. Ultimately, they employed the mutual information maximization method to differentiate between the multiple lesions. 50% of the images are taken from the public databases DRIVE, ROCh, STARE, and DIARETDB1, yielding an average accuracy of 97.71%. In (Zhang et al., 2019) work, a custom-made standard deep neural network was combined with CNNss (CNNs) and labeled by registered practitioners of retinopathy. They used the image dataset—13,767 pictures of 1872 patients—that the Sichuan Provincial Peoples Hospital in Chengdu and the Sichuan Academy of Medical Sciences had provided. The first step of the proposed supervised system involves allowing the dark images to undergo histogram equalization and contrast stretch operation, and extracting multiple features for training. Nine statistical metrics were used to evaluate their system, and the results showed 98.1% sensitivity and 98.9% specificity.

The importance of an automated image assessment system based on deep learning for the successful classification of DR images has been presented by (Liu et al. 2019). They put forth a brand-new classification strategy known as multiple weighted path into CNN (WP-CNN), in which back propagation is used to optimize the weight coefficients. By averaging the multiple path weight coefficients, they were able to achieve fast convergence and reduce the redundancy of the data. Utilizing the STARE dataset (91 images), they reported 94.23% accuracy, 95.74% specificity, and 90.94% sensitivity. Deep learning framework of (Elswah D.K et al., 2020) consists of three stages: the fundus image is preprocessed, a ResNet CNNs model is used to grade it, and the grade of DR is detected and determined. The ISBI'2018 Indian Diabetic Retinopathy Image Dataset (IDRiD), which has been balanced to eliminate training bias, is used to train the framework. With an overall classification accuracy of 86.67%, the system performs better than related techniques when compared to related techniques using the same data.

Using the dropout concept, (Lee C.H. et al. 2021), proposed a way to categorize the severity of DR. Data pre-processing is done using contrast-limited adaptive histogram equalization (CLAHE), and the VGG-16 and ResNet-50 models are adjusted. To address training over-fitting and data imbalance, data expansion is used. In the IDRiD database, the model achieves an average sensitivity of over 70% and specificity of over 90%. Its accuracy is assessed using a confusion matrix. The works of (Pamadi A M et. al 2022) proposes a CNNs (CNN) model based on multi-modal classification. Gaussian filtered fundus photos enhance the identification of diagnoses by enhancing the visibility of small features such as dots or edges (Thaseen, A.,2023)

DenseNet-based strategic deep learning algorithms to automate the diagnosis of DR is proposed by (Saranya et al. 2022). Their classification model processes pre-processed retinal images without additional feature enhancements. To enhance the accuracy of DR detection, minimal preprocessing is applied to the noisy images. This approach achieved peak accuracy and precision of 0.83 on the Kaggle APTOS database. Bilal A. et al. (2022) introduced a two-stage DR detection system that combines Optic Disc (OD) and Blood Vessel (BV) segmentation with transfer learning. During preprocessing, they applied green channel extraction, uniform resizing, top-bottom hat transformation, and segmentation. DIARETDB0, EyePACS-1, Messidor-2, and other datasets that are freely available were used to train the transfer learning model, Inception-V3. Their research, which achieved an average accuracy of 91.4%, a sensitivity of 92.5%, and a specificity of 90.5% on the MESSIDOR2 database, demonstrated Inception-V3's promising potential for clinical use. The accuracy of a multinomial classification is further increased to 78% through machine learning on a previously trained MobileNetV2 model. Using the Unet encoder

Efficientnet, mask, and IDRID dataset, the study of (Padmasini S et. al., 2023) presents an automatic semantic multiclass segmentation method for classifying retinal anomalies into multiple groups. With a loss of 0.0969 and an IoU score of 88.26%, the method yielded 99.65% accuracy and 99.33% precision.

RESNET-152, a 152-layer neural network that is excellent at capturing intricate image features, to create a deep learning model was used by (Rai B K et. al 2024). Using the Kaggle dataset, this model is used to categorize images of DR. Their research yielded an accuracy rate of 72.6%, indicating the model's ability to discriminate between various stages. This demonstrates how cutting-edge deep learning methods can be used for early diagnosis and detection in medical image analysis. One of the most important network models, ResNet, was introduced in 2015 and substantially enhanced CNN's image classification capabilities.

Overall Drawbacks of Existing Methods

(i) Small Sample Sizes

A significant limitation of many current techniques for DR classification is their reliance on small sample sizes. Often, these methods are tested on restricted or private datasets, which limits the extent to which the findings can be generalized. Models trained on limited data may perform well on specific datasets but may not be as effective when applied to broader or more diverse populations. This restricted applicability can lead to models that are overfitted to the particular characteristics of the training data, which can adversely affect their performance on new or varied datasets. The inability to generalize across different demographic groups, geographic locations, and image qualities can result in reduced accuracy and potentially overlooked diagnoses in real-world scenarios. To develop robust and reliable diagnostic tools, it is crucial to use large and diverse datasets that capture the full range of variability in DR presentations.

(ii) Computational Requirements

Many advanced techniques for DR classification come with substantial computational demands. Sophisticated methods, especially deep learning models like CNNss (CNNs), often require significant computational resources for both training and inference. This need typically involves high-performance hardware, such as Graphics Processing Units (GPUs) or specialized processors, which can be costly and may not be accessible in all clinical or research environments. The computational burden also includes the time and energy required for model training, which can be a limiting factor for institutions with limited computational infrastructure. As such, there is a need for more efficient algorithms and optimization strategies that provide high performance without imposing excessive computational costs.

(iii) Complexity and Implementation Challenges

The complexity inherent in advanced models such as ResNet and Inception Net V3 presents its own set of challenges. While these models are highly effective, their implementation can be quite intricate and requires specialized knowledge and expertise. Setting up, fine-tuning, and deploying these models involves navigating numerous hyperparameters and sophisticated network architectures, which can be daunting for those without a strong background in deep learning. Moreover, these models often require specialized hardware and software, adding further complexity to their implementation. This complexity can limit the adoption of such models to well-resourced institutions with the capability to manage advanced technologies.

(iv) Lack of Standardization and Validation

A notable drawback of many existing methods is the lack of standardization in evaluation metrics, testing protocols, and validation procedures. This lack of uniformity makes it difficult to compare different techniques and assess their relative performance effectively. The inconsistency in testing and validation approaches can lead to varying results, complicating the process of identifying the most effective DR classification methods. Establishing standardized benchmarks and validation protocols is essential for ensuring consistent evaluation and reliable comparison of different models, ultimately facilitating better-informed decisions about model adoption and implementation.

(v) Limited Interpretability

The constrained accessibility of many sophisticated mathematical models presents another difficulty. Even though deep learning methods are very accurate, they frequently function as "black boxes," offering little information about the decision-making process. In healthcare environments, where trust-building with clinicians and patients depends on an understanding of the justification behind a model's predictions, this lack of openness may pose a problem. Interpretability is important for validating the model's findings, ensuring that they are based on meaningful and clinically relevant features, and making informed decisions about patient care. Models that do not offer clear explanations for their predictions may face obstacles in clinical adoption and integration.

Future research and development efforts can address these shortcomings and concentrate on enhancing the methods' robustness, scalability, and generalizability for the detection of DR and other medical imaging applications.

3 PROPOSED METHOD

Inception Net V3, a cutting-edge deep learning architecture, has shown considerable success in classifying DR from retinal images. Its design optimizes both computational efficiency and feature extraction, making it particularly effective for this task. The architecture utilizes several advanced techniques, including factorized convolutions, aggressive regularization, and dimension reduction, to enhance performance while managing computational demands. Factorized convolutions are a key component of Inception Net V3, allowing the network to decompose complex convolution operations into simpler, more efficient components. This approach improves the network's ability to extract intricate features from retinal images without excessive computational overhead. Additionally, aggressive regularization techniques are employed to minimize the risk of overfitting, ensuring that the model generalizes well to new and diverse datasets. Dimension reduction further contributes to performance optimization by decreasing the number of parameters and computational requirements, facilitating the efficient processing of large-scale image data.

The application of Inception Net V3 in DR classification involves several important steps, beginning with image preprocessing. This phase includes resizing retinal images to a consistent size, normalizing pixel values for uniformity, and applying methods to enhance the model's ability to generalize across varied images. Effective preprocessing is crucial for improving classification accuracy and ensuring that the network can handle the variability encountered in real-world retinal images. Inception Net V3's architecture features multiple inception modules, which perform parallel convolutional and pooling operations. These modules are designed to capture and analyze multi-scale information from retinal images, allowing the network to identify and classify different DR stages with high accuracy. By leveraging these modules, Inception Net V3 can efficiently handle the complexities of DR classification. However, despite its strengths, Inception Net V3 faces challenges such as the need for extensive annotated datasets and significant computational resources during the training phase. Large annotated datasets are essential for effectively training the model, while the training process itself demands considerable computational power and time, which can be a limitation in resource-constrained settings.

Inception Net V3 is a sophisticated deep learning architecture that excels in image classification tasks, including the classification of DR from retinal images. The architecture is designed to handle the complexities of analysing medical images by leveraging several advanced techniques that enhance computational efficiency and feature extraction. The process begins with the input layer, where retinal images are fed into the network. These images are typically pre-processed to ensure consistency in size and quality; they are resized to a standard resolution and normalized to standardize pixel values. This preprocessing step is crucial for maintaining uniformity and preparing the images for effective analysis by the network. Following preprocessing, the initial convolutional layer performs a series of convolution operations with large kernels to capture fundamental features from the retinal images. This layer is essential for extracting low-level details, such as edges and textures, which form the basis for more complex feature extraction in subsequent layers. Batch normalization is often applied here to stabilize and accelerate the training process.

3.1 Proposed InceptionNet V3 classifier workflow

The core of Inception Net V3 consists of multiple inception modules. These modules are designed to capture multi-scale information by applying different types of convolutions in parallel. Specifically, the inception modules use 1x1 convolutions to capture fine details and reduce dimensionality, 3x3 convolutions to detect medium-sized features, and 5x5 convolutions to identify larger patterns. Pooling layers within the inception modules extract spatial features and further reduce the dimensionality of the data. This parallel processing approach allows the network to efficiently handle diverse aspects of DR, such as microaneurysms, hemorrhages, and exudates. A notable feature of Inception Net V3 is its use of factorized convolutions. These convolutions break down larger operations (such as 5x5 convolutions) into smaller, sequential operations (such as two 3x3 convolutions). This method reduces computational complexity while maintaining the ability to capture intricate features. Aggressive regularization techniques are also employed to prevent overfitting, ensuring that the model generalizes well to new data.

After feature extraction, the network employs global average pooling. This pooling layer reduces the entire feature map to a single value per channel by averaging, converting the high-dimensional data into a fixed-size vector. This vector is then processed by fully connected (dense) layers, which perform the final classification. The fully connected layers interpret the extracted features and output a vector of class scores. The final classification step is achieved through the softmax layer, which applies the softmax activation function to convert the output scores into probabilities for each possible DR stage. This probabilistic output allows the network to classify retinal images into specific DR stages, such as healthy, mild NPDR, moderate NPDR, severe NPDR, or PDR.

Figure 3. Proposed DR classification model work flow

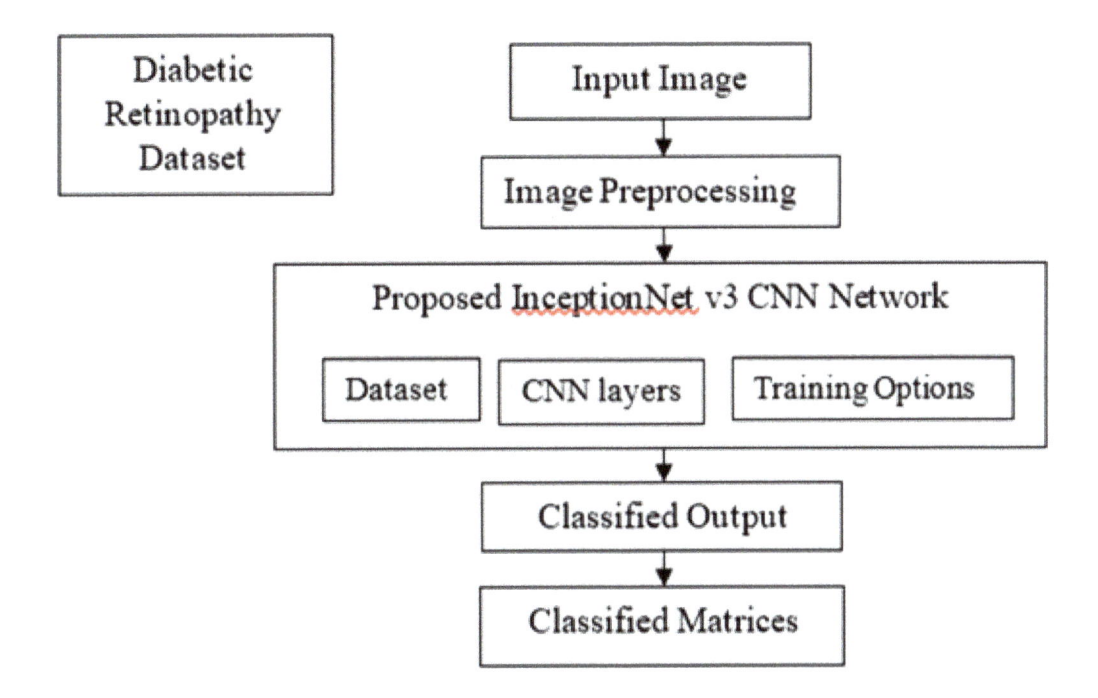

Despite its strengths, Inception Net V3 faces challenges related to the need for large annotated datasets and significant computational resources. Training the model requires substantial computational power and time, which can be a limitation in environments with constrained resources. Additionally, the effectiveness of the model is heavily dependent on the quality and quantity of the annotated training data. It provides a powerful framework for DR classification, but addressing the challenges related to dataset size and computational requirements is crucial for optimizing its application in practical scenarios. The proposed method leverages CNNs for imprecise classification of DR stages, aiming to diminish early detection and intervention. The framework comprises a randomly-designed CNN architecture tailored to the intricacies of retinal image analysis. Figure 3, presents the proposed classifying process's workflow. This method involves excessively preparing the retinal pictures to improve their characteristics. Initial, a pre-processing step extracts significant features from retinal images, including non-existent microaneurysms, exudates, and hemorrhages and then the proposed Inception Net V3 model is trained.

3.2 Requirements

The dataset is essential in the preparation, validation, testing, and comparison of various frameworks, acting as a critical benchmark for assessing the effectiveness of different systems. For this study, we carefully utilize an open-source dataset from the Kaggle Database [Kaggle 2024], focusing on selecting high-quality images to serve as the foundation for training our classification models. This dataset is crucial for developing and refining models that can accurately identify and categorize the stages of DR. It is a comprehensive collection of retinal images designed to support the development and evaluation of models for detecting and classifying DR. It includes 88,702 color fundus images, all resized to a uniform resolution of 512x512 pixels. The dataset, originally derived from the EyePACS and Messidor-2 datasets, is widely used in medical imaging research to train and validate machine learning models for automated DR detection and classification. Its large size, diverse cases, and consistent image format make it a valuable resource for advancing research in this area.

Table 1. Distribution of images according to the presence of DR

Category	No. of images	Labels
Healthy	40	1
Mild_DR	45	2
Moderate_DR	48	3
Proliferate_DR	37	4

Each image in the dataset is evaluated for the severity of DR and classified into one of four categories, ranging from 1 to 4: (i) Healthy, indicating no signs of DR; (ii) Mild_DR, showing early symptoms; (iii) Moderate_DR, indicating a more advanced stage; and (iv) Proliferate_DR, representing the most severe form. The dataset comprises 170 images, evenly distributed across these four stages, offering a comprehensive overview of DR's progression. This diverse and well-curated dataset is vital in ensuring that the classification models developed in this study are robust, reliable, and capable of performing accurately in various scenarios and patient conditions (Table.I).

Figure 4 illustrates the various aspects and key components of the proposed CNNss (CNNs). A significant part of the CNN design involves the use of padding techniques, such as zero-value pixels and reflection padding, which are essential for handling the edge pixels during convolution operations. These padding methods ensure that the CNN can effectively process the image borders without losing crucial information. Another important feature is the use of stride-2 convolutions, which reduce the output dimensions by half, resulting in a more compact and computationally efficient representation. However, this downsampling also leads to a rounded output, which may slightly impact the precision of feature detection. The process begins with an essential pre-processing step, which extracts important features from the retinal images. This step focuses on identifying key retinal features, including microaneurysms, exudates, and hemorrhages, which are critical indicators of DR. Following this feature extraction, the proposed model, which is based on the Inception Net V3 architecture, is trained. Inception Net V3 is particularly effective for this task due to its deep and sophisticated structure, which enables it to capture complex patterns within the retinal images. The combination of thorough pre-processing and the robust CNN architecture aims to improve the model's accuracy in classifying different stages of DR.

Figure 4. Proposed InceptionNet V3 CNN architecture

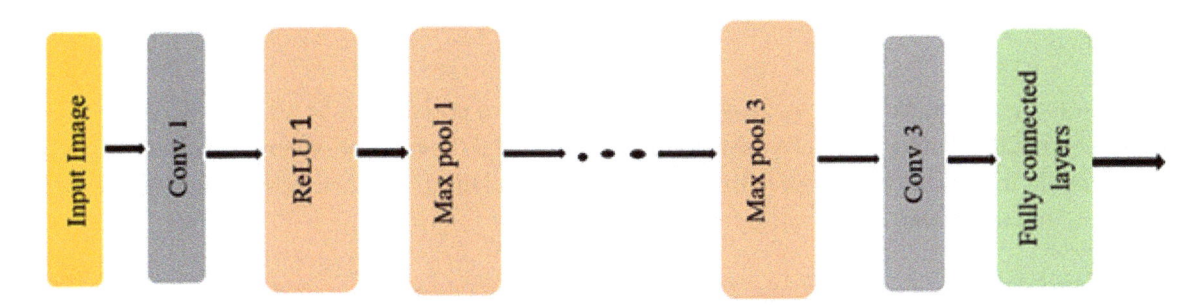

Image input layers create data normalization, convolutional layers apply filters, and dilated convolution separates filter elements. Zero padding adjusts layer output size. Rectified Linear Unit (ReLU) reduces overfitting and speeds up training by improving consistency. CNNs use ReLU to create down-sampled feature maps in fixed-size frames. The proposed method improves DR stage classification, enhances automated diagnostic tools, improves patient care, and aids medical image analysis. ANNs are used for categorization tasks like word prediction and image classification. The CNN building piece consists of input, hidden, and output layers, with input layers processing data and hidden layers calculating probability scores for each class. The next stage, referred to as feed forward, involves feeding the model's input so that each layer's output can be collected. Next, an error function is prone to determine error; common examples of error functions include square loss error and cross entropy. Next, by computing the variations, we backpropagate into the model. The goal of this stage, known as back propagation, is to reduce the loss as much as possible.

3.3 Statistical Metrics

Evaluating supervised classifiers with statistical metrics is essential for a comprehensive understanding of their performance and practical implications. Although accuracy gives a general idea of the model's performance, it might only be fully representative when datasets are balanced. To evaluate the model's efficacy in detecting pertinent cases, recall and precision are essential. Recall concentrates on identifying real positives, while precision evaluates the accuracy of positive predictions. Combining recall and precision, the F1 score provides a balanced assessment that is particularly useful for unbalanced data. By displaying the amounts of true positives, false positives, true negatives, and false negatives, the confusion matrix helps to pinpoint specific areas of error and offers detailed insights. The model's capacity to distinguish between classes at various thresholds is demonstrated by the ROC curve and AUC, with the AUC indicating overall performance. Statistical significance metrics, such as confidence intervals and p-values, assess whether observed performance improvements are meaningful or due to random chance. Collectively, these metrics offer a thorough assessment of a classifier's effectiveness, guiding model selection, tuning, and deployment to ensure reliable performance on new, unseen data. The proposed system is statistically assessed using the following metrics

Accuracy: The percentage of properly categorized and incorrectly classified samples is referred as accuracy.

Accuracy =

$$\frac{TP + TN}{(TP + TN + FP + FN)} \quad (1)$$

Accuracy indicates the percentage of predictions that are correct across all classes. While it is a simple and intuitive metric, it can be misleading in cases of class imbalance, where one class dominates.

Precision: It gives the link between true positive values and the total of true positive and false positive estimates, and the quality of a positive forecast.

Precision =

$$\frac{TP}{(TP + FP)} \quad (2)$$

Precision is important when the cost of false positives is high, such as in medical diagnostics where a high precision means that when a positive result is given, it is more likely to be correct.

Recall: It evaluates how effectively the model detects good examples. This is the total of correctly categorized factual positive cases.

Recall =

$$\frac{TP}{(TP + FN)} \quad (3)$$

Recall is crucial when the cost of missing a positive case is high. For example, in medical screening, high recall means that most patients with a disease are identified, reducing the risk of missed diagnoses.

F1 Score: It is a measurement of average harmonic of accuracy and recall.

F1 score =

$$\frac{2 * precision * recall}{precision + recall} \quad (4)$$

The F1 score balances precision and recall, providing a more comprehensive measure of a model's performance when both false positives and false negatives are important. It is particularly valuable when there is a trade-off between precision and recall.

Because accuracy indicates the percentage of correctly classified instances, it offers a broad indicator of a model's overall performance. For unbalanced datasets, on the other hand, where certain classes are noticeably underrepresented, it might not be the ideal metric. When the expense of false positives is significant, as in the case of medical diagnostics, precision—which concentrates on the accuracy of positive predictions—becomes crucial. Conversely, recall assesses a model's capacity to detect all pertinent positive cases and is especially crucial in situations where the value of false negatives is high, such as in the detection of diseases where failing to detect a case could have grave repercussions. By understanding and appropriately applying these metrics, one can better evaluate and select models based on the specific needs and constraints of the problem at hand.

4 EXPERIMENTAL RESULTS

Utilizing the cross-entropy loss function, the proposed model is trained using an appropriate optimization procedure. To enhance model performance and achieve more efficient training, this study employs a combination of learning rate scheduling and other optimization techniques and is developed in MATLAB R2023a script. Learning rate scheduling is a crucial strategy for managing the learning rate over time, which helps in adjusting the step size of the optimization process. By carefully altering the learning rate during training (Figure 5), the model can converge more effectively to a minimum of the loss function, potentially accelerating the learning process and improving the overall performance. In this study, the learning rate is scheduled to remain constant at 0.001 throughout the training process. This approach ensures stability in the learning rate schedule, which is vital for maintaining consistent training dynamics and avoiding abrupt changes that could disrupt convergence. The constant learning rate of 0.001 is chosen based on preliminary experiments to balance between sufficiently large updates and stability, thus fostering steady and reliable learning.

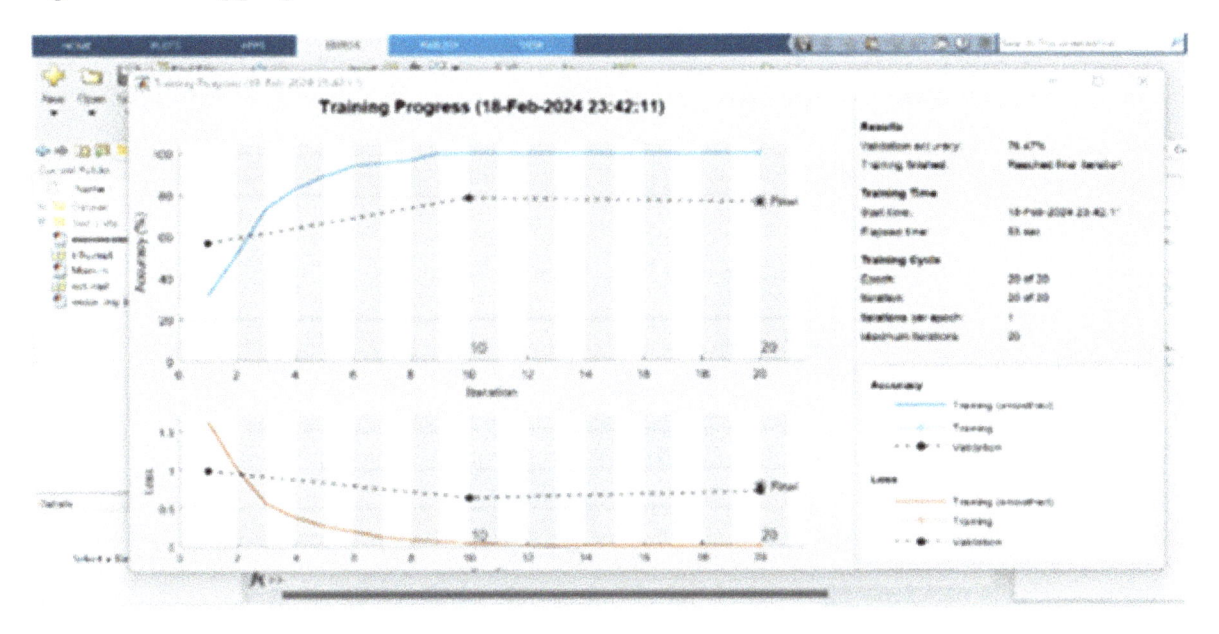

Figure 5. Training progress

Additionally, to address the issue of overfitting, early stopping is implemented. Early stopping monitors the model's performance on a validation set and halts training if no significant improvement is observed for a predefined number of epochs. This technique helps prevent the model from overfitting to the training data by stopping the training process before the model starts to memorize the data rather than generalizing from it. The training process involves executing one iteration per epoch across a total of 20 epochs. This setup ensures that the model is trained sufficiently while maintaining simplicity and control over the training dynamics. The use of learning rate scheduling in conjunction with early stopping aims to refine the optimization process, enhance convergence rates, and prevent overfitting, thereby improving the robustness and efficacy of this model. The training process involves executing one iteration per epoch across a total of 20 epochs. This setup ensures that the model is trained sufficiently while maintaining simplicity and control over the training dynamics. In conjunction with early stopping aims to refine the optimization process, enhance convergence rates, and prevent overfitting, thereby improving the robustness and efficacy of the model.

The confusion matrix is a crucial tool for evaluating the performance of classification models, including Inception Net V3. It provides a detailed summary of predicted versus actual classifications by presenting true positives, false positives, true negatives, and false negatives. This matrix not only reveals the overall accuracy of the model but also helps in understanding how well it distinguishes between different classes. It is essential for calculating key metrics such as precision, recall, and F1 score, which offer deeper insights into the model's performance, especially in cases of class imbalance. Additionally, the confusion matrix aids in error analysis by highlighting specific classes that are often misclassified, which can guide model improvements. Overall, it serves as an invaluable tool for assessing and enhancing classifier performance by providing a comprehensive view of its accuracy and error patterns. It is a N*N matrix table with N total targeted classifications that are used to assess how well a categorization model performs. It functions as an overview of the results for the counts of TN, TP, FN, and FP. It makes it easier to figure out whether the system is conflating two classifications. With 28 images predicted to be in class 1 and no images in the confused stage, Figure 6 illustrates that there are two to four classes.

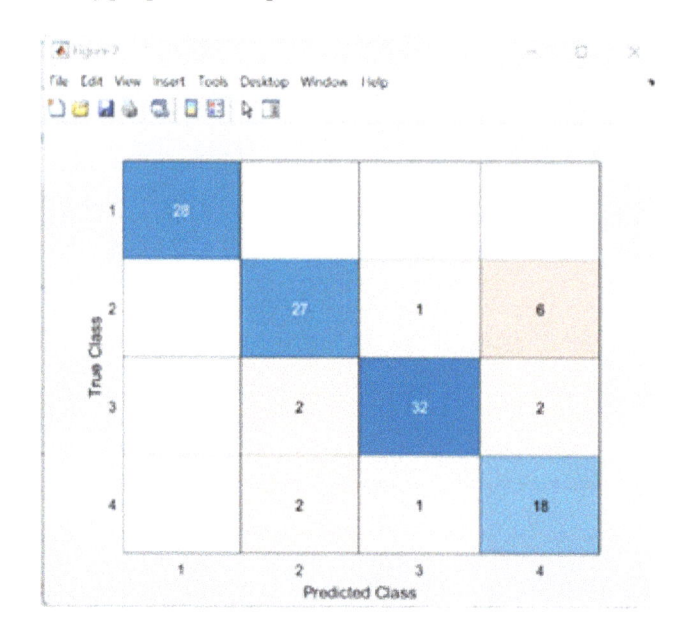

Figure 6. Confusion matrix of proposed inception net v3

The training analysis of the Inception Net V3 model offers a detailed look at its performance across several key parameters. Training was carried out over a designated number of epochs, with each epoch comprising multiple iterations where the model processed batches of data. The time elapsed during training was recorded to gauge the model's efficiency and the computational resources required. Mini-batch accuracy was a critical metric, reflecting how well the model performed on small subsets of the training data during each iteration. This measure provided insight into the model's learning progress and how effectively it was adjusting its parameters. Validation accuracy was also monitored to assess the model's performance on a separate validation dataset that wasn't used in training, offering a view of its ability to generalize beyond the training data. Validation loss, which measures the discrepancy between the model's predictions and the actual labels on the validation set, was another crucial parameter. A decreasing validation loss indicated that the model was refining its predictions over time. The base learning rate, an essential hyperparameter, was kept constant throughout the training to ensure stable and consistent learning. By evaluating these parameters, the effectiveness and efficiency of the Inception Net V3 training process were comprehensively assessed.

Figure 7. Training analysis

```
Command Window
    Training on single CPU.
    Initializing input data normalization.
|=======================================================================================================|
| Epoch | Iteration | Time Elapsed | Mini-batch | Validation | Mini-batch | Validation | Base Learning |
|       |           | (hh:mm:ss)   | Accuracy   | Accuracy   | Loss       | Loss       | Rate          |
|=======================================================================================================|
|    1  |     1     | 00:00:04     | 10.94%     | 29.41%     | 1.7863     | 2.2680     | 0.0010        |
|   10  |    10     | 00:00:26     | 82.81%     | 56.86%     | 0.5187     | 2.7182     | 0.0010        |
|   20  |    20     | 00:00:51     | 98.44%     | 62.75%     | 0.0487     | 2.4258     | 0.0010        |
|=======================================================================================================|
```

The training analysis of the Inception Net V3 classifier involves several critical steps to ensure effective learning and performance. Initially, prepare a diverse dataset of retinal images, including various DR stages, and preprocess the data by resizing, normalizing, and augmenting it. Configure the model by setting up its architecture, adjusting hyperparameters, and selecting an appropriate loss function and optimizer. During training, monitor the model's progress across epochs, evaluating performance using metrics such as accuracy, precision, recall, and F1 score, along with analyzing the confusion matrix. Validate the model through techniques like cross-validation and assess its final performance on a separate test set. Refine the model by tuning hyperparameters, implementing early stopping to prevent overfitting, and applying regularization methods to enhance generalization. This comprehensive approach ensures that the Inception Net V3 classifier is effectively trained to accurately classify DR stages and perform reliably in practical scenarios.

Figure 7 shows how the training analysis is done. It is evident that the attained validation accuracy is 29.41% at the first epoch, with a validation loss of 2.2680, and 98.44% at the twentieth epoch, with a loss of 0.0487 and a constant base learning rate. Thirty percent of each stage's data is set aside for testing, with the remaining seventy percent being the training data. The network training process was carefully executed, with each stage undergoing 20 epochs of training. This iterative approach allowed the model to gradually enhance its ability to classify different stages of DR, resulting in marked performance improvements. A key achievement from this training regimen is the model's impressive accuracy, which reached 86%. This high accuracy level highlights the effectiveness of the approach, demonstrating that the model is well-optimized for accurately identifying and classifying DR stages from retinal images. In addition to achieving high accuracy, the training process also focused on minimizing the loss function, a critical metric that indicates the model's overall performance. Through meticulous adjustments and fine-tuning, the loss function was successfully reduced to 0.6061. This decrease in loss signifies the model's enhanced predictive capabilities and its ability to make more accurate classifications with fewer errors.

Moreover, these successful outcomes were attained using a constant base learning rate throughout the training process. Maintaining a consistent learning rate was crucial for ensuring stable and effective learning, enabling the model to converge towards an optimal solution. In summary, the combination of systematic training, effective loss reduction, and a stable learning rate contributed significantly to the model's robust performance in classifying DR stages.The performance matrices, or accuracy, recall, precision, and F1score, of the InceptionnetV3 model for four classes—Healthy-DR, Mild, Moderate, and PDR are shown in Table 2.

Table 2. Result of inception NetV3 model on all the classes of DR

Model	Class	Label	Accuracy %	Recall %	Precision %	F1 score %
Inception Net V3	Healthy	1	86	100	85.7	92
	Mild	2	93.25	76.3	93.5	84
	Moderate	3	80	93.1	79.4	85
	Proliferate	4	88.24	85.50	87.25	87.78
Average			**88.24**	**87.25**	**85.50**	**87.78**

The Inception Net V3 model demonstrates strong overall performance in classifying different stages of DR, as evidenced by its high accuracy and robust evaluation metrics. The model achieves an average accuracy of 88.24% across the DR stages, indicating effective classification. For individual classes, the model performs as follows: it reaches an accuracy of 86% for the Healthy stage, 93.25% for Mild DR, 80% for Moderate DR, and 88.24% for Proliferate DR. This variation in accuracy reflects the model's proficiency in distinguishing between the different stages of DR. In terms of recall, which measures the model's ability to identify all relevant positive instances, the Inception Net V3 model shows excellent performance with a perfect recall of 100% for the Healthy stage, meaning it accurately identifies all non-DR cases. However, the recall for the Mild DR stage is lower at 76.3%, suggesting that some Mild DR cases may be missed by the model. Recall values for Moderate and Proliferate stages are 93.1% and 85.50%, respectively, indicating a strong capability to identify these stages but with some room for improvement.

Precision, which evaluates the accuracy of the model's positive predictions, reveals that the model is particularly effective for the Mild DR class with a precision of 93.5%, and for Proliferate DR with 87.25%. This indicates that when the model predicts these stages, it is often correct. Precision for the Healthy class is 85.7%, which shows a good level of accuracy for non-DR predictions. However, the Moderate DR class has a lower precision of 79.4%, suggesting a higher rate of false positives in this category. The F1 score, which combines precision and recall into a single metric to balance the two, is highest for the Healthy class at 92, reflecting an excellent balance between precision and recall. The F1 score for Mild DR is 84, indicating that while recall is lower, precision compensates somewhat to maintain a balanced score. The Moderate DR class has an F1 score of 85, showing strong performance but with a notable gap between precision and recall. The Proliferate DR stage achieves the highest F1 score of 87.78%, highlighting its balanced and robust classification performance.

Overall, the Inception Net V3 model excels in classifying DR stages, particularly for Healthy and Proliferate cases, with high accuracy and F1 scores. While it performs well, there is room for enhancement in the classification of Mild and Moderate DR stages. Addressing these areas can further refine the model's ability to detect and categorize DR stages accurately, leading to improved diagnostic outcomes and better management of the disease. The model's ability to combine high precision, recall, and F1 scores across most DR stages underscores its effectiveness as a diagnostic tool, with the potential for further optimization to address specific weaknesses in detecting Mild and Moderate DR.

CONCLUSION

The integration of CNNss (CNNs) into the classification of DR represents a pivotal advancement in leveraging artificial intelligence for healthcare applications. This study underscores the transformative potential of CNNs in improving early detection and management of DR, a condition that can lead to significant vision impairment if not addressed promptly. Our in-house developed CNN model has demonstrated exceptional efficacy and precision in differentiating between the various stages of DR, showcasing its capability to analyze retinal images with high accuracy. By detecting subtle patterns and intricate details within the images, our algorithm enables a highly sensitive staging process, which is crucial for timely intervention and preventing the progression of the disease. The successful implementation of our CNN model highlights the promising role of deep learning technologies in enhancing diagnostic procedures. Early detection facilitated by our model can significantly mitigate the risk of severe visual loss and improve patient outcomes. The ability of our CNN to deliver precise and reliable classifications not only enhances diagnostic accuracy but also paves the way for more personalized and effective treatment strategies.

As we continue to refine and expand our model, incorporating advanced machine learning techniques into healthcare has the potential to revolutionize the diagnosis and treatment of various medical conditions. This progress emphasizes the importance of adopting state-of-the-art technology to effectively address complex health challenges. The successful implementation of our CNN model for DR classification demonstrates the significant impact that tailored artificial intelligence solutions can have on medical innovation. By harnessing advanced AI, we not only enhance the accuracy of DR diagnosis but also set a benchmark for future healthcare applications. Over the long term, such technological advancements are expected to greatly improve patient care, drive better health outcomes, and advance healthcare practices. The ongoing development and application of these technologies will play a crucial role in shaping the future of medical diagnostics and treatment.

REFERENCES

Bhatkar, A. P., & Kharat, G. (2015). Detection of Diabetic Retinopathy in Retinal Images Using MLP Classifier. In *Proceedings of the IEEE International Symposium on Nanoelectronic and Information Systems*, Indore, India, pp. 331–335. DOI: 10.1109/iNIS.2015.30

Bilal, A., Zhu, L., Deng, A., Lu, H., & Wu, N. (2022). AI-Based Automatic Detection and Classification of Diabetic Retinopathy Using U-Net and Deep Learning. *Symmetry*, 14(7), 1427. DOI: 10.3390/sym14071427

Bloom, D. E., Cafiero, E. T., Jané-Llopis, E., Abrahams-Gessel, S., Bloom, L. R., Fathima, S., ... (2011)., The global economic burden of non-communicable diseases, Geneva: Harvard School of Public Health and World Economic Forum.

DeFronzo, R. A., Ferrannini, E., Zimmet, P., ... (2015). International Textbook of Diabetes Mellitus, Wiley-Blackwell, 2 (4).

Elswah, D. K., Elnakib, A. A., & Moustafa, H. E. d (2020). Automated diabetic retinopathy grading using resnet; *Proceedings of the 2020 37th National Radio Science Conference (NRSC)*; Cairo, Egypt. 8–10; pp. 248–254. DOI: 10.1109/NRSC49500.2020.9235098

Evans, J. M., Newton, R. W., Ruta, D. A., MacDonald, T. M., & Morris, A. D. (2000). Socio-economic status, obesity and prevalence of type 1 and type 2 diabetes mellitus. *Diabetic Medicine*, 17(6), 478–480. DOI: 10.1046/j.1464-5491.2000.00309.x PMID: 10975218

Frank, K. J., & Dieckert, J. P. (1996). Clinical review of diabetic eye disease: A primary care perspective. *Southern Medical Journal*, 89(2), 463–470. DOI: 10.1097/00007611-199605000-00002 PMID: 8638169

Gang, L., Chutatape, O., & Krishnan, S. M. (2002). Detection and measurement of retinal vessels in fundus images using amplitude modified second-order Gaussian filter. *IEEE Transactions on Biomedical Engineering*, 49(2), 4–37. DOI: 10.1109/10.979356 PMID: 12066884

GBD 2015 Risk Factors Collaborators (2016). Global, regional, and national comparative risk assessment of 79 behavioural, environmental and occupational, and metabolic risks or clusters of risks, 1990-2015: a systematic analysis for the Global Burden of Disease Study 2015. Lancet; 388: 1659-1724; DOI: http://dx.doi.org/ (16)31679-8.DOI: 10.1016/S0140-6736

International Diabetes Federation. IDF Diabetes Atlas (2021), 10th Ed Brussels, Belgium. Available at: https://www.diabetesatlas.org; Last accessed on 03.02.2024

Kar, S. S., & Maity, S. P. (2018). Automatic Detection of Retinal Lesions for Screening of Diabetic Retinopathy. *IEEE Transactions on Biomedical Engineering*, 65(3), 1–9. DOI: 10.1109/TBME.2017.2707578 PMID: 28541892

Lee, C. H., & Ke, Y. H. (2021). Fundus images classification for Diabetic Retinopathy using Deep Learning; *Proceedings of the 2021 The 13th International Conference on Computer Modeling and Simulation*; Melbourne, Australia. 25–27; pp. 264–270. DOI: 10.1145/3474963.3475849

Litjens, G., Kooi, T., Bejnordi, B. E., Setio, A. A. A., Ciompi, F., Ghafoorian, M., van der Laak, J. A. W. M., van Ginneken, B., & Sánchez, C. I. (2017). A survey on deep learning in medical image analysis. *Medical Image Analysis*, 42, 60–88. DOI: 10.1016/j.media.2017.07.005 PMID: 28778026

Y. P. Liu, Z. Li, C. Xu, J. Li, and R. Liang (2019). Referable diabetic retinopathy identification from eye fundus images with weighted path for convolutional neural network. Artif. Intell. Med. 99 101694, doi: . artmed. 2019. 07. 002DOI: 10. 1016/j

Medhi, N., & Dandapat, S. (2016). An effective fovea detection and automatic assessment of diabetic maculopathy in color fundus images. *Computers in Biology and Medicine*, 74, 30–44. DOI: 10.1016/j.compbiomed.2016.04.007 PMID: 27174686

Padmasini, N., Krithika, G. K., Lithiga, P., & Akshaya, S. J. (2023). Automatic Detection and Segmentation Of Retinal Manifestations Due To Diabetic Retinopathy. *International Conference on Signal Processing, Computation, Electronics, Power and Telecommunication (IConSCEPT)*, Karaikal, India, pp. 1-6. DOI: 10.1109/IConSCEPT57958.2023.10170621

Pamadi, A. M., Ravishankar, A., Nithya, P. A., Jahnavi, G., & Kathavate, S. (2022). Diabetic Retinopathy Detection using MobileNetV2 Architecture; *Proceedings of the 2022 International Conference on Smart Technologies and Systems for Next Generation Computing (ICSTSN)*; Villupuram, India. 25–26 March 2022; pp. 1–5.

Rai, B. K., Ojha, H., & Srivastava, I. (2024, March). Diabetic Retinopathy Detection using Deep Learning Model ResNet15. In *2024 2nd International Conference on Disruptive Technologies (ICDT)* (pp. 1361-1366). IEEE. DOI: 10.1109/ICDT61202.2024.10489478

Ravindraiah, R., & Reddy, S. C. M. (2020). An Instinctive Application of Spatially Weighted Possibilistic Clustering Methods for the Detection of Lesions in Diabetic Retinopathy Images in Multi-dimensional Kernel Space. *Wireless Personal Communications*, 113(1), 223–240. DOI: 10.1007/s11277-020-07186-5

Sandra. M, Kjersti. E, Valery. N and Adrian. C (2017). Retinal Diabetes Screening through Local binary patterns. IEEE Journal of Biomedical and Health Informatics (Volume: 21, Issue: 1), pp 184 – 192, .DOI: 10.1109/JBHI.2015.2490798

Saranya, P., Devi, S. K., & Bharanidharan, B. (2022). Detection of Diabetic Retinopathy in Retinal Fundus Images using DenseNet based Deep Learning Model; *Proceedings of the 2022 International Mobile and Embedded Technology Conference (MECON)*; Noida, India. 10–11 March 2022; pp. 268–272. DOI: 10.1109/MECON53876.2022.9752065

Thaseen, A., Unnisa, R., Sultana, N., & Madhavi, K. R., NagaJyothi, G., & Kirubakaran, S. (2023, March). Breast Cancer Detection Using Deep Learning Model. In *Proceedings of Third International Conference on Advances in Computer Engineering and Communication Systems: ICACECS 2022* (pp. 669-677). Singapore: Springer Nature Singapore. DOI: 10.1007/978-981-19-9228-5_57

Thomas, E. R., Brackenridge, A., Kidd, J., Kariyawasam, D., Carroll, P., Colclough, K., & Ellard, S. (2016). Diagnosis of monogenic diabetes: 10-Year experience in a large multi-ethnic diabetes center. *Journal of Diabetes Investigation*, 7(3), 332–337. DOI: 10.1111/jdi.12432 PMID: 27330718

Wong, E., Backholer, K., Gearon, E., Harding, J., Freak-Poli, R., Stevenson, C., & Peeters, A. (2013). Diabetes and risk of physical disability in adults: A systematic review and meta-analysis. *The Lancet. Diabetes & Endocrinology*, 1(2), 106–114. DOI: 10.1016/S2213-8587(13)70046-9 PMID: 24622316

Wong, T. Y., Cheung, C. M. G., Larsen, M., Sharma, S., & Simó, R. (2016). Diabetic retinopathy. *Nature Reviews. Disease Primers*, 2, 1–16. PMID: 27159554

Zhang, W. et al (2019). Automated identification and grading system of diabetic retinopathy using deep neural networks. *Knowledge-Based Syst., 175*, 12–25. . knosys. 2019. 03. 016DOI: 10. 1016/j

Chapter 12
A Diabetes Mellitus Detection Using Fusion of IoMT, Generative AI, and eXplainable AI:
Diabetes Classification Using IoMT

G. Varun
https://orcid.org/0009-0006-4738-8999
Sri Ramachandra Institute of Higher Education and Research, India

B. V. Arun Krishna
https://orcid.org/0009-0002-9469-8333
Sri Ramachandra Institute of Higher Education and Research, India

S. Sarveswaran
Sri Ramachandra Institute of Higher Education and Research, India

M. C. Nidhisheshwin
Sri Ramachandra Institute of Higher Education and Research, India

S. Shreeshaa
Sri Ramachandra Institute of Higher Education and Research, India

P. Ashokkumar
https://orcid.org/0000-0003-2531-1326
Sri Ramachandra Institute of Higher Education and Research, India

ABSTRACT

Diabetes Mellitus (DM) is a metabolic disorder when the sugar level in the blood is elevated consistently. The presence of Diabetes Mellitus is one of the global health challenges, several research works focusing on the early detection and management of innovative machine learning technologies were developed in recent years. In this book chapter, we introduce a novel approach to classify diabetes mellitus by leveraging the Internet of Medical Things (IoMT) and generative AI models. IoT devices continuously monitor critical health data and transmit them to a central machine learning model for analysis and preprocessing is done. The preprocessed data act as the input for the machine learning models to predict diabetes. The imbalanced dataset is converted into a balanced one using two generative AI models called VAE and GAN. We used five ML classification models kNN, SVM, DT, LR and RF with boosting. Hard voting is performed to determine the final class. Our experiment result shows that the proposed ensemble model produces an accuracy of 81% which outperformed other model's accuracy

DOI: 10.4018/979-8-3693-6180-1.ch012

1 INTRODUCTION

In this subsection, we give an introduction to using IoMT, machine learning, and generative AI in diabetes classification.

1.1 Introduction of IoMT

Introduction of IoMT In the past few years, there has an exponential growth in the amount of medical data extraction in the healthcare industry [Patel et al., 2024]. The majority of the data is extracted through the integration of Internet of Things (IoT) devices. IoT devices play an important role in the medical healthcare industry [Alwahedi et al., 2024]. This technology allows the communication of health-related information across various devices, people, and nodes using the internet. Communication is done automatically without the need for human-to-human or computer-to-computer [Ashfaq et al., 2022]. The IoT network can store, transmit, process, and analyze the data from one connected node to another. In most cases, the nodes are connected to the wireless sensor networks which can easily monitor and track important health parameters such as glucose level, heart rate, and so on [Messinis et al., 2024]. The recorded data can be processed for classification tasks. The integration of IoT devices and the medical healthcare industry led to the establishment of a new subdomain known as the Internet of Medical Things (IoMT) [Wal et al., 2022]. In IoMT, the professionals make use of one or more wearable sensors that can gather and transmit data to a central ecosystem. These wearable sensors are autonomous, self-contained devices [Al-Turjman et al., 2020]. This technology has been integrated into almost all medical fields such as diabetes prediction, liver disease classification, skin cancer, and so on. The development of advanced IoT devices such as wearable devices make the integration into smart healthcare systems [Neto et al., 2024].

The use of IoMT in the medical industry offers many benefits such as improved patient care, high operational efficiency, assisting in many research works [Sujith et al., 2022]. The devices can continuously monitor the patient's health information such as glucose level, blood pressure, and so on. This allows a medical expert to track the patient's health in real-time and provide continuous patient monitoring and care [Manivannan, 2024]. Early detection of some abnormal incidents can be monitored, and timely interventions are done to prevent complex health issues. Even these devices can transmit the data to a remote location so that re-admission to the hospital can be prevented and the patient feels comfortable at home under the supervision of doctors [Rotbei et al., 2024]. IoMT devices are connected to a data analytics algorithm as it collects vast amounts of data, a comprehensive picture of the patient needs to be summarized. Sometimes, the machine learning models are also integrated into the devices so that the hidden patterns and found and enhanced diagnostics can be provided [Motwani et al., 2022]. As many patients may use IoMT for tracking their data and getting timely help from the medical industry, in many cases, personalized treatment is required. Data from these devices can be structured to build personalized treatment plans for individuals based on their specific needs and health conditions [Chatrati et al., 2022]. Personalized treatment is more effective in the betterment of the patient's health. One more advantage of using IoMT is operational efficiency, as the workload of medical staff is reduced significantly by automating many routine tasks. Many traditional hospital operations can also be streamlined so that the overall efficiency is increased [Ziwei et al., 2024].

The use of IoMT can also decrease the operational cost as early preventive steps can be taken before an alarming situation, this reduces the expensive treatment cost and hospital stays. Even frequent hospital visits can be reduced significantly by using IoMT [Kakhi et al., 2022].

One of the major advantages of IoMT is it aids in enhanced research and development. The devices generate large amounts of data which can be easily pre-processed by a data analysis algorithm and can be used for new research works in the field of medical science [Upreti et al., 2024]. A well-structured Electronic Health Records (EHRs) can be developed by using IoMT [Nti et al., 2023].

Self-management such as a patient or his close relatives can monitor the health status with the help of user-friendly interfaces (such as mobile phone apps, and websites). This is helpful in patient engagement to track their data. Even patients residing in rural and underserved areas can benefit from IoMT [Mbunge et al., 2021].

1.2 Introduction to Machine Learning

Machine learning (ML) is a subset of Artificial Intelligence (AI) which can identify the patterns in the data and predict new outcomes [Habib et al., 2022]. ML has been used in various domains and healthcare is one of them. All the sectors which use ML have observed significant revolution and success after its implementation. In healthcare, the ability of the ML models to understand the data identify proper patterns between the features, and make accurate decisions saves many lives and improves the way the patients are treated. The timely decision-making ability of ML makes a significant impact on the diagnostics of patients [Lv et al., 2021]. In many works, ML has proven that it can identify diseases more accurately than many traditional methods. For example, a well-trained ML model can be used to detect abnormalities in medical data such as CT scans, X-rays, and MRI images and find the presence of tumors with high accuracy. These ML models outperform the diagnostic capabilities of a human expert in the medical field [Mahadevkar et al., 2022].

Apart from the normal detection of diseases, ML models can also predict the likelihood of a disease that can attack a patient shortly. For example, several input features such as blood pressure, BMI, age, lifestyle factors, climate factors, and history of diabetes in a patient's family can be used to find the risk level for a patient to become diabetic. Early identification of these diseases can save many people's lives and money. ML can help in real-time patient monitoring, by using IoT devices and wearable devices, the patient data is closely monitored without any human intervention. In diabetes management, blood sugar levels can be monitored continuously by IoT devices, and a warning system can be built if the sugar level falls below target, and insulin dosage can be recommended [Das et al., 2022]. This improves the overall disease management system and quality of patient care. This can also reduce or completely avoid the number of days the patient is admitted to the hospital, this makes the hospital available for other needy patients. A few of the limitations that an ML model faces the data privacy, health-related information is very sensitive and confidential, and ensuring privacy is the supreme priority. On the other hand, the ML model requires lots of data to train. A perfectly trained ML model is essential in providing good accuracy. Hence the data that is used by the ML model is regulated by various policies such as the Health Insurance Portability and Accountability Act (HIPAA). Another big challenge that an ML model faces is the interpretation of the model. Many ML models are black boxes by nature. These ML models lack the transparency behind how the predictions are made. Much research works focused on providing explainability to ML models to make the predictions easy to understand and build a trust over it. Integrating ML models into the health industry also introduces learning challenges as health professionals resist adopting new technologies in their workflow. Proper teaching methodology can be introduced to the healthcare stakeholders to teach them how to use these ML models can be helpful to overcome the resistance [Vaccari et al., 2022].

Classification is one of the types of machine learning models where the main task is assigning labels or classes to the data points based on their feature values. They are used in many applications such as the medical field, intrusion detection, image processing, natural language processing, and so on. The objective of the classification models is to assign a class to unseen data correctly based on the training data [Alshammari, 2024]. Classifications are classified into three types, binary classification, multiclass classification, and multilabel classification.

In binary classification, there are only two classes. A data point can either be mapped to the first class or the second class [Massari et al., 2022]. For example, classifying an email as spam or not is a binary classification. In multiclass classifications, there are more than two classes. A data point may be mapped to any of the N classes. For example, identifying the species of a flower is a multiclass classification. The last type of classification is multilabel classification, in this classification, the classifier assigns more than one class to a data point. This type of classification is relevant to many real-world problems where data belongs to more than one group [Saleem et al., 2024]. For example, a cat can be mapped to an animal class and a domesticated class at the same time. The assigned classes can be independent also, that is they can be mutually exclusive too.

1.2 Ensemble Machine Learning Methods

Instead of depending on a single machine learning classifier, an ensemble-based classifier aggregates the output of multiple classifiers to make the final classification decision. Ensembling can be done in three ways, which includes bagging, boosting and stacking. Bagging allows a model to train on different data subsets, boosting corrects errors from previous trained model and stacking merges the different model strengths. There are some advantages of using ensemble methods such as reduced overfitting and increased performance [Yang G et al., 2024].

2. RELATED WORKS

IoMT plays an important role in monitoring, collecting, and transmitting highly sensitive medical data in the healthcare domain. However, there are a few challenges faced by the IoMT devices such as energy efficiency, interference, latency problems, and a few security issues. Research done by [Lazrek et al., 2024] focuses on addressing these issues by introducing an innovative IoMT model to reduce the interference from one device to another during transmission using hospital settings. The proposed model makes use of an interference avoidance distributed deep learning model which uses the Lagrange optimization technique to find the optimal distance between the interfering node and the medical receptions. This makes sure that the system achieves the required signal-to-interference plus noise ratio without losing energy efficiency and data transfer speed. A CNN-based deep learning model is developed to maintain a low computational cost and increase energy efficiency. The deep learning model predicts the optimal interference distance. The results show that the proposed method excels in various environments and balances the system performance requirements while maintaining the energy efficiency and data rate. The experiment shows that the interference distance can vary based on a factor's transmission power; when the power levels are high, the interference distance is low. The interference distance is also predicted with the given power level.

The use of advanced methods of IoMT technology enhances the quality of life across various sectors, especially in healthcare. Type 1 patients' details of more complex than type 2 which involves studying lifestyles, diet, insulin intake, and so on. As diabetes mellitus requires continuous blood glucose monitoring, pattern identification, and prediction of glycemic levels to determine the insulin dosage recommendation, IoMT devices are used by [Osman, 2024], since the use of normal computer-based methods is slightly risky, some advanced level of diagnosis is used such as IoMT, machine learning and so on. Their study uses IoMT for monitoring Diabetes Mellitus without any interruption. Machine learning-based wearable devices are reliable for short-term glucose prediction. Nearly 40 patients are used in the study and the random forest is used to predict the glucose level within a 3-minute horizon with an average error of 18.6 mg/dL for six-hour data and an error of 26.21 mg/dL for a 45-minute prediction horizon. These results are validated by the data of 1 type 2 patients.

Saudi Arabia is one of the countries that is rapidly developing in the field of IoMT and it is currently competing with other developed nations such as the United States, the United Kingdom, Australia, and so on. The pharmaceutical and biotechnology industries are focusing on developing and adopting novel IoMT products. A review paper by [Mathkor et al., 2024] highlighted many key technologies such as Artificial Intelligence, blockchain, and their integration of IoMT in the medical industry. Important challenges of IoMT such as patient standards, network energy management, transmission range management, working in heterogeneous backgrounds, increasing the quality of service, and increasing the security of the system. The authors compare and evaluate many IoMT designs in the field of medical domain.

Machine learning models have gained prominence in this field of early diabetes prediction. SVM is one of the models which has been used in various classification tasks notably. The authors in [Reza et al., 2023] use an enhanced nonlinear kernel for SVM to improve the type 2 diabetes classification. They combine the radial basis function and the RBF city block kernels. This allows the classifier to learn more complex decision boundaries. The missing values are imported using the median impute strategy. The outliers are removed before the classification and the class imbalance problem is addressed using a robust synthetic-based oversampling (SMOTE) method. An experiment is conducted by comparing the proposed kernel functions and the existing kernel functions and the results show that the proposed kernel outperforms all the existing kernels with improved performance metrics of accuracy of 85.5%, recall of 87.0%, precision of 83.4%, and F1-score of 85.2% and AUC of 85.5%. Along with the standard comparison of the kernel and the existing kernel, a simulation study is conducted to further validate the strength of the proposed kernel. In the clinical settings, as promising results are obtained in both early detection and management of individual risk, the authors also recommended the use of the proposed kernel for increasing the predictive performance in the field of diabetes classification.

Missing values in the dataset can significantly reduce the learning skill of a machine learning model in the training phase. This causes a decreased performance in the testing set and a drop in classification accuracy. To mitigate this issue, the authors in [Palanivinayagam and Damaševičius, 2023] use a popular regression model called a support vector machine (SVM) repressor for finding and imputing the missing values in the training dataset. In addition to this, a two-level classification model is proposed to reduce the classification errors made by the classifier. The PIMA Indian dataset is used for this study and the performance of five classifiers are compared. The five classifiers are Naive Bayes (NB), Support Vector Machine (SVM), k-nearest Neighbors (KNN), Random Forest (RF), and Linear Regression (LR). The experiment results show that the SVM classifier achieved the highest performance in terms of accuracy when compared with the other four classifiers. The maximum accuracy recorded by the SVM is 94.89%.

As IoMT rapidly grows in healthcare offering efficient and effective services to patients and healthcare stakeholders, it is having lots of security challenges. Novice IoMT stakeholders often lack experience in handling the security flaws in the system that lead to the exposure of data and other possible healthcare attacks. These security issues need to be addressed by cyber security algorithms to implement the IoMT system in healthcare. One research done by [Kumar et al., 2022], addresses these issues with the implementation of a security enhancement method using rooted elliptic curve cryptography with vigenere cipher. There are three main components in the proposed system, which are privacy preservation, data sensitivity, and secure data transmission. In the first stage, the privacy of the data is preserved using a special algorithm called the K-anonymity algorithm. This algorithm makes it difficult for hackers to differentiate the real user information from the anonymized data. This allows unauthorized persons to find the real user information in the system. The second stage is responsible for data sensitivity. An improved Elman neural network (IENN) is introduced to examine the level of sensitivity in the data. IENN is a form of a recurrent neural network (RNN) that is specialized for use in this application. The Gaussian mutated chimp is used to further increase the performance of the IENN by updating optimal weights in the model. The introduction of this optimization helps the IENN to learn better and improve its efficiency, leading to better sensitivity analysis of data. Finally, the last stage uses the RECC-VC method for securely transmitting the health data to the cloud storage. A cryptographic approach is used to encrypt the data. A mix of rooted elliptical curve cryptography with the Vigenere cipher is used to provide a robust security mechanism. To provide an additional level of security the stored data in the cloud server is protected using blockchain technology. This adds more data integrity and immutability of the data in the cloud storage. In the experiment, the authors obtained an accuracy of 96% using the IENN model and it is compared with other state-of-the-art methods. The proposed model also attained a 98% security level significantly increasing the security standards when compared to other existing methods.

The Use of wearable devices in IoMT is very prevalent. These devices often have very limited computing power and limited storage capacity. The data stored in these devices are not sufficient enough to train the machine learning model, hence, to overcome this issue a federated learning-based concept is introduced. The authors of [Ni et al., 2024] propose a new method called a federated split learning framework which allows collaborative healthcare data analytics across multiple wearable IoMT devices. As federated learning does not need the entire data to be transmitted across the nodes in the network, the IoMT devices are allowed to keep the private and sensitive data of the user in their local storage, thus increasing user privacy as it is not required to transmit the raw data in the network. Moreover, their proposed systems are specialized in the IoMT domain as small devices can also participate in the model training process. The experiment results show that their methods work well in the medical image data and robust and effective model training is performed with diverse healthcare data.

To overcome the imbalance problem, the authors [V, K. et al., 2024] used three ensemble models InceptionV3+DenseNet-BC-121-32 + Xception, ResNet50V2+DenseNet-BC-121-32, and ResNet-50V2+ResNet50. The ensembling of these models shows an increased performance of 97.89% for InceptionV3, Xception, DenseNet-BC-121-32 ensemble method. The authors in [Khezri, S et al., 2024] solves the concept drift by comparing 21 ensemble models with 30 synthetic datasets. The pros and cons of each ensemble model are discussed.

3 DEVICES

The expeditious development of the Internet of Things (IoT) has transformed many sectors, particularly healthcare industries. Medical devices equipped with IoT sensors allow continuous monitoring of various health parameters, providing necessary data for pre diagnosis and treatment. In this chapter, we will explore some of the advanced sensors used in health monitoring for diabetic patients including their function and applications. The following subsections explain about the sensors used.

3.1 Sensors

The section covers the usage of various sensors in the system.

3.1.1 Load Cell with HX711 Sensor

A load cell is an electro-mechanical sensor that converts mechanical force into electrical signals. It plays a major role in measuring body weight, a rudimentary health parameter for diabetic patients. The load cell is connected with an hx711 sensor, an analog digital converter that converts the analog signal to digital signal specifically designed for weighing scales.

3.1.2 Ultrasonic Sensor

An ultrasonic sensor is a device that generates and senses ultrasound waves. It measures the distance of the object by emitting the sound waves and computes the time taken to return back. In healthcare, it is used to measure the height of the patients.

3.1.3 Gas Sensor

Gas sensor is mainly used to detect the chemical compounds in the surrounding air. In healthcare, it is used to predict the insulin level by measuring the acetone level in breath exhale.

3.1.4 VL53L0X Sensor

The VL53L0X sensor works under the 'time of flight' principle. It measures the distance of the object from the sensor by emitting a laser pulse. The sensor calculates the distance by calculating the time taken for the laser pulse to reflect back from the surface. This sensor is used to measure the skin thickness af diabetic patients.

3.1.5 Blood Pressure Sensor

Blood pressure is an essential health parameter of diabetic health. Blood pressure sensors are made to measure the force exerted by blood on the walls of arteries. These sensors are incorporated with inflatable cuffs that restrict the blood flow as the cuff deflates a pressure transducer to measure the oscillation in the arterial wall that allows the device to calculate both systolic and diastolic pressure.

In this section, we will discuss how the automated health data collection system works and how it captures the data and stores the various health parameters in mongodb cloud db, cloud accessibility

3.2 Weight Measurement Using Load Cell with HX711 Sensor

The process begins when patients step onto the weight machine which is designed with a load cell and hx711 sensor. The load cell will convert the force exerted by the person's weight to electrical signal and hx711 will amplify the signal and convert it into digital signal making it understandable for the microcontroller. Then the microcontroller sends the data to MongoDB cloud database and local host website. This weight of patients will be measured and stored in cloud database for further analysis.

Figure 1. Circuit diagram of node MCU with load cell

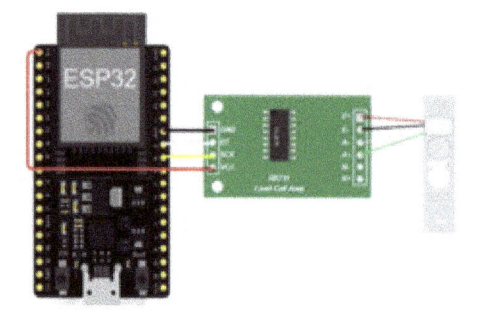

3.3 Height Measurement Using Ultrasonic Sensor

Next, the patient has to stand in the height measuring zone where height is measured using an ultrasonic sensor, which emits sound waves towards the top of the patient's head and measures the time taken for the echo to return. This time is used to calculate the distance between the sensor and the head and the calculated height is sent to the microcontroller. Then the microcontroller sends the data to MongoDB cloud database and local host website. The height of patients will be measured and stored in a cloud database for further analysis.

Figure 2. Circuit diagram of node MCU with ultrasonic sensor

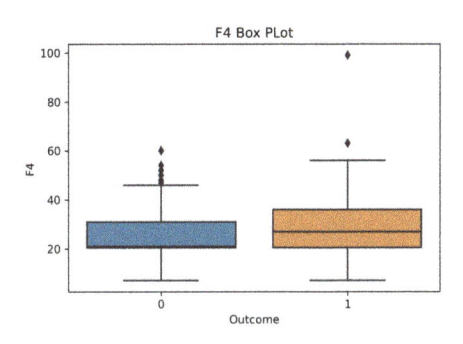

3.4 BMI Calculation

With both height and weight data collected from the sensors discussed above, the system will automatically compute the Body Mass Index (BMI), an essential health parameter to determine if the person has a healthy body weight for a given height. BMI is calculated using the formula at eq (1):

$$\text{BMI} = \frac{\text{Weight (kg)}}{\text{Height (m)}^2} \qquad (1)$$

The calculated BMI is then stored in the MongoDB database and local host website for further analysis.

3.5 Skin Thickness Measurement Using VL53L0X Sensor

The vl53lox sensor is used to measure the tricep skinfold thickness of patients. The sensor is fused with a tricep measuring scale. It emits a laser pulse when a patient places his/her triceps in the measuring scale. The thickness of the skin is measured by calculating the time taken for the laser pulse to reflect back. This data is automatically recorded in the microcontroller. The microcontroller sends this data to MongoDB cloud database and the local host website for further analysis.

Figure 3. Circuit diagram of node MCU with VL56L0X sensor

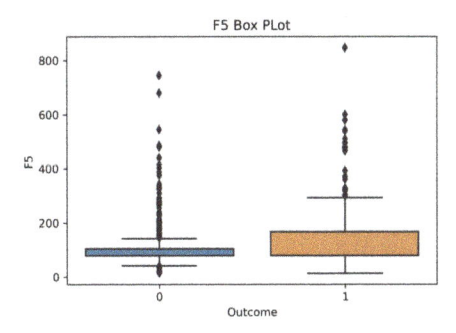

3.6 Blood Pressure Measurement Using Blood Pressure Sensor

Blood pressure is measured using a blood pressure sensor with the help of a nurse. This sensor records both systolic and diastolic pressure reading by inflating a cuff around the patient's arms and measures the force of blood against the artery walls as the cuff deflates and this data is recorded in the microcontroller, which sends the data to MongoDB cloud database and local host website for further analysis.

Figure 4. Circuit diagram of node MCU with blood pressure sensor

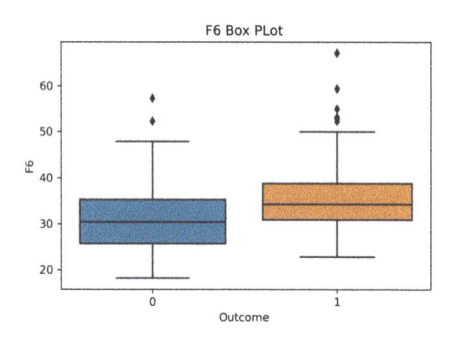

3.7 Insulin Prediction Using Gas Sensor

To determine the most important health parameter (Insulin), the patient has to exhale in a glucose prediction device designed with a gas sensor. This device will detect the acetone level and give the acetone content in breath, which indicates the insulin or glucose level in the patient's body. This insulin or glucose level is sent to the microcontroller, which further sends the data to MongoDB cloud database and local host website for further analysis.

Figure 5. Circuit diagram of node MCU with gas sensor

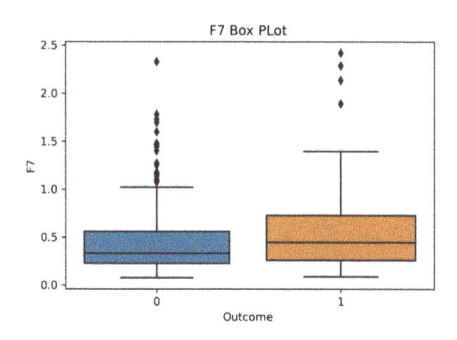

3.8 Cloud Storage in MongoDB

The data from the microcontrollers is transmitted to cloud-based storage mongo db (no sgl database), it handles various data generated by iot medical devices. The microcontroller sends the collected data to the cloud using wifi, cellular or other iot protocols and these collected data are stored as documents in excel are jason etc… in mongodb and these stored data documents are used for further the analysis and prediction.

3.9 Data Accessibility and Use

Once the data is stored in the cloud, the data becomes accessible to healthcare professionals through secure interfaces such as custom-built applications or dashboard connected to MongoDB database. This enables real-time access and analysis. Data can also be accessed through localhost website, when medical devices connected to same Wi-Fi network this provides real time data monitoring without need of the cloud

4 ARCHITECTURE

Figure 6. Architecture

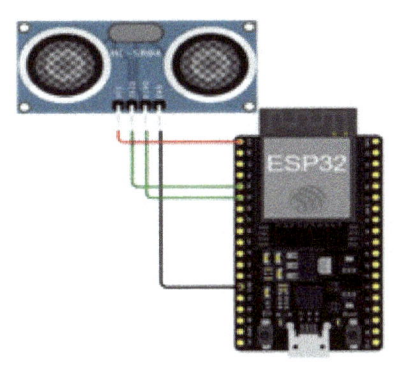

Diabetes is a chronic disease that affects millions of people worldwide. Management and prevention of complications are all about early detection and continuous monitoring. With the advent of the Internet of Things, Artificial Intelligence, and advanced machine learning in healthcare, diagnosis and treatment of diabetes have been revolutionized. Overall holistic detection model for diabetes with IoT sensors, GANs, VAEs, and ensemble machine learning models is shown above in the diagram. The process has been divided into a few steps and all those steps are crucial for proper diagnosis and prediction.

Step 1: IoT Sensors for Data Collection

The process starts with the patient with different types of IoT sensors monitoring different parameters of the patient. These devices will collect key health data which includes glucose levels, blood pressure, heart rate, and other relevant physiological parameters. These sensors are embedded in wearable devices like smartwatches or dedicated medical devices that will monitor the body's vital parameters unobtrusively. Data from these IoT end devices will provide real-time accurate information to make decisions about the patient's health condition.

Step 2: Data Aggregation and Processing

Data after collection from IoT sensors is sent to endpoint devices for aggregation and preliminary processing. These endpoint devices act as an intermediary between sensors and data analysis models. Raw data is cleaned, normalized, and structured into a format for further analysis. Then it is fed to the system and combined with the PIMA dataset, a well-known dataset in medical applications, especially in diabetes research.

Step 3: Data enhancement with GAN and VAE

Data is processed with the help of two latest AI models, Generative Adversarial Network (GAN) and Variational Autoencoder to get a balanced dataset that represents the entire population.

- Generative Adversarial Network: GANs are one type of AI model; it consists of two neural networks; one is a generator and the other is a discriminator. The generator creates synthetic data which looks real, and the discriminator identifies the fake data by distinguishing between original and synthetic. GANs create realistic and diverse synthetic data that can be used to augment the original dataset and solve the problem of data imbalance.
- Variational Autoencoder: This is another way of creating new data points within the neural network. VAE is different from GAN in the sense that it takes the given input data maps it to a hidden variable space and then decodes it back to its original form with some variations. That's how new data points—which are statistically similar to the original data—are created and diversity is brought in.

With GAN and VAE, it creates balanced data so that model bias is prevented, and machine learning algorithms are fed with a dataset that is practical and representative.

Step 4: Model Training Using Ensemble Learning

This involves getting a balanced dataset and then training multiple machine-learning models with the dataset to predict diabetes. This system uses an ensemble learning model. An ensemble learning model is one in which multiple models are trained and the predictions from all such models are aggregated to make a better forecast with more accuracy and robustness. The ensemble learning models used in this experiment are:

1. Logistic Regression
2. Support Vector Machine
3. K-Nearest Neighbor
4. Decision Tree
5. Random Forest

All these models are trained on the balanced dataset and the predictions from all are combined to get the final output. Ensemble learning reduces variance and bias.

Step 5: Generate Prediction and Results

The models we create in these stages help us predict data from IoT sensors. This tells us if a patient has diabetes or not. When we get new patient data, we run it through our combined models. The result shows if the diabetes test is positive (+VE) or negative (-VE). We then send this result back to the devices. This lets healthcare staff and the patient see the outcome.

5 MACHINE LEARNING MODELS

Machine Learning is a field of AI where we create algorithms that allow computers to learn from data and make decisions. There are five models used in our experiment, they are Support Vector Machine (SVM), k-nearest neighbor (k-NN), Logistic Regression (LR), Decision Tree (DT), and Random Forest (RF). The details of the models are as follows

5.1 Support Vector Machines (SVM)

Support Vector Machines (SVM) are a class of supervised learning algorithms used primarily for classification tasks but can also be adapted for regression. The fundamental goal of an SVM is to find the optimal hyperplane that separates different classes with the maximum margin. In simpler terms, it searches for the best boundary that divides data into distinct classes while maximizing the distance between the boundary and the nearest data points from each class. These nearest points are called support vectors. The SVM algorithm is highly effective, especially in high-dimensional spaces, thanks to its ability to create complex decision boundaries through the kernel trick. This trick allows SVM to handle non-linearly separable data by transforming it into a higher-dimensional space where a linear separation is possible. By solving a convex optimization problem, SVM ensures a globally optimal solution, making it both powerful and efficient. SVMs are widely used in various applications, including image recognition, text classification, and bioinformatics, due to their robustness and ability to handle high-dimensional data effectively.

5.2 K-Nearest Neighbors (k-NN)

K-Nearest Neighbors (k-NN) is a flexible and versatile algorithm for classification and regression tasks in supervised learning. The basic idea is to determine the class or value of the new data point by examining the 'k' nearest data points in the training set. For classification purposes, additional points are assigned to the class most likely to lie within the 'k' of its nearest neighbors. The prediction of the regression is the average of the values of these 'k' neighbors. Typically, the distance between data points is measured in terms of Euclidean distance, but depending on the context, other metrics can also be used. The choice of 'k'—the number of neighbors to consider—significantly affects the performance of the model. Smaller 'k's may make the model more sensitive to noisy data, while larger 'k's may simplify predictions but ignore smaller local trends Although indicated k-NN is appreciated for its simplicity and effectiveness it can be computationally demanding in large data sets, due to distance computation for each forecast It is important.

5.3 Logistic Regression (LR)

Logistic regression (LR) is a statistical technique used for binary classification problems, where the objective is to determine the probability that a given input belongs to one of the two classes Regardless of the name, logistic regression is used for classification rather than regression. It models the relationship between the independent variables and the binary outcome using a logistic function, also known as the sigmoid function. This function maps each real-valued number to 0 to 1 possibilities. The logistic regression model estimates the probability that the default class (usually specified as 1) depends on input characteristics by applying a logistic function to the linear combination of these features. The model is trained using maximum likelihood estimation, which searches for the best-fitting parameters to the observed data. Logistic regression is popular for its simplicity, explanation, and effectiveness in situations where the relationship between factors and outcomes is nearly linear. Devices such as one-vs-rest or softmax regression Can be extended to multiclass classification problems.

5.4 Decision Tree (DT)

Decision tree (DT) is a versatile and flexible machine learning algorithm used for both classification and regression tasks. It models decision-making and potential outcomes in a tree-like structure, similar to a flow chart. Each node of the tree represents a decision based on a factor, each branch represents the outcome of that decision, and each leaf node represents a class label or value persistent in the case of the regression. The return of the data group based on the feature values of each node is used in the decision-building.minimum Number of samples. Decision trees are popular for their explicability and intuitive logic, as decision rules are visually represented. But they are too suitable, especially for deep woods. Typically pruning and trimming techniques, such as random forests and gradient boosting, are used to deal with overloading and improve performance.

5.5 Random Forest (RF)

Random forest (RF) is a powerful cluster learning technique for classification and regression tasks. It creates multiple decision trees to create a robust and accurate model. Each tree in the forest has been trained on random data and features, helping to reduce overfitting and improving generalization

Random forestry steps:
- Bootstrapping: Create multiple training datasets by sampling with replacements from the original dataset. Each tree is raised in a small group, giving the trees diversity.
- Feature Randomness: Only a small random subset of features is considered for each split in the decision trees. This randomness helps distinguish each tree from the others, resulting in a more robust model overall.

6 METHODOLOGY

We have used the PIMA Indian dataset to train the machine learning model. The trained ML model is then deployed in a central system where IoMT devices are connected. Once the data from the various IoT devices are received, the pre-trained model starts its classification. Finally, the ensemble operation is performed to complete the classification. The PIMA Indian dataset consists of nine features out of which 8 features are independent features and one feature is a binary dependent feature. The value of 0 represents a normal healthy patient and the value of 1 represents that the patient is having diabetes.

The dataset itself is highly imbalanced because there are a total of 268 instances belonging to diabetes diabetes-positive class and the remaining 500 instances belonging to the negative class, that is the healthy set of patients. As there is a huge difference in the number of instances between these two datasets, the dataset is termed as an imbalanced dataset. The ratio of healthy and diabetes-infected patients is 67:125. We have used two generative AI models called Variational Autoencoder and Generative Adversarial Networks to generate synthetic samples in the minority class and convert the dataset into a balanced dataset. This balanced dataset is used to train five machine-learning models. The details of the dataset are tabulated in Table 1.

Table 1. Description of the feature

Sno	Feature Name	Name used in this chapter	Description of the feature
1	Pregnancies	F1	This feature represents how many times the patient had become pregnant in the past
2	Glucose	F2	An oral glucose tolerance test is performed for 2 hours and the plasma glucose concentration is observed.
3	blood pressure	F3	The value of Diastolic blood pressure (mm Hg)
4	SkinThickness	F4	The value of the skin fold thickness in millimeters of triceps
5	Insulin	F5	The serum insulin measured in 2 hours in the unit mu U/ml
6	BMI	F6	The ratio of weight and height of the patient
7	DiabetesPedigreeFunction	F7	The family history of the patient
8	Age	F8	The age of the patient during the study
9	Outcome	F9	A binary variable that denotes 0 for healthy patients and 1 for diabetes patients.

Despite the various advantages of machine learning, people still have lots of trust issues as no one knows how the decision is made. Explainable AI is one of the techniques that make everyone understand how machine learning classification models work and the reason behind how the classification is made. To provide insights into how various decisions are made, and the lack of transparency has created the need for explainable AI. In healthcare systems, the ML model may produce high accuracy but still, medical professionals hesitate to trust the process and act on the recommendations provided by the model due to its lack of explainability.

7 RESULTS AND DISCUSSION

This section explains about the results in detail

7.1 Dataset Description

The properties of each features are listed below.

7.1.1 Feature 1

The feature named Pregnancies has a correlation value of 0.25, with a maximum value of 17 and a minimum value of 1. The standard deviation is 2.98. The 25th, 50th, and 75th percentiles are 1, 2, and 3.85, respectively. Table 2 presents the statistical values of the feature, and Figure 7 displays the box plot of the feature. There are 111 instances which having missing values in this feature.

Table 2. Description of feature 1

	Mean	Standard deviation	0% Quantile	25% Quantile	50% Quantile	75% Quantile	100% Quantile
Feature 1 - F1	4.4	2.98	1	2	3.85	6	17

Figure 7. F1 box plot

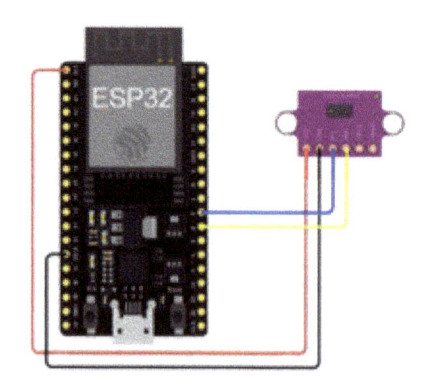

7.1.2 Feature 2

Glucose, a feature in the dataset, shows a correlation of 0.49. Its values range from a minimum of 44 to a maximum of 199. The standard deviation is 30.44. The quantiles at 25%, 50%, and 75% are 99.75, 117, and 140.25, respectively. The statistical values of the feature are shown in Table 3, while the box plot of the feature is illustrated in Figure 8. Five instances have missing value of this feature.

Table 3. Description of feature 2

	Mean	Standard deviation	0% Quantile	25% Quantile	50% Quantile	75% Quantile	100% Quantile
Feature 2- F2	121.68	30.44	44	99.75	117	140.25	199

Figure 8. F2 box plot

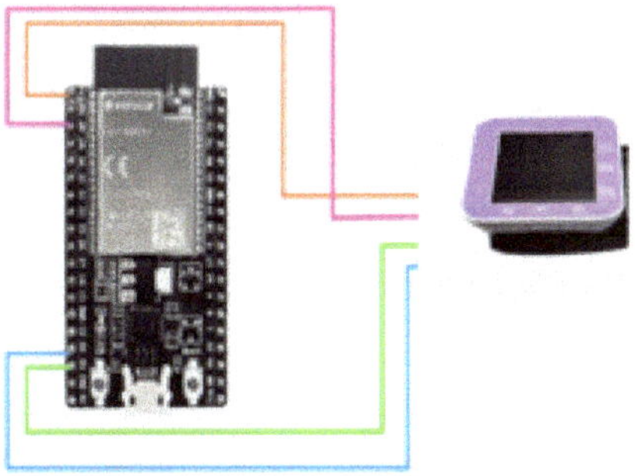

7.1.3 Feature 3

The Blood Pressure feature exhibits a correlation value of 0.16, with a range from 24 to 122. It has a standard deviation of 12.12. The 25th, 50th, and 75th percentiles are 64, 72, and 80, respectively. In Table 4, you can find the statistical values of the feature, and Figure 9 shows its corresponding box plot. 35 instances in the dataset have missing values for this feature.

Table 4. Description of feature 3

	Mean	Standard deviation	0% Quantile	25% Quantile	50% Quantile	75% Quantile	100% Quantile
Feature 3- F3	72.25	12.12	24	64	72	80	122

Figure 9. F3 box plot

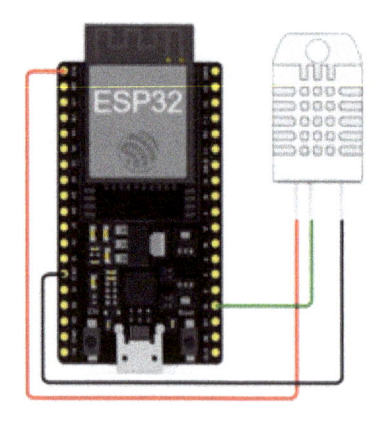

7.1.4 Feature 4

With a correlation of 0.18, the Skin Thickness feature spans from 7 to 99. Its standard deviation is 9.63. The values for the 25th, 50th, and 75th quartiles are 20.54, 23, and 32, respectively. The feature's statistical values are detailed in Table 5, with its box plot depicted in Figure 10. 227 instances contain missing values for this feature.

Table 5. Description of feature 4

	Mean	Standard deviation	0% Quantile	25% Quantile	50% Quantile	75% Quantile	100% Quantile
Feature 4- F4	26.61	9.63	7	20.54	23	32	99

Figure 10. F4 box plot

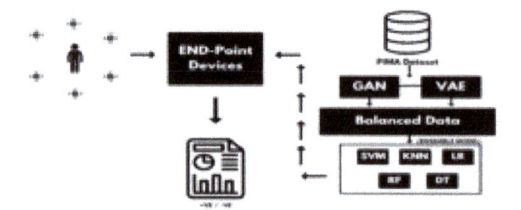

7.1.5 Feature 5

The feature Insulin has a correlation coefficient of 0.18. It ranges between 14 and 846, with a standard deviation of 93.08. The 25%, 50%, and 75% quantiles are 79.8, 79.8, and 127.25, respectively. Table 6 contains the statistical values of the feature, and Figure 11 depicts the box plot of the feature. This feature contains the highest number of instances with missing values. The total number of instances with missing values is 374. In the negative class, 236 instances contain missing values and 138 instances from the positive class contain missing values.

Table 6. Description of feature 5

	Mean	Standard deviation	0% Quantile	25% Quantile	50% Quantile	75% Quantile	100% Quantile
Feature 5- F5	118.66	93.08	14	79.8	79.8	127.25	846

Figure 11. F5 box plot

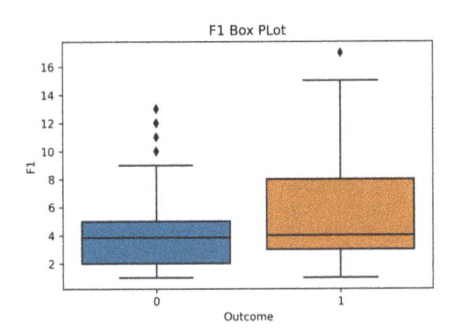

7.1.6 Feature 6

BMI has a correlation value of 0.31, with its values ranging from 18.2 to 67.1. The standard deviation is 6.88. The 25th, 50th, and 75th quartiles are at 27.5, 32, and 36.6, respectively. The statistical data of the feature is summarized in Table 7, and its box plot is shown in Figure 12. There are 11 instances with missing values for these features where 9 of them belong to the negative class and 2 of them belong to the majority class.

Table 7. Description of feature 6

	Mean	Standard deviation	0% Quantile	25% Quantile	50% Quantile	75% Quantile	100% Quantile
Feature 6- F6	32.45	6.88	18.2	27.5	32	36.6	67.1

Figure 12. F6 box plot

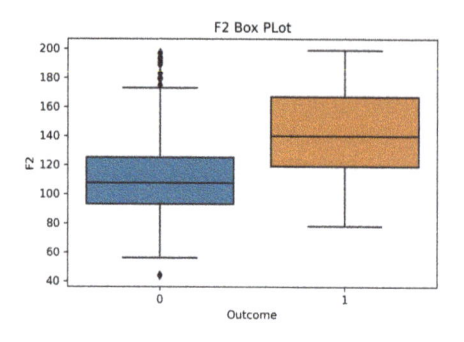

7.1.7 Feature 7

The feature named Diabetes Pedigree Function, having a correlation value of 0.17, varies between 0.08 and 2.42. It has a standard deviation of 0.33. The 25th, 50th, and 75th percentiles are 0.24, 0.37, and 0.63, respectively. Statistical values for the feature are presented in Table 8, and the box plot can be seen in Figure 13. No instances have a missing value for this feature.

Table 8. Description of feature 7

	Mean	Standard deviation	0% Quantile	25% Quantile	50% Quantile	75% Quantile	100% Quantile
Feature 7- F7	0.47	0.33	0.08	0.24	0.37	0.63	2.42

Figure 13. F7 box plot

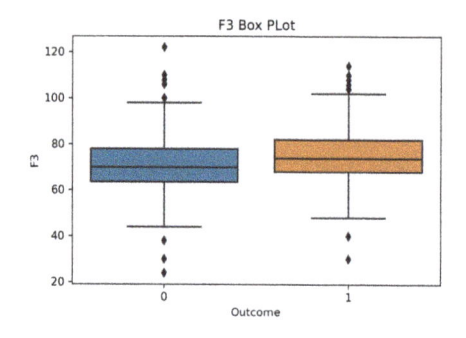

7.1.8 Feature 8

The Age feature in the dataset shows a correlation of 0.24. It ranges from a minimum of 21 to a maximum of 81, with a standard deviation of 11.76. The 25th, 50th, and 75th quartiles are 24, 29, and 41, respectively. Table 9 illustrates the statistical values of the feature, while Figure 14 displays its box plot. No instances have a missing value for this feature.

Table 9. Description of feature 8

	Mean	Standard deviation	0% Quantile	25% Quantile	50% Quantile	75% Quantile	100% Quantile
Feature 8- F8	33.24	11.76	21	24	29	41	81

Figure 14. F8 box plot

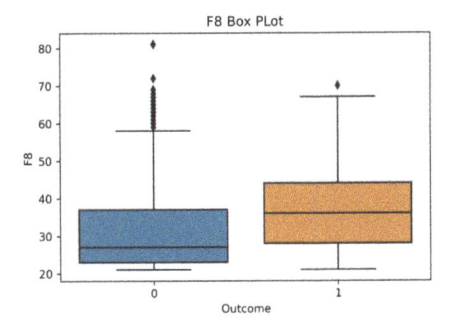

7.2 Preprocessing the Dataset

The dataset used in the experiment contains lots of missing values, with the insulin feature being the most affected. Specifically, 374 out of 768 instances in the insulin feature alone contain missing values, this accounts for 47.58% of the total dataset. The missing values should be resolved for better machine learning training. If the number of instances with missing values is significantly less, then deleting them can be a good strategy, however, the number of instances with at least one missing value is which accounts for % of the total instances in the dataset. To address the missing value issue, we employed mean imputation to handle the missing values. In this method, the mean of each feature is calculated, and the calculated value is replaced with all the missing values in the respective feature. The mean imputation ensures that the dataset remains complete and ready for the training of the classifier.

We make use of five distinct classification models in our experiments, they are k-nearest Neighbors (KNN), Support Vector Machine (SVM), Naive Bayes (NB), Random Forest (RF), and Decision Tree (DT). These five models are chosen to increase the strength of the classification by providing diverse methods and a broad range of perspectives on the data. To train the models, we have used a 70-30 split, with 70% of the instances used for training the model and the rest 30% of the instances used for testing. This splitting methodology allows for a balanced testing of classifiers on the unseen data.

After fixing the experimental variables and the perfect hyperparameters for all the models, we conducted a feature selection and feasibility study on all the features and determined the list of features that were most relevant for the classification task. As a result of the selection, it was determined that except the feature number 4 and feature number 7, all other features are used for building and training the classifiers.

Finally, to conclude the final result of the classification and to enhance the reliability of the models, we employed an ensemble method using hard voting. The classification results of all the five models are used in the hard voting process and the final classification result leverages the strength of each model.

7.3 The Imbalance Problem

The PIMA Indian dataset is imbalanced. That is the distribution of instances across the classes is highly different. The majority class (negative class) has 500 instances whereas the positive class is the minority class of only 268 instances. When the classifier is trained using the dataset, the learning will not be appropriate. The classifier will learn more about the negative class and learn very little about the positive class because only a few instances are given in the training stage. To address the class imbalance problem, a combination of Generative Adversarial Networks (GANs) and Variational Autoencoders (VAEs) is employed to generate synthetic samples of the minority class, the main objective of GAN and VAE in this experiment is to balance the dataset by an equal number of instances in both the classes.

7.3.1 Balancing the Dataset

Once the synthetic samples are generated, half of them from GAN and half of them from VAE are picked stochastically causing a balance between the count of majority and minority class instances

7.4 Model Parameters

The hyperparameters for each model used in this experiment are listed below. These hyperparameters are selected by grid search CV method which picks the best combination of hyperparameters in respect to accuracy.

7.4.1 KNN

n neighbors = 11, weights = uniform, algorithm = brute, p = 1

7.4.2 SVM

C = 1, kernel = rbf, gamma = 0.01, degree = 2

7.4.3 DT

criterion = gini, splitter = best, max depth = None, min samples split = 2, min samples leaf = 4, max features = log2

7.4.4 RF

n estimators = 50, criterion = gini, max depth = 30, min samples split = 10, min samples leaf = 2, max features = sqrt, bootstrap = True

7.4.5 LR

penalty = l1, C = 1, solver = liblinear, max iter = 100, l1_ratio = None

7.5 Performance Evaluation Metrics

Performance metrics for a classifier are very crucial for evaluating the model. To evaluate the performance of the classifiers, we have used four standard performance metrics. They are

1. *Accuracy:* Accuracy measures the proportion of the correctly classified instances out of all the instances in the dataset.
2. *Precision:* this is the measure of how well the model avoids the false positive rate.
3. *Recall:* sometimes, this is known as sensitivity. This indicates the measure of how well the model captures the positives.
4. *F1 score:* it is the harmonic mean of precision and recall.

Table 10, Table 11, Table 12, Table 13, Table 14 And Table 15 shows the confusion matrix of, kNN, SVM, DT, RF, LR and ensemble model.

Table 10. Confusion matrix of the kNN model

Actual Values		Predicted Values	
		Positive	Negative
	Positive	139	18
	Negative	30	44

Table 11. Confusion matrix of the SVM model

Actual Values		Predicted Values	
		Positive	Negative
	Positive	138	19
	Negative	35	39

Table 12. Confusion matrix of the DT model

Actual Values		Predicted Values	
		Positive	Negative
	Positive	127	30
	Negative	32	42

Table 13. Confusion matrix of RF model

Actual Values		Predicted Values	
		Positive	Negative
	Positive	140	17
	Negative	29	45

Table 14. Confusion matrix of LR model

Actual Values		Predicted Values	
		Positive	Negative
	Positive	139	18
	Negative	37	37

Table 15. Confusion matrix of the ensemble model

Actual Values		Predicted Values	
		Positive	Negative
	Positive	142	15
	Negative	28	46

The kNN model got an accuracy of 0.79 a precision of 0.76 a recall of 0.82 and an F1 score of 0.79. The Figure 15 shows the performance result of the kNN model.

Figure 15. Performance of kNN

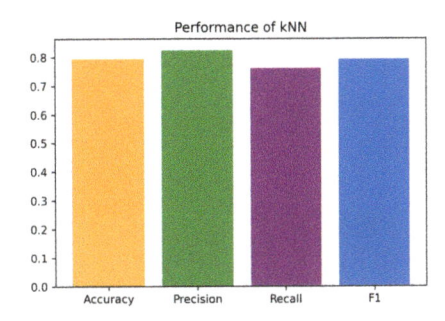

For the SVM model, the accuracy is 0.77, the precision is 0.8, the recall stands at 0.78 and the F1 score is 0.79. The Figure 16 displays the performance of the SVM model.

Figure 16. Performance of SVM

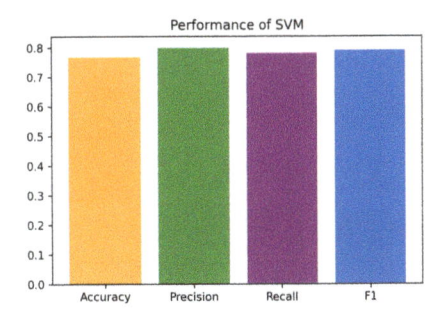

The performance of the DT classifier is marked by an accuracy of 0.73, a precision of 0.8, a recall of 0.75, and an F1 score of 0.77. Figure 17 exhibits the performance of the DT.

Figure 17. Performance of DT

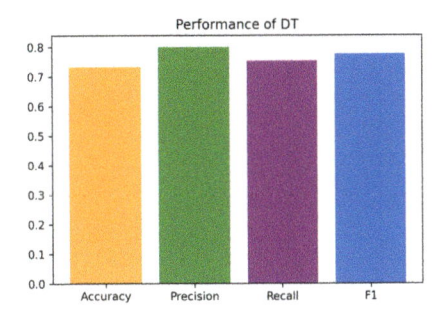

RF shows an accuracy of 0.8, a precision of 0.83, a recall reaching of 0.76, and an F1 score of 0.79. The performance of the RF model is displayed in Figure 18. Random forest is the model that produces the highest accuracy.

Figure 18. Performance of RF

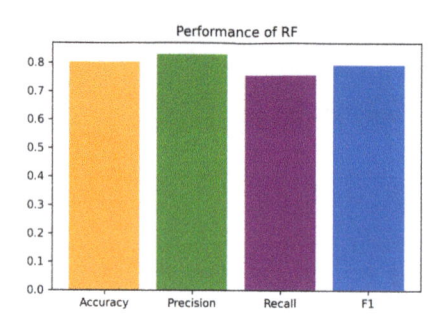

The LR algorithm delivered an accuracy of 0.76, with precision at 0.79, recall at 0.79, and an F1 score also at 0.79. Figure 19 presents the results of the LR model.

Figure 19. Performance of LR

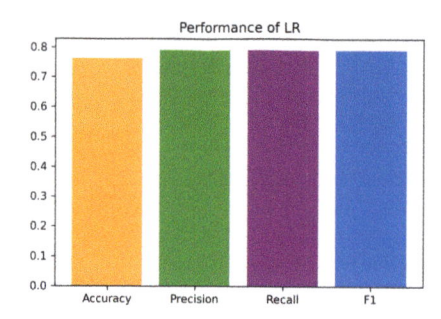

The ensemble classification results include an accuracy of 0.81, a precision of 0.84, a recall of 0.76, and an F1 score of 0.79. Figure 20 presents the Ensemble model.

Figure 20. Performance of ensemble

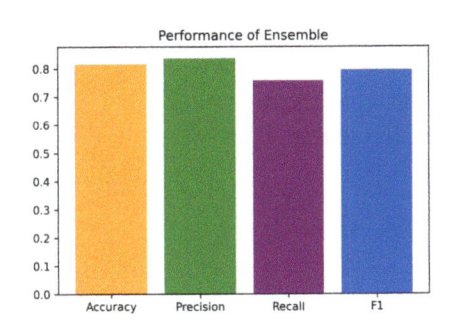

The table 16 presents the evaluation metric values of each classifier. Table 17 presents the accuracy comparison of the selected hyperparameter vs the default hyper parameters.

Table 16. Evaluation metrics of each classifier

Model	Accuracy	Precision	Recall	F1 Score
kNN	0.79	0.82	0.76	0.79
SVM	0.77	0.8	0.78	0.79
DT	0.73	0.8	0.75	0.77
RF	0.8	0.83	0.76	0.79
LR	0.76	0.79	**0.79**	0.79
Ensemble	**0.81**	**0.84**	0.76	**0.79**

Table 17. Accuracy comparison of selected hyperparameters vs default hyperparameters

Model	Accuracy (Selected best hyperparameters)	Accuracy (default hyperparameters)
kNN	0.79	0.63
SVM	0.77	0.7
DT	0.73	0.66
RF	0.8	0.66
LR	0.76	0.72
Ensemble	**0.81**	**0.78**

7.6 Explainability Using SHAP

SHAP (Shapley Additive Explanations) is an algorithm that is used popularly in game theory. The SHAP algorithm can be used to pick the feature importance based on how much they are contributing towards the classification of target variables. It can easily list out the features according to their contributions (either negative or positive). If a feature is contributing more to the target class, then the SHAP value will be high.

7.6.1 kNN Explainability

Figure 21 shows the feature importance according to the SHAP method. It says that glucose is positively correlated with the value 0.6, followed by BMI with a positive correlation of 0.03, the age is negatively correlated with -0.03. Figure 22 explains the overall summary of the kNN classification.

Figure 21. SHAP Values using kNN

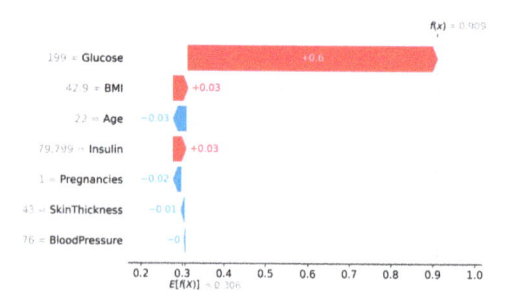

Figure 22. Summary of kNN Classification

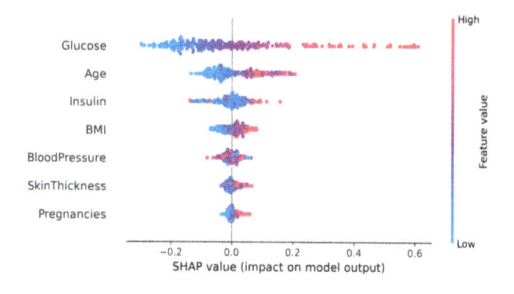

8 CONCLUSION AND FUTURE WORK

In this chapter, we presented a IoMT based system to classify diabetes mellitus by integrating with generative AI. Two models VAE and GANs are used to generate a balanced dataset and develop efficient trained machine learning models. By using ensemble approach an accuracy of 81% is obtained. Future work could explore increasing the accuracy by training larger samples and extend the application of this approach to other diseases. We are planning to create specialized training for different geographical areas in the future.

REFERENCES

Al-Turjman, F., Nawaz, M. H., & Ulusar, U. D. (2020). Intelligence in the Internet of Medical Things era: A systematic review of current and future trends. *Computer Communications*, 150, 644–660.

Alshammari, T. S. (2024). Applying machine learning algorithms for the classification of sleep disorders. *IEEE Access : Practical Innovations, Open Solutions*, 12, 36110–36121. DOI: 10.1109/ACCESS.2024.3374408

Alwahedi, F., Aldhaheri, A., Ferrag, M. A., Battah, A., & Tihanyi, N. (2024). Machine learning techniques for IoT security: Current research and future vision with generative AI and large language models. *Internet of Things and Cyber-Physical Systems*, 4, 167–185. DOI: 10.1016/j.iotcps.2023.12.003

Ashfaq, Z., Rafay, A., Mumtaz, R., Hassan Zaidi, S. M., Saleem, H., Raza Zaidi, S. A., Mumtaz, S., & Haque, A. (2022). A review of enabling technologies for the Internet of Medical Things (IoMT) ecosystem. *Ain Shams Engineering Journal*, 13(4), 101660. DOI: 10.1016/j.asej.2021.101660

Chatrati, S. P., Hossain, G., Goyal, A., Bhan, A., Bhattacharya, S., Gaurav, D., & Tiwari, S. M. (2022). Smart home health monitoring system for predicting type 2 diabetes and hypertension. *Journal of King Saud University. Computer and Information Sciences*, 34(3), 862–870. DOI: 10.1016/j.jksuci.2020.01.010

Das, P. K., A, D. V., Meher, S., Panda, R., & Abraham, A. (2022). A systematic review of recent advancements in deep and machine learning-based detection and classification of acute lymphoblastic leukemia. *IEEE Access : Practical Innovations, Open Solutions*, 10, 81741–81763. DOI: 10.1109/ACCESS.2022.3196037

Habib, M., Wang, Z., Qiu, S., Zhao, H., & Murthy, A. S. (2022). Machine learning-based healthcare system for investigating the association between depression and quality of life. *IEEE Journal of Biomedical and Health Informatics*, 26(5), 2008–2019. DOI: 10.1109/JBHI.2022.3140433 PMID: 34986108

Kakhi, K., Alizadehsani, R., Kabir, H. D., Khosravi, A., Nahavandi, S., & Acharya, U. R. (2022). The internet of medical things and artificial intelligence: Trends, challenges, and opportunities. *Biocybernetics and Biomedical Engineering*, 42(3), 749–771. DOI: 10.1016/j.bbe.2022.05.008

Khezri, S., Tanha, J., & Samadi, N. (2024). An experimental review of the ensemble-based data stream classification algorithms in non-stationary environments. *Computers & Electrical Engineering*, 118, 109420. DOI: 10.1016/j.compeleceng.2024.109420

Kiruthika, V., Shoba, S., Sendil, M., Nagarajan, K., & Punetha, D. (2024). Hybrid ensemble-deep transfer model for early cassava leaf disease classification. *Heliyon*, 10(16).

Kumar, M., Kavita, , Verma, S., Kumar, A., Ijaz, M. F., & Rawat, D. B. (2022). Anaf-it: A novel architectural framework for IoT-enabled smart healthcare system by enhancing security based on reccvc. *IEEE Transactions on Industrial Informatics*, 18(12), 8936–8943. DOI: 10.1109/TII.2022.3181614

Lazrek, G., Chetioui, K., Balboul, Y., Mazer, S., & El bekkali, M. (2024). An rfe/ridge-ml/dl based anomaly intrusion detection approach for securing iomt system. *Results in Engineering*, 23, 102659. DOI: 10.1016/j.rineng.2024.102659

Lv, Z., Qiao, L., Wang, Q., & Piccialli, F. (2021). Advanced machine-learning methods for brain-computer interfacing. *IEEE/ACM Transactions on Computational Biology and Bioinformatics*, 18(5), 1688–1698. DOI: 10.1109/TCBB.2020.3010014 PMID: 32750892

Mahadevkar, S. V., Khemani, B., Patil, S., Kotecha, K., Vora, D. R., Abraham, A., & Gabralla, L. A. (2022). A review on machine learning styles in computer vision—Techniques and future directions. *IEEE Access : Practical Innovations, Open Solutions*, 10, 107293–107329. DOI: 10.1109/ACCESS.2022.3209825

Manivannan, D. (2024). Recent endeavors in machine learning-powered intrusion detection systems for the internet of things. *Journal of Network and Computer Applications*, 229, 103925. DOI: 10.1016/j.jnca.2024.103925

Massari, H. E., Sabouri, Z., Mhammedi, S., & Gherabi, N. (2022). Diabetes prediction using machine learning algorithms and ontology. *Journal of ICT Standardization*, 10(2), 319–337. DOI: 10.13052/jicts2245-800X.10212

Mathkor, D. M., Mathkor, N., Bassfar, Z., Bantun, F., Slama, P., Ahmad, F., & Haque, S. (2024). Multirole of the internet of medical things (iomt) in biomedical systems for managing smart healthcare systems: An overview of current and future innovative trends. *Journal of Infection and Public Health*, 17(4), 559–572. DOI: 10.1016/j.jiph.2024.01.013 PMID: 38367570

Mbunge, E., Muchemwa, B., Jiyane, S., & Batani, J. (2021). Sensors and healthcare 5.0: Transformative shift in virtual care through emerging digital health technologies. [Special issue on Intelligent Medicine Leads the New Development of Human Health.]. *Global Health Journal (Amsterdam, Netherlands)*, 5(4), 169–177. DOI: 10.1016/j.glohj.2021.11.008

Messinis, S., Temenos, N., Protonotarios, N. E., Rallis, I., Kalogeras, D., & Doulamis, N. (2024). Enhancing internet of medical things security with artificial intelligence: A comprehensive review. *Computers in Biology and Medicine*, 170, 108036. DOI: 10.1016/j.compbiomed.2024.108036 PMID: 38295478

Motwani, A., Shukla, P. K., & Pawar, M. (2022). Ubiquitous and smart healthcare monitoring frameworks based on machine learning: A comprehensive review. *Artificial Intelligence in Medicine*, 134, 102431. DOI: 10.1016/j.artmed.2022.102431 PMID: 36462891

Neto, E. C. P., Dadkhah, S., Sadeghi, S., Molyneaux, H., & Ghorbani, A. A. (2024). A review of machine learning (ml)-based iot security in healthcare: A dataset perspective. *Computer Communications*, 213, 61–77. DOI: 10.1016/j.comcom.2023.11.002

Ni, W., Ao, H., Tian, H., Eldar, Y. C., & Niyato, D. (2024). Fedsl: Federated split learning for collaborative healthcare analytics on resource-constrained wearable iomt devices. *IEEE Internet of Things Journal*, 11(10), 18934–18935. DOI: 10.1109/JIOT.2024.3370985

Nti, I. K., Adekoya, A. F., Weyori, B. A., & Keyeremeh, F. (2023). A bibliometric analysis of technology in sustainable healthcare: Emerging trends and future directions. *Decision Analytics Journal*, 8, 100292. DOI: 10.1016/j.dajour.2023.100292

Osman, R. A. (2024). Internet of medical things (iomt) optimization for healthcare: A deep learning-based interference avoidance model. *Computer Networks*, 248, 110491. DOI: 10.1016/j.comnet.2024.110491

Palanivinayagam, A., & Damaševičius, R. (2023). Effective handling of missing values in datasets for classification using machine learning methods. *Information (Basel)*, 14(2), 92. DOI: 10.3390/info14020092

Patel, H., Shah, H., Patel, G., & Patel, A. (2024). Hematologic cancer diagnosis and classification using machine and deep learning: State-of-the-art techniques and emerging research directives. *Artificial Intelligence in Medicine*, 152, 102883. DOI: 10.1016/j.artmed.2024.102883 PMID: 38657439

Reza, M., Hafsha, U., Amin, R., Yasmin, R., & Ruhi, S. (2023). Improving svm performance for type ii diabetes prediction with an improved non-linear kernel: Insights from the pima dataset. *Computer Methods and Programs in Biomedicine Update*, 4, 100118. DOI: 10.1016/j.cmpbup.2023.100118

Rotbei, S., Tseng, W. H., Merino-Barbancho, B., Haleem, M. S., Montesinos, L., Pecchia, L., Fico, G., & Botta, A. (2024). Evaluating impact of movement on diabetes via artificial intelligence and smart devices systematic literature review. *Expert Systems with Applications*, 257, 125058. DOI: 10.1016/j.eswa.2024.125058

Saleem, M. A., Javeed, A., Akarathanawat, W., Chutinet, A., Suwanwela, N. C., Asdornwised, W., & Kaewplung, P. (2024). Innovations in stroke identification: A machine learning-based diagnostic model using neuroimages. *IEEE Access : Practical Innovations, Open Solutions*.

Sujith, A., Sajja, G. S., Mahalakshmi, V., Nuhmani, S., & Prasanalakshmi, B. (2022). Systematic review of smart health monitoring using deep learning and artificial intelligence. [Multimedia-based Emerging Technologies and Data Analytics for Neuroscience as a Service] [NaaS]. *Neuroscience Informatics (Online)*, 2(3), 100028. DOI: 10.1016/j.neuri.2021.100028

Upreti, D., Yang, E., Kim, H., & Seo, C. (2024). A comprehensive survey on federated learning in the healthcare area: Concept and applications. CMES -. *Computer Modeling in Engineering & Sciences*, 140(3), 2239–2274. DOI: 10.32604/cmes.2024.048932

Vaccari, I., Carlevaro, A., Narteni, S., Cambiaso, E., & Mongelli, M. (2022). explainable and reliable against adversarial machine learning in data analytics. *IEEE Access : Practical Innovations, Open Solutions*, 10, 83949–83970. DOI: 10.1109/ACCESS.2022.3197299

Wal, P., Wal, A., Verma, N., Karunakakaran, R., & Kapoor, A. (2022). Internet of medical things – the future of healthcare. *The Open Public Health Journal*, 15(1), 15. DOI: 10.2174/18749445-v15-e221215-2022-142

Yang, G., Wu, D., Mao, J., & Du, Y. (2024). Comprehensive resilience assessment of bridge networks using ensemble learning method. *Advances in Engineering Software*, 198, 103774. DOI: 10.1016/j.advengsoft.2024.103774

Ziwei, H., Dongni, Z., Man, Z., Yixin, D., Shuanghui, Z., Chao, Y., & Chunfeng, C. (2024). The applications of internet of things in smart healthcare sectors: A bibliometric and deep study. *Heliyon*, 10(3), e25392. DOI: 10.1016/j.heliyon.2024.e25392 PMID: 38356528

Chapter 13
Prediction of Thyroid Disease Using Machine Learning Models

N. Krishnamoorthy
Vellore Institute of Technology, India

V. Vinoth Kumar
Vellore Institute of Technology, India

Bryan Samuel James
Vellore Institute of Technology, India

ABSTRACT

In recent decades, thyroid dysfunction has become a widespread illness that affects millions of individuals worldwide, mostly women between the ages of 17 to 54. TSH (Thyroid-Stimulating Hormone) that are too high or too low may be a sign of a thyroid problem. The extreme stage of thyroid results in heart problem, depression, etc. Here implements the proactive system to predict the thyroid at its earliest stage is done. This will reduce the death rate and other side effects due to thyroid problems. The techniques used in this work include logistic regression, KNN (k-nearest neighbors) and Decision trees, and these was selected for its different method. These algorithms are the best and most suitable to deal with the prediction of thyroid disease at the earliest stage with less complexity and more accuracy in the implementation. Based on the results obtained, the logistic regression is better and, hence used for the problem in the thyroid disease.

I. INTRODUCTION

Thyroid gland is a gland which present near the front of the neck that wraps around the trachea. It is shaped like a butterfly with a smaller center and has two broad wings that wrap over the side of your throat. The body is made up of glands, which generate and release substances that allow various bodily

DOI: 10.4018/979-8-3693-6180-1.ch013

Copyright ©2025, IGI Global. Copying or distributing in print or electronic forms without written permission of IGI Global is prohibited.

functions to take place. The thyroid gland generates hormones that contribute in the regulation of several critical body processes.

FTI is the free thyroxine hormone which helps in the determination of the thyroid disease. Two hormones are available in the thyroid i.e., total serum thyroxin (T4) and total serum triiodothyronine (T3) which control the metabolism of the body and increase or decrease in the hormone levels lead to the thyroid disease. These hormones help in the functioning of cells, tissue, and organ in good way, helps in energy yield.

Men, women, children, teenagers, and even the elderly can get thyroid illness. When the people get older (especially after menopause in women), it can occur. It can also be present at birth. An estimated 25 million Americans are thought to have a thyroid issue, making it one of the most widespread diseases. A thyroid issue is around five to eight times more likely to be diagnosed in women than in men.

Treating it seriously and coming up with a proactive method are therefore imperative if we want to prevent this. To predict the thyroid in its earliest stage, we have deployed the proactive algorithm in this instance. This will lessen thyroid-related deaths and other negative effects. The methods employed in this study include decision trees, logistic regression, and KNN, each of which was chosen for its own advantages. With less complexity and greater accuracy in the early stages of thyroid illness prediction, these algorithms are the best and most practical.

1.1 Machine Learning (ML)

In current days the data plays the major role in every field like medicine, technology, science, math's etc. With the help of the existing data the new things can be developed further. If the large amount of data is provided, the analysis of the data is easy. Machine learning is one of the technologies in IT industry to make the research and it can be done in many fields in the above mentioned. The large amount of data provides the researcher to make the more accurate prediction. In this machine learning plays a vital role. Machine learning contains many types like supervised, unsupervised, reinforcement learning, and it is one of the branches in artificial intelligence and it done with the statistical data. In this paper various algorithm are firstly described and then some algorithm addressed our work and methodology are also described.

II. LITERATURE SURVEY

Pavya, K & Srinivasan B (2017) Improved feature extraction and used the Support Vector Machine algorithm to offer a new way for identifying thyroid illness. The authors wanted to improve the accuracy of thyroid illness diagnosis and reduce misdiagnosis rates. Jha, R., et.al (2022) Thyroid illness prediction model based on an improved K-Nearest Neighbor (KNN) algorithm was suggested. The study was conducted using clinical data of patients with thyroid disease. Prochazka, A., et.al (2019) Proposed a novel method for diagnosing thyroid nodules based on an improved support vector machine and Gray level co-occurrence matrix algorithm. Authors aimed to improve the accuracy of thyroid nodule diagnosis.

Zhang, X. et.al (2022) the study was conducted using ultrasound images of thyroid nodules for the early detection of thyroid diseases.

Xu, J et.al (2023) proposed an intelligent diagnosis model for thyroid nodules based on support vector machine and convolutional neural network algorithms. They have evaluated 17 epidemiological results using Deep Learning algorithms. Chen, W et.al (2021) author's first used algorithm is convolutional neural network to collect the data from different scales of the images. Proposed an improved model for thyroid nodule diagnosis based on Transfer Learning. Lee, E et.al (2019) proposed a new intelligent diagnostic model for thyroid nodules based on algorithm like convolutional neural network and random forest. Authors first used a CNN to extract features from the images, and then used an RF (Random Forest) algorithm to classify the nodules into benign or malignant categories. Xu, L et.al (2020) introduced am step by step systematic approach with computer aided diagnosis of thyroid symptoms prediction. Lee, K. S., & Park, H. (2022) conducted a review by comparing traditional classification methods with other, proposed a new thyroid nodule classification model based on the summarization on the limitation identified.

Xie, J et.al (2020) the authors wanted to increase thyroid nodule diagnosis accuracy and reduce misdiagnosis. The ultrasound scans of thyroid nodules were used in the investigation with the hybrid Deep Leaning Models. Iqbal, N et.al (2021) Deep learning and the gray-level co-occurrence matrix (GLCM) were used to develop a new approach for diagnosing thyroid nodules Liu, Z. et.al (2021) suggested a hybrid deep learning-based strategy for thyroid illness classification. The scientists wanted to create an accurate and dependable diagnostic tool for thyroid illness utilizing ultrasound pictures of the thyroid gland. Krishnamoorthy, N et.al (2021) author identified the disease prediction using rice plant leaves. Ongole, D., & Saravanan, S. (2023) Color based segmented images with FCM and K-means clustering identified the symptoms of thyroid diseases. Natarajan, K et.al (2024) authors used an efficient disease prediction using an ensemble firefly algorithm. Krishnamoorthy, N et.al (2024) proposed Myers-Briggs Type Indicator Using Machine Learning to predict the personality of a person. Krishnamoorthy, N et.al (2024) suggested the different models for employee Attrition Prediction with ML. Ranjith, C et.al (2023) introduced feature-based analysis with segmented medical images. Habchi et.al (2024) proposed method coupled features retrieved from a pre-trained convolutional neural network (CNN) with a texture-based feature extraction method with medical images. Natarajan, K et.al (2024) has adopted ensemble methods with firefly optimization to predict heart diseases. Ezhilarasi, K et.al (2023) used BERT techniques for crop information retrieval. Wang, R et.al (2022) had introduced a pulmonary nodule diagnosis.

III. PROBLEM DESCRIPTION

Thyroid disease has been increased in recent years across the world, and it primarily affects women. Thyroid gland plays a major role in the regulating the metabolism. Thyroid gland irregularities can result in a variety of disorders. Due to this various malfunction in human body occurs which lead to experiencing anxiety, irritability and nervousness, trouble sleeping, losing weight, heart disease, depression etc. The existing system is taken with less field attributes and with dataset range was also less. The accuracy was less, which leads to the wrong predictions.

IV. PROPOSED WORK

In this system, machine learning models predict and analyze thyroid-related issues. There are a number of classifiers involving K-Nearest Neighbors (KNN), Decision Trees (DT), and Logistic Regression (LR) used for the dataset in predicting thyroid disease. Firstly, the relevant libraries and dataset have been imported. Thereafter, data cleaning and exploratory analysis are performed. This involves creating a Correlation Matrix and a Heatmap that is viewed to comprehend any possible relationship between the features. From this, it will be possible to know which features are strongly correlated and how each affects the target variable of interest. The feature importance is evaluated after splitting the data into training and testing sets. Finally, the performances of these three algorithms: Logistic Regression, Decision Tree, and KNN will be compared to determine which model has yielded the highest prediction accuracy of thyroid disease.

V. DATA COLLECTION

The dataset contains nearly 7500 records with several attributes like TSH, TT4, TT3, FTI, etc. Each attribute consists of the several numerical values and the non-numerical values are also present in it. Non-numerical values like it contains true, false etc. and also non-numerical dataset contain the attribute like tumor, goiter, sick, etc. has been illustrated in the Figure 1.

Figure 1. Features considered from the dataset

	TSH	T3	TT4	T4U	FTI	Binary	Goitre	TBG	Lithium	Tumor	onthyroxine	T3_measure	FTI_measure
0	20	0.85	35	0.89	6.0	P	f	0.09	400	f	f	f	f
1	72	1.56	15	0.29	32.0	P	f	0.03	322	f	f	f	f
2	66	1.96	34	0.72	30.0	P	f	0.09	384	f	f	t	f
3	55	0.58	31	2.01	37.0	P	f	0.04	197	f	f	t	f
4	80	1.57	26	108.83	15.0	P	f	0.04	293	f	f	f	t

VI. DATA PREPROCESSING AND ANALYZING

In this the data pre-processing done with making feature and convert categorical to non-categorical is shown in Figure 2.

Figure 2. Dataset and pre-processing

```
 #   Column        Non-Null Count   Dtype
---  ------        --------------   -----
 0   TSH           7447 non-null    int64
 1   T3            7447 non-null    float64
 2   TT4           7446 non-null    float64
 3   T4U           7446 non-null    object
 4   FTI           7446 non-null    float64
 5   Binary        7447 non-null    object
 6   Goitre        7447 non-null    object
 7   TBG           7447 non-null    object
 8   Lithium       7447 non-null    object
 9   Tumor         7447 non-null    object
10   onthyroxine   7447 non-null    object
11   T3_measure    7447 non-null    object
12   FTI_measure   7447 non-null    object
13   TTH_measure   7447 non-null    object
14   TT4_measure   7447 non-null    object
15   TSH_measure   7445 non-null    object
16   TBG_measure   7447 non-null    object
17   sick          7447 non-null    object
dtypes: float64(3), int64(1), object(14)
```

VII. EVALUATION METRICS

Several parameters are used to make the comparison to obtain the results. The results are obtained based on the relation among the parameters.

Precision

Precision is used in the parametric evaluation. It consists of true positive values and false

$$\text{Precision} = \frac{TP}{TP + FP}$$

positive values which plays important role in the calculation of precision. It is the calculation of true positive values to the addition of the tp and fp.

Recall

Recall also used in the parametric evaluation. It is calculated through diving the true positive values by total addition of true positive values and false positive values.

$$\text{Recall} = \frac{TP}{TP + FN}$$

F1 Score

F1 score is also used in the parameter evaluation. It consists of P which represent the precision and

$$\frac{2(P * R)}{P + R}$$

R represents the recall. F1 score is the calculation of precision and recall multiplication by two and divided by addition of precision and recall values.

More accuracy gives the more correct prediction, and the accuracy can be calculated through the evaluation metrics like precision, recall etc. In this the precision and recall values can be calculated through the false positive values, true positive values, true negative values and false negative values and the more tp values gives the more accuracy prediction. For example, thyroid disease is present, and the predicted values is thyroid which is come under the true positive category. The predicted value is negative but the actual value is true which comes under true negative like that false positive and false negative follows and correct prediction of false negative also gives more accuracy and correct prediction of false negative which predict the thyroid disease is negative. Other metrics can also use evaluate like specificity and sensitivity. These metrics also based on the positive and negative values.

Confusion matrix is represented in the table format or graph format and it consists of several attributes like true positive and negative and false positive and negative. It calculates the classification performance.

VIII. IMPLEMENTATION PLATFORM AND LANGUAGE

Python is the interpreted language, high level language etc., used to build software, conduct analysis etc. It consists of several libraries which is used for to conduct the research analysis.

Python consists of the several libraries like NumPy, matplotlib, pandas etc. NumPy which is worked with the arrays and matrices. Matplotlib is used for mapping the graph representation. It consists other several inbuilt function like Sklearn, logistic regression etc. Many algorithms are there in the machine learning which helps to make prediction and the accuracy can be determined. Machine learning consists of several data like structured and unstructured. Excel sheet format or csv file are example of structured dataset and video, text in images, image are example of unstructured data and audio can also be included. In this structured dataset is taken and it consists of several categorical and numeric values etc. Data pre-processing is the technique which is used to convert the data into usable that is raw data to usable format. Data pre-processing is the which is used in machine learning, and it consists of missing values, unrelated data etc. The pre-processing technique done encoding the categorical data, splitting the data into training and testing, feature scaling etc. Data cleaning is also done, and several inbuilt functions are also used for the data pre-processing like label-encoder, one-hot-encoder etc. and before pre-processing several steps are done like collecting the dataset related to the project. Some problems may arise in pre-processing due to insufficient data collection. The missing values can be filled with various techniques like by taking mean values, imputation methods etc. In this the comparison analysis of the different evaluation metrics like precision, recall, f1-score are shown below and in this precision which is calculation of ratio of true positive and false positive in which KNN precision is higher and the F1-score for the logistic regression is high. The F1-score, recall values for the decision tree is lower than the other algorithm. The comparison between the different evaluations is shown below in the bar graph. In this the decision tree algorithm evaluation metrics lower for the precision, recall, f1-score. Correlation is the method which interrelate the different attribute in the data for example the hormones values like tt4 tt3, fti, are taken for the correlation etc. The variation may happen in this for example if one attribute increased and other attribute is decreased, or both may decrease or increase. It consists of the mathematical problems. The correlation is observed for different attributes. So that the understanding between the attributes is determined.

Figure 3. Correlation between attributes

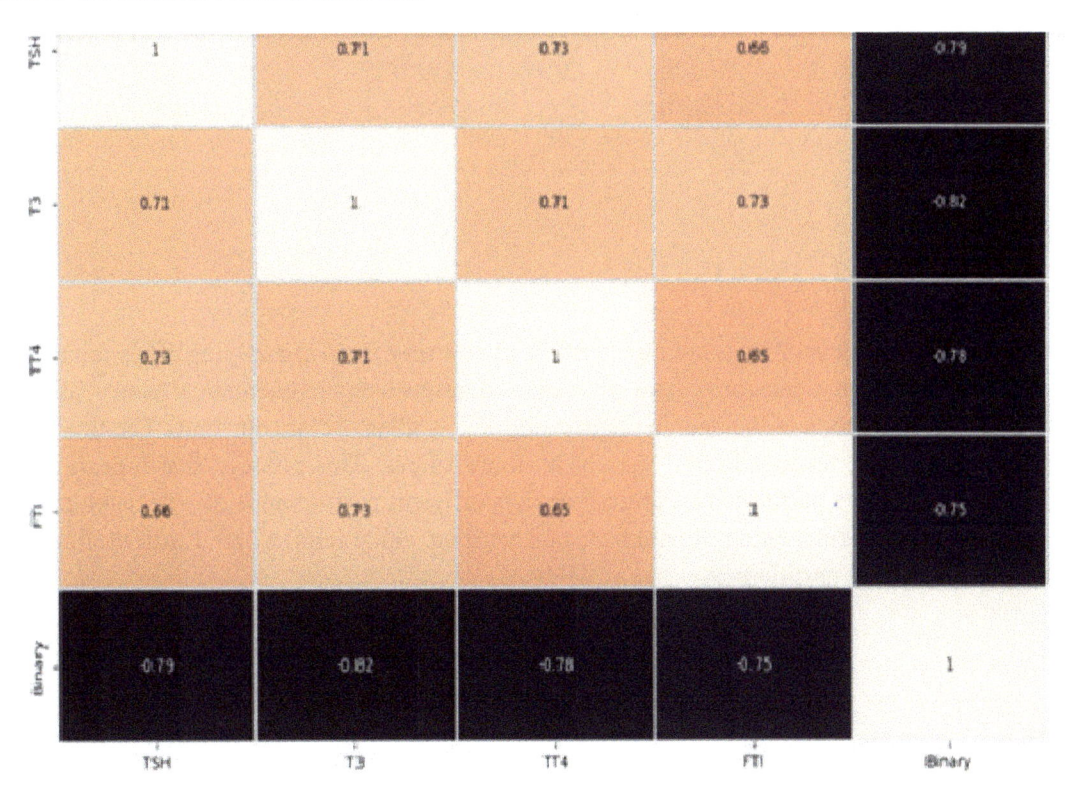

IX. CLASSIFICATION TECHNIQUES

• **Logistic Regression** - In machine learning algorithms logistic algorithm consists of different aspect. It is supervised learning algorithm and used to forecast. It is used for prediction of the categorical value using the independent categorical values. Logistic regression output is categorical values and values can be numeric or categorical and the values is 0 or 1 and yes or no and true or false. It depends on the data provided. It may give the statistical or probabilistic values in between 0 and 1. The sigmoid function is used in this algorithm. The logistic regression and linear regression are mostly similar, but it is different how it is used. Logistic regression is mostly for classification problems and linear regression is mostly for the regression problem and the same technique is given in the Figure 4.

Figure 4. Logistic regression technique

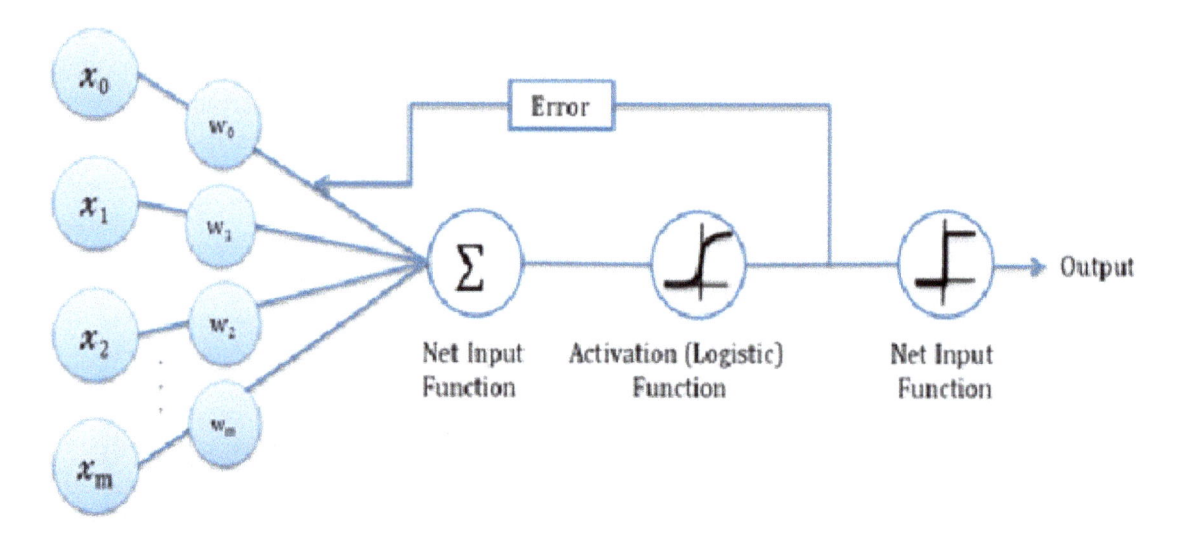

• **Decision Tree** – Decision trees are highly efficient and very rapid in applying. They are a method of data mining that classify, categorize, and generalizes datasets using mathematical as well as computational methods. Each node of the data in the decision tree is given a class attribute. The tree "learns" by subdividing the data set based upon tests of attribute values. This process, that repeats for each subset, is called recursive partitioning. Figure 5 depicts efficient performance of a decision tree. Tree construction involves segmentation of data based on attribute value tests, where further refinement at each level uses recursive partitioning.

Figure 5. Decision tree technique

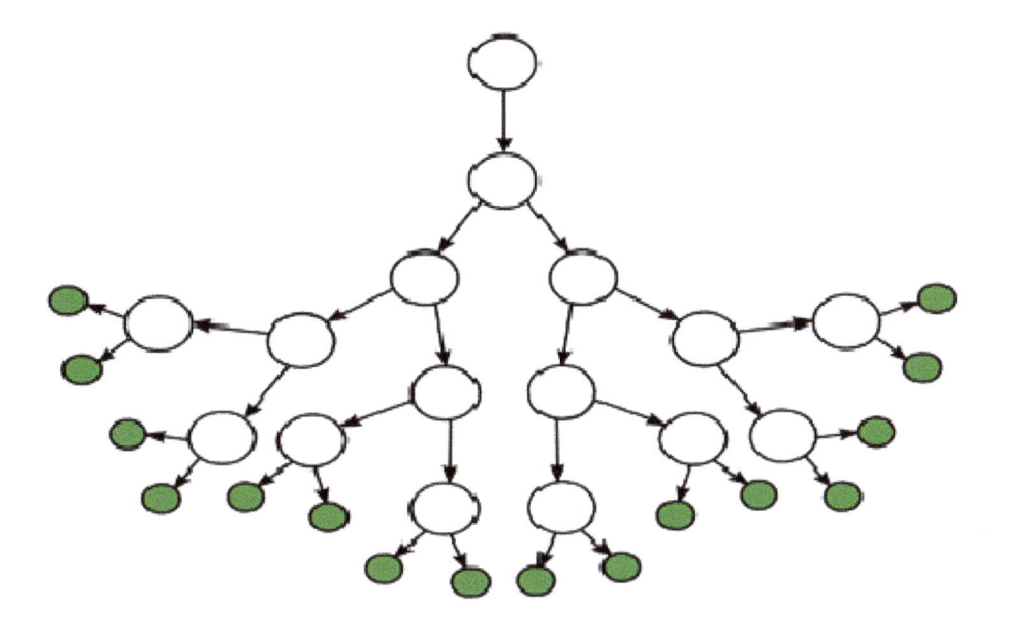

• **K-Nearest Neighbor (KNN)** — KNN is a supervised ML algorithm mainly used for classification as well as regression tasks. Works by matching new data points with that of the existing one and based on its similarity to the known cases, it assigning them into a category. This algorithm generally identifies nearest neighbors by using the distance metric (Euclidean distance formula) to calculate proximity. The Euclidean distance formula used in KNN algorithm is given below:

$$dis = \sqrt{\sum_{i=0}^{n}(x_{1i} - x_{2i})^2 + (y_{1i} - y_{2i})^2 + \cdots} \quad (1)$$

Where *dis* represents Euclidean Distance, *xi* denotes the value of the x-variable in the sample data, *yi* indicates the corresponding value of the y-variable in the sample, and *n* refers to the total number of data points.

For every instance in the X_test dataset, KNN algorithm finds out the k nearest neighbors present in TR dataset. The algorithm that calculates the distances between samples in TR and X_test, as shown in Figure 6 is performed by KNN and uses either the Manhattan distance or more commonly used Euclidean distance. The k value is vital to this method as its choice determines the performance of the method and how well it can handle noise.

Figure 6. K- nearest neighbor technique

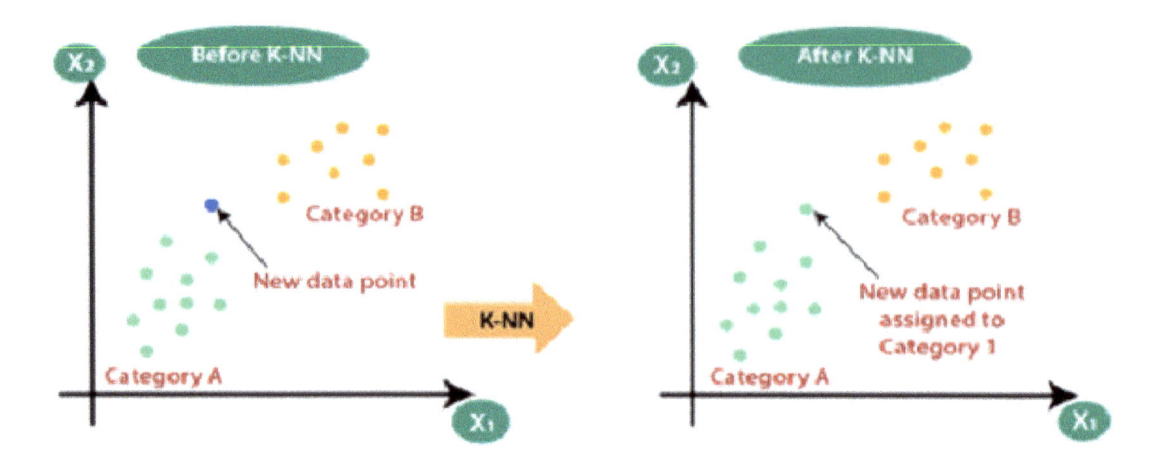

X. DETAILED DESIGN

The design process begins with data collection and preprocessing, followed by data exploration, feature extraction, and the application of the four classification techniques, such as Decision Tree, KNN, and Logistic Regression. The complete workflow is illustrated in Figure 7.

Figure 7. Process flow

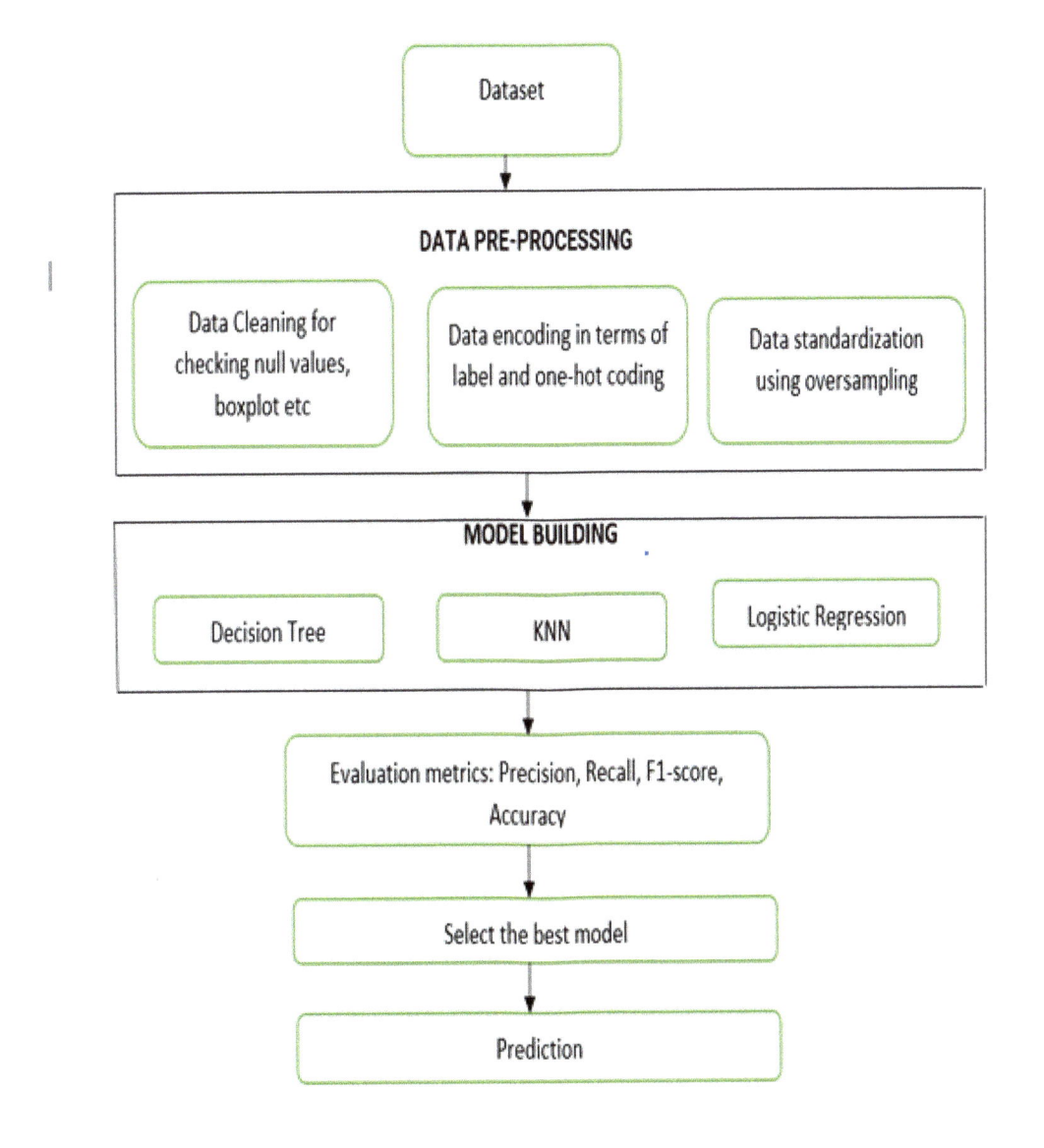

XI. RESULT AND DISCUSSION

This study demonstrates the prediction of thyroid disease by utilizing several classification algorithms, such as the Decision Tree Classifier (DT), Logistic Regression Classifier, and K- Neighbors (KNN).

In KNN algorithm which gives accuracy of 92% and the other decision tree with 88% and logistic regression with 93%. The early prediction of thyroid disease can be done with the provided input. The input values consist of the TSH, tt4, t3, t4, fti values etc. The result will give whether the patient has thyroid disease or not based on the input. The confusion matrix, AUC curve is provided.

Figure 8. Accuracy comparison

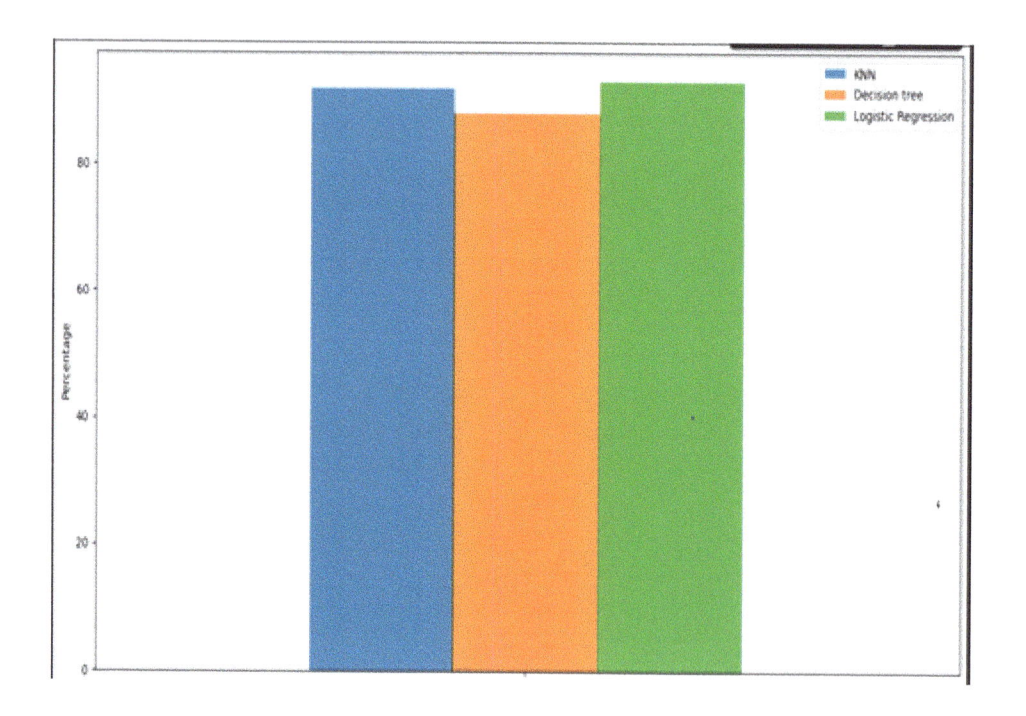

Figure 9. TD Confusion matrix for KNN

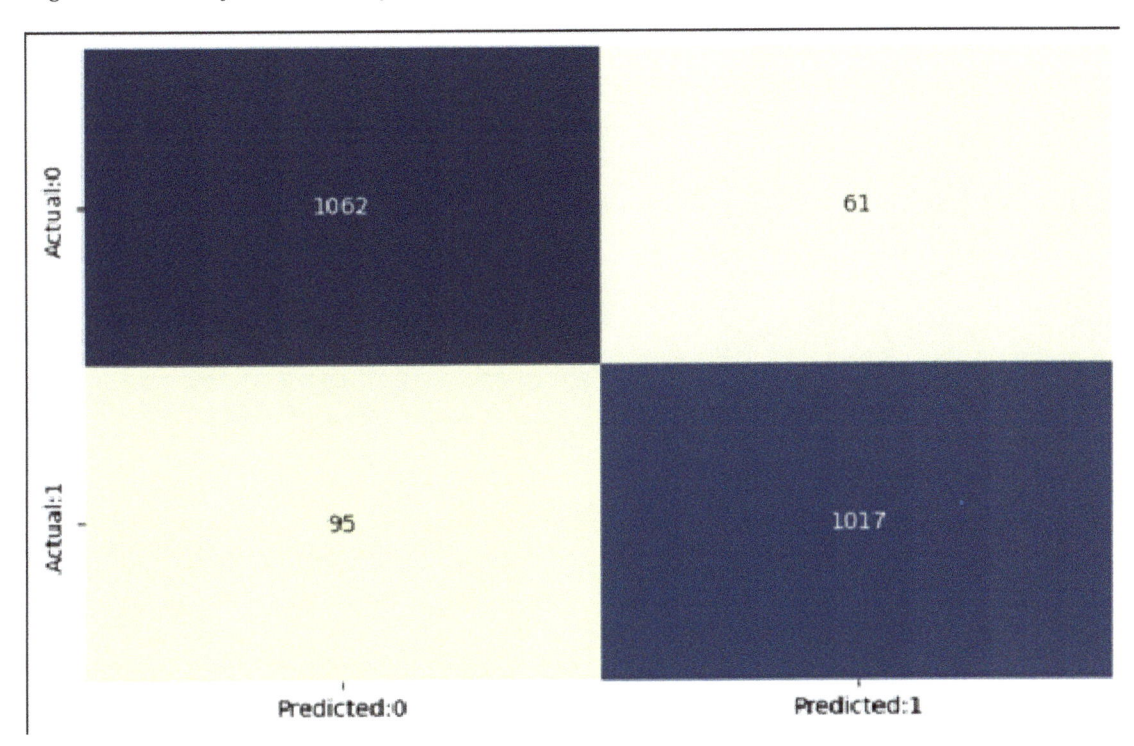

	Predicted:0	Predicted:1
Actual:0	1062	61
Actual:1	95	1017

In the above the confusion matrix for the KNN algorithm which contain the truer positive values and after that true negative values are there and false positive values is lesser than the false negative in this matrix.

Figure 10. Confusion matrix for logistic regression in TD

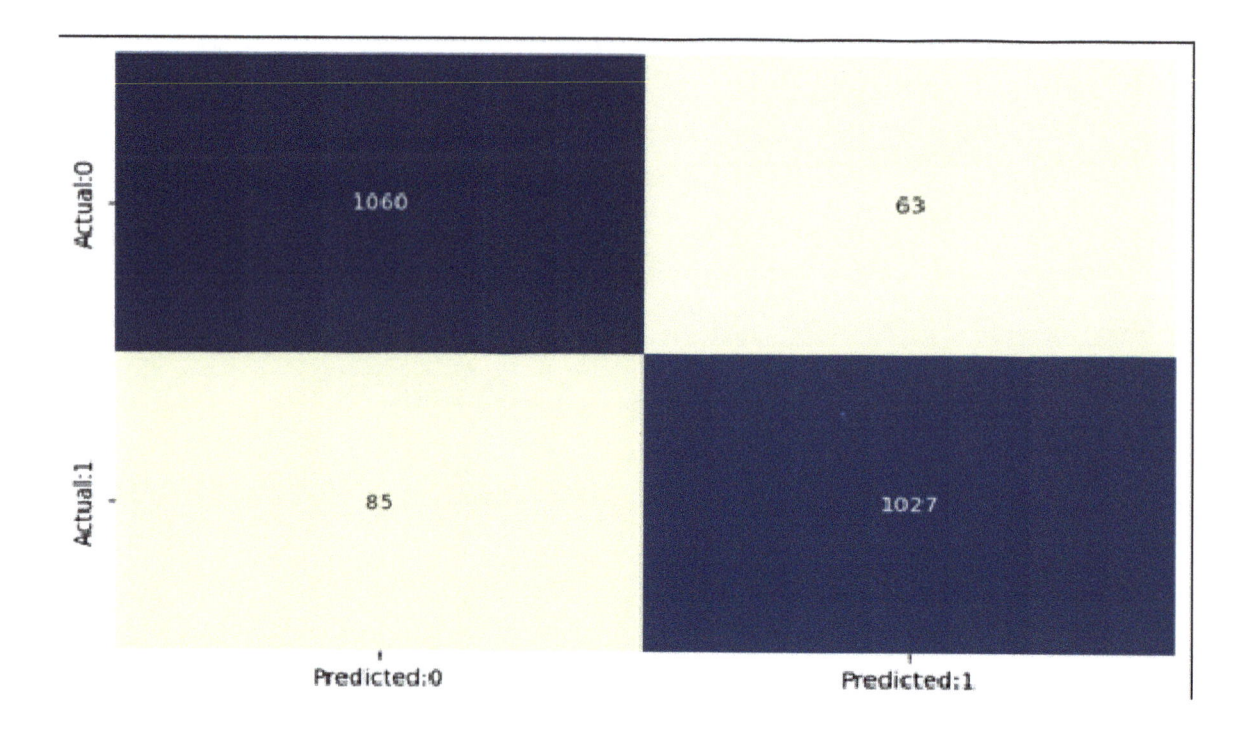

	Predicted:0	Predicted:1
Actual:0	1060	63
Actual:1	85	1027

The confusion matrix for logistic regression is displayed in the above Figure 10, and it has the same ratio of false positive values and false negative values, and true positive values are larger in KNN, and the true negative ratio is lower in logistic regression than in decision tree.

Figure 11. Precision-recall for logistic regression

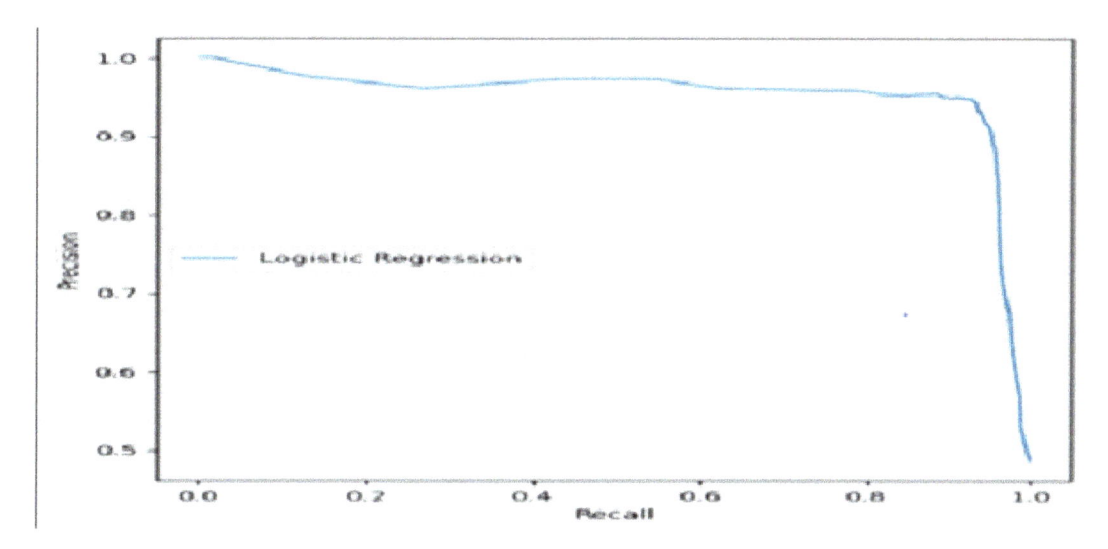

The graph for the precision and recall comparison graph is presented in the above picture, as is the graph for the logistic regression. In it, precision is used to calculate evaluation metrics.

Figure 12. Precision-recall for KNN in TD

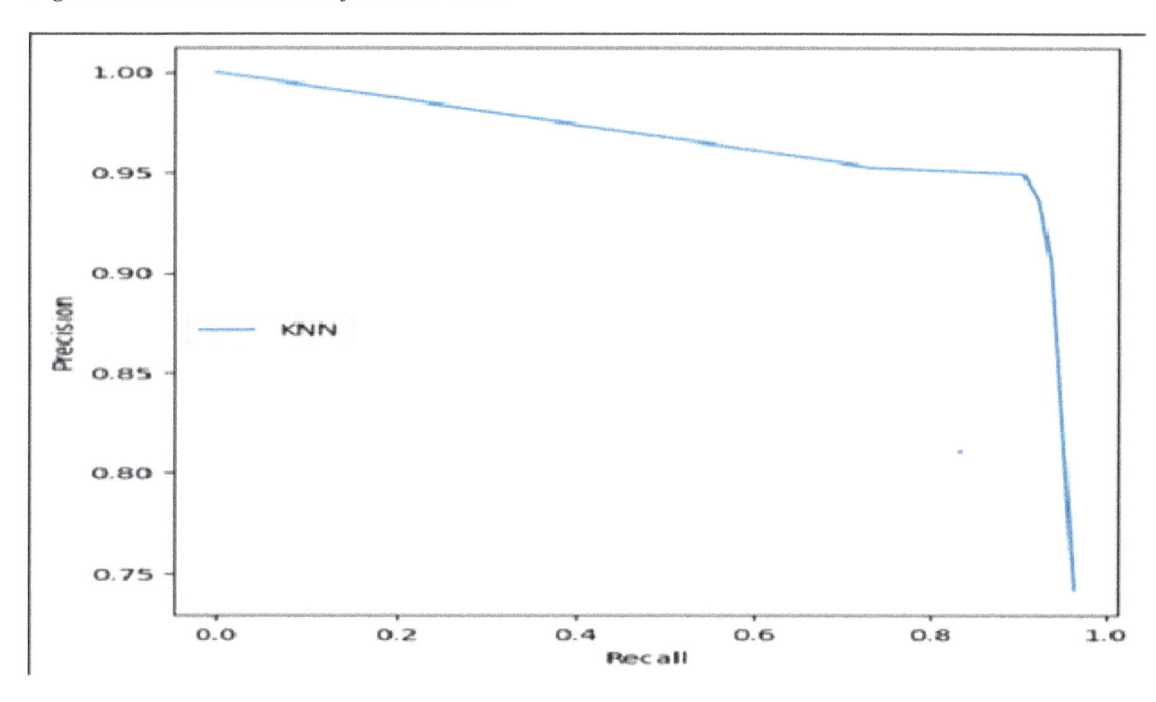

In the above Figure 12 the graph for the precision and recall comparison graph is drawn and the graph is shown for the KNN.

XII. CONCLUSION AND FUTURE WORK

The machine learning algorithms is adopted for thyroid prediction in people. So that the doctors can be able to give treatment at the early stage itself and further development of the thyroid disease is prevented, and the patient can easily cure from this disease easily with the initial treatment and with the medicines and the complication of the thyroid treatment is avoided. The thyroid treatment may lead to various side effects in the human body and the thyroid patient may affect from the various malfunction in the human organs. This can be avoided by the early prediction of the disease in thyroid. The different machine learning algorithms in the future can also be implemented to improve the accuracy and the large number of the datasets can be taken with more attributes related to the thyroid disease. The web-based application can also be implemented for the thyroid prediction. The deep learning algorithms can also be implemented to improve the accuracy.

REFERENCES

Chen, W., Gu, Z., Liu, Z., Fu, Y., Ye, Z., Zhang, X., & Xiao, L. (2021). A new classification method in ultrasound images of benign and malignant thyroid nodules based on transfer learning and deep convolutional neural network. *Complexity*, 2021(1), 6296811. DOI: 10.1155/2021/6296811

Ezhilarasi, K., Hussain, D. M., Sowmiya, M., & Krishnamoorthy, N. (2023). Crop information retrieval framework based on LDW-ontology and SNM-BERT techniques. *Information Technology and Control*, 52(3), 731–743. DOI: 10.5755/j01.itc.52.3.31945

Habchi, Y., ... "Machine learning and vision transformers for thyroid carcinoma diagnosis: A review." arXiv preprint arXiv:2403.13843 (2024).

Iqbal, N., Mumtaz, R., Shafi, U., & Zaidi, S. M. H. (2021). Gray level co-occurrence matrix (GLCM) texture based crop classification using low altitude remote sensing platforms. *PeerJ. Computer Science*, 7, e536.

Jha, R., Bhattacharjee, V., & Mustafi, A. (2022). Increasing the prediction accuracy for thyroid disease: A step towards better health for society. *Wireless Personal Communications*, 122(2), 1921–1938. DOI: 10.1007/s11277-021-08974-3

Krishnamoorthy, N., Kumar, V. V., Nair, C., Maheswari, A., Mishra, S., & Sinha, A. (2024). HR Analytics and Employee Attrition Prediction Using Machine Learning. In Emerging Advancements in AI and Big Data Technologies in Business and Society (pp. 79-96). IGI Global. DOI: 10.4018/979-8-3693-0683-3.ch004

Krishnamoorthy, N., Prasad, L. N., Kumar, C. P., Subedi, B., Abraha, H. B., & Sathishkumar, V. E. (2021). Rice leaf diseases prediction using deep neural networks with transfer learning. *Environmental Research*, 198, 111275. DOI: 10.1016/j.envres.2021.111275 PMID: 33989629

Krishnamoorthy, N., Venkatesan, V. K., Swapna, B., Rawal, D., Dutta, D., & Sushil, S. (2024). Personality Prediction Based on Myers-Briggs Type Indicator Using Machine Learning. In Emerging Advancements in AI and Big Data Technologies in Business and Society (pp. 353-368). IGI Global.

Lee, E., Ha, H., Kim, H. J., Moon, H. J., Byon, J. H., Huh, S., Son, J., Yoon, J., Han, K., & Kwak, J. Y. (2019). Differentiation of thyroid nodules on US using features learned and extracted from various convolutional neural networks. *Scientific Reports*, 9(1), 19854. DOI: 10.1038/s41598-019-56395-x PMID: 31882683

Lee, K. S., & Park, H. (2022). Machine learning on thyroid disease: A review. *Frontiers in Bioscience (Landmark Edition)*, 27(3), 101. DOI: 10.31083/j.fbl2703101 PMID: 35345333

Liu, Z., Zhong, S., Liu, Q., Xie, C., Dai, Y., Peng, C., Chen, X., & Zou, R. (2021). Thyroid nodule recognition using a joint convolutional neural network with information fusion of ultrasound images and radiofrequency data. *European Radiology*, 31(7), 5001–5011. DOI: 10.1007/s00330-020-07585-z PMID: 33409774

Natarajan, K., Vinoth Kumar, V., Mahesh, T. R., Abbas, M., Kathamuthu, N., Mohan, E., & Annand, J. R. (2024). Efficient Heart Disease Classification Through Stacked Ensemble with Optimized Firefly Feature Selection. *International Journal of Computational Intelligence Systems*, 17(1), 1–14. DOI: 10.1007/s44196-024-00538-0

Ongole, D., & Saravanan, S. (2023). Colour-based segmentation using FCM and K-means clustering for 3D thyroid gland state image classification using deep convolutional neural network structure. *International Journal of Imaging Systems and Technology*, 33(5), 1814–1826. DOI: 10.1002/ima.22900

Pavya, K., & Srinivasan, B. (2017). Feature selection algorithms to improve thyroid disease diagnosis. In 2017 International conference on innovations in green energy and healthcare technologies (IGEHT) (pp. 1-5). IEEE. DOI: 10.1109/IGEHT.2017.8094070

Prochazka, A., Gulati, S., Holinka, S., & Smutek, D. (2019). Patch-based classification of thyroid nodules in ultrasound images using direction independent features extracted by two-threshold binary decomposition. *Computerized Medical Imaging and Graphics*, 71, 9–18. DOI: 10.1016/j.compmedimag.2018.10.001 PMID: 30453231

Ranjith, C. P., Natarajan, K., Madhuri, S., Ramakrishna, M. T., Bhat, C. R., & Venkatesan, V. K. (2023). Image Processing Using Feature-Based Segmentation Techniques for the Analysis of Medical Images. *Engineering Proceedings*, 59(1), 100.

Wang, R., Zhang, Y., & Yang, J. (2022, October). TransPND: A Transformer Based Pulmonary Nodule Diagnosis Method on CT Image. In Chinese Conference on Pattern Recognition and Computer Vision (PRCV) (pp. 348-360). Cham: Springer Nature Switzerland DOI: 10.1007/978-3-031-18910-4_29

Xie, J., Guo, L., Zhao, C., Li, X., Luo, Y., & Jianwei, L. (2020, December). A hybrid deep learning and handcrafted features based approach for thyroid nodule classification in ultrasound images. [). IOP Publishing.]. *Journal of Physics: Conference Series*, 1693(1), 012160.

Xu, J., Xu, H. L., Cao, Y. N., Huang, Y., Gao, S., Wu, Q. J., & Gong, T. T. (2023). The performance of deep learning on thyroid nodule imaging predicts thyroid cancer: A systematic review and meta-analysis of epidemiological studies with independent external test sets. *Diabetes & Metabolic Syndrome*, 17(11), 102891. DOI: 10.1016/j.dsx.2023.102891 PMID: 37907027

Xu, L., Gao, J., Wang, Q., Yin, J., Yu, P., Bai, B., Pei, R., Chen, D., Yang, G., Wang, S., & Wan, M. (2020). Computer-aided diagnosis systems in diagnosing malignant thyroid nodules on ultrasonography: A systematic review and meta-analysis. *European Thyroid Journal*, 9(4), 186–193. DOI: 10.1159/000504390 PMID: 32903956

Zhang, X., Lee, V. C., Rong, J., Liu, F., & Kong, H. (2022). Multi-channel convolutional neural network architectures for thyroid cancer detection. *PLoS One*, 17(1), e0262128. DOI: 10.1371/journal.pone.0262128 PMID: 35061759

Chapter 14
The Evolution of Artificial Intelligence in Healthcare:
Transforming Personalized Medicine and Biosensor Engineering

Seneha Santoshi
https://orcid.org/0000-0001-8893-2221
Amity University, Noida, India

Hina Bansal
https://orcid.org/0000-0003-1683-1581
Amity University, Noida, India

Banashree Bondhopadhyay
https://orcid.org/0000-0002-6679-7791
Amity University, Noida, India

Palak Maurya
https://orcid.org/0009-0001-0008-6823
Amity University, Noida, India

ABSTRACT

Artificial Intelligence (AI) has become an unprecedented force in healthcare with significant impact on personalized medicine and Biosensor Engineering. This chapter discusses the evolution of AI in healthcare from the early Expert Systems to the advanced Machine Learning (ML) algorithm in practice. Integration of AI in personalized medicine has revolutionized Genomic Analysis, Predictive Analytics, and Drug Discovery and Manufacture with customized treatment. The advancement of AI and AI empowered Biosensor Engineering Technologies has brought future of real time health management and diagnosis by the development of wearable and implantable devices with advanced technologies like ML. The research reveals that AI improves diagnostic accuracy, shortens the time to treatment, and streamlines the drug development process. Additionally, progress in AI-driven biosensor engineering has led to innovations in real-time health monitoring and diagnostics, particularly through the creation of wearable and implantable devices that leverage machine learning technologies.

DOI: 10.4018/979-8-3693-6180-1.ch014

INTRODUCTION

With each and every passing day, Artificial Intelligence (AI) is being seen as a groundbreaking technology which has shown its competencies in almost every sector; healthcare industry being no exception. The prospect of AI in revolutionizing healthcare industry is absolutely enormous and widespread, which consists of enhancing diagnostic precision, treatment plans based on the patient, poop's drug discovery and improving biosensor technology. AI aids healthcare contributors to take prudent actions and make a much better decision by analyzing and examining large datasets and altering the constructing practices of healthcare in turn, directly favoring the patient's results (Obermeyer & Emmanuel, 2016). The inception of AI in healthcare can be first seen during the time when expert systems were being built in the era of 1970's and 1980's. The expert systems were developed to replicate human expertise or decision-making process, one of them being IBM's MYCIN which was essentially created as a tool for diagnosing bacterial infections, and then helping the doctor choose the right antibiotic treatment (Shortliffe & Buchanan, 1975). These experiments and tests were very limited, they were heavily reliant on knowledge which was manually put in and rule-based algorithm which was determined.

In healthcare, machine learning (ML) and big data analytics being introduced made a breakthrough in artificial intelligence (AI). Machine learning capacities of gaining knowledge from data and improve by self could further the analysis of the complex medical datasets to classify patterns and make predictions. (Esteva et al., 2017) wanted to prove how appropriate is deep neural networks to distinguish skin cancer from dermatologist-level accuracy by collecting and annotating 129,450 clinical images of skin diseases, including 2,032 different diseases. Indeed, it is deep convolutional neural networks that can be informed in large sets of data, which were applied in the field of skin cancer. AI used to be a tool to support authenticatronics in medical diagnosis to show itself with machine learning.

Among various AI technologies, Natural Language Processing (NLP) plays an important role in healthcare. Algorithms of NLP are able to capture valuable information in unstructured data sources, for instance, clinical notes and research articles. For example, (Beam and Kohane, 2018) mentioned the use of NLP in detecting adverse drug reactions through Electronic Health Records (EHRs) and Social media posts, offering early warnings thus increasing patient safety.

The possibilities for AI in healthcare are numerous—especially as advanced techniques like reinforcement, transfer, and federated learning are being used. Personalized treatment strategies are being developed using algorithms trained through the traditional method of trial and error, as well as this emerging kind of training. At the same time, AI models are benefiting from "knowledge transfer." They learn from earlier work in AI and from other fields, too. Finally, an approach called "federated learning" allows the training of very large models on decentralized data. This allays concerns about both privacy and security. (Kaushal, Bates, & Poon, 2003).

AI's effect on personalized medicine has been especially strong, and for good reason. The cutting-edge approach to patient care seeks to use a person's unique characteristics—genomic, environmental, and lifestyle factors, for instance—to tailor what can be an incredibly complex series of medical treatments. (Poplin et al., 2018) And the revolution that AI has brought to what's known medically underlies the very foundation of that approach, with genomic medicine being on the forefront. At the most basic level, for instance, AI is now used to improve the accuracy of finding really rare variants in the repeats of the genomic code and for the more commonplace but hard-to-find single letter variants, too.

In personalized medicine, artificial intelligence (AI) has found an application in "predictive analytics." This term refers to using various types of data to make predictions—for instance, predicting which people will develop a certain medical condition. One thing that predictive analytics does especially well is comb through "big data" to find patterns and associations between various conditions and events. Thanks to algorithms in IBM's Watson computer system, for example, many patients today can benefit from evidence-based, personalized cancer treatment plans (Ferrucci et al., 2013).

The drug discovery area has seen rapid acceleration thanks to AI. This technology has not only expedited the search for potential drug candidates but has also made predictions about their efficacy and safety. Traditional drug discovery methods are both time-consuming and expensive, but AI can help to serve as a compass in the otherwise perplexing world of biology and chemistry. Capable of identifying potential compounds, the technology of AI shows nothing if not promise in an emergent field like that of health crises such as COVID-19 (Zhavoronkov et al., 2019).

The field of biosensor engineering has greatly profited from advancements in artificial intelligence (AI) and wearable technology. (Bumgarner et al., 2018) With these new tools, we can create smarter biosensors that have the ability to continuously monitor physiological signals. This is quite important, because in truth, our hearts even manage signals. So with these powerful new wearable platforms, we have the possibility of catching diseases like atrial fibrillation much earlier than today.

Biosensors enhanced by artificial intelligence serve point-of-care diagnostics, allowing doctors to carry out rapid and precise tests in a wide range of locations, including relatively poor and inaccessible settings. . (Erdem, Morales-Narváez, and Dincer., 2020) These devices are essentially portable laboratories that make use of AI's pattern recognition powers to analyze physiological samples, instantly producing a verdict on what's going right—or wrong—inside the body. The imminent question: When AI is added to the mix in this way, does it actually improve healthcare access? That's the unanswerable question we set out to explore.

Although numerous benefits can be derived from using artificial intelligence (AI) in healthcare, there are several challenges and ethical considerations that need to be surmounted. One of the core issues is data privacy and security because the health arena is a delicate one. Patients need to trust that their data isn't going to be handled inappropriately. (Kaushal, Bates, & Poon, 2003) In previous ages, the big issue was the security of paper records (and it still is). Now, the core issue is how to maintain security in a world of almighty interconnected networks. In no uncertain terms, we need to do so because, without patient trust, this whole effort is for naught.

To integrate artificial intelligence (AI) successfully into the clinical setting, we must first overcome the resistance that healthcare professionals may have to using these technologies. This means, at its core, understanding the dynamics and power structures of clinical practice and also understanding the working mindset of clinicians. We must make the intelligence of these AI tools understandable, if not to the regulators, as promises or proofs of enhanced quality and safety, then certainly to the doctors and nurses who'd be using them. Once the resistance obstacle is partially cleared, the reliability and accuracy of AI tools must be demonstrated through validation studies. (Char, Shah, & Magnus, 2018)

1. PERSONALIZED MEDICINE

The past few years have seen medicine transformed in a way that few had anticipated—not only by recent advances in information technology (IT) but also by a new vision of what patients could expect from their healthcare. For the first time in decades, this vision has introduced to us a path toward miracle-like forecasts. Nowadays, projections for when cures for major diseases might be found are much more optimistic than what we've seen in recent history. The reason? Healthcare has turned its attention toward a new frontier: artificial intelligence (AI). The experiments and projections being carried out under the umbrella of AI in healthcare are reformers' dreams. Why? Because they're enabling unprecedented tailoring of medical interventions to patients. That's what precision or personalized medicine is all about—distinctively and individually treating patients, not as a group but as unique members of society.

The collection of data, along with the use of machine learning, enables the formation of a strong framework that enhances the accuracy of the diagnoses and treatments in the field of medicine. **Figure 1** shows they are interconnected and work together. We are taking data collection and using that for our machine learning algorithms down the line. And then we can take the predictions from those algorithms and put them to use in serving patients—enhancing their outcomes, mostly in the realm of our smart treatments, enhanced kind of healthcare provision.

Figure 1. Investigating the interrelatedness of data gathering, algorithms, and edge AI in the provisioning of healthcare

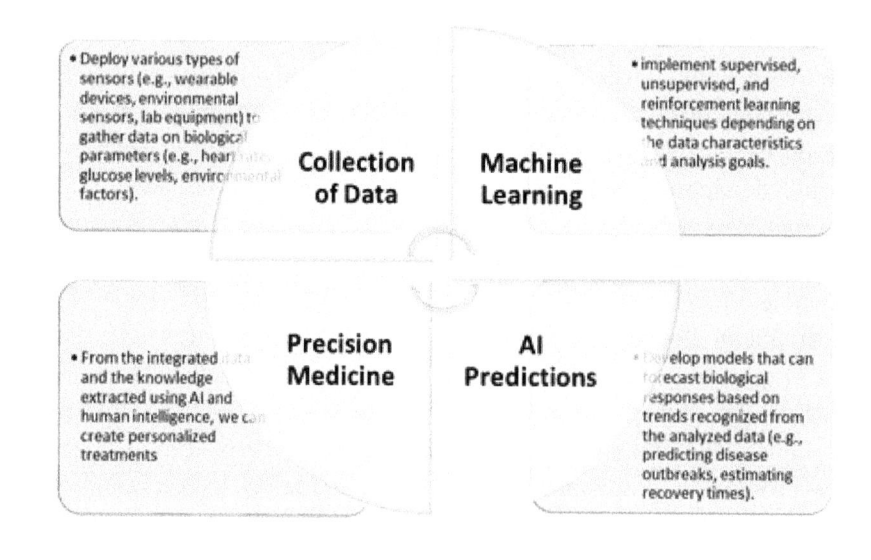

1.1 AI in Genomic Analysis

Personalized medicine has seen considerable benefits from artificial intelligence. One of the shining stars in this area is the genome. It is the unique constellation of a person's genes that can give us these critical insights. The science of genomic analysis is rapidly progressing. Researchers have moved from looking at individual genes to observing how they interact with others and their environment. This, too, is now made possible with the help of AI—an exceptional meld of humans working alongside their smart algorithms. When it comes to AI in genomics, one widely-used tool that's almost a household name is Google's DeepVariant. (Poplin et al., 2018).

The capacity to rapidly and precisely comprehend the full instructions present in genomes has a very significant effect on one of the most prized aspects of medicine—its personalization. Thanks to their proficiency in detecting the many direct and indirect variants that lead to disease, today's AI technologies can do a remarkable job in this area. They properly discern both pathogenic and nonpathogenic variations with a 1-in-20-million rate of false positives. These tools can tell you at the moment of diagnosis that you have the BRCA1 or BRCA2 mutations that are associated with a much higher rate of breast and ovarian cancers. (Collins & Varmus, 2015).

1.2 Predictive Analytics

Another area where AI has significantly advanced personalized medicine is in the field of predictive analytics. Massive amounts of patient data, including a growing pool of electronic health records (EHRs), have given AI researchers a remarkable resource to mine for new healthcare insights.

Parsing EHRs reveals a wealth of information that medical experts had never before had access to, including patterns and correlations in patient histories, medication outcomes, and disease progression, which can be crucial for developing more accurate diagnostic and treatment strategies. By running that same data through their algorithms, AI researchers can use it to create health models that can not only understand how health conditions develop but also predict, with a remarkable degree of accuracy, who will ultimately fall ill and when.

IBM Watson for Oncology is an AI-driven technology that can rifle through mountains of patient data swiftly and accurately. Watson can then recommend treatments that are right for individual patients (Ferrucci et al., 2013). IBM's AI has ingested myriad forms of knowledge—from the FINISH (Federal, Inherited, Natural, Substantial, and High) set, AACR Project GENIE, and medical literature to clinical trial information and even an encyclopedia of medical treatments. Watson then generates this coherent narrative around the pile of data and publishes it as treatment recommendations for specific cases.

The role that predictive analytics plays in managing chronic diseases cannot be overstated. Artificial intelligence algorithms can study the data gathered from wearable devices while they are continuously monitoring patients' health. These same AI algorithms can also make predictions about conditions that might possibly crop up later. One AI-driven device that has shown real promise is the continuous glucose monitor (CGM) used in diabetes management. CGMs have the ability to look ahead, make predictions, and help patients decide what to do next. All of this constitutes a significantly upgraded quality of life for patients and a dramatic reduction in the time, effort, and resources devoted to what we think of today as routine health checks (Veiseh et al., 2015).

1.3 AI in Drug Discovery

Discovering new drugs can be an exceedingly slow and expensive process, sometimes taking over ten years and billions of dollars for a single new medicine to reach the market. Yet there is great promise in artificial intelligence (AI) for revolutionizing this process, potentially cutting both the time it takes and the enormous cost associated with getting a new drug ready for humans to use. With AI and its subset machine learning (ML), for instance, drug formulators can look to much vaster amounts of data and can expect much more reliable results.

Moreover, the second AI also changes drugs for therapeutics. Using AI during the coronavirus pandemic, for example, permitted researchers to rapidly screen existing drugs without dangerous Sars-CoV-2 co-infecting them. (Zhavoronkov et al., 2019) This led to a number of potential therapeutics that have since carried forward into preclinical studies. Drug development using AI and MA has the added value not just of being faster, but also of offering a sort of sandbox within which to envision development.

2. BIOSENSOR ENGINEERING

Biosensor engineering is a multidisciplinary field that converges biology, chemistry, physics, and engineering to create devices that can detect biological signals. By combining artificial intelligence (AI) with biosensor engineering, healthcare can be revolutionized, making the small, affordable devices capable of sending health, disease, and research signals far morpotent. This revolution can rest on several key aspects.

The first is real-time analysis and interpretation of the kind of massive data that biosensors generate. AI algorithms can read this data in a fraction of the time it takes human analysts. Moreover, AI can "see" in the data; it can find patterns and correlations that are elusive to our biological detective skills. More accurate diagnostics should naturally follow from this.

The second aspect is the design and optimization of biosensors themselves. In this instance, AI can be understood to mean not just artificial intelligence but also the use of intelligent human researchers. We can use AI as a tool to help us improve sensor aspects ranging from their materials to how well they can detect certain signals under a variety of conditions. We can even use AI to help us "think" through the many possibilities for how to do all of these tasks better and more reliably.

The other major aspect of using AI in biosensor situations has to do with the physical arrangement of the two: the biosensor and the human body, or the biosensor and the environment being monitored. We can use AI to tell us how to construct wearable biosensors, e.g., devices embedded in smart clothes, to do health monitoring in a signal-detecting way and not to miss so many health-related signals. We can—along these same lines—arrange for the inhabitation of biosensors in the environment and for them to do so in a way that will allow us to get as many useful environmental-detecting signals as we can without destroying the biosensors or the places in which we have put them. **Figure 2** gives the idea of an AI-Powered Biosensor System for the Analysis and Oversight of Biological Information for biosensor deployment and maintenance.

Figure 2. Creation of an AI-powered biosensor system for the analysis and oversight of biological information

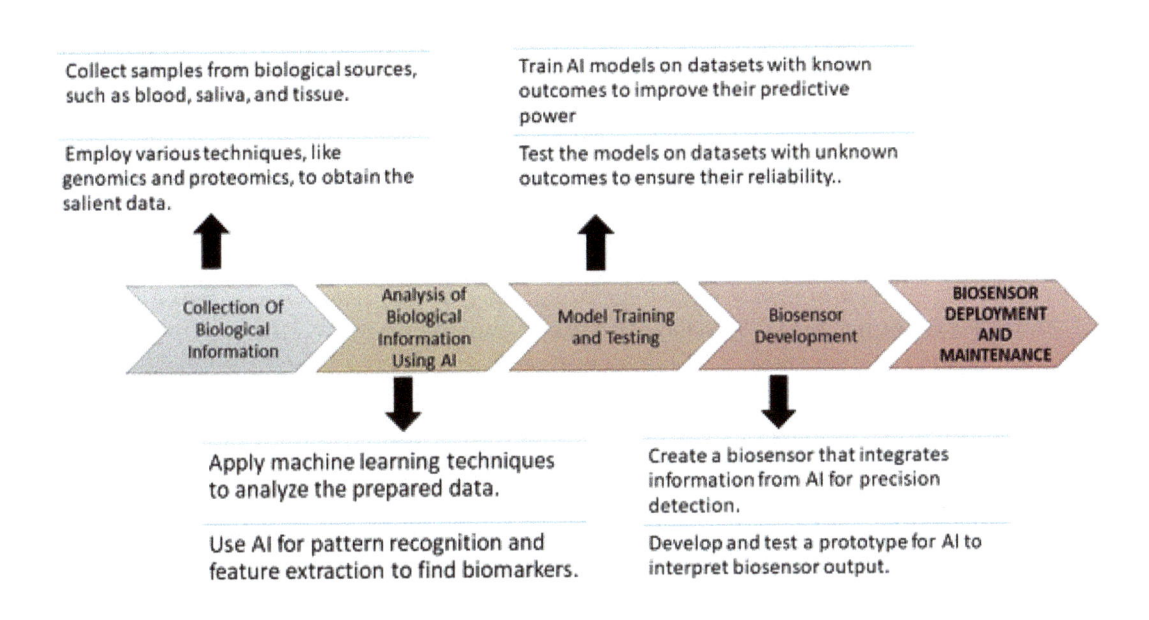

2.1 AI-Enhanced Wearable Devices

Over the past few years, wearable gadgets stuffed with biometric tools that monitor a person's health and fitness have become all the rage. These devices keep tabs on all sorts of vital signs, such as heart rate, glucose levels in the blood, and the patterns of our activities. That's a lot of very personal data, of course, and these gadgets allow individuals to collect that data over long periods of time, providing us with a wealth of information about ourselves. And the great thing about physiological data is that it is amenable to all sorts of AI-based analyses: algorithms can pick out health problems, make predictions about what might go wrong with our bodies in the future, or tell us when we've been siting around way too much and need to move.

The Apple Watch's ECG feature is an excellent illustration of this change. AI enables the watch to use sensors to, basically, see into your heart. And those AI-read signals have so far proven to be pretty accurate, as well. To this end, the Apple Watch—which some claim is the closest thing we've got to a bona fide "killer app" for wearable tech—has actually saved lives. There have been multiple instances where it has detected dangerous, even life-threatening, arrhythmias that might not have been spotted in time to avoid Afib's (Atrial fibrillation) potential for causing a stroke .(Bumgarner et al., 2018)

2.2 AI in Implantable Biosensors

Artificial intelligence advancements have also been advantageous for implantable biosensors, which are devices that are inserted into the body and monitor essential health metrics without interruption. These biosensors pick up changes in levels of liquids or gases in the body and wirelessly send them to doctors for remote analysis. Still, these changes in substances that could signal health issues have to be sorted somehow. That's where AI comes in—to crunch the data and give doctors a warning when there's something unclear.

Take continuous glucose monitors (CGMs) as an instance. They use artificial intelligence to get better at predicting how much glucose a person is going to have in their blood and what to do about it. They are carried on a person and take glucose levels quite frequently throughout the day and night—about every five minutes or so. They use lots of data to learn what pattern of glucose leads to what kind of condition in a person. They try to find the pattern that helps them to know what to do. So they don't just present what your number is right now and leave it to you and your healthcare team to figure out what to do.

2.3 Point-of-Care Diagnostics

The use of AI-enabled biosensors is becoming more widespread in point-of-care diagnostics. These devices, often small and inexpensive, carry out complex biochemical analyses; for example, they can "read" the tiny electric currents produced by molecules of interest, such as those indicating the presence of a tumorous or infectious microorganism. But to make that readout meaningful and actionable, you need AI to interpret it. These devices use machine learning to analyze the results of a test, yielding treatment-relevant information.

Paper-based plasmonic biosensors powered by AI can identify infectious diseases quickly and efficiently. AI can sift through the massive amounts of data these sensors produce and detect the presence of various biomarkers for diseases like COVID-19. The plasmonic part of the sensor is a tiny, light-responsive structure that can detect biomarkers at very low concentrations. By converting the signal, the biomarker produces to a color-luminescent or dark-path, the plasmonic structure makes the presence of the biomarker noticeable to the naked eye.

3. SIGNIFICANCE AND IMPACT

3.1 Enhancing Patient Outcomes

AI in medicine and biosensors can combine to elevate the services rendered by healthcare personnel to a level that produces improved patient outcomes. Using AI and machine learning to identify cancers missed by human sight is a prospect both exciting and a bit unnerving. On one hand, algorithms that improve the images produced by MRI, CT, and PET/MRI scanners and identify minute changes are a potential game-changer in diagnosing diseases earlier in their development. Artificial intelligence algorithms have the capability of recognizing structures in medical images that might go unnoticed or be very hard for human clinicians to discern. Consequently, the push to utilize them in early disease detection for things like cancer is on the upswing. (Smith et al., 2021)

Therapies are more effective when they're personalized, and they're truly personalized when, in addition to learning about someone's health history, you can use the person's genetic makeup to sort out the factors that may put them at risk for disease or influence how they'll respond to treatments.

Just as exciting as the idea of using genetic profiling to get a more precise handle on the state of someone's health—allowing healthcare professionals to catch potential problems while they're still in the early stages and a little easier to deal with—the idea of continuous monitoring is really coming into its own.

3.2 Healthcare Expenses

The promise of artificial intelligence (AI) technology to reduce healthcare costs lies in its ability to increase the efficiency of healthcare services and to prevent illnesses from progressing to serious and expensive-to-treat stages. Much of the present and most of the future use of AI in healthcare is and will be in the area of diagnostics. AI is currently being used to develop more efficient diagnostic tests, such as lung cancer tests, which are cheaper and more accurate than what has been available until now (White & Davis, 2020). The effectiveness of artificial intelligence lies in optimizing treatment plans. This helps guarantee that patients are receiving the most suitable treatments, which can potentially help them recover faster and at reduced costs. AI can also serve to streamline the daunting administrative processes of healthcare, which can help save time and resources for clinicians who can instead focus on patient care. Furthermore, AI holds the potential for operational cost savings, resource allocation improvements, and as the upshot, better access to superb healthcare (Jones & Peterson, 2020).

3.3 Enhancing the Reach of Healthcare

Biosensors that are boosted by AI can fulfill a vital role in making healthcare accessible to everyone in society. They do this by being remotely monitorable and by allowing "high touch" telemedicine when patients can't get to a doctor in person. Consider what happens when a patient in a remote or underserved region sends their health data to a clinician. That doctor is potentially hundreds or thousands of miles away. Still, they can work their usual magic thanks to AI. When you have a powerful tool like that, you can give care with real-time medicine the same way you do with "normal medicine." The remote monitoring of patients made possible by artificial intelligence and biosensors is one of the most profound effects of these enhanced devices. They allow continuous monitoring of the vital signs of telehealth patients. AI algorithms analyze the data gathered by the sensors, and thus the algorithms can tell the difference between a patient who is healthy and one who is not. The systems in the hospital mostly rely on human judgment to interpret the data. With these new devices, the human element is reduced because the AI-driven algorithms can be trusted to "see" everything that the warm-bodied human has the capacity to "see." The systems can also be more accurately and effectively "heard" because of the biosensors and the AI-driven alerts and warnings that accompany these devices.

3.4 Endorsing Preventive Medicine

The focus of preventive medicine is on warding off diseases before they strike, and artificially intelligent biosensors are aiding this approach. These monitor health indicators in real time and can alert individuals if something seems amiss. They're a bit like the medical equivalent of the smoke detector—always on, always watching, but only alarming when absolutely necessary. Take, for instance, the biosensor wristband. It's kind of a fitbit, but with far greater significance. In the near future, it could do things like monitor the wearer's EKG and call for help if the pattern changes in a way that suggests the person might be having a heart attack.

Biosensors augmented by artificial intelligence will also have a significant part in what is known as "lifestyle medicine," which focuses on the use of biosensors to assist with health-driven, day-to-day decision-making. Think of them as writing one's health "data life" in a way that the individual can understand and use. These devices are already providing something close to an on-the-body quantum of signal intelligence. And they are doing it in real time and largely at the level of the individual. In this regard, fitness trackers are the forerunners. Also serving an essential role in helping us lead healthier lives that are conducive to preventive medicine. These sensors give us immediate real-time information about the state of our bodies that can nudge us in the right direction. For example, my Apple Watch tells me my current heart rate and also notifies me when my heart rate is above or below normal, serving as an early warning and—effectively—keeping me in line with my heart-healthy lifestyle.

4. CHALLENGES AND ETHICAL CONSIDERATIONS

4.1 Data Privacy and Security

Integrating artificial intelligence into healthcare carries great challenges, especially when it comes to data privacy and security. It's necessary for healthcare providers to follow the rules laid down in certain regulations, such as the more recent General Data Protection Regulation (GDPR) and the slightly older Health Insurance Portability and Accountability Act (HIPAA), which, in the United States, are designed to foster and protect the privacy and security of personal health information (Kaushal, Bates, & Poon, 2003). Nonetheless, the use of AI in healthcare often relies on the collection and interpretation of massive amounts of personal health information.

The possibility of data breaches is a primary concern. Of course, if such an event occurs, sensitive and private patient information could fall into the wrong hands. To see that AI systems are, for the most part, secure, many of the same systems and practices already in place for digital security and privacy must be extended. Strong encryption methods and access controls are two ways that systems can be made more secure and keep data well out of the reach of anyone who should not have it. And regular, open, and public security audits should be conducted to ensure that vulnerabilities are detected before they can be used maliciously (Rieke et al., 2020).

4.2 Bias and Fairness

The problem of bias in AI models is crucial in terms of the disparities it can create in the delivery of healthcare. When you train an AI system on biased data, you're almost guaranteed to produce biased results. That can mean unfairly diagnosing one group over another or not diagnosing one group altogether. It can also mean an unfair distribution of healthcare resources. (Obermeyer et al., 2019).

If an AI model is primarily trained on data from one demographic, it may not perform accurately for other groups. Consequently, this could result in misdiagnoses or treatment recommendations that aren't as effective as they could be.

To tackle bias, it is necessary to meticulously create training datasets that reflect the varied appearances and expressions of the human populace. Even then, developers must fashion algorithms that are sensitive to the concept of fairness (Char, Shah, & Magnus, 2018). Moreover, programmers have to use equitable algorithms that identify and alleviate unfairness in the development phase. They must monitor the models they create and ensure that they work justly in diverse patient populations.

4.3 Integration with Clinical Practice

There are many tough aspects to incorporating AI into healthcare, and one of the hardest compromises that implementers must make involves the very human part of our work. Most successful AI tools aren't really all that human-like, and many that are fallible seem to try too hard to appear human. Many of our tools are developed with this in mind and with the idea that the physician will be the ultimate decisionmaker, with the AI tool being designated as solely advisory.

In addition, it's necessary to put AI systems through a strict validation process to make sure they work reliably and with precision. That means not just doing a little testing but, rather, testing a lot and in many different ways—especially the ways that result in the "right" decisions when using AI (Holmes & Durbin, 2020). Clearing up what AI can and cannot do is basic to facilitating its acceptance and also avoiding any unwarranted handovers of control to another—or, rather, to an anything but infallible—intelligence.

4.4 Regulatory and Legal Challenges

AI is an evolving matter of regulation in healthcare; the Food and Drug Administration (FDA) and the European Medicines Agency (EMA) are both developing frameworks for evaluating the algorithms of AI. These frameworks share a focus on transparency, interpretability, and robustness, which are all ways of ensuring that AI systems meet high standards of safety and efficacy (Char, Shah, & Magnus, 2018). Regulating agencies have difficulty keeping up with fast-moving technology like artificial intelligence.

To make certain that artificial intelligence (AI) is reasonably safe and used ethically in healthcare, it is necessary to establish some straightforward rules for its development and deployment. And this is precisely what the National Academy of Medicine (NAM) (formerly the Institute of Medicine) has done. They have taken the necessary and welcome step of articulating in a document called "Artificial Intelligence in Health Care: Anticipating Challenges and Opportunities for Ethical Deployment" a series of rules, principles, and considerations that should be kept in mind along every step of AI's journey in healthcare.

5. FUTURE DIRECTIONS AND COLLABORATIVE EFFORTS

The future of AI in healthcare is very bright, and it is predicted to make major advances in two specific areas: genomic medicine and biosensor technologies. These two areas have the potential to enormously improve the healthcare landscape. They will revolutionize medicine and personalize treatments (Topol, 2019). Biosensors that are powered through AI will provide more in-depth real-time information that can be used in numerous health applications for the average patient.

It will be of utmost importance to discuss and confront the ethical and social dimensions of artificial intelligence in healthcare as AI increasingly infiltrates clinical practice. Keeping the innovation of AI in line with societal values and fair practices demands regular communication among core stakeholders, including but not limited to healthcare providers, patients, policymakers, and AI developers (Char, Shah, & Magnus, 2018). As shown in **Figure 3** AI has endless future trends in various section and future modifications are required in these fields.

Figure 3. Future trends of AI in healthcare and biosensor technology and advancement in ML, sensor technology and healthcare system

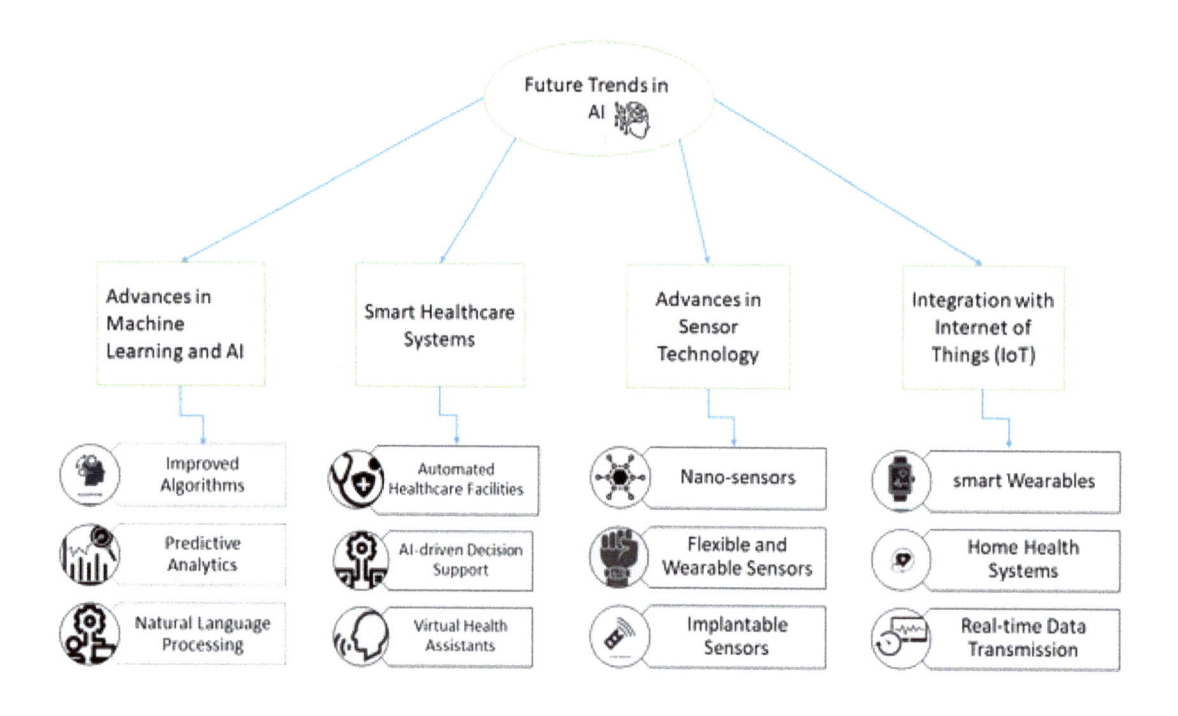

5.1 AI-Driven Genomic Medicine

We anticipate that AI-driven genomic medicine will continue to make enormous leaps forward. They promise to enable us to finally understand what makes illnesses like cancer so inherently complex on the cellular level, thus leading to the development of treatments that truly work.

AI will become even more useful in the future when scientists integrate the large, often disparate sets of data that pour in from different platforms and technologies. These data include not only genomics, proteomics, and metabolomics but also imaging and molecular-cellular measurements in various formats. In the future, multi-omics data will be increasingly integrated in AI pipelines, with the ultimate potential of providing a more complete view of complex disease mechanisms and of the various combinations of factors that drive them (Topol, 2019). Artificial intelligence is expected to have a major impact on the development of personalized vaccines and the field of precision oncology (Mamoshina et al., 2016).

5.2 Advanced Biosensor Technologies

The future of biosensor engineering will produce even more sophisticated wearable and implantable devices capable of continuous and real-time monitoring of a far wider variety of our body's functions and contents.

A typical biosensor has three main components: a bio-recognition element, a transducer, and an electronic system that includes a signal amplifier, a signal processor, and a display. The bio-recognition element, which can be an enzyme, an antibody, a nucleic acid, or a cell, specifically interacts with the analyte of interest. The transducer converts the interaction into a measurable signal. The signal processor takes the result and makes sense of it. The final step is for the display to show the signal in a form that is understandable to the operator (Chen et al., 2021).

Artificial Intelligence will precisely better the sensors' accuracy and capabilities and enable proactive health management. Changes in materials and nanotechnology for the sensor will also help by miniaturizing the size and increasing the compatibility of the biosensor; hence its increase in use within the healthcare sector (Lundervold & Lundervold, 2019).

5.3 AI in Healthcare Delivery

The part AI plays in transforming healthcare will keep changing, especially as it becomes more integrated into telemedicine, remote patient monitoring, and clinical decision support systems. And on top of that, virtual health assistants and chatbots that are powered by AI are really starting to be something else. These things will undoubtedly change patient engagement and the entirely impersonal nature of telemedicine, which is very much a first hire in terms of curbside.

The use of AI in healthcare will also improve patient care and decrease costs. It will facilitate all aspects of healthcare, from the administration of healthcare organizations to the very practice of medicine (Thompson et al., 2018).

5.6 Collaborative Research and Development

The future of AI in healthcare will be driven by the coming together of academia, industry, and healthcare institutions. Amplification of AI solutions will take place with interdisciplinary research initiatives and public-private partnerships. Organizations will share data and resources while following ethical guidelines which will lead to AI models that are more powerful, repeatable and will improve patient's lives throughout the world (Jha & Topol, 2021).

Advanced biosensor technologies are rapidly evolving and integrating with artificial intelligence. The collaborative research and development (R&D) undertaken by these three sectors—academia, industry, and healthcare—propels the full realization of innovative technology with a feasible application in today's world. This is the pathway that leads from potential to function. And when it comes to the integration of AI with biosensors, that path is well marked and heavily trafficked.

5.6.1 Partnerships Between Academia and Industry

AI-enhanced biosensor technologies are largely the result of academic-industry partnerships. The participating academic researchers supply the essential knowledge of biosensor design, AI algorithms, and the almost limitless biomedical applications of these component technologies. The industrial partners—the ones who might eventually manufacture the devices and regulate their use—provide the resources, the direction, and the motivation both to develop the devices and, when necessary, to abide by the rules of the regulatory road to their large-scale implementation (Smith et al., 2021). One instance of an effective public-private partnership is when universities and research institutions join forces with technology companies. These agreements are often systematic and long-term. The University of California, San Francisco, and Stanford University, for example, have specifically collaborated with tech firms, like Google, to develop artificial intelligence for healthcare applications—AI that has the power, they say, to revolutionize the industry. These collaborations produce star-studded research papers and grant access to state-of-the-art laboratory facilities; they're also a clear vector for the rapidly advancing technology of biosensors for disease diagnosis and monitoring.

5.6.2 The Organizations of the Government and the Non-Profit Sector

The collaborative research and development that is critical to the merging of artificial intelligence and biosensor technologies is underwritten, primarily, by government agencies and non-profit organizations. They do this by providing the money necessary to conduct the kind of research that most businesses, including those in the biosensor industry, cannot afford; by establishing the research priorities that lead to the most beneficial results; and by setting up the public-private partnerships that allow various stakeholders—from small and medium-sized enterprises to academic researchers and healthcare providers—to work together in an integrated way (Wang & Zhang, 2023).

In addition, nonprofit organizations frequently aim at tackling particular health problems and help find innovative solutions through collaborations. For example, foundations devoted to diabetes research might fund projects that develop AI-enhanced wearable biosensors for nonstop glucose monitoring, ensuring that these biosensors (and the glucose they monitor) are used in populations that socioeconomic forces often keep underserved.

CONCLUSION

A transformative tipping point in the healthcare landscape stems from integrating artificial intelligence (AI) into personalized medicine and biosensor engineering. AI's capability to analyze enormous and multivariate data sets enables healthcare providers to achieve diagnostics at an unprecedented level of precision, to tune treatments far more accurately, and to monitor patient health in real-time to an unprecedented degree. These advances establish the potential not only to enrich individual patient outcomes, but also to reframe on a macroscopic scale healthcare systems. Yet, for all its promise, AI presents significant hurdles that must be thoughtfully cleared. Issues of patient privacy, algorithmic biases amplifying disparities in care, and guaranteeing compliance with the rigors of regulatory standards loom large. Tackling these obstacles in a responsible way necessitates collaboration among AI researchers, healthcare providers, policymakers, and even patients themselves. Only together can they plot a course that integrates AI safely into medical delivery, reaping the benefits while minimizing the downsides. When we look to the future of healthcare, what we see is AI evolving to become a seamless part of it. This integration will give rise to a new age of healthcare that is more precise in with its diagnostics, more targeted in its treatments, and altogether more effective. As AI evolves and expands its current limited applications, collaboration across fields and dialects is more important than ever if we are to make the best use of AI's health-enhancing and health-optimizing potential.

REFERENCES

Ardila, D., Kiraly, A. P., Bharadwaj, S., Choi, B., Reicher, J. J., Peng, L., Tse, D., Etemadi, M., Ye, W., Corrado, G., Naidich, D. P., & Shetty, S. (2019). End-to-End Lung Cancer Screening with Three-Dimensional Deep Learning on Low-Dose Chest Computed Tomography. *Nature Medicine*, 25(6), 954–961. DOI: 10.1038/s41591-019-0447-x PMID: 31110349

Beam, A. L., & Kohane, I. S. (2018). Big data and machine learning in health care. *Journal of the American Medical Association*, 319(13), 1317–1318. DOI: 10.1001/jama.2017.18391 PMID: 29532063

Bhalla, N., Jolly, P., Formisano, N., & Estrela, P. (2016). Introduction to biosensors. *Essays in Biochemistry*, 60(1), 1–8. DOI: 10.1042/EBC20150001 PMID: 27365030

Bumgarner, J. M., Lambert, C. T., Cantillon, D. J., Cantillon, D., Rooney, L., Tarakji, K. G., & Wazni, O. M. (2018). Assessing the accuracy of an artificial intelligence–based ECG algorithm for detecting atrial fibrillation. *American Heart Journal*, 207, 94–100.

Califf, R. M. (2018). Biomarker definitions and their applications. *Experimental Biology and Medicine*, 243(3), 213–221. DOI: 10.1177/1535370217750088 PMID: 29405771

Char, D. S., Shah, N. H., & Magnus, D. (2018). Implementing machine learning in health care—Addressing ethical challenges. *The New England Journal of Medicine*, 378(11), 981–983. DOI: 10.1056/NEJMp1714229 PMID: 29539284

Collins, F. S., & Varmus, H. (2015). A new initiative on precision medicine. *The New England Journal of Medicine*, 372(9), 793–795. DOI: 10.1056/NEJMp1500523 PMID: 25635347

De Fauw, J., Ledsam, J. R., Romera-Paredes, B., Nikolov, S., Tomasev, N., Blackwell, S., & Suleyman, M. (2018). Clinically applicable deep learning for diagnosis and referral in retinal disease. *Nature Medicine*, 24(9), 1342–1350. DOI: 10.1038/s41591-018-0107-6 PMID: 30104768

Dincer, C., Bruch, R., Kling, A., Dittrich, P. S., & Urban, G. A. (2017). Multiplexed point-of-care testing – xPOCT. *Trends in Biotechnology*, 35(8), 728–742. DOI: 10.1016/j.tibtech.2017.03.013 PMID: 28456344

Dinges, S. S., Hohm, A., Vandergrift, L. A., Nowak, J., Habbel, P., Kaltashov, I. A., & Cheng, L. L. (2019). Cancer Metabolomic Markers in Urine: Evidence, Techniques and Recommendations. *Nature Reviews. Urology*, 16(6), 339–362. DOI: 10.1038/s41585-019-0185-3 PMID: 31092915

Erdem, A., Morales-Narváez, E., & Dincer, C. (2020). Paper-based plasmonic biosensors for point-of-care applications. *Chemical Reviews*, 120(17), 8832–8853.

Esteva, A., Kuprel, B., Novoa, R. A., Ko, J., Swetter, S. M., Blau, H. M., & Thrun, S. (2017). Dermatologist-level classification of skin cancer with deep neural networks. *Nature*, 542(7639), 115–118. DOI: 10.1038/nature21056 PMID: 28117445

Ferrucci, D. A., Levas, A., Bagchi, S., Gondek, D., & Mueller, E. T. (2013). Watson: Beyond jeopardy! *Artificial Intelligence*, 199, 93–105. DOI: 10.1016/j.artint.2012.06.009

Goldstein, B. A., Navar, A. M., Pencina, M. J., & Ioannidis, J. P. A. (2017). Opportunities and challenges in developing risk prediction models with electronic health records data: A systematic review. *Journal of the American Medical Informatics Association : JAMIA*, 24(1), 198–208. DOI: 10.1093/jamia/ocw042 PMID: 27189013

Holmes, J. H., & Durbin, D. R. (2020). Emergency medical services: Using data to advance pediatric emergency care. *Pediatrics*, 145(Supplement_2), S111–S117.

Huynh, T. P., & Haick, H. (2016). Self-Healing, Fully Functional, and Multiparametric Flexible Sensing Platform. *Advanced Materials*, 28(1), 138–143. DOI: 10.1002/adma.201504104 PMID: 26551539

Jalal, A. H., Alam, F., Roychoudhury, S., Umasankar, Y., Pala, N., & Bhansali, S. (2018). Prospects and Challenges of Volatile Organic Compound Sensors in Human Healthcare. *ACS Sensors*, 3(7), 1246–1263. DOI: 10.1021/acssensors.8b00400 PMID: 29879839

Javaid, M. A., Ahmed, A. S., Durand, R., & Tran, S. D. (2016). Saliva as a Diagnostic Tool for Oral and Systemic Diseases. *Journal of Oral Biology and Craniofacial Research*, 6(1), 67–76. DOI: 10.1016/j.jobcr.2015.08.006 PMID: 26937373

Jha, S., & Topol, E. J. (2021). Adapting to Artificial Intelligence: Radiologists and Pathologists as Information Specialists. *Journal of the American Medical Association*, 316(22), 2353–2354. DOI: 10.1001/jama.2016.17438 PMID: 27898975

Kaushal, R., Bates, D. W., & Poon, E. G. (2003). Health information technology: A national imperative. *Health Affairs*, 22(4), 117–126.

Lee, B. G., & Chung, W. Y. (2017). Wearable Glove-Type Driver Stress Detection Using a Motion Sensor. *IEEE Transactions on Intelligent Transportation Systems*, 18(7), 1835–1844. DOI: 10.1109/TITS.2016.2617881

Lee, J., Little, T. D., & Helal, S. (2018). Adopting a remote patient monitoring system: Application to congestive heart failure monitoring. *Computers in Biology and Medicine*, 98, 89–96.

Lundervold, A. S., & Lundervold, A. (2019). An overview of deep learning in medical imaging focusing on MRI. *Zeitschrift für Medizinische Physik*, 29(2), 102–127. DOI: 10.1016/j.zemedi.2018.11.002 PMID: 30553609

Mahadevaiah, G., Rv, P., Bermejo, I., Jaffray, D., Dekker, A., & Wee, L. (2020). Artificial Intelligence-Based Clinical Decision Support in Modern Medical Physics: Selection, Acceptance, Commissioning, and Quality Assurance. *Medical Physics*, 47(5), 228–235. DOI: 10.1002/mp.13562 PMID: 32418341

Majumder, S., & Deen, M. J. (2019). Smartphone Sensors for Health Monitoring and Diagnosis. *Sensors (Basel)*, 19(9), 2164. DOI: 10.3390/s19092164 PMID: 31075985

Mamoshina, P., Vieira, A., Putin, E., & Zhavoronkov, A. (2016). Applications of deep learning in biomedicine. *Molecular Pharmaceutics*, 13(5), 1445–1454. DOI: 10.1021/acs.molpharmaceut.5b00982 PMID: 27007977

Obermeyer, Z., & Emanuel, E. J. (2016). Predicting the future—Big data, machine learning, and clinical medicine. *The New England Journal of Medicine*, 375(13), 1216–1219. DOI: 10.1056/NEJMp1606181 PMID: 27682033

Obermeyer, Z., Powers, B., Vogeli, C., & Mullainathan, S. (2019). Dissecting racial bias in an algorithm used to manage the health of populations. *Science*, 366(6464), 447–453. DOI: 10.1126/science.aax2342 PMID: 31649194

Poplin, R., Chang, P. C., Alexander, D., Schwartz, S., Colthurst, T., Ku, A., Newburger, D., Dijamco, J., Nguyen, N., Afshar, P. T., Gross, S. S., Dorfman, L., McLean, C. Y., & DePristo, M. A. (2018). A universal SNP and small-indel variant caller using deep neural networks. *Nature Biotechnology*, 36(10), 983–987. DOI: 10.1038/nbt.4235 PMID: 30247488

Rajpurkar, P., Irvin, J., Ball, R. L., Zhu, K., Yang, B., Mehta, H., & Ng, A. Y. (2018). Deep learning for chest radiograph diagnosis: A retrospective comparison of the CheXNeXt algorithm to practicing radiologists. *PLoS Medicine*, 15(11), e1002686. DOI: 10.1371/journal.pmed.1002686 PMID: 30457988

Shortliffe, E. H., & Buchanan, B. G. (1975). A model of inexact reasoning in medicine. *Mathematical Biosciences*, 23(3-4), 351–379. DOI: 10.1016/0025-5564(75)90047-4

Smith, A., Nugent, C., & McClean, S. (2002). Implementation of Intelligent Decision Support Systems in Health Care. *Journal of Management in Medicine*, 16(2/3), 206–218. DOI: 10.1108/02689230210434943 PMID: 12211346

Smith, D.. (2021). Deep learning in medical imaging: A comprehensive review. *NeuroImage*, 222, 117254. DOI: 10.1016/j.neuroimage.2020.117254

Smith, D., Johnson, K., & Williams, P. (2021). Deep learning in medical imaging: A comprehensive review. *NeuroImage*, 222, 117254.

Thompson, R. F., Valdes, G., Fuller, C. D., Carpenter, C. M., Morin, O., Aneja, S., & Deasy, J. O. (2018). Artificial intelligence in radiation oncology: A specialty-wide disruptive transformation? *Radiotherapy and Oncology : Journal of the European Society for Therapeutic Radiology and Oncology*, 129(3), 421–426. DOI: 10.1016/j.radonc.2018.05.030 PMID: 29907338

Topol, E. J. (2019). High-performance medicine: The convergence of human and artificial intelligence. *Nature Medicine*, 25(1), 44–56. DOI: 10.1038/s41591-018-0300-7 PMID: 30617339

Veiseh, O., Tang, B. C., Whitehead, K. A., Anderson, D. G., & Langer, R. (2015). Managing diabetes with nanomedicine: Challenges and opportunities. *Nature Reviews. Drug Discovery*, 14(1), 45–57. DOI: 10.1038/nrd4477 PMID: 25430866

Wang, B., Cancilla, J. C., Torrecilla, J. S., & Haick, H. (2014). Artificial Sensing Sntelligence with Silicon Nanowires for Ultraselective Detection in the Gas Phase. *Nano Letters*, 14(2), 933–938. DOI: 10.1021/nl404335p PMID: 24437965

Wang, Y., & Zhang, L. (2023). AI-driven biosensors for healthcare: Current trends and future perspectives. *Trends in Biotechnology*, 41(3), 230–242. DOI: 10.1016/j.tibtech.2022.11.008

Wang, Y., & Zhang, L. (2023). AI-driven biosensors for healthcare: Current trends and future perspectives. *Trends in Biotechnology*, 41(3), 230–242.

White, R., & Davis, L. (2020). AI-driven predictive analytics in healthcare: Applications and challenges. *Journal of Predictive Analytics*, 14(3), 129–137. DOI: 10.1080/15228053.2020.1776158

Zhavoronkov, A., Aliper, A., Kazennov, A., Zhebrak, A., Zagribelnyy, B., Lee, L. H., & Aspuru-Guzik, A. (2019). Potential COVID-19 therapeutics identified by deep learning model. *Computers & Chemical Engineering*, 140, 106973.

Zhavoronkov, A., Ivanenkov, Y. A., Aliper, A., Veselov, M. S., Aladinskiy, V. A., Aladinskaya, A. V., Terentiev, V. A., Polykovskiy, D. A., Kuznetsov, M. D., Asadulaev, A., Volkov, Y., Zholus, A., Shayakhmetov, R. R., Zhebrak, A., Minaeva, L. I., Zagribelnyy, B. A., Lee, L. H., Soll, R., Madge, D., & Aspuru-Guzik, A. (2019). Deep learning enables rapid identification of potent DDR1 kinase inhibitors. *Nature Biotechnology*, 37(9), 1038–1040. DOI: 10.1038/s41587-019-0224-x PMID: 31477924

Chapter 15
Artificial Intelligence and Machine Learning-Assisted Internet of Medical Things:
Approaches Drug Discovery

Zuber Peermohammed Shaikh
Savitribai Phule Pune University, India

ABSTRACT

IoMT devices, also referred to as healthcare IoT, enable human intervention-free healthcare monitoring by integrating automation, interfacial sensors, and machine learning-based artificial intelligence. IoMT technologies aid in reducing unnecessary hospital stays and thereby the associated health costs by facilitating wireless monitoring of health parameters. In this review, we discuss importance of AI in improving capabilities of IoMT in Drug design and development will continue to be an early user of new and growing experimental and computational tools. Among the challenges is deciding whether to use these technologies to improve the existing pipeline and processes or to reengineer the processes in light of these technologies. These research chapter elaborates drug discovery and formulation optimization through Big data, digital healthcare, remote monitoring, and genomics will increase the need to investigate how computational and reasoning approaches might be used to improve the process in terms of clinical significance as well as cost reduction.

INTRODUCTION OF ARTIFICIAL INTELLIGENCE AND IOMT IN PHARMACEUTICAL INDUSTRY

Artificial intelligence (AI) has become more prevalent in a number of societal fields, most notably the pharmaceutical industry. In this review, we focus on how AI is being used in a variety of pharmaceutical industry fields, such as drug discovery and development, drug repurposing, increasing pharmaceutical productivity, and clinical trials, among others. This use of AI lessens the workload of human workers while also achieving goals quickly. A interesting and expanding field is artificial intelligence (AI). Because of the large and growing volume of data, AI techniques are becoming indispensable for the full evaluation of information underlying data. AI is being used to accelerate progress and improve decision making

DOI: 10.4018/979-8-3693-6180-1.ch015

in various sectors and disciplines of drug discovery and development, including medicinal chemistry, upscaling, molecular and cell biology, pharmacology, pharmacokinetics, formulation development, and toxicity. In clinical testing, AI plays a critical role in raising success rates by improving trial design (biomarkers, efficacy parameters, dose selection, trial duration), target patient population selection, patient stratification, and patient sample evaluation. We also explore crosstalk between AI tools and methodologies, current issues and solutions, and the future of AI in the pharma industry.(Awad A., 2021)

Introduction of AI and IoMT in Drug Design and Discovery

In the pharmaceutical market, data digitization has increased dramatically in recent years. However, the challenge of gathering, evaluating, and utilizing knowledge to solve complicated clinical problems arises with digitalization. This encourages the adoption of AI, which can manage massive amounts of data with greater automation. AI is a technology-based system that use a variety of advanced tools and networks to simulate human intelligence. At the same time, it does not threaten to totally replace human physical presence. AI employs systems and software that can read and learn from input data in order to make independent judgments for achieving certain goals. As stated in this review, its applications in the pharmaceutical industry are constantly being expanded. According to the McKinsey Global Institute, rapid breakthroughs in AI-guided automation are likely to totally transform society's work culture.

Artificial Intelligence in Life Cycle Product

AI can be imagined assisting in the development of a pharmaceutical product from the bench to the bedside because it can aid in rational drug design, decision making, determining the right therapy for a patient, including personalized medicines, and managing clinical data generated and using it for future drug development. E-VAI is an analytical and decision-making AI platform developed by Eularis that uses machine learning (ML) algorithms and an easy-to-use user interface to create analytical roadmaps based on competitors, key stakeholders, and currently held market share to predict key drivers in pharmaceutical sales, allowing marketing executives to allocate resources for maximum market share gain, reversing poor sales, and anticipating where to make investments.(Dash S., 2019)

Figure 1. Artificial Intelligence (AI) is being used in various areas of the pharmaceutical drug discovery sector

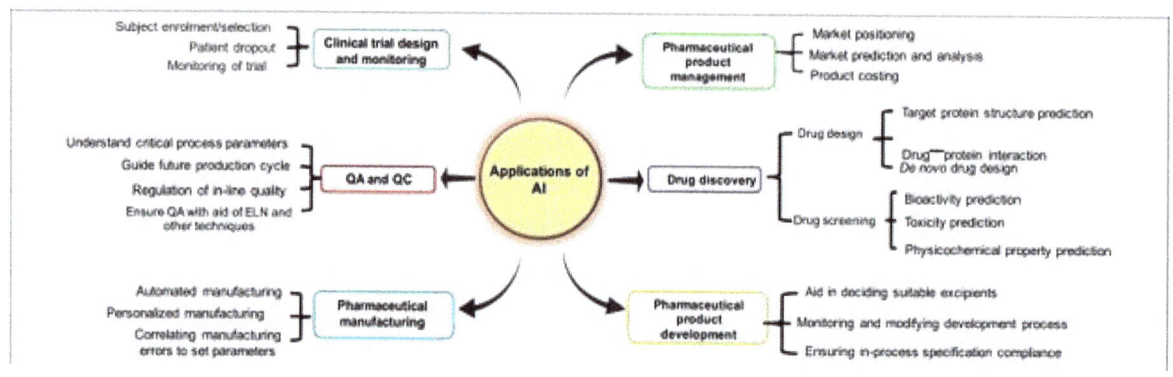

2. LITERATURE REVIEW OF ARTIFICIAL INTELLIGENCE IN IOMT DRUG DISCOVERY

The enormous chemical space, which contains >1060 compounds, encourages the synthesis of a huge number of pharmacological molecules. The lack of new technology, on the other hand, delays the medication development process, making it a time consuming and expensive task that can be handled by applying AI. AI can identify hit and lead compounds, as well as provide faster validation of the drug target and optimization of drug structure design.

Figure 2. Applications of AI in drug discovery and development

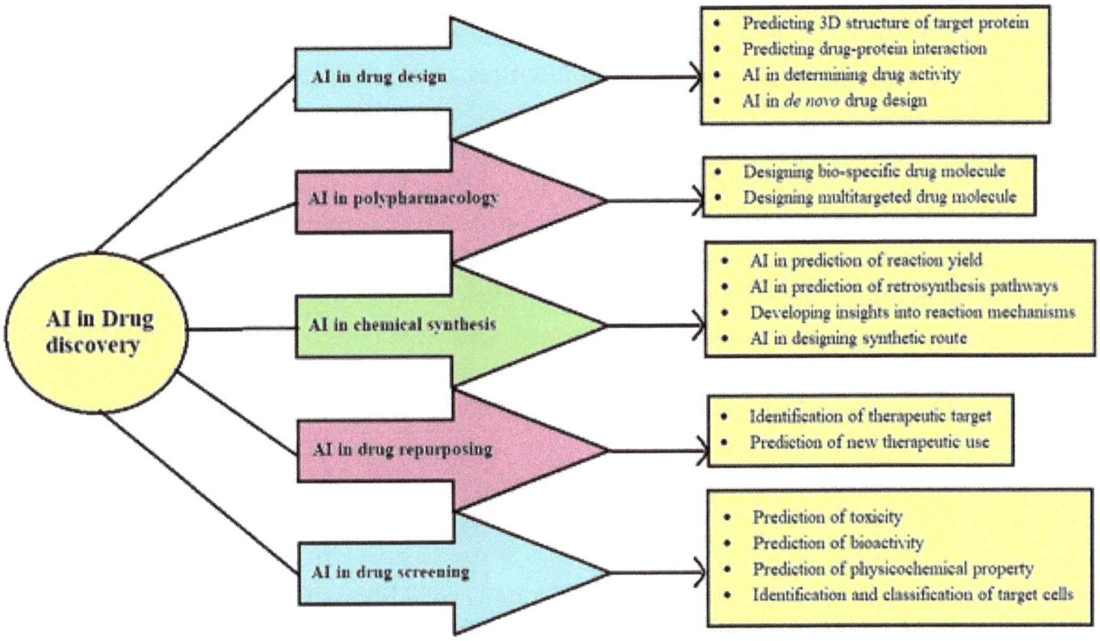

2.1 Artificial Intelligence (AI) in Drug Discovery

AI has the potential to help in several areas of drug discovery, including drug design, chemical synthesis, drug screening, polypharmacology, and drug repurposing. Despite its benefits, AI has substantial data difficulties, such as data volume, growth, diversity, and uncertainty. Traditional ML algorithms may be unable to deal with the data sets accessible for drug discovery in pharmaceutical organizations, which might include millions of molecules. A computational model based on the quantitative structure-activity relationship (QSAR) can swiftly predict a large number of chemicals or simple physicochemical characteristics like log P or log D. However, these models fall short of predicting complicated biological features such as chemical activity and side effects. Furthermore, QSAR-based models encounter issues such as short training sets, experimental data error in training sets, and a lack of experimental validations. To address these issues, recently emerging AI tools, such as Deep learning (DL) and relevant modelling studies, can be used to evaluate the safety and efficacy of medicinal compounds using big data modelling and analysis. Merck sponsored a QSAR ML competition in 2012 to investigate the benefits of DL in the drug discovery process in the pharmaceutical business. For 15 drug candidate absorption, distribution, metabolism, excretion, and toxicity (ADMET) data sets, DL models outperformed classic ML approaches in terms of predictability.(*Ding B., 2018*)

2.2 Distributions of Molecules

By depicting the ***distributions of molecules*** and their attributes, the virtual chemical space resembles a geographical map of molecules. The goal behind the chemical space visualization is to collect positional information about molecules inside the space in order to search for bioactive compounds; hence, virtual screening (VS) aids in the selection of relevant molecules for subsequent testing. Several chemical spaces, including PubChem, ChemBank, DrugBank, and ChemDB, are open to the public. Numerous in silico methods for virtual screening compounds from virtual chemical spaces, as well as structure and ligand-based methodologies, allow superior profile analysis, faster elimination of nonlead compounds, and therapeutic molecule selection at a lower cost. To pick a lead ingredient, drug design techniques such as coulomb matrices and molecular fingerprint recognition examine the physical, chemical, and toxicological profiles. To forecast the intended chemical structure of a substance, several characteristics such as predictive models, molecule similarity, the molecule generation process, and the usage of in silico methodologies can be used. Pereira et al. presented DeepVS, a new docking method for 40 receptors and 2950 ligands that demonstrated remarkable performance when 95000 decoys were tested against these receptors. A multi-objective automated replacement algorithm was used in another study to enhance the potency profile of a cyclin-dependent kinase-2 inhibitor by examining its form similarity, biochemical activity, and physicochemical features.

2.3 QSAR Modeling

The use of ***QSAR modelling*** tools has led to the development of AI-based QSAR techniques, including decision trees, support vector machines, random forests, and linear discriminant analysis (LDA), which can be used to accelerate QSAR analysis. When King et al. evaluated the capacity of six AI algorithms to rank anonymous substances in terms of biological activity with that of conventional techniques, they discovered a minimal statistical difference.(*Estrela V. V., 2018*)

3. BACKGROUND OF ARTIFICIAL INTELLIGENCE IN DRUG SCREENING

3.1 Prediction of Physicochemical Properties

When developing a new medicine, physicochemical characteristics including solubility, partition coefficient (logP), degree of ionization, and intrinsic permeability of the drug must be considered because they have an indirect impact on its pharmacokinetics and target receptor family. It is possible to predict physicochemical properties using a variety of AI-based methods. For example, ML uses large data sets created during earlier compound optimization to train the software. Molecule descriptors, such as SMILES strings, potential energy readings, electron density around the molecule, and coordinates of atoms in 3D, are used in drug design algorithms to produce feasible molecules via DNN and thus forecast its properties. The Estimation Program Interface (EPI) Suite is a quantitative structure-property relationship (QSPR) process developed by Zang et al. to ascertain the six physicochemical properties of environmental chemicals received from the Environmental Protection Agency (EPA). The lipophilicity and solubility of different substances have been predicted using neural networks based on the ADMET predictor and ALGOPS software. The solubility of molecules has been predicted using DL techniques like undirected graph recursive neural networks and graph-based convolutional neural networks (CVNN). The acid dissociation constant of substances has been predicted using ANN-based models, graph kernels, and kernel ridge-based models in a number of cases. Similar to this, data on cellular permeability of a wide range of molecules has been generated using cell lines, such as Madin-Darby canine kidney cells and human colon adenocarcinoma (Caco-2) cells and is then fed to AI assisted predictors. In order to predict the intestinal absorptivity of 497 compounds, Kumar et al. developed six predictive models, including SVMs, ANNs, k-nearest neighbor algorithms, LDAs, probabilistic neural network algorithms, and partial least square (PLS), using 745 compounds for training. These models took into account parameters such as molecular surface area, molecular mass, total hydrogen count, molecular refractivity, molecular volume, logP, total polar surface area, the sum of E- states indices, solubility index (log S), and rotatable bonds. In a similar vein, in silico models based on RF and DNN were created to estimate human intestinal absorption of various chemical substances. As a result, AI plays a crucial role in the creation of a medicine by predicting both the needed bioactivity and the intended physicochemical qualities. (Shapiro *SC., 1992)*

3.2 Prediction of Bioactivity

The affinity of drug molecules for the target protein or receptor determines their efficacy. Drug molecules that do not bind with or have affinity for the targeted protein will not be able to provide the therapeutic response. In rare cases, therapeutic compounds may interact with unwanted proteins or receptors, resulting in toxicity. As a result, drug target binding affinity (DTBA) is essential for predicting drug-target interactions. AI-based approaches can calculate a drug's binding affinity by taking into account the traits or similarities between the drug and its target. To determine the feature vectors, feature-based interactions recognize the chemical moieties of the medication and the target. In contrast, similarity-based interaction takes into account the similarity between medication and target, and it is assumed that similar compounds will interact with the same targets. For predicting drug-target interactions, web application such as ChemMapper and the similarity ensemble technique (SEA) are available. Many ML and DL-based techniques, including as KronRLS, SimBoost, DeepDTA, and PADME, have been utilized to determine DTBA. To determine DTBA, ML-based techniques such as Kronecker-regularized least squares (KronRLS) analyze the similarity between medicines and protein molecules. SimBoost, on the other hand, uses regression trees to predict DTBA and takes into account both feature-based and similarity-based interactions. SMILES drug characteristics, ligand maximum common substructure (LMCS), extended connectivity fingerprint, or a mix of these can all be evaluated.DL approaches have shown improved performance compared with ML because they apply network-based methods that do not depend on the availability of the 3D protein structure. DeepDTA, PADME, WideDTA, and DeepAffinity are some DL methods used to measure DTBA. DeepDTA accepts drug data in the form of SMILES, whereby, the amino acid sequence is entered for protein input data and for the 1D representation of the drug structure. WideDTA is CVNN DL method that incorporates ligand SMILES (LS), amino acid sequences, LMCS, and protein domains and motifs as input data for assessing the binding affinity. Deep-Affinity and Protein and Drug Molecule Interaction Prediction (PADME) are techniques comparable to those published previously. Deep-Affinity is an interpretable deep learning model that employs both RNN and CNN, as well as unlabeled and labelled data. In the structural and physicochemical aspects, it considers the compound in SMILES format and protein sequences. (*Dasta JF., 1992*)

PADME is a DL-based platform that predicts drug target interactions using feed-forward neural networks (DTIs). It takes as input data the combination of medication and target protein properties and anticipates the intensity of the interaction between the two. The SMILES representation and the protein sequence composition (PSC) are used to illustrate the drug and the target, respectively. Unsupervised machine learning techniques, such as MANTRA and PREDICT, can be used to forecast the therapeutic efficacy of drugs and target proteins of known and unknown pharmaceuticals, which can then be extrapolated to the application of drug repurposing and interpreting the therapeutics' molecular mechanism. Using a CMap data set, MANTRA classifies substances based on comparable gene expression profiles and clusters those anticipated to have a shared mode of action and biological pathway. A drug's bioactivity also contains ADME data. AI-based techniques such as XenoSite, FAME, and SMARTCyp are used to determine the drug's sites of metabolism. Additionally, tools like CypRules, MetaSite, MetaPred, SMARTCyp, and WhichCyp were utilized to pinpoint individual CYP450 isoforms that control a given drug's metabolism. SVMbased predictors performed the clearance pathway analysis of 141 authorized medicines with high accuracy. (*Goldberg D., 1989*)

3.3 Prediction of Toxicity

It is crucial to predict the toxicity of any drug molecule in order to avoid negative effects. The frequent use of cell-based in vitro tests as preliminary studies, followed by animal trials to ascertain a compound's toxicity, raises the price of creating new medications. A number of web-based applications, such as LimTox, pkCSM, admetSAR, and Toxtree, can assist reduce the cost. Advanced AI-based techniques examine similarities between compounds or estimate a compound's toxicity based on input features. The Tox21 Data Challenge was organized by the National Institutes of Health, the Environmental Protection Agency (EPA), and the US Food and Drug Administration (FDA) to test various computational techniques for predicting the toxicity of 12 707 environmental chemicals and medicines. By identifying static and dynamic features within the chemical descriptors of the molecules, such as molecular weight (MW) and Van der Waals volume, a machine learning algorithm called DeepTox outperformed all other methods and was able to accurately predict the toxicity of a molecule based on predefined 2500 toxicophoric features.

4. METHODOLOGY OF CURRENT CONTEXT OF RESEARCH: ARTIFICIAL INTELLIGENCE IN DESIGNING DRUG MOLECULES

4.1 Prediction of the Target Protein Structure

In order to treat patients effectively, choosing the appropriate target during therapeutic molecule development is essential. Several overexpressed proteins are involved in the development of the disease. Therefore, in order to specifically target disease, it is essential to predict the structure of the target protein while creating the drug molecule. AI can assist in structure-based drug development by predict the 3D protein structure since the design is in accordance with the chemical environment of the target protein location. This makes it easier to predict a compound's impact on the target and safety concerns prior to its synthesis or manufacture. By comparing the distances between nearby amino acids and the corresponding angles of the peptide bonds, the AI tool AlphaFold, which is based on DNNs, was used to predict the 3D target protein structure. With 25 out of 43 structures correctly predicted, this method produced excellent results. RNN was used to predict the protein structure in a study by AlQurashi. The author considered a recurrent geometric network (RGN), which consists of three stages: computation, geometry, and assessment. The basic protein sequence was encoded in this case, and the torsional angles for a certain residue and a partially finished backbone derived from the geometric unit upstream of this were then taken into account as input and gave a new backbone as output. The result from the final unit was a 3D structure. The distance based root mean square deviation (dRMSD) metric was used to evaluate the variance between anticipated and experimental structures. The RGN settings were tuned to minimize the dRMSD between the predicted and experimental structures. AlQurashi projected that his AI approach would predict the protein structure more quickly than AlphaFold. While predicting protein structures with sequences comparable to those of the reference structures, AlphaFold is probably more accurate. In a study, a nonlinear three-layered NN toolbox based on a feed-forward supervised learning and backpropagation error algorithm was used with MATLAB to predict the 2D structure of a protein. The input and output data sets were trained in MATLAB, and the NNs served as learning algorithms and performance judges. The prediction of the 2D structure was accurate to 62.72%.*(Holmes J, 2004)*

4.2 Predicting Drug Protein Interaction

Drug-protein interactions are crucial to a therapy's effectiveness. To understand a medicine's efficacy and effectiveness, predict how it will interact with a receptor or protein is crucial. This also enables drug repurposing and avoids polypharmacology. The accurate prediction of ligand-protein interactions made possible by a variety of AI techniques has improved therapeutic efficacy. In order to find nine new compounds and their interactions with four important targets, Wang et al. described a model utilizing the SVM approach that was constructed based on primary protein sequences and structural properties of small molecules and trained on 15 000 protein-ligand interactions. Yu et al. used two RF models to predict potential drug-protein interactions by combining pharmacological and chemical data and validating them with excellent sensitivity and specificity against well-known platforms, such as SVM. Additionally, these modes could forecast drug-target relationships, which could then be expanded to anticipate associations between target-disease and targettarget, accelerating the drug discovery process. The Neighborhood Cleaning Rule and the Synthetic Minority Over-Sampling Technique were used by Xiao et al. to collect optimum data for the creation of iDrugTarget. This is a mixture of four sub-predictors (iDrug-GPCR, iDrug-Chl, iDrug-Enz, and iDrug-NR) for figuring out how a drug interacts with G-protein-coupled receptors (GPCRs), ion channels, enzymes, and nuclear receptors, in that order. Target-jackknife tests were used to compare this predictor to other predictors, and the former outperformed the latter in terms of consistency and prediction accuracy.*(Miles JC, 2006)*

4.3 Artificial Intelligence in Quality Control and Quality Assurance

A balance of different criteria must be achieved throughout the production of the desired product from raw materials. It takes human intervention to maintain batch-to-batch consistency and conduct quality control testing on the products. This illustrates the need for AI implementation at this time and may not be the optimal strategy in every situation. By implementing a "Quality by Design" approach, the FDA modified Current Good Manufacturing Practices (cGMP) in order to better understand the crucial process and precise standards that determine the ultimate quality of the pharmaceutical product. Gams et al. created decision trees using a combination of human effort and artificial intelligence (AI) by analyzed preliminary data from production batches. The operators further turned them into rules and examined them in order to direct the manufacturing cycle going forward. Goh et al. used ANN to analyze the dissolution profile of theophylline pellets, a sign of batch-to-batch consistency, and they found that it accurately predicted the dissolution of the tested formulation with an error of only 8%. AI can also be used to regulate in-line manufacturing processes in order to attain the target product standard. The freeze-drying process is monitored using an ANN-based method that employs a combination of self-adaptive evolution, local search, and backpropagation algorithms. This can be utilized to anticipate the temperature and desiccated-cake thickness at a future time point (t + t) for a specific set of operating circumstances, thereby assisting in the quality control of the final product. An automated data input platform, such as an Electronic Lab Notebook, combined with advanced, intelligent algorithms can ensure product quality. Furthermore, data mining and various knowledge discovery techniques in the Total Quality Management expert system can be employed as valuable approaches in making difficult judgments, resulting in the development of new technologies for intelligent quality control.(*Wirtz BW, 2019*)

4.4 Artificial Intelligence in Pharmaceutical Product Management

4.4.1 Artificial Intelligence in Market Positioning

Market positioning is the process of establishing a product's identity in the market in order to persuade customers to acquire it, making it a key component in almost all business strategies for enterprises to build their own distinct identity. This strategy was employed in the promotion of the pioneer brand Viagra, which was marketed not only for the treatment of erectile dysfunction in males, but also for other disorders impacting quality of life. Companies can now achieve natural brand recognition in the public realm with the use of technology and e-commerce as a platform. Companies use search engines as one of the technology platforms to get a prominent place in online marketing and aid in product positioning, as affirmed by the Internet Advertising Bureau. Companies are constantly attempting to rank their websites higher than those of other companies in order to gain attention for their brand in a short amount of time. Other techniques, such as statistical analysis methods and particle swarm optimization algorithms used in conjunction with NNs, produced a more accurate picture of markets. They can assist in determining the product's marketing strategy based on accurate consumer demand prediction.

4.4.2 Artificial Intelligence Market Prediction and Analysis

A company's success is determined by the constant expansion and growth of its business. Despite having access to large funding, R&D production in the pharmaceutical business is declining due to companies' failure to adopt new marketing technologies. The 'Fourth Industrial Revolution' in digital technologies is assisting innovative digitalized marketing through a multicriteria decision-making approach, which collects and analyses statistical and mathematical data and implements human inferences to make AI-based decision-making models explore new marketing methodology. AI also aided in a full examination of a product's core requirements from the customer's perspective, as well as analyzing market demand, which aids in decision-making using prediction tools. It can also forecast sales and conduct market research. AI-based software engages customers and raises physician awareness by providing adverts that connect them to the product site with a single click. Furthermore, these strategies employ natural language processing tools to examine keywords entered by clients and associate them with the likelihood of purchasing the goods. Several business-to-business (B2B) companies have introduced self-service solutions that enable free browsing of health items, which can be easily located by providing specifications, placing orders, and tracking their shipping. Pharmaceutical companies are also launching online programmers such as 1 mg, Medline, Netmeds, and Ask Apollo to meet patients' unmet requirements. Market prediction is also important for various pharmaceutical distribution organizations that can apply AI in the sector, such as 'Business clever Smart Sales Prediction Analysis', which employs a combination of time series forecasting and real-time application. This enables pharmaceutical companies to forecast product sales in advance, avoiding the expenditures of excess stock or client loss due to shortages.(*Smith RG, 2000*)

5. RESULT OF CURRENT CONTEXT OF RESEARCH

AI has also been used to help reuse already-approved drugs and avoid polypharmacology because of its potential to predict drugtarget interactions. A drug that has been repurposed is immediately qualified for Phase II clinical trials. Releasing an outdated medication results in financial savings because doing so only costs $8.4 million as opposed to $41.3 million to release a completely new pharmacological entity. A fresh connection between a drug and a disease can be predicted using the "guilt by association" strategy, which can be knowledge-based or computationally driven. In networks that are computationally driven, the ML methodology—which uses techniques like SVM, NN, logistic regression, and DL—is widely used. Logistic regression platforms like PREDICT, SPACE, and other ML techniques consider drug-drug, disease-disease, target-molecule, chemical structure, and gene expression profiles when repurposing a medicine. Drug-protein interactions can also foretell the likelihood of polypharmacology, or a drug's propensity to interact with many receptors and cause unintended side effects. In order to create safer medicinal compounds, AI can build a novel molecule using the principles of polypharmacology. Multiple substances can be linked to a variety of targets and off-targets using AI systems like SOM and the enormous databases that are already available. The pharmacological characteristics of medications and potential targets can be connected using Bayesian classifiers and SEA algorithms.(*Lamberti MJ, 2019*)

5.1 De Novo Medication Design With AI

De novo drug design has been popular in recent years as a method for creating therapeutic compounds. De novo drug design is being replaced by emerging DL approaches since the former has drawbacks including difficult synthesis routes and problematic bioactivity prediction of the novel molecule. Thousands of distinct synthesis paths can be predicted for each of the millions of structures that can be produced using computer-aided synthesis planning. Because of its many benefits, including online learning, optimization of previously learned data, and suggestions for potential synthesis routes for compounds, the use of AI in the de novo design of molecules can be advantageous to the pharmaceutical industry and result in quick lead design and development.

5.1 Artificial intelligence in Advancing Pharmaceutical Product Development

The subsequent inclusion of a novel therapeutic molecule into an appropriate dosage form with the requisite delivery properties is necessary. The traditional method of trial and error can be replaced in this area by AI. With the use of QSPR, a variety of computational methods can be used to overcome concerns with stability, dissolution, porosity, and other aspects of formulation design. Decision-support tools operate through a feedback mechanism to monitor the entire process and sporadically adjust it. They employ rule-based systems to choose the type, nature, and quantity of the excipients based on the physicochemical parameters of the medicine. Guo et al. combined expert systems (ES) and artificial neural networks (ANN) to produce a hybrid method for the production of piroxicam direct-filling hard gelatin capsules that adhere to the parameters of its dissolution profile.

5.2 Model Expert System

Based on the input parameters, the MODEL EXPERT SYSTEM (MES) generates decisions and suggestions for formulation development. Contrarily, ANN makes formulation development simple by using backpropagation learning to connect formulation parameters to the intended response, which is jointly regulated by the control module. The influence of the powder's flow property on the die-filling and tablet compression process has been studied using a variety of mathematical tools, including computational fluid dynamics (CFD), discrete element modelling (DEM), and the Finite Element Method. The effect of tablet geometry on its dissolution profile can also be studied using CFD. The quick manufacture of pharmaceutical items may benefit greatly from the integration of these mathematical models with AI. *(Duch W, 2007)*

5.3 Artificial Intelligence in Pharmaceutical Manufacturing

Modern manufacturing systems are attempting to impart human knowledge to machines as a result of the growing complexity of production processes, as well as the growing desire for efficiency and greater product quality. The pharmaceutical industry may profit from the use of AI in manufacturing. Utilizing the automation of many pharmaceutical activities, tools like computational fluid dynamics (CFD) use **Reynolds-Averaged Navier-Stokes solvers technology** to examine the effects of agitation and stress levels in various pieces of equipment (such stirred tanks). Similar systems, such big eddy simulations, and direct numerical simulations, use sophisticated techniques to address challenging flow problems in manufacturing. The innovative Chemputer platform aids digital automation for molecule synthesis and manufacture by including numerous chemical codes and working through the use of a scripting language known as Chemical Assembly. With yield and purity very similar to manual synthesis, it has been used to successfully synthesize and produce sildenafil, diphenhydramine hydrochloride, and rufinamide. AI technology can effectively complete the estimated granulation in granulators with capacities ranging from 25 to 600l. ***Neuro-fuzzy logic and technology*** were used to correlate key factors with their answers. In order to anticipate the proportion of granulation fluid to be supplied, the necessary speed, and the diameter of the impeller in both geometrically identical and dissimilar granulators, they developed a polynomial equation. (*Blasiak A, 2020*)

Table 1. Artificial Intelligence (AI), and Machine Learning (ML) in pharmaceutical drug discovery applications

Parameters	Applications of Pharmaceutical Drug Discovery.
Drug discovery	Screening of drug compounds, prediction of the success rate of a drug, drug target identification and validation, multi-target drug discoveries, drug repurposing and biomarker identification.
Diagnostics	FDA granted Bayer and Merck & Co with Breakthrough Device Designation for AI pattern recognition software that analyses images from cardiac, lung perfusion and pulmonary vessels. This software will support radiologists by identifying signs of Chronic Thromboembolic Pulmonary Hypertension (CTEPH), a rare form of pulmonary hypertension.
In Formulation	Modelling pharmaceutical formulations. Three-dimensional plots of massing time, compression pressure and crushing strength, or drug release, massing time and compression pressure in an attempt to maximize tablet strength or to select the best lubricant.
In Product Development	The combination of Self-learning AI platforms like Artificial Neural Network (ANN) and Design of Experiment (DoE) provides more flexibility, powerful results, supports in composition and process optimization. It helps in developing a quality drug product, as it provides a better clarity between formulation ingredients/process parameters and quality target product profile.
In Genomics	verge Genomics has developed a platform technology that maps genes which are responsible for causing disease and then maps the drug molecule that target them to provide cure. Currently, the platform is being used to discover molecules for treatment of neurological diseases.
In Drug repurposing	AI helps to match the available data of drug molecules to new targets.
In Personalized medicine	AI can be used to stratify patients, initiate specific tailored treatments, and thus increase response rates, reduce adverse effects and medical errors.
In Rare disease identification	Using AI, body scans can be done to detect cancer and other diseases early and as well as predict health issues based on genetics. AI can use a patient's medical information and history to optimize a personalized treatment plan.
IN clinical trial research	AI can monitor a patient's movement via smartphone camera and determine the severity of the symptoms. It can allow a doctor to monitor patient remotely, adjust dose and fix appointment for the patient.
In data management	Maintenance of medical records using a sensor or mobile application, beneficial for patients in whom adherence is an issue and for clinical trials.
Betterment in patient care	Artificial Intelligence is on target to wholly alter the longer term of healthcare. With the mixing of AI into the work of both medical professionals and hospital systems, expect to ascertain dramatic changes in both patient health outcomes and within the operational efficiency of hospitals.AI help to people in health care system - The "open AI ecosystem" is one among the highest 10 promising technologies in 2016. It is useful to gather and compare the info from social awareness algorithms. In healthcare system vast information is recorded which incorporates patient medical record and treatment data from childhood thereto age. This enormous data can be analyzed

6 DISCUSSION OF CURRENT CONTEXT OF RESEARCH

The pharmaceutical industry has used DEM extensively, for example, to investigate the segregation of powders in a binary mixture, the effects of varying blade speed and shape, predict the potential path of the tablets during coating, and analyze the amount of time that tablets spend in the spray zone. In order to decrease tablet capping on the production line, ANNs and fuzzy models investigated the relationship between machine settings and the capping problem. AI tools like the meta-classifier and tablet-classifier are used to control the final product's quality standard by flagging potential production errors in tablets. A patent application demonstrates a system that employs a processor that receives patient information to determine the ideal drug and dose regimen for each patient, then constructs the appropriate transdermal patch in accordance with that information.

6.1 Artificial Intelligence in Clinical Trial Design

Clinical trials take 6-7 years and a significant financial investment to establish the safety and efficacy of a medicinal product in people for a specific illness condition. However, just one out of every ten molecules that enter these trials is approved, resulting in a substantial loss for the industry. These failures might occur as a result of poor patient selection, a lack of technological needs, or a lack of infrastructure. However, with the large amount of digital medical data available, these failures can be decreased by the use of AI. Enrolling participants consumes one-third of the clinical study timeline. The enrollment of suitable patients ensures the success of a clinical study, which otherwise results in 86% of failure cases. AI can help in the selection of a specific diseased population for enrollment in Phase II and III clinical trials by applying patient-specific genome-exposome profile analysis, which can aid in the early prediction of possible therapeutic targets in the patients chosen. Preclinical molecule discovery and prediction of lead compounds prior to the start of clinical trials using other aspects of AI, such as predictive ML and other reasoning techniques, aid in the early prediction of lead molecules that would pass clinical trials with consideration of the selected patient population. Drop out of patients from clinical trials accounts for 30% of clinical trial failure, resulting in additional recruiting requirements for the trial's completion, resulting in a waste of time and money. This can be avoided by closely monitoring the patients and assisting them in adhering to the clinical trial procedure. AiCure developed mobile software to track regular medication intake by patients with schizophrenia in a Phase II trial, which boosted patient adherence by 25%, assuring the clinical trial's successful completion.*(Baronzio G, 2015)*

6.2 Artificial Intelligence Based Nanorobots for Drug Delivery

Nanorobots are primarily composed of integrated circuits, sensors, power supplies, and secure data backup, all of which are maintained using computational technologies such as AI. They are engineered to avoid collisions, identify targets, detect and attach, and then excrete from the body. Nano/microrobot advancements allow them to go to the desired region based on physiological parameters such as pH, boosting efficacy and lowering systemic adverse effects. The development of implantable nanorobots for controlled drug and gene delivery necessitates consideration of characteristics such as dose modification, sustained release, and control release, and drug release necessitates automation controlled by AI tools such as NNs, fuzzy logic, and integrators. Microchip implants are utilized for both programmed release and detecting the implant's position in the body.

6.3 Artificial Intelligence in Emergence of Nanomedicine

Nanomedicines combine nanotechnology and medicine to diagnose, treat, and monitor complicated diseases such as HIV, cancer, malaria, asthma, and inflammatory diseases. Nanoparticle-modified drug delivery has become essential in the field of therapeutics and diagnostics in recent years due to improved efficacy and therapy. Many formulation development difficulties could be solved by combining nanotechnology and AI. A methotrexate nanosuspension was computationally created by evaluating the energy released by the drug molecules' interaction and monitoring the variables that could lead to formulation aggregation. Coarse-grained simulation, in conjunction with chemical calculations, can help determine drug-dendrimer interactions and assess drug encapsulation within the dendrimer. Furthermore, tools such as LAMMPS and GROMACS 4 can be utilized to investigate the effect of surface chemistry on nanoparticle internalization into cells. AI aided in the development of silicasomes, which are composed of iRGD, a tumor-penetrating peptide, and irinotecan-loaded multifunctional mesoporous silica nanoparticles. This boosted silicasomes uptake three to fourfold because iRGD enhances silicasomes transcytosis, resulting in improved treatment outcome and overall survival.(*Mak KK, 2019*)

6.4 Pharmaceutical Market of Artificial Intelligence

To reduce the monetary cost and chances of failures that accompany VS, pharmaceutical businesses are shifting towards AI. The AI market grew from US$200 million in 2015 to US$700 million in 2018, and it is predicted to grow to $5 billion by 2024. AI is expected to disrupt the pharmaceutical and medical sectors, with a 40% estimated rise from 2017 to 2024. Various pharmaceutical corporations have made and continue to make investments in AI, as well as cooperated with AI companies to build critical healthcare technologies. DeepMind Technologies, a Google company, collaborated with the Royal Free London NHS Foundation Trust to help people with acute renal injury. Major pharmaceutical companies and AI players are detailed.(*Mishra V., 2018*)

6.5 AI Drug Discovery

AI can play an important role in initial screening of drug compounds, prediction of the success rate of a drug and more specifically, it may play a role in drug target identification and validation, multi-target drug discoveries, drug repurposing, and biomarker identification. Ideally, this would also translate to lower drug costs for patients, all while offering them more treatment choices. Many pharma companies, in collaboration with AI companies, have developed cloud-based AI platforms to accelerate their drug discovery programs. These platforms look for pattern in data and make use of algorithms that can make accurate predictions about the potential drug molecules based on computational structure analysis, drug target and data from in-vivo cell line studies. For instance, Watson Health and Pfizer announced a collaboration to accelerate Pfizer's immuno-oncology discovery program using cloud-based Watson's machine-learning system. The IBM Watson platform will aid in identification of new drug targets, fixed-dose combinations to be studied and provide assistance in selecting patients for trials. Similarly, UK-based AI drug discovery company Exscientia signed one of the biggest AI drug discovery deal with Celgene to accelerate its small molecule discovery program in oncology and autoimmunity segment. In addition to it, Exscientia is also supporting drug discovery program of Sanofi, GlaxoSmithKline, Sumitomo, Evotec, etc, using its artificial intelligence algorithms.

6.5.1 In Formulation: a) Controlled Release Tablets

The first work in the use of neural networks for modelling pharmaceutical formulations was performed by Hussain and co-workers at the University of Cincinnati (OH, USA). In various studies they modelled the in vitro release characteristics of a range of drugs dispersed in matrices prepared from various hydrophilic polymers. In all cases, neural networks with a single hidden layer were found to offer reasonable performance in the prediction of drug release. In general, the results were comparable with those generated through the use of statistical analysis, but when predictions outside the limits of the input data were attempted performance was poor. No attempt was made to optimize the formulations using genetic algorithms, but the results generated did lead the researchers to propose the concept of computer aided formulation design based on neural networks. In a more recent study involving the formulation of diclofenac sodium from a matrix tablet prepared from cetyl alcohol, personnel from the pharmaceutical company KRKA dd (Smerjeska, Slovenia) and the University of Ljubljana (Slovenia) have used neural networks to predict the rate of drug release and to undertake optimization using two- and three-dimensional response surface analysis. Non-linear relationships were found between the release rate and the amounts of the ingredients used in the formulation, suggesting the possibility of the production of several formulations with the same release profile. (*Sellwood MA, 2018*)

6.5.2 Immediate Release Tablets

add this area began only around three years ago with two studies. One by Turkoglu and associates from the University of Marmara (Turkey) and therefore the University of Cincinnati used both neural networks and statistics to model tablet formulations of hydrochlorothiazide. The networks produced were wont to prepare three-dimensional plots of either massing time, compression pressure and crushing strength, or drug release, massing time and compression pressure in an effort to maximize either tablet strength or to pick the simplest lubricant. Although trends were observed but no optimal formulations got. The trends were like those generated by statistical procedures. Comparable neural network models were generated then optimized using genetic algorithms.it had been found that the optimum formulation trusted the constraints applied to ingredient levels utilized in the formulation and therefore the relative importance placed on the output parameters. A high tablet strength and low friability could only be obtained at the expense of disintegration time. Altogether cases lactose was the well-liked diluents and fluidized bed was the well-liked granulating technique.

6.5.3 In Product Development

The pharmaceutical development process may be a multivariate optimization problem. It involves the optimization of formulation and process variables. one among the foremost useful properties of artificial neural networks is their ability to generalize. These features make them suitable for solving problems within the area of optimization of formulations in pharmaceutical development.(*Zhu H., 2020*)

6.5.4 Self-Learning AI Platforms Like Artificial Neural Network (ANN)

and style of Experiment (DoE) helps in understanding inter-parameter interactions and further supports in composition and process optimization. It helps in developing a multivariate correlation to get a top quality drug product, supported understanding of cause-effect relationship between formulation ingredients/process parameters and quality target product profile. ANNs provided a useful gizmo for the event of microemulsion-based drug-delivery systems during which experimental effort was minimized. ANNs were used to predict the phase behavior of quaternary microemulsion-forming systems consisting of oil, water and two surfactants. ANN was also used to simulate aerosol behavior, with a view to employing this type of methodology in the evaluation and design of pulmonary drug-delivery systems. For controlling and decision-making, symbolic logic may be a very powerful problem-solving technique. It provides very useful rules from input data, in the form of "if... so... then". Fuzzy logic can be combined with neural networks as neuro fuzzy logic. This combination provides more flexibility and capability to the technique and provides powerful results ANN (Artificial Neural Network) models showed better fitting and predicting abilities in the development of solid dosage forms in investigations of the effects of several factors (such as formulation, compression parameters) on tablet properties (such as dissolution).*(Ciallella HL, 2019)*

6.5.5 In Genomics

Currently, the platform is being used to discover molecules for treatment of neurological diseases. Additionally, Broad Institute of MIT and Harvard offering to welcome sequencing, genotyping and expression projects. They currently offer access to the platforms like Human Whole Exome Sequencing, Human Whole Transcriptome Sequencing, Data Analysis etc. HealNet is one of the largest and complex database systems available for existing drugs for rare diseases. This database is developed by Healx and it contains more than billion documented interactions among patients, existing drug molecules and rare diseases. It uses machine learning and AI to repurpose drug molecules for curing rare diseases. Also, Ligand Express, a cloud-based platform from Cyclica, leverages biophysics and AI to identify drug target, mechanism of action, elucidation of adverse effect and repurposing of small molecules.*(Chan HS, 2019)*

6.5.6 In Personalized Medicine

All individuals are not same with respect to physical structure, rate of metabolism, genetic makeup etc, and therefore the therapy/dose needs to be personalized based on individual requirement. Methods like artificial intelligence and the underlying machine learning can provide the framework to stratify patients, initiate specific tailored treatments and thus increase response rates, reduce adverse effects and medical errors. GNS Healthcare's "Reverse Engineering and Forward Simulation" (REFS), a machine-learning and simulation platform, aids in finding and validating potential new drug candidates based on patient response marker and thus leading to personalized treatments that are better match to individual patients.*(Brown N., 2015)*

6.5.7 In Rare Disease Identification

Using AI, body scans can detect cancer and other diseases early, as well as predict health issues people might face based on their genetics. Although far from perfect, IBM Watson for Oncology is currently the leader in AI for personalized treatment decisions in the oncology space. It uses each patient's medical information and history to optimize the treatment decision-making. Recently, Watson correctly diagnosed a rare form of leukemia in a patient originally thought to have acute myeloid leukemia. It reportedly examined millions of oncology research papers in 10 minutes after which it successfully diagnosed the patient and recommended a personalized treatment plan.(*Pereira JC, 2016*)

6.5.8 In Clinical Trial Research

Tencent Holdings, along with Medopad, has developed AI algorithms for patients suffering from Parkinson's disease. AI monitors patient's movement via smartphone camera and determines the severity of the symptoms. Further, it also permits the doctor to monitor patient remotely, adjust dose and fix doctor's appointment.

6.5.9 In Data Management

This includes management of medical records. Using a sensor or mobile application like AiCure, a patient's medication use are often monitored in real-time by AI. This could be especially beneficial for patients in whom adherence is an issue and for clinical trials. IoT and its integration with various wearables to have the real time data sent over to a centralized processing center can help monitor the patients without being physically present. (*Firth NC, 2015*)

6.5.10 Betterment in Patient Care

Artificial Intelligence is on track to wholly alter the future of healthcare. With the integration of AI into the work of both medical professionals and hospital systems, one can expect to see dramatic changes in both patient health outcomes and in the operational efficiency of hospitals. The "open AI ecosystem" is one among the highest 10 promising technologies in 2016. It is useful to gather and compare the info from social awareness algorithms. In healthcare system vast information is recorded which incorporates patient medical record and treatment data from childhood thereto age. This enormous data can be analyzed by the ecosystems and gives suggestions about lifestyle and habits of the patient.

6.5.11 Internet of Medical Things (IoMT)

Earlier, due to different information formats for different methods in a medication manufacturing plant, data access and understanding posed a significant challenge for operative communication. IoT technologies based on various underlying communication protocols for example NFC, Bluetooth, Ultra Wide Band and 5G empower calibration within a pharmaceutical manufacturing plant by meritoriously connecting network, equipment, and schemes across the plant. Moreover, using IoT, pharma companies can gain access to instantaneous data and prominence of operations through the whole manufacturing process. The Internet of Things (IoT) has a massive effect on many industries universal. But, the pharmaceutical industry has been relatively conservative in implementing technological variation, so the belongings haven't been felt as powerfully across the pharmaceutical and medical industry yet. However, the IoT has unbelievable potential to help pharma and device companies recover superiority output, reduce costs, and even change the way that medication is delivered to the prescribers.(*Zhang L, 2017*)

6.6.12.1 Industrial Mechanics and Maintenance

Although the use of industrial monitoring devices is already widespread in the pharmaceutical industry, real-time status information is yet to be widely available. Using pharma IoT monitoring sensors, companies can instantaneously feed all relevant facility data into a single dashboard and can alert a supervisor in case of any abnormal conditions or urgent maintenance requirements. IoT in pharmaceutical manufacturing will also enable handling critical conditions remotely.

6.6.12.2 Managing Pharma Supply Chain

Once the drugs leave the manufacturing plant, they travel through different modes of transport and may be subject to varying temperatures and weather conditions. Although in most cases care is undertaken to maintain the packages within the prescribed temperatures, chances of variations during transit cannot be completely ruled out. IoT can be helpful in such situations to provide real-time data to manufacturers with improved supply chain visibility. The temperature changes or any damage to the products will be immediately notified to the manufacturers to determine whether the drugs are fit to sell or not.(*Gupta S, 2015*)

6.6.12.3 Controlling Drug Manufacturing Environment

In pharmaceutical manufacturing, sub-optimal environmental conditions can often prove to be fatal. However, this obstacle can be easily overcome using IoT. Pharma IoT establishes transparency in drug production and storage environment by allowing multiple sensors to monitor environmental indicators such as temperature, humidity, radiation, and light in real time.

6.6.12.4 Smart Pills and Implanted Devices

Leading pharmaceutical companies are using smart devices to administer medications and monitor their effect on patients. This includes the delivery of medications or medical monitors in "smart pills." One use is simply to check whether patients, especially ones with lapses in memory, are taking their medications on schedule. If they miss a dose or consultation, it will give them a prompt reminder on their phone to help get them back on track. If they fall too far behind schedule, it can notify their physician to step in. Smart pills or implanted devices can also detect changes in a patient's condition. For example; if there is a serious event, such as a hypoglycemic episode, the device can immediately alert a physician or paramedic.

7. APPLICATION OF AI, ML, AND IOMT IN PHARMACEUTICAL DRUG DISCOVERY

Internet of Things is a reality in today's era of digitization and, therefore, it deems fit that Pharma companies adopt it at the earliest. Though IOT is still in its nascent stages of development and adoption across industries, it is imperative for Pharma companies to include IOT as part of their strategic focus. This will help them start exploring and implementing IOT applications across value chain components that are ailing and are potential candidates for IOT adoption. This would require companies to take reformative steps such as rehauling systems and processes and transforming business models using nextgen architectures. On one hand, IoT offers added quality, agility and value to the business; on the other hand, it promises tremendous opportunities for innovation and can lead to a new era of transformation in Pharma.

7.1 Machine Learning

Machine Learning in pharma and medicine could generate a value of up to $100B annually, based on better decision making, optimized innovation, improved efficiency of research/clinical trials, and new tool creation for physicians, consumers, insurers, and regulators. Research and development (R&D); physicians and clinics; patients; caregivers; etc. The array of (at present) disparate origins is part of the issue in synchronizing this information and using it to improve healthcare infrastructure and treatments. Hence, the present-day core issue at the intersection of machine learning and healthcare: finding ways to effectively collect and use lots of different types of data for better analysis, prevention, and treatment of individuals. Burgeoning applications of ML in pharma and medicine are glimmers of a potential future in which synchronicity of data, analysis, and innovation are an everyday reality. We provide a breakdown of several of these pioneering applications, and provide insight into areas for continued innovation.

7.2 Disease Identification/Diagnosis

Disease identification and diagnosis of ailments is at the forefront of ML research in medicine. According to a 2015 report issued by Pharmaceutical Research and Manufacturers of America, more than 800 medicines and vaccines to treat cancer were in trial. In an interview with Bloomberg Technology, Knight Institute Researcher Jeff Tyner stated that while this is exciting, it also presents the challenge of finding ways to work with all the resulting data. "That is where the idea of a biologist working with information scientists and computation lists is so important," said Tyner. It's no surprise that large players were some of the first to jump on the bandwagon, particularly in high-need areas like cancer identification and treatment. In October 2016, IBM Watson Health announced IBM Watson Genomics, a partnership initiative with Quest Diagnostics, which aims to make strides in precision medicine by integrating cognitive computing and genomic tumor sequencing.

7.3 Personalized Treatment/ Behavioral Modification

Personalized medicine, or more effective treatment based on individual health data paired with predictive analytics, is also a hot research area and closely related to better disease assessment. The domain is presently ruled by supervised learning, which allows physicians to select from more limited sets of diagnoses, for example, or estimate patient risk based on symptoms and genetic information.

7.4 Drug Discovery/Manufacturing

The use of machine learning in preliminary (early-stage) drug discovery has the potential for various uses, from initial screening of drug compounds to predicted success rate based on biological factors. This includes R&D discovery technologies like next-generation sequencing. Precision medicine, which involves identifying mechanisms for "multifactorial" diseases and in turn alternative paths for therapy, seems to be the frontier in this space. Much of this research involves unsupervised learning, which is in large part still confined to identifying patterns in data without predictions (the latter is still in the realm of supervised learning).

7.5 Clinical Trial Research

Machine learning has several useful potential applications in helping shape and direct clinical trial research. Applying advanced predictive analytics in identifying candidates for clinical trials could draw on a much wider range of data than at present, including social media and doctor visits, for example, as well as genetic information when looking to target specific populations; this would result in smaller, quicker, and less expensive trials overall. ML can also be used for remote monitoring and real-time data access for increased safety; for example, monitoring biological and other signals for any sign of harm or death to participants. According to McKinsey, there are many other ML applications for helping increase clinical trial efficiency, including finding best sample sizes for increased efficiency; addressing and adapting to differences in sites for patient recruitment; and using electronic medical records to reduce data errors (duplicate entry, for example).

7.6 Radiology and Radiotherapy

In an October 2016 interview with Stat News, Dr. Ziad Obermeyer, an assistant professor at Harvard Medical School, stated: "In 20 years, radiologists won't exist in anywhere near their current form. They might look more like cyborgs: supervising algorithms reading thousands of studies per minute." Until that day comes, Google's DeepMind Health is working with University College London Hospital (UCLH) to develop machine learning algorithms capable of detecting differences in healthy and cancerous tissues to help improve radiation treatments.

7.7 Smart Electronic Health Records

Document classification (sorting patient queries via email, for example) using support vector machines, and optical character recognition (transforming cursive or other sketched handwriting into digitized characters), are both essential ML-based technologies in helping advance the collection and digitization of electronic health information. MATLAB's ML handwriting recognition technologies and Google's Cloud Vision API for optical character recognition are just two examples of innovations in this area: Artificial Neural Network using MATLAB – Handwritten Character Recognition The MIT Clinical Machine Learning Group is spearheading the development of next-generation intelligent electronic health records, which will incorporate built-in ML/AI to help with things like diagnostics, clinical decisions, and personalized treatment suggestions. MIT notes on its research site the "need for robust machine learning algorithms that are safe, interpretable, can learn from little labeled training data, understand natural language, and generalize well across medical settings and institutions."(*King RD, 1995*)

7.8 Epidemic Outbreak Prediction

ML and AI technologies are also being applied to monitoring and predicting epidemic outbreaks around the world, based on data collected from satellites, historical information on the web, real-time social media updates, and other sources. The opioid epidemic is a direct example of AI technology being utilized today. Support vector machines and artificial neural networks have been used, for example, to predict malaria outbreaks, taking into account data such as temperature, average monthly rainfall, total number of positive cases, and other data points.

7.9 IoMT-Based-Drug-Discovery Models

have shown their worth in pharmaceutical and healthcare industries by improving the efficiency in therapeutic drug manufacturing, real-time health monitoring, and predictive forecasting. AI has already shown its promise in drug discovery and is being implemented in different phases, from ***drug design to drug screening***. In 2020, the DL model "Alphafold" solved a 50-year-old problem by accurately predicting the structure of a protein from its amino acid sequence. Alphafold performed better with 0.7 and higher TM scores for 24 out of 43 free modeling domains compared to the second best protein-structure prediction method. AI has proven to be a potential tool in the early-stage detection of Alzheimer's, cancer, diabetes, and cardiac diseases, even in the asymptomatic stages. The review reports on the recent developments and advancements made mainly in AI-supported IoMT devices for efficient biosensing needed for successful disease management. In support of aspects of AI and IoMT, we have discussed the significance of nanotechnology in the IoMT platform for developing next-generation biomedical devices such as e-skin, e-nose, and e-textiles. AI-integrated IoMT devices are important in crucial medical areas such as cardiac monitoring, surgeries, diabetes, and cancer monitoring. Through cloud computing, AI has shown promise in monitoring cardiac electrophysiology and imaging. The innovations made by AI in the surgery sector are noteworthy. One such remarkable invention is the Davinci surgical system, a robotic-assisted surgical system. AI interfacing established a quantum shift in diabetes and cancer management in a personalized manner. Apparently, AI cannot do multiple jobs at a time, and the complete replacement of a physician is still yet to be developed. Despite this shortcoming, AI has proven its excellence in the medical field with continuous evolvement. The outcome of this review motivates young researchers to promote and investigate combinational approaches involving nano-enabled sensing, AI, and IoMT for efficient biosensing needed for disease control and management in a personalized manner.(*Wang Y, 2015*)

8. CONCLUSION AND FUTURE SCOPE

Lower success rate in drug discovery phase with huge speculation of money and time, is one of the most critical reasons for decline in number of NCEs being discovered. In order to conflict these challenges, many pharma companies have already adopted AI in their research program. Both IoT and AI are powerful and are capable of making your business smarter. And if you combine these two technologies, it will enable enterprises to achieve even greater digital transformation. There are tons of domains that can harvest the advantages of the coexistence of both technologies. Uptake in pharmaceutical industry has been relatively slow compared to others. But in order to stay relevant the industry will need to adapt faster. AI can play a critical role in health industry, like exploring the unmet medical needs of healthcare sector, meeting the pace with which resistance is being developed for molecules such as anti-tuberculosis, and matching the rate at which new diseases are being identified. The traditional drug discovery approach can take up to 10 to 15 years and about $2.5 billion investment to bring a molecule from conceptual stage to market.

REFERENCES

Awad, A., Trenfield, S. J., Pollard, T. D., Ong, J. J., Elbadawi, M., McCoubrey, L. E., Goyanes, A., Gaisford, S., & Basit, A. W. (2021). Connected healthcare: Improving patient care using digital health technologies. *Advanced Drug Delivery Reviews*, 178, 113958. DOI: 10.1016/j.addr.2021.113958 PMID: 34478781

Baronzio, G., Parmar, G., & Baronzio, M. (2015, July 23). Overview of methods for overcoming hindrance to drug delivery to tumors, with special attention to tumor interstitial fluid. *Frontiers in Oncology*, 5, 165. DOI: 10.3389/fonc.2015.00165 PMID: 26258072

Blasiak, A., Khong, J., & Kee, T. (2020, April 1). CURATE. AI: Optimizing personalized medicine with artificial intelligence. *SLAS Technology*, 25(2), 95–105. DOI: 10.1177/2472630319890316 PMID: 31771394

Brown, N. (2015). *In silico medicinal chemistry: computational methods to support drug design*. Royal Society of Chemistry.

Chan, H. S., Shan, H., Dahoun, T., Vogel, H., & Yuan, S. (2019). Advancing drug discovery via artificial intelligence. *Trends in Pharmacological Sciences*, 40(8), 592–604.

Ciallella, H. L., & Zhu, H. (2019, March 14). Advancing computational toxicology in the big data era by artificial intelligence: Data-driven and mechanism-driven modeling for chemical toxicity. *Chemical Research in Toxicology*, 32(4), 536–547. DOI: 10.1021/acs.chemrestox.8b00393 PMID: 30907586

Dash, S., Shakyawar, S. K., Sharma, M., & Kaushik, S. (2019). Big data in healthcare: Management, analysis and future prospects. *Journal of Big Data*, 6(1), 1–25. DOI: 10.1186/s40537-019-0217-0

Dasta, J. F. (1992). Application of artificial intelligence to pharmacy and medicine. *Hospital Pharmacy*, 27(4), 312–315.

Ding, B. (2018). Pharma Industry 4.0: Literature review and research opportunities in sustainable pharmaceutical supply chains. *Process Safety and Environmental Protection*, 119, 115–130. DOI: 10.1016/j.psep.2018.06.031

Duch, W., Swaminathan, K., & Meller, J. (2007, May 1). Artificial intelligence approaches for rational drug design and discovery. *Current Pharmaceutical Design*, 13(14), 1497–1508. DOI: 10.2174/138161207780765954 PMID: 17504169

Estrela, V. V., Monteiro, A. C. B., França, R. P., Iano, Y., Khelassi, A., & Razmjooy, N. (2018). Health 4.0: applications, management, technologies and review: array. *Medical Technologies Journal*, 2(4), 262–276.

Firth, N. C., Atrash, B., Brown, N., & Blagg, J. (2015, June 22). MOARF, an integrated workflow for multiobjective optimization: Implementation, synthesis, and biological evaluation. *Journal of Chemical Information and Modeling*, 55(6), 1169–1180. DOI: 10.1021/acs.jcim.5b00073 PMID: 26054755

Golberg, D. E. (1989). Genetic algorithms in search, optimization, and machine learning. Addion wesley, 1989(102), 36.

Gupta, S., Sapre, N., & Sapre, N. S. (2015). In silico de novo design of novel NNRTIs: A bio-molecular modelling approach. *RSC Advances*, 5(19), 14814–14827. DOI: 10.1039/C4RA15478A

Holmes, J., Sacchi, L., & Bellazzi, R. (2004). Artificial intelligence in medicine. *Annals of the Royal College of Surgeons of England*, 86(5), 334–338. DOI: 10.1308/147870804290 PMID: 15333167

King, R. D., Hirst, J. D., & Sternberg, M. J. (1995, March 1). Comparison of artificial intelligence methods for modeling pharmaceutical QSARS. *Applied Artificial Intelligence*, 9(2), 213–233. DOI: 10.1080/08839519508945474

Lamberti, M. J., Wilkinson, M., Donzanti, B. A., Wohlhieter, G. E., Parikh, S., Wilkins, R. G., & Getz, K. (2019, August 1). A study on the application and use of artificial intelligence to support drug development. *Clinical Therapeutics*, 41(8), 1414–1426. DOI: 10.1016/j.clinthera.2019.05.018 PMID: 31248680

Mak, K. K., & Pichika, M. R. (2019, March 1). Artificial intelligence in drug development: Present status and future prospects. *Drug Discovery Today*, 24(3), 773–780. DOI: 10.1016/j.drudis.2018.11.014 PMID: 30472429

Miles, J. C., & Walker, A. J. (2006, September). The potential application of artificial intelligence in transport. In IEE proceedings-intelligent transport systems (Vol. 153, No. 3, pp. 183-198). IET Digital Library.

Mishra, V. (2018, May 30). Artificial intelligence: The beginning of a new era in pharmacy profession. [AJP]. *Asian Journal of Pharmaceutics*, 12(02).

Pereira, J. C., Caffarena, E. R., & Dos Santos, C. N. (2016, December 27). Boosting docking-based virtual screening with deep learning. *Journal of Chemical Information and Modeling*, 56(12), 2495–2506. DOI: 10.1021/acs.jcim.6b00355 PMID: 28024405

Sellwood, M. A., Ahmed, M., Segler, M. H., & Brown, N. (2018, September). Artificial intelligence in drug discovery. *Future Medicinal Chemistry*, 10(17), 2025–2028. DOI: 10.4155/fmc-2018-0212 PMID: 30101607

Shapiro, S. C. (1992). Artificial intelligence. Encyclopedia of Artificial intelligence: Vol. 1. *2ndedn*. Wiley.

Smith, R. G., & Farquhar, A. (2000). The road ahead for knowledge management: An AI perspective. *AI Magazine*, 21(4), 17–17.

Wang, Y., Guo, Y., Kuang, Q., Pu, X., Ji, Y., Zhang, Z., & Li, M. (2015, April). A comparative study of family-specific protein–ligand complex affinity prediction based on random forest approach. *Journal of Computer-Aided Molecular Design*, 29(4), 349–360. DOI: 10.1007/s10822-014-9827-y PMID: 25527073

Wirtz, B. W., Weyerer, J. C., & Geyer, C. (2019, May 19). Artificial intelligence and the public sector—Applications and challenges. *International Journal of Public Administration*, 42(7), 596–615. DOI: 10.1080/01900692.2018.1498103

Zhang, L., Tan, J., Han, D., & Zhu, H. (2017, November 1). From machine learning to deep learning: Progress in machine intelligence for rational drug discovery. *Drug Discovery Today*, 22(11), 1680–1685. DOI: 10.1016/j.drudis.2017.08.010 PMID: 28881183

Zhu, H. (2020, January 1). Big data and artificial intelligence modeling for drug discovery. *Annual Review of Pharmacology and Toxicology*, 60(1), 573–589. DOI: 10.1146/annurev-pharmtox-010919-023324 PMID: 31518513

KEY TERMS AND DEFINITIONS

Artificial Intelligence: AI is defined as computer systems able to perform tasks that normally require human intelligence. It comprises three distinct types: human-created algorithms, machine-learning, and deep learning.

Approaches of AI: Artificial Intelligence (AI) is the branch of engineering science which deals with creating and implementing intelligent computer programs which make the machines capable of making intelligent decisions during operation.

Applications of AI: It refers to the ability of a computer or a robotic computer enabled system to process the given information and produce outcomes in a manner similar to the attention process of humans in learning, deciding and solving problems.

Genomics: It has developed a platform technology that maps genes which are responsible for causing disease and then maps the drug molecule that target them to provide cure.

Internet of Medical Things (IoMT): It has the supremacy to modernize pharmaceutical manufacturing in processes ranging from drug discovery to secluded patient access and monitoring. Numerous top pharma companies from around the gradually adopting IoT technologies in their developed plants to accomplish optimization and improve development efficiency.

Applications of AI in Drug Discovery: AI is being used to accelerate progress and improve decision making in various sectors and disciplines of drug discovery and development, including medicinal chemistry, upscaling, molecular and cell biology, pharmacology, pharmacokinetics, formulation development, and toxicity.

Chapter 16
Healthcare Monitoring System Driven by Machine Learning and Internet of Medical Things (MLIoMT)

Kutubuddin Sayyad Liyakat Kazi
https://orcid.org/0000-0001-5623-9211
Brahmdevdada Mane Institute of Technology, India

ABSTRACT

The primary objective of the project is to develop an ML-based healthcare system that can quickly and accurately diagnose a variety of diseases. Seven machine learning classification algorithms were used in this work to forecast nine deadly diseases, such as kidney disorders, hepatitis, diabetes, and blood pressure: adaptive boosting, Random Forest, DT, Support Vector Machines, Naïve Bayes, Artificial Neural Networks, and K-Nearest Neighbour. Performance metrics including Precision, Accuracy, and Recall are used to assess the suggested model's effectiveness. The performance of the classifiers is evaluated using four metrics: accuracy, precision, recall, and precision. For every ailment, the current healthcare model achieves a minimum accuracy of 82.3% and a maximum accuracy of 95.7%. There are minimal and maximum precision and recall values for each disease: 81.4% and 95.7%, respectively, and 64.3% and 90.3%, respectively. This ML driven IoMT approach we call as DL approach.

INTRODUCTION

Given that healthcare is a basic human right in every society, there is an increasing demand for an effective healthcare system (Nagare, 2014, 2015). Advancements in technology led by Kazi K S (2022, 2023) have made healthcare monitoring systems an indispensable instrument for raising the standard of healthcare delivery.

A healthcare monitoring system is an all-inclusive and integrated framework that sends data to a central database from a variety of medical equipment and sensors, including blood pressure, glucose, and heart rate monitors. Following processing, Kutubuddin S. L. (2022a), Kazi (2022) utilize this data to track a person's health, spot possible problems, and assess how well a treatment is working.

DOI: 10.4018/979-8-3693-6180-1.ch016

One of a healthcare monitoring system's primary advantages is its ability to deliver data in real time. This implies that medical specialists can keep eyes on patients from a distance and respond quickly to treat them when needed. This is especially important for those who need ongoing care due to chronic conditions. By providing patients with prompt medical attention, a healthcare monitoring system lowers the incidence of problems and improves overall health outcomes.

Healthcare monitoring systems could be helpful in spotting possible health problems before they worsen. These technologies allow for the discovery of data patterns and trends across time that can point to a possible health issue. This lowers the likelihood of hospitalization and enhances the quality of life for patients by empowering medical professionals to take preventative actions and offer early interventions by Ravi (2022).

Enhancing patient engagement and self-care is another benefit of healthcare monitoring systems. Patients can easily track their personal health information and maintain communication with their healthcare professionals by utilizing wearable technologies and smartphone applications (Altaf, 2023). This gives people the ability to take charge of their health and enables medical experts to keep their eyes on their progress and deliver individualized care.

The quality and cost-effectiveness of healthcare services can both be enhanced via healthcare monitoring systems. By utilizing these technologies, the time and costs associated with in-person visits and hospital stays can be reduced for both patients and healthcare providers. Patients who live in isolated or rural locations and do not have easy access to medical services would particularly benefit from this.

Healthcare monitoring systems will assist medical professionals in treating patients as well as efficiently managing their workload and resources. These technologies can free up healthcare workers' time so they can concentrate on giving their patients high-quality care by automating data collecting and processing.

According to Sultanabanu(2024a)(2024b)(2024c), Kazi K(2024b), Healthcare monitoring systems have difficulties, just like any other technology. Two of the most important ones are patient data security and privacy. Since these systems gather this kind of information, it is crucial to make sure that adequate safeguards are in place to stop the misuse of private health information.

Integrating these systems into the current healthcare system presents another difficulty. The range of medical equipment and software used by healthcare facilities makes it difficult to combine data into a single, centralized system suggested by Sultanabanu(2024m)(2024l), Kazi K S(2024c). The healthcare practitioners, IT specialists, and vendors must carefully plan and organize this.

All things considered, by enhancing patient outcomes, raising productivity, and cutting expenses, healthcare monitoring systems have the potential to completely transform the healthcare sector. These systems will keep developing as long as technology does since they are essential to delivering high-quality healthcare. To ensure that these technologies are successfully implemented and utilized in the healthcare industry, it is imperative that the issues and obstacles surrounding them are addressed by Pradeepa (2022).

Within the field of artificial intelligence-AI, machine learning-ML is the branch of study that focuses on teaching algorithms to learn from data and act in a certain way even when they are expressly designed to make judgments or predictions. The broad range of applications this profession provides across many different industries has led to its current surge in popularity. According to Veena (2023), Kazi K (2024), K S L (2018), and K S (2017), machine learning(ML) has completely changed how data is handled, analyzed, and used, making it a vital tool for both individuals and organizations. Figure 1 depicts the possible use of machine learning in 2024, based on published research.

Data analysis is one of machine learning's main uses. Data is growing exponentially in the digital age, making traditional data analysis techniques labor-intensive and outdated. However, ML algorithms can process massive volumes of data fast and effectively, allowing for the extraction of significant patterns and insights. Businesses like marketing, finance, and healthcare—where data analysis is crucial to decision-making—have benefited most from this, according to Kazi K S (2024).

Natural language processing (NLP) is an intriguing field in which machine learning is being used. The area of AI called natural language processing (NLP) focuses on how human and computer languages work together. The development of apps like chatbots, virtual assistants, and language translation tools is made possible by ML algorithms' capacity to comprehend and analyze human language. According to Kazi K, these devices have become an indispensable aspect of our daily existence due to their enhanced efficacy in communication and information retrieval (2022).

Furthermore, machine learning has made significant advancements in the field of CV-computer vision. The ability of computer systems to analyze and comprehend visual input, such as pictures and videos, is known as computer vision. ML techniques have made it possible for computers to recognize and categorize items in photos and videos with accuracy. This makes it possible to develop applications like self-driving automobiles, facial recognition software, and object detection technologies. These applications have the potential to improve security and efficiency in a number of industries, including manufacturing, transportation, and security, claims Kazi K S (2024).

The developments in machine learning have also been extremely beneficial to the healthcare sector. By analyzing enormous volumes of patient data for possible health issues, ML algorithms allow physicians to accurately identify patients. As a result, medical treatments are now shorter and less expensive while maintaining the same level of care. Furthermore, Pardeshi has been able to offer patients more precise and effective care since ML has been applied to drug discovery and personalized treatment plans (2022).

Furthermore, the way that a variety of products and services feel to use has been profoundly altered by machine learning. Recommender systems, which are based on ML algorithms, are frequently used by businesses like Netflix and Amazon to provide their customers with personalized recommendations. This has not only improved customer satisfaction but also generated revenue for these businesses by enticing clients to purchase pertinent goods and services from Kutubuddin (2022), Kazi K S (2023), Liyakat (2023) (2024), and K K S (2023).

Machine learning has been applied in the banking sector to activities such as fraud detection, investment forecasting, and risk evaluation. A lot of financial data can be analyzed using ML algorithms. In order to reduce risks, they can also help identify fraudulent activity and spot questionable tendencies. Additionally, machine learning (ML) has been used to construct trading algorithms that can accurately foresee and make judgment calls, which will assist investors in making better judgments.

All things considered, machine learning has completely changed the way we handle and evaluate data, making it a vital tool for a wide range of sectors. Its uses in data analysis, CV, natural language processing (NLP), healthcare, user experience, and finance have shown to be quite advantageous. In the future, these applications could totally change a variety of different industries. We should anticipate additional state-of-the-art ML apps that will improve the convenience and effectiveness of our daily lives as technology develops.

Internet of Things (IoT), a rapidly evolving technology, is fundamentally altering the way we live and work. It is an automated internet-based network of interconnected hardware, software, and sensors that have communicate with each other without the need for human intervention. According to Wale (2019) and Mishra (2024b), the aforementioned technology has potential to completely transform markets, increase efficiency, and provide new opportunities for commerce and consumers.

Even though the concept of the IoT like artificial intelligence, big data, and cloud computing by Prasad(2024). Massive amounts of data that are now able to be gathered, saved, and analyzed are at the heart of the IoT Mishra (2024a) Kasat (2023).

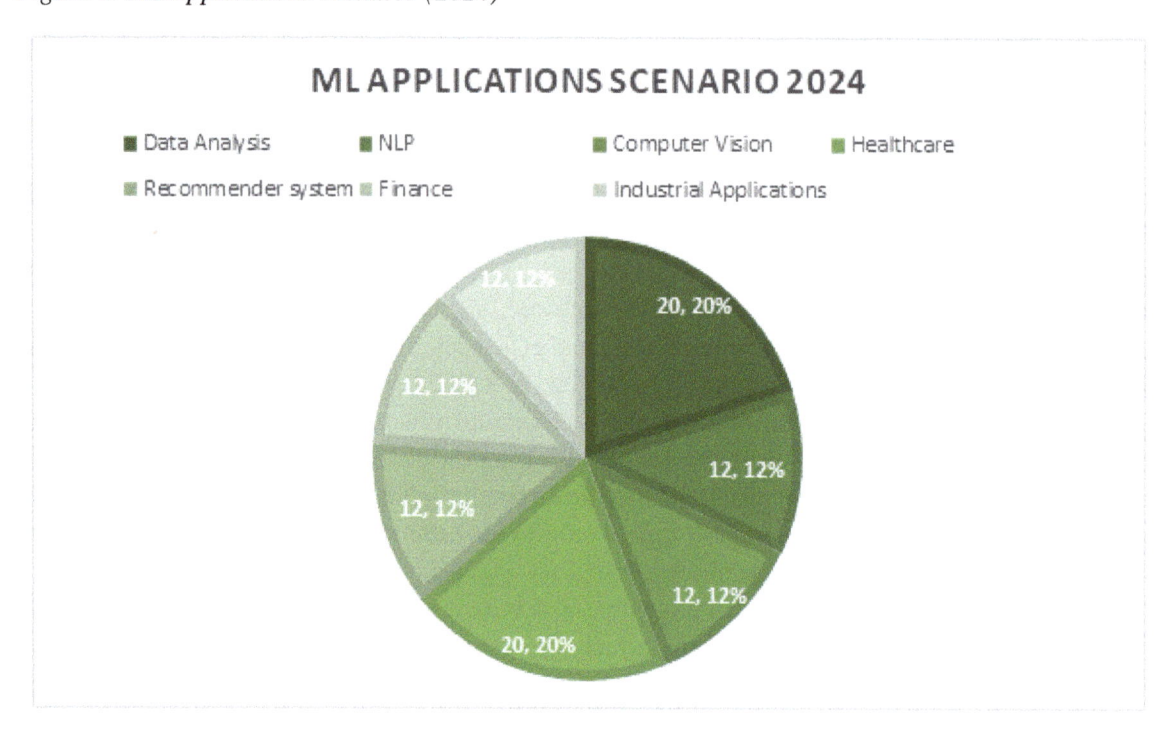

Figure 1. ML applications scenario (2024)

IoT can transform almost every aspect of our life and has a plethora of applications, according to Kutubuddin (2022b). Figure 2 lists some of the most significant applications of the IoT, from industrial automation to smart homes:

1. **Smart Homes:** Homeowners may now monitor and manage their properties from a distance thanks to IoT. By handling anything from turning on lights and altering the temperature to managing home appliances and security systems, IoT-enabled devices have increased our lives' convenience and security by Kazi K S L (2022).
2. **Healthcare:** IoT is transforming the healthcare industry by offering remote patient monitoring, real-time vital sign tracking, and prescription administration. Furthermore, Kazi Kutubuddin(2023a,2023b) is using it to monitor and improve the performance of medical equipment, reducing downtime and improving patient care (Megha(2024)).

3. **Industrial Automation:** This IoT is transfiguring the manufacturing sector by empowering real-time monitoring and management of industrial advancements. Thanks to this technology, businesses have been able to increase overall productivity, reduce costs, and improve efficiency by Sultanabanu(2023a), (2023b), (2023c), (2023d), and (2023e).
4. **Transportation:** The use of IoT in this industry has led to an increase in smart cars, trains, and airplanes. The sensors and software integrated into these vehicles, which collect data on fuel consumption, maintenance needs, and traffic conditions by KKS(2022), Nikita(2022), and Kazi K(2024), enable better navigation and enhanced safety.
5. **Agriculture:** This industry is rapidly modernizing thanks to IoT. With the use of sensors and analytics, farmers can keep an eye on crop health, soil moisture content, and weather patterns, leading to more effective farming methods and higher yields by K K(2022), Wale(2019).
6. **Retail:** This IoT is transforming the retail sector by providing analytical data on consumer behavior and preferences. By using this data, retailers may enhance the general shopping experience, manage inventories more effectively, and target marketing campaigns more precisely (Karale, 2023; Vahida2023) by Kazi K S(2024a, 2024b).
7. **Energy Management:** Energy use in homes, buildings, and communities is maximized through the use of IoT. According to K Kazi (2022), smart energy meters, connected appliances, and smart lighting systems are examples of IoT-enabled energy cost and utilization savings.
8. **Smart Cities:** This IoT can be used to build smart cities by assimilating various systems, such as energy, transportation, and public services. According to Kasat (2023) and Sultana (2023f), this technology improves the quality of life for residents, reduces the negative environmental effects of urban areas, and enables better resource management.

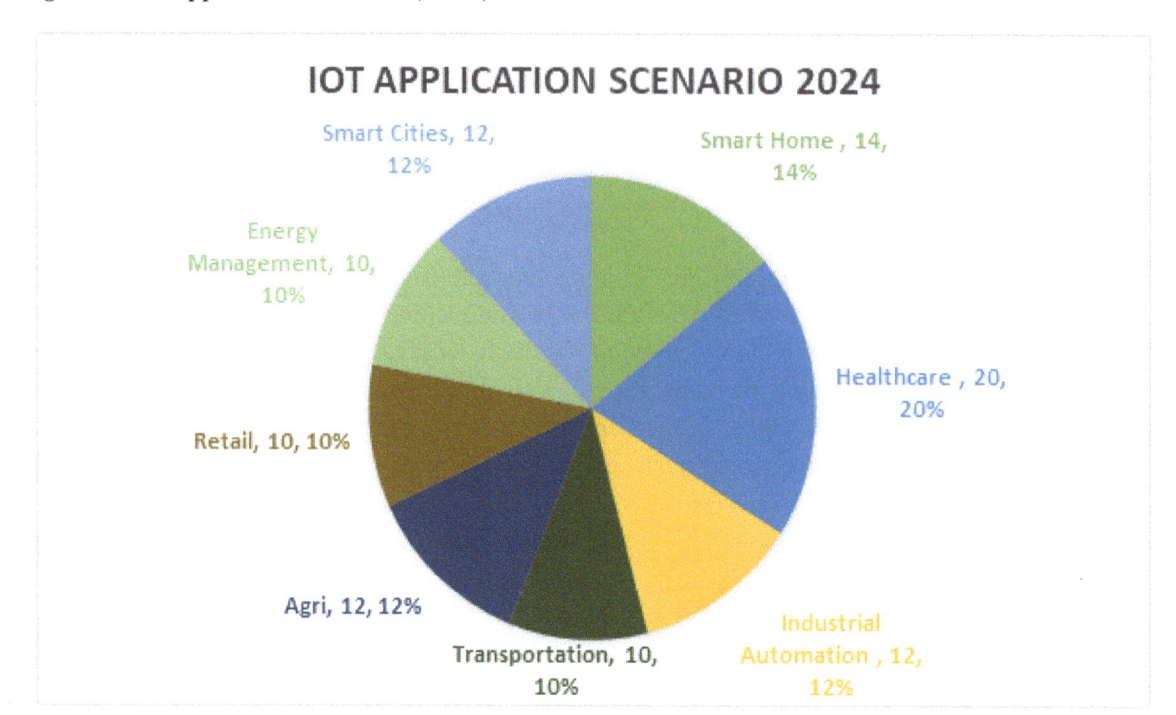

Figure 2. IoT application scenario (2024)

IOT APPLICATION SCENARIO 2024

- Smart Cities, 12, 12%
- Smart Home, 14, 14%
- Energy Management, 10, 10%
- Healthcare, 20, 20%
- Retail, 10, 10%
- Agri, 12, 12%
- Transportation, 10, 10%
- Industrial Automation, 12, 12%

The uses of IoT are constantly expanding, and its potential is limitless. As more devices become connected, the amount of data generated will increase quickly, leading to even more innovative uses for this sort of technology by K S (2023).

The widespread use of IoT raises anxieties about privacy and data security. Because there are lakhs of devices associated to the internet, there is a possibility of data breaches and cyberattacks. Accordingly, it is crucial that people and businesses implement the right security measures to safeguard their information and gadgets by Halli (2022), K. Kazi (2017). To overcome this disadvantage of insecurity, we suggest KK approach suggested by Dr. Kazi Kutubuddin (2024) for WSN and IoT networks by Liyakat(2024).

Taking everything into account, IoT with the globe. Its numerous applications could lead to the creation of a future that is more efficient, sustainable, and integrated. As we continue to employ this technology and work to realize all of its potential for the benefit of society, it is imperative that we resolve any problems that may come up (Sultanabanu, 2023f).

A network of medical devices, sensors, and systems that are connected to the internet is referred to as "Internet of Medical Things," or IoMT. These devices can collect and send data, which makes it possible to do data analysis, real-time intervention, and remote monitoring. This data can be used to speed up medical operations and improve patient care, as well as to enable new medical applications.

IoMT gadgets range in complexity from simple fitness trackers or intelligent insulin pumps to complex remote patient monitoring systems and intelligent insulin pumps. They can be used in a range of healthcare settings, including homes, clinics, and hospitals.

Benefits of IoMT

The application of IoMT is expected to yield significant benefits for the healthcare industry.

- One of the primary advantages is the ability to collect and analyze medical data in real time. Healthcare professionals who use this information to make well-informed decisions about patient care may see improved outcomes.
- Furthermore, IoMT can improve the efficiency of medical treatments. By deploying connected devices, medical personnel can monitor patients remotely, reducing the need for frequent hospital visits. This saves time for patients and medical staff while also lowering healthcare expenses.
- IoMT also makes possible previously unachievable novel medical uses. For example, remote patient monitoring systems can alert healthcare providers if a patient's vital signs show any abnormalities, allowing for early intervention and the prevention of serious health issues.

The Problems of IoMT

- IoMT has many potential benefits, but there are also certain disadvantages that need to be taken into account. Security and privacy of patient data are two of the main issues. As with any internet-connected device, there is a risk of data breaches and unauthorized access to personal health information. This illustrates the need for robust security measures to protect patient data. For IoT security, we recommend the KK method.
- Another challenge relates to interoperability amongst different IoMT systems and devices. With so many platforms and devices, it can be difficult to ensure that they can all connect with one other without interruption. Data silos could arise from this, preventing IoMT from realizing its full potential.

IoMT's Future

As long as technology continues to advance and improve, IoMT seems to have a bright future.

- Acknowledgements to developments in artificial intelligence and machine learning, IoMT devices are now able to analyze and interpret patient data more effectively and intelligently. This could lead to more precise and individualized healthcare.
- In addition, the increasing prevalence of telemedicine—especially since the COVID-19 pandemic—has raised awareness of the potential applications of IoMT. By facilitating remote consultations and monitoring, it increases patient convenience and accessibility to healthcare.
- The healthcare sector could undergo a transformation thanks to the IoMT, which could potentially contribute to better patient outcomes. Through real-time data collection and analysis, IoMT can enable more individualized and efficient healthcare. However, we must address the problems and ensure the security and interoperability of these devices. As technology advances, IoMT will only become more and more exciting, offering great possibilities for the future of healthcare.
- Recent years have seen a major impact on the healthcare industry from technological advancements. One of the most significant developments in this sector is the fusion of machine learning and IoT to create the powerful healthcare monitoring system known as MLIoT.

- The grouping of two cutting-edge technologies in DL approach suggested by Dr. Kazi Kutubuddin as Dilshad-Liyakat approach, ML and the IoT, or MLIoT, will revolutionize the healthcare industry. ML is a subset of AI, which uses statistical models and algorithms to analyze and learn from data, whereas IoT is a networked system of physical things that exchange and gather data by Kazi K (2024).
- In the healthcare sector, these two technologies have been combined to build automated, data-driven, intelligent systems that can monitor and assess patients' health in nearly real time. Healthcare services are now far more efficient, effective, and reasonably priced as a result.

The key benefit of MLIoMT –DL approach in the healthcare sector is its ability to collect and analyze massive amounts of patient data in real time. Wearable's, sensors, and Intelligent Medical Equipment are samples of IoT gadgets that can be used to continuously monitor and transfer patients' vital indicators, such as heart rate, blood pressure, and SO_2 level, to a central database. Subsequently, machine learning algorithms scrutinize this data to detect any patterns or irregularities in the patient's health, facilitating prompt detection and intervention.

Studies have demonstrated that persistent conditions including diabetes, heart-disease, and asthma can significantly benefit from this ongoing monitoring and assessment of patient data. These conditions require continuous monitoring and timely intervention, which can be efficiently offered by an MLIoMT-based healthcare system. Patients can also be notified of any changes in their health, which enables them to seek out preventative care and avoid hospitalization.

Furthermore, MLIoMT-based healthcare systems are increasing the accuracy and potency of treatment and diagnosis. With the help of ML algorithms, medical professionals may quickly review patient data and arrive at an accurate diagnosis. By doing this, doctors can design tailored treatment plans which take into account patient's medical past-info and information while also reducing the risk of a misdiagnosis.

The many notable advantages of MLIoMT for the healthcare sector is remote patient monitoring. This may be especially helpful for patients with long-term conditions or those who live in remote areas with limited access to medical services. IoT devices enable real-time patient data transmission to medical specialists and allow for remote patient monitoring. This allows for timely action and reduces the need for multiple hospital visits.

MLIoMT-based healthcare systems have the potential to improve the overall efficacy of healthcare services. Healthcare professionals can automate many activities, including as data collection, analysis, and communication, to free up time and focus on providing patients with high-quality treatment. It also eases the burden on the medical industry, enhancing its sustainability and affordability.

However, concerns over privacy and data security are growing as technology advances. Healthcare systems based on MLIoMT manage sensitive patient data, and a data leak could have disastrous consequences. According to Halli(2023a)(2023b), it is crucial to ensure that these systems have robust security measures in place to secure patient information. For security purpose, author suggests KK approach for IoT networks.

In our opinion, the combination of machine learning and IoT has resulted in a significant transformation of the healthcare industry. Since MLIoMT-based healthcare systems have improved the caliber, availability, and efficacy of healthcare services, they are now a vital tool for managing and preventing diseases. As technology advances, we might expect more developments in this field, which will enhance patient outcomes globally.

Problem Statement

Statement of the Problem: The fast growth of medical technologies has resulted in an influx of data, which presents opportunities as well as obstacles in the management of healthcare. The traditional healthcare system frequently has difficulties in successfully monitoring the health of patients in real time, which results in treatment plans that are reactive rather than ones that are proactive. This limitation is made much more difficult by the growing prevalence of chronic diseases, which necessitate ongoing monitoring and interventions at the appropriate time. Furthermore, the fragmented nature of healthcare information systems can be a barrier to the integration of vital patient data, which can lead to inadequate care delivery and bad outcomes for patients. As a consequence of this, there is an immediate demand for creative solutions that are able to make use of cutting-edge technologies in order to improve the monitoring of patients and the management of their health.

Goal

Establishing a comprehensive, real-time health monitoring framework that is powered by Machine Learning (ML) and the Internet of Medical Things (IoMT) is the fundamental objective of the Healthcare Monitoring System (HMS), which aims to achieve this objective. The Health Management System (HMS) is designed to provide continuous tracking of important health metrics through the integration of wearable devices, smart sensors, and powerful analytics. This would therefore make it possible to deliver prompt interventions and individualized care. The ultimate goal of this system is to strengthen the delivery of healthcare by facilitating the proactive management of patient health, lowering the number of hospital admissions, and improving the quality of life for individuals in general.

Objective of Study

The HMS will contain a number of important objectives, including the following:

- In order to provide a comprehensive view of a patient's health, data integration involves the seamless aggregation and analysis of data from a variety of Internet of Medical Things (IoMT) devices and electronic health records.
- Utilize machine learning algorithms to perform an analysis of both historical and real-time data in order to perform predictive analytics. This allows for the early detection of health deteriorations and promotes the implementation of preventative care measures.
- User engagement involves the creation of user interfaces that are easy to use for both patients and healthcare providers. These interfaces should encourage active participation in health management by means of alerts, reminders, and individualized health recommendations.
- Scalability and Interoperability: The system should be designed to be scalable and compatible with the healthcare infrastructures that are already in place. This will ensure that it is widely adopted and effectively integrated across a variety of healthcare settings.
- Enhanced Decision-Making: Make use of advanced analytics to better assist medical personnel in making well-informed decisions, which will ultimately lead to improved clinical outcomes through the utilization of data-driven insights.

- By concentrating on these goals, the Healthcare Monitoring System intends to usher in a new age of patient-centered care that not only tackles the issues that are currently being faced in the healthcare industry but also anticipates the expectations that will be placed on it in the future.

LITERATURE SURVEY

The application of ML by Heart Healthcare System is explained by Priya et al. (2023). In both developed and developing countries, cardiovascular diseases (CVD) currently cause more fatalities than all other causes combined. Early identification of cardiac problems and ongoing skilled care can lower the death rate. However, because it takes more thought, energy, and experience, it is still impractical to accurately diagnose cardiac problems in all situations and to provide 24-hour medical consultation. This research presented an underlying idea towards machine learning (ML)-based platform that employs ML approaches to estimate the probability of acquiring heart illness and identify heart disease in the not-too-distant future. Despite the growing number of empirical studies on the subject, especially from emerging nations, this discipline has less synthesized research publications. In the current era of rapidly expanding data availability, predictive modeling is becoming an increasingly important tool for services related to human safety and heart wellbeing. Heart-care organizations can make more educated decisions about how to best support their clients by using this cutting-edge technology, which uses data from past events to forecast future patterns and outcomes. Predictive analytics must be used properly, just like any other data-driven technology, to ensure moral and practical corporate operations. The analysis's featured papers center on ML-based heart healthcare system (HHS) forecasting. They used K-means Elbow for registration and notification, a decision tree for HHS, and MySQL for immunization reminders.

Sunita et al. provide an explanation of ML and IoT with reference to fruit and food quality for food safety (2023). This paper describes ML and IoT approach for tracking perishable goods. The recommended approach is to use IoT devices to upload high-resolution camera photographs to a distant server. Before being uploaded to cloud server, K-means clustering was utilized to segment these photographs. After PCA is used to extract attributes from the photos, trained ML algorithms are applied to classify the images. This proposed method used IoT, ML, and image processing to track perishable food.

Niraja et al.'s (2024) Hand Gesture Recognition System makes use of Ml. Human-computer interaction can be made intuitive and natural by using hand gestures. In order to maximize hand motion recognition for mouse action, our method combines well-established techniques of skin color-based ROI segmentation and Haar-like feature-based object detection. Using the left or right mouse button to click while dragging the pointer around is the essence of mouse operation. This study initially establishes the ROI using color, a robust feature. Then, utilized the AdaBoost Learning technique and Haar-like properties, hand postures within this ROI were detected. By merging several poor classifiers, the AdaBoost learning technique significantly improves performance and produces a trustworthy cascaded classifier.

Pradeepa et al. (2022) explain the application of ML & IoT for students' health perdition. Since more and more students live unsupervised and are spread out over wide geographic areas, it is imperative to keep an eye on their health. This work proposed IoT-based approach to health management for students that continuously monitors their vital signs and used cutting-edge medical methods to identify biological and behavioral anomalies. This method entails the IoT module gathering crucial data, which is subsequently assessed using NN models to pinpoint any risks to students' altered physiology and behavior. The results of the experiments demonstrated that the proposed model was reliable and accurate way to assess the students' states. The suggested model was evaluated, the SVM achieved a perfect performance of 99.1%, fulfilling our goals. Furthermore, the outcomes outperformed methods utilizing decision trees, random forests, and multilayer perceptron neural systems.

By Kazi (2018), the used of ML in aquatic research is explained. Using color matching reduces both the total color correction and the color differences between neighboring photographs. Author applied linear correction and gamma correction, respectively, to the brightness and chrominance components of the original pictures (marine), for aquatic image applications. The problem of color consistency in 360^0 panoramic images were addressed by color correspondence and color difference distribution techniques. The article combines the stitching process into an automated panoramic imaging system to generate high-quality, high-resolution panoramic photographs for mobile-phones.

Ravi et al. (2022) provide an explanation of the IoT application on LOVE. A method is needed so that they can express their love and closeness to one another through their memories. These days, mail or phone calls are still the only ways to communicate closeness. As such, we will use contemporary methods like the IoT to express our love and remembering. Author presents this sensor-driven, IoT-based system.

METHODOLOGY

Internet of Medical Things(IoMT) links millions of somatic techniques to collect and share patient healthcare information online. A range of software and sensors for healthcare and biotechnology make up IoMT. It connects mobile devices, other used physical gadgets, and equipment located remotely via wireless communication protocols. Healthcare models are substantially advanced by the IoMT. A multitude of both external and internal sensors are used to collect patient data. While the eternal sensor collects the patient's exterior and ambient data, body-implanted (Bio) sensors collect the patient's internal data. Physicians evaluate the information provided by Sultanabau (2023g) to forecast illness.

To distinguish between those who are physically healthy and those who are not, the model is constructed using many ML classification techniques to categorize the gathered information. Diseases are consistently and early classified by ML. Three types of patient data are gathered through IoT in the suggested model:

• Details about patients under quarantine: Patients in this group of data have inexpensive, readily accessible IoT devices. These IoMT sensors gather patient health data and transmit it to an IoT assistant so that Kazi K(2022)(2023) can further analyze it.

• Labs or clinical patient information: In this scenario, the patient goes to clinics and laboratories, but even with all the resources at their disposal, no physicians are there to help them with their problems. The patient data was gathered by K K (2022) and the medical aid staff.

• Remote patient information: In this case, the patient resides distant from the hospitals or in a remote place. IoMT sensors gather patient data and instantly provide it to physicians so they can give patients better care.

Any IoMT device is used to collect data relevant to healthcare, which is subsequently uploaded to a hospital or cloud server for Sayyad Liyakat's extra analysis (2023a, 2023b). The fog server uses categorization techniques to analyze the data. In order to facilitate early patient diagnosis, the data is sent to power storage facilities and physicians via a cloud server. Using ML classification algorithms, such as DT-Decision Tree, SVM-Support Vector Machine, NB-Naïve Bayes, AB-Adaboost, RF-Random

Forest, ANN-Artificial Neural Network, and KNN-K-Nearest Neighbor, is the focus of healthcare model development, according to Ravi A. (2022) and Vinay (2022).

These algorithms are used on a dataset comprising information about blood pressure, diabetes, hepatitis, and kidney diseases. The expected model's framework is shown in Figure 3. The expected paradigm in DL approach includes ML and IoMT as key elements. The first parameter, IoT, allows anything to be connected to the internet. Kazi S (2023), Shaikh(2023) acquire and process patient data in real-time, ensuring that it is delivered to the appropriate parties on time. The ML-machine learning parameter uses the gathered data to produce timely results. AI and IoT technologies efficiently manage massive volumes of data.

Figure 3. MLIoMT (DL approach) based proposed system

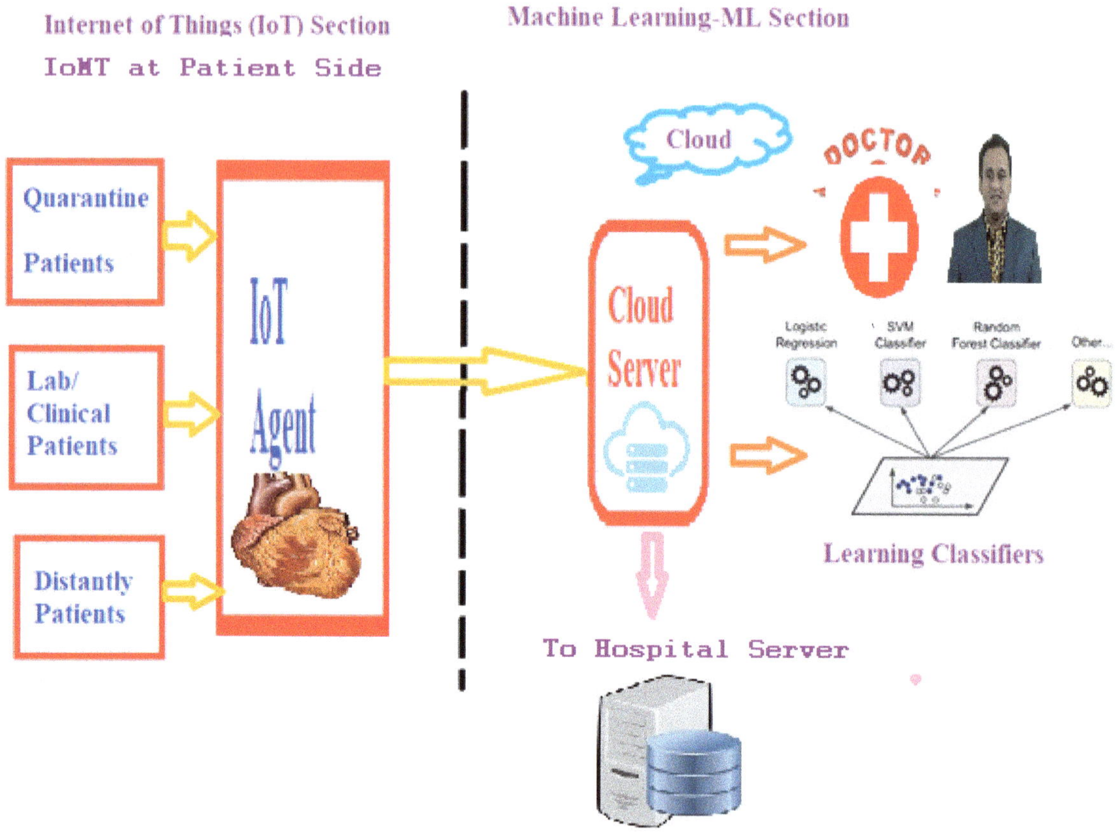

There are three stages to the work. The steps consists of data collecting, pre-processing, and computing. In the final phase, the results are saved on an online server and made available to physicians or end users.

1. **Data Collection:** To do this, patient data is gathered from a variety of sources, including remote information and information from the patient's home, lab, or clinic. Real-time patient data collection is accomplished through the use of a range of sensors and IoT devices. The necessary range of sensors has been positioned for patients who are receiving care at home. The IoT agent receives

the clinical and lab data from the lab technicians. Patients in outlying areas are outfitted with an array of sensors. The data is gathered by these sensors and delivered to an IoT agent for additional processing.
2. **Data Pre-Processing and Computation:** Filtering and missing value checking are two aspects of pre-processing the data that is provided. Following the completion of pre-processing, the data is transferred to a cloud server for processing. The data is computed and classified using seven ML classifiers (DT, SVM, NB, AB, RF, ANN, and K-NN).

I. Decision Trees

This approach, commonly referred to as DTs, is well-liked and frequently applied in the field of machine learning. These tools are quite popular because they are simple to use, easy to interpret, and can handle both categorical and numerical data. They are highly adaptable and efficient. Decision trees have been used successfully for regression and classification analysis in a variety of fields, such as marketing, finance, and healthcare.

So, what exactly is a DT-decision tree? It's a structure that looks like a tree and shows a sequence of options and possible results. The structure is made up of internal nodes, branches, and leaves. The internal nodes indicate a test run on a characteristic, and the branches display the test's outcome. The leaves, also known as terminal nodes, contain the choice or outcome of the classification or regression task. Recursively dividing information into smaller groups according to attribute values is how DT algorithm operates. Making branches that best divide the classes or forecast the target variable is the aim. Recursive partitioning is the term for this process, which keeps going until the final subsets are pure or only contain one class. To put it another way, DT algorithm generates a set of human-friendly if-then rules.

Decision trees' capacity to handle both numerical and categorical data without the need for previous data preprocessing is one of their main features. They are quite well-liked among researchers and data scientists because of this feature. Decision trees are appropriate for real-world applications because they can accept missing values while functioning well on huge datasets.

The interpretability of DT is another important advantage. Decision trees, in contrast to other sophisticated algorithms like neural networks, generate an easily interpreted graphical representation. This is so that consumers can easily see the reasoning behind the decisions taken, as every branch on the tree indicates a decision made because of a certain attribute. In the event that there are any mistakes, this interpretability also aids in debugging and model improvement.

In addition, nonlinear interactions among both the input and the output variables can be handled by decision trees. This implies that they don't require any transformation in order to identify intricate patterns in the data. Additionally, they have a high degree of prediction accuracy, particularly when combined with different DTs in an ensemble setting, as in random forests.

When all is said and done, DTs are a powerful and well-liked technique in the machine learning field. Their outstanding projected accuracy, interpretability, and ability to handle both numerical and categorical data make them a preferred choice for a wide range of applications. Trimming and group procedures, however, can aid in getting above their limitations. Given the continuous advancements in machine learning, decision trees are expected to play an increasingly significant role in problem-solving and decision-making processes.

II. SVM, or Support Vector Machine

This well-liked ML technique is applied to regression and classification problems. This provides support for a supervised learning method with applications in image recognition, text categorization, and bioinformatics, among other domains. SVM is a powerful and adaptable technique that works well for solving challenging classification issues.

SVM is a non-probabilistic binary linear classifier that divides data points into discrete groups using a hyperplane. In order to categorize the input points consistently, SVM looks for the best hyperplane with the biggest margin between the two categories. This margin, commonly known as the maximum margin hyperplane, is the most important part of SVM. The capacity of SVM to cope with both non-linear and linear data is one of its main advantages. SVM has the ability to map data into higher dimensions, which allows it to be possible to discover a hyperplane that can accurately separate the data points, in contrast to other algorithms which are limited to handling linearly separable data. This is accomplished by converting the data onto a higher-dimensional space using a technique known as the kernel trick, which makes it simpler to identify a hyperplane that can divide the classes. SVM's capacity to handle big datasets effectively is another benefit. Most ML algorithms have a tendency to perform poorly as the number of features rises. Nevertheless, SVM makes use of a subset of training points known as support vectors, which aids in simplifying the issue and increases its effectiveness when working with big datasets.

In addition, SVM features a special cost function called the hinge loss function that aids in locating the optimal hyperplane. Better separation among both categories is achieved as a result of the cost function's harsher penalty for misclassified points. When compared to other algorithms, this makes SVM more resilient and less susceptible to outliers.

All things considered, SVM is a strong and adaptable ML algorithm which has shown to be quite successful in resolving challenging classification issues. Data scientists and ML practitioners frequently use it because of its versatility in handling both linear and non-linear data, resilience to outliers, and strong theoretical underpinnings. SVM keeps developing and getting better because to technological breakthroughs, which makes it a vital tool in the machine learning industry.

III. Using Naïve Bayes (NB)

It is a popular and widely used classification algorithm in ML. Because it is simple to use and efficient, this technique is widely used for sentiment analysis, text categorization, spam filtering, and other data analysis and classification tasks. In this post, we will discuss Naïve Bayes's principles, operation, and applications.

The Naïve Bayes probabilistic algorithm is based on the Bayes theorem, which measures the probability of an event occurring based on historical data. The algorithm is known as supervised learning since it gains knowledge from labelled training data. The 'naïve' aspect originates from the presumption that elements within a dataset are unrelated to each other, an assumption that may not hold true in practical scenarios. Despite this oversimplifying premise, Naïve Bayes has shown to be a successful algorithm for a range of classification applications. Using the Bayes theorem, NB determines the likelihood that a data point belongs to a specific class. Based on an analysis of the data point's attributes, the algorithm determines the likelihood of each class. The data point is then allocated to the class having the highest likelihood.

The straightforward yet potent NB classification algorithm has shown its worth in a number of practical uses. Data scientists and ML practitioners use it extensively because, in most circumstances, it performs well despite its simplifying assumptions. It is a well-liked option for text classification assignments and other applications due to its scalability and ease of implementation. Selecting the appropriate NB classifier given a specific dataset and being aware of its limits are crucial, just like any other ML technique.

IV. Adaptive Boosting

Also referred to as AB, this well-liked ML method has numerous applications across a range of sectors. This kind of ensemble learning technique produces a strong learner by combining several weak learners, which improves predicted performance. Because AB can handle complicated datasets and yield precise answers, it has becoming more and more popular. It is a potent algorithm that enhances the model's overall performance by repeatedly changing the weights of cases that are erroneously identified. The boosting concept, which combines several weak learners to produce a powerful learner, is the foundation of the method.

The basic classifier, namely is a straightforward and unreliable learning algorithm, is created by AB. A portion of the initial data set is used to train this base classifier, and it's efficacy is assessed. Subsequently, the method trains another classifier on the identical dataset by giving the erroneously classified examples larger weights. Until the required degree of accuracy is attained, this process is repeated. The capacity of AB to handle intricate and high-dimensional datasets is one of its main advantages. Because AB does not need feature engineering or data preprocessing, unlike other ML techniques, it is a preferred option among data scientists and ML practitioners. Moreover, AB is quite resilient to noisy data, which makes it a great option for practical uses.

AB's capability to evolve and gain information from its failures is one of its most important characteristics. The approach modifies the weights of cases that are erroneously identified, making them more significant in the subsequent iteration, as it iteratively trains new classifiers. With each iteration, AB is able to consistently enhance its performance thanks to this adaptive process, producing a robust and precise model.

All things considered, adaptive boosting represents a potent ML method that has grown in favor because of its capacity to manage noisy data, complex datasets, and class imbalances. Data scientists and ML practitioners favor it because of its adaptable nature and capacity for constant performance improvement. AB is anticipated to have a big impact on ML and AI in the future as the need for precise and effective predictive models grows.

V. Random Forest (RF)

It is a well-liked ML method that has been well-known and used in a number of industries, including natural language processing, banking, and healthcare. Several decision trees are combined in this potent ensemble learning technique to produce a more reliable and accurate model. We will examine the idea of Random Forest, how it operates, and its uses in this post.

A supervised ML technique called RF builds numerous DTs and aggregates them to produce predictions that are more reliable and accurate. It is regarded as an ensemble learning technique since it builds upon multiple foundational models to produce a more potent one. It is predicated on the notion that several, largely uncorrelated models (trees) functioning as a committee will perform better than any one of the individual models that make up the model. Since each decision tree is constructed using a random subset of features along with information points, the approach is known as "Random Forest" because it reduces the likelihood of overfitting in the model.

The way Random Forest operates is by training an enormous amount of DTs on a randomized portion of the training set. The two main strategies used by the algorithm are feature randomness and bagging. Using replacement, each DT is trained on a random subset of the training data using a technique called bagging (also known as bootstrap aggregation) to lower the variance of the model. As a result, certain data points can appear more than once in an identical tree, whereas other ones might not appear at all. This reduces the model's sensitivity to noise and outliers in the training set.

In contrast, feature randomness selects a subset of characteristics at each decision tree node at random. As a result, the model is more resilient and less likely to overfit by generating a diversified set of trees.

Following the training of each decision tree, the RF algorithm uses a majority vote procedure to integrate the predictions made by each tree. This indicates that the majority vote from each decision tree is the basis for the final prediction. This procedure aids in lowering the model's variance and raising its overall accuracy.

Because of its accuracy and resilience, Random Forest is a potent ML algorithm which has grown in popularity. It has demonstrated promising outcomes in handling complicated issues and is widely employed in many different fields. The model performs better and is less prone to overfitting thanks to the application of bagging and feature randomization approaches. In the future of ML, RF_Random Forest is anticipated to be extremely important due to the increasing volume of data.

VI. Artificial Neural Networks (ANN)

Because of their potential to completely transform a number of industries, they have been creating waves throughout the tech community. Voice recognition software and self-driving automobiles are only two examples of how ANN are enabling machines to absorb information and adapt like the human brain. However, what are ANNs really, and how do they operate?

A class of ML algorithms called ANN is modeled after the composition and operation of the human brain. Millions of linked neurons make up the human brain, which functions as a single unit that helps process information, make decisions, and regulate behavior. Comparably, an ANN consists of networked units, or artificial neurons, that collaborate to solve complicated issues.

An input layer, hidden layers, and output layer make up an ANN's fundamental structure. After data is received by the input layer, it undergoes processing and analysis in the hidden layers. According to the investigation carried out by the hidden layers, the output layer subsequently generates the intended outcome. The foundation of ANNs learning is the process of backpropagation, which modifies the weights allocated to the connections between the neurons.

ANN learn in a manner akin to that of human beings. Our brains absorb new information, and depending on how important the information is, the connections between neurons become stronger or weaker. Similar to this, an ANN learns and becomes more efficient over time by adjusting the relative weights on the connections according to its input information and the intended output.

Notwithstanding these drawbacks, ANNs have a lot of potential, and scientists are always trying to advance the field. ANNs are growing more and more powerful and are being employed in a wide range of applications because to advances in processing power and data availability. They have the power to revolutionize entire sectors by increasing machine intelligence, automating repetitive processes, and enhancing decision-making.

All things considered, ANN have demonstrated a lot of potential in the area of ML and are anticipated to have a big impact on the future. ANNs have the power to transform the way we engage with technology and improve our lives through their self-learning and complex data handling capabilities. To guarantee their accountable and ethical use, it is necessary to overcome the difficulties and constraints associated with ANNs. ANNs will surely be at the forefront of innovation and technological advancement as we strive to expand the envelope.

VII. K-Nearest Neighbor, or KNN

K-Nearest Neighbor(K-NN) technique is the most prevalent and adaptable algorithms in the discipline of ML. It is a straightforward approach that works well for both regression and classification problems. Since K-NN constitutes a non-parametric technique, it doesn't assume anything about the distribution of the underlying data. It is extensively employed in many different applications, including text categorization, image recognition, and recommendation systems.

Since K-NN relies supervised learning algorithm, its ability to provide predictions is dependent on labeled training data. The number of closest neighbors that are utilized to generate predictions is indicated by the letter "K" in K-NN. Comparable data points were closer to one another in the feature space, which is how K-NN operates. As a result, the K-NN method takes a given data point and discovers the K closest data points, labeling the new data point with most of its neighbors. Put another way, a new data point will be assigned to the same class if the majority of its closest neighbors are also members of that class.

Like every algorithm, K-NN is not without its limits, though. The computational cost of the K-NN technique is one of its main disadvantages, particularly when dealing with huge datasets. The time required to produce predictions rises with the amount of the dataset. Its sensitivity to outliers, which have the potential to materially alter the distance estimations, is another drawback.

There are many uses for the K-NN method, even with its drawbacks. Recommendation systems—which use K-NN to suggest products or offerings based on user behavior and preferences—are among the most common applications of K-NN. In computer vision and image recognition applications, such handwritten digit identification and object detection in photos, it is also extensively utilized. K-NN is used in the medical field to categorize diseases according to a patient's medical history and symptoms. Applications for credit scoring and fraud detection systems also use it.

All things considered, the K-NN algorithm is a strong and adaptable ML technique that is frequently employed in a variety of settings. Data scientists choose it because of its ease of use, adaptability, and capacity for handling data that is numerical as well as categorical. To get the best results, you must, however, take into account its restrictions and select the right number for K. Future developments in computer power and data availability should lead to an increase in the number of applications utilizing the K-NN method.

RESULTS ACCESSIBILITY

In this subsection, computed data is transferred via the cloud server to physicians and end users, allowing the cloud server to start treating patients right away. Physicians use the findings to reply to patients about course of treatment. The received record, which includes the patient's current medical care and billing information, is kept on a cloud server for later use.

Assessment of a Classifier's Effectiveness

A classifier is an ML approach that divides data into numerous groups or classes. It is a crucial tool for machine learning and is applied in many different contexts, including predictive modeling, picture recognition, and text analysis. One of the main determinants of a classifier's efficacy in tackling real-world situations is its performance. This article will go over the various measures that are employed in the process of evaluating a classifier's performance.

By comparing the expected and actual outputs, one may assess the performance of the classifier. This method is called performance evaluation or model evaluation. Determining the classifier's accuracy in classifying new data is the primary objective of this evaluation. A classifier's performance needs to be assessed in order to weigh its advantages and disadvantages and make the necessary corrections.

The effectiveness of a classifier can be assessed using a variety of criteria. The most commonly utilized metrics are recall, accuracy, and precision. Let's take a closer look at these metrics.

1. **Accuracy:** Accuracy is the most basic metric used to evaluate a classifier's performance. It measures the %(percentage) of right predictions finished by classifier. It is premeditated by dividing number of correct predictions by total number of predictions. E.g., if a classifier makes 81 correct predictions out of 90, its accuracy would be 90%.

$$Accuracy = \left(\frac{TP + TN}{TP + FP + TN + FN}\right) * 100 \tag{1}$$

2. **Precision:** Precision measures the percentage of correct positive predictions made by the classifier. It is calculated by dividing the number of true positives (correctly classified positive instances) by the total number of positive predictions (both true positives and false positives). A high precision indicates that the classifier is good at identifying the relevant instances.

$$Sensitivity/Precision = \left(\frac{TP}{TP + FN}\right) * 100 \tag{2}$$

3. **Recall:** Also known as sensitivity, measures the percentage of correct positive predictions made by the classifier out of all actual positive instances. It is calculated by dividing the number of true positives by the total number of positive instances in the dataset. A high recall indicates that the classifier is good at identifying all the relevant instances.

$$Specificity/Recall = \left(\frac{TN}{TN + FP}\right) * 100 \tag{3}$$

where as, TP- true positives, TN-true negatives, FP- false positives, and FN- false negatives predicted by the classifier for proposed Heathcare system.

RESULTS AND DISCUSSION –

The experimental findings of various classification methods, such as DT, SVM, NB, AB, RF, ANN, and K-NN, are discussed here. Numerous disease datasets, including those concerning blood pressure, kidney disease, hepatitis A, B, and C, Type I and Type II diabetes, and hepatitis C, have been used. The dataset that was used with several samples is shown in Table 1.

Table 1. Dataset utilized for experimentation

Sr. No.	Dataset	Number of Samples
1	BP	750
2	High-Diabetes	750
3	Kidney disease	300
4	Hepatitis	100

The dataset is split into two ratios for this investigative work: 80% and 20% shown in Figure 4. Twenty percent of the data set is used for testing, while the remaining eighty percent is used to create classification algorithms. We assess each of the seven classifiers' sensitivity, specificity, and accuracy. The seven different classifiers' performance indicators for BP. Figure5 displays the accuracy, precision, and recall of the seven classifiers for the BP dataset.

Figure 4. Dataset division for working

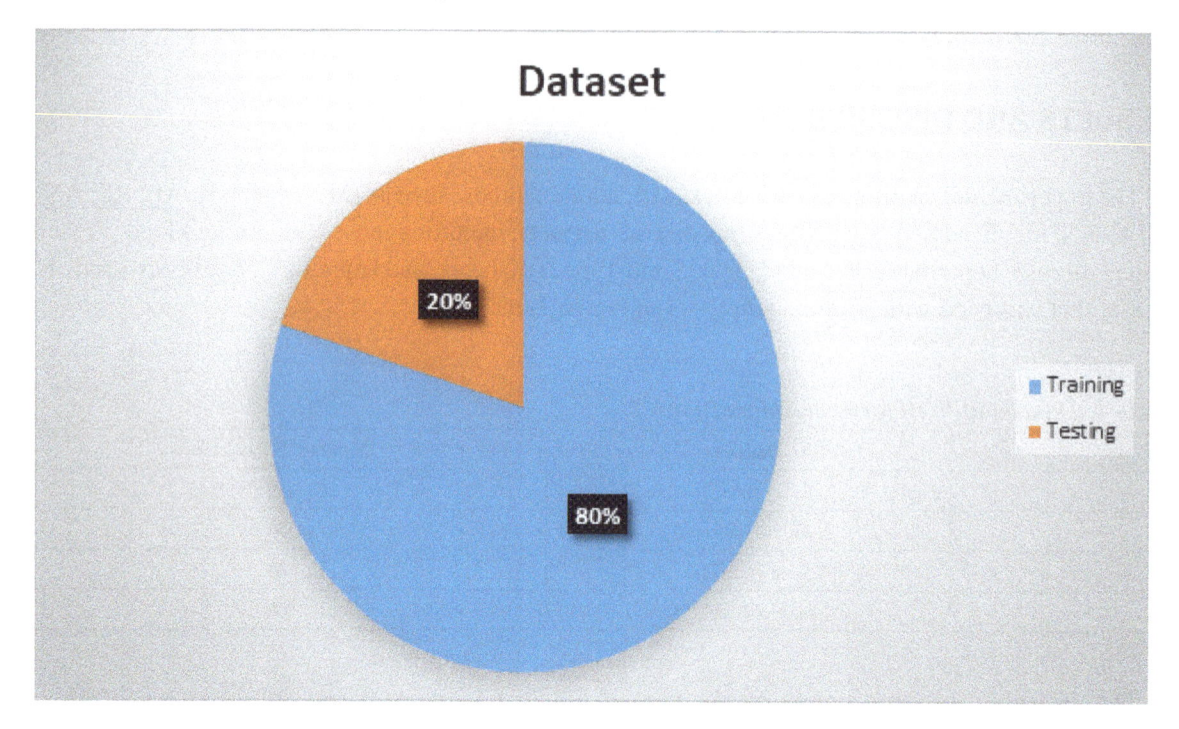

Figure 5. 7 Different classifiers for BP dataset

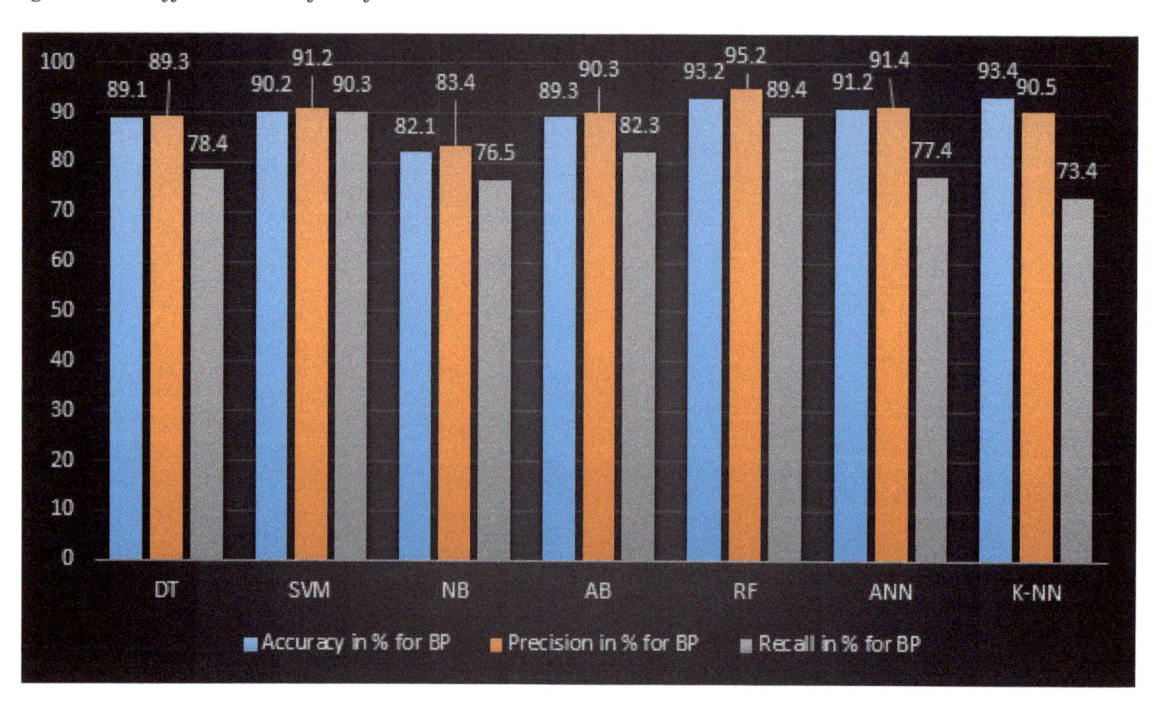

The seven different classifiers' performance parameters for Diabetes. Figure 6 displays the results of the seven classifiers for accuracy, precision, and recall for High-Diabetes dataset.

Figure 6. 7 Different classifiers for high-diabetes dataset

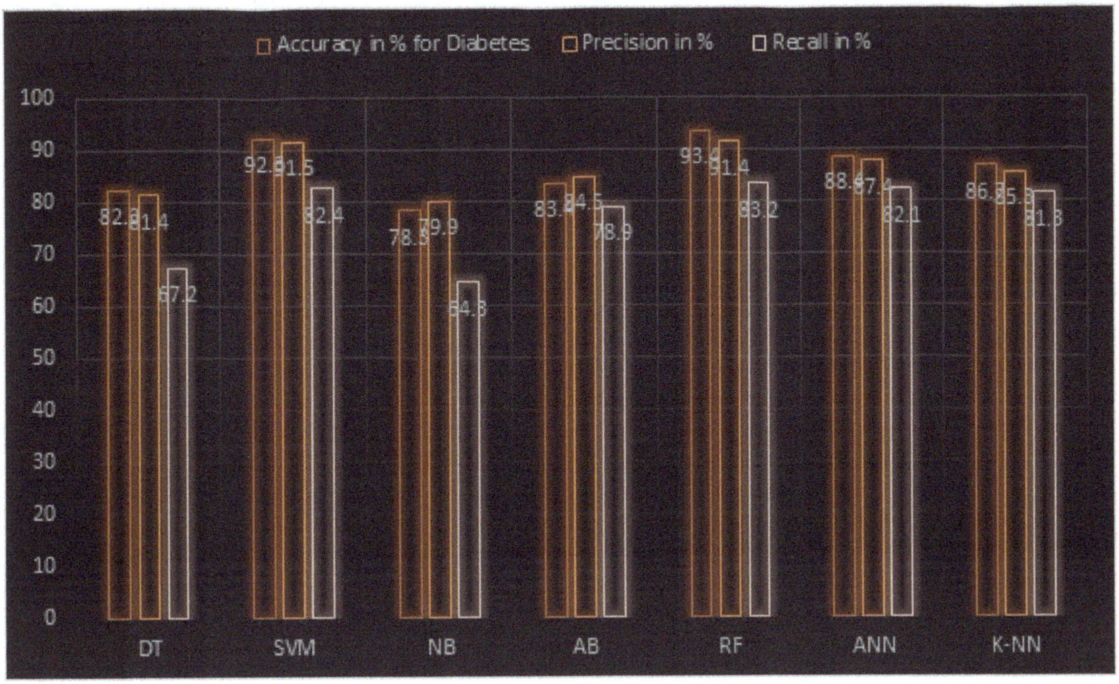

The seven different classifiers' performance parameters for Kidney Diseases. Figure 7 displays the results of the seven classifiers for accuracy, precision, and recall for Kidney Diseases dataset.

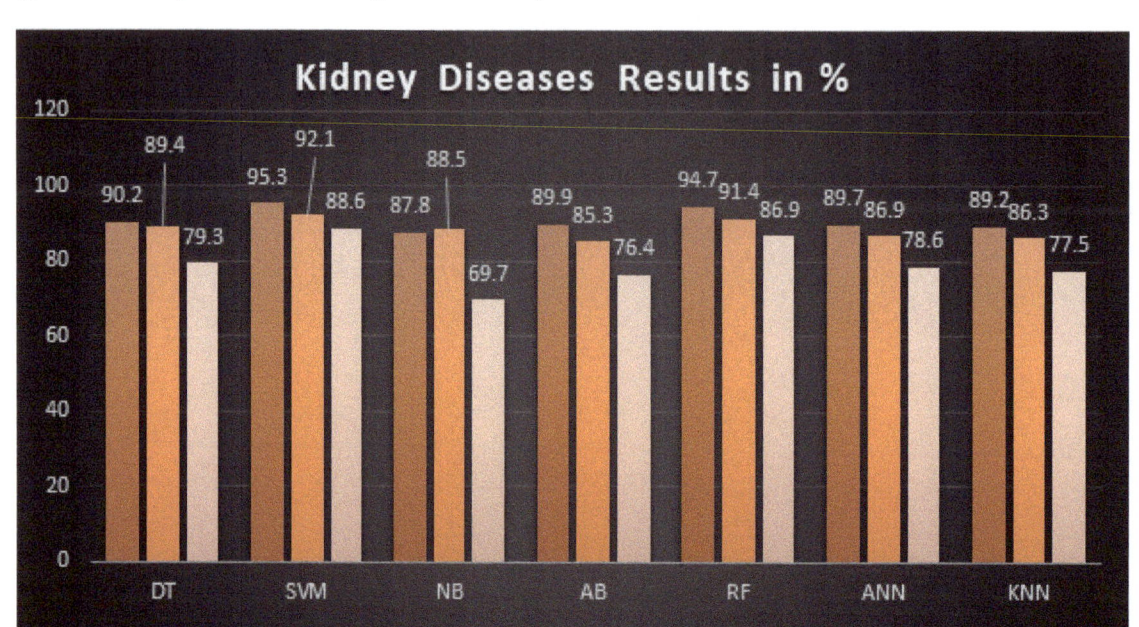

Figure 7. Kidney diseases results for all 7 classifiers

[Bar chart titled "Kidney Diseases Results in %" showing Accuracy, Precision, and Recall for seven classifiers:
- DT: 90.2, 89.4, 79.3
- SVM: 95.3, 92.1, 88.6
- NB: 87.8, 88.5, 69.7
- AB: 89.9, 85.3, 76.4
- RF: 94.7, 91.4, 86.9
- ANN: 89.7, 86.9, 78.6
- KNN: 89.2, 86.3, 77.5]

The seven different classifiers' performance parameters for Hepatitis. Figure 8 displays the results of the seven classifiers for accuracy, precision, and recall for Hepatitis dataset.

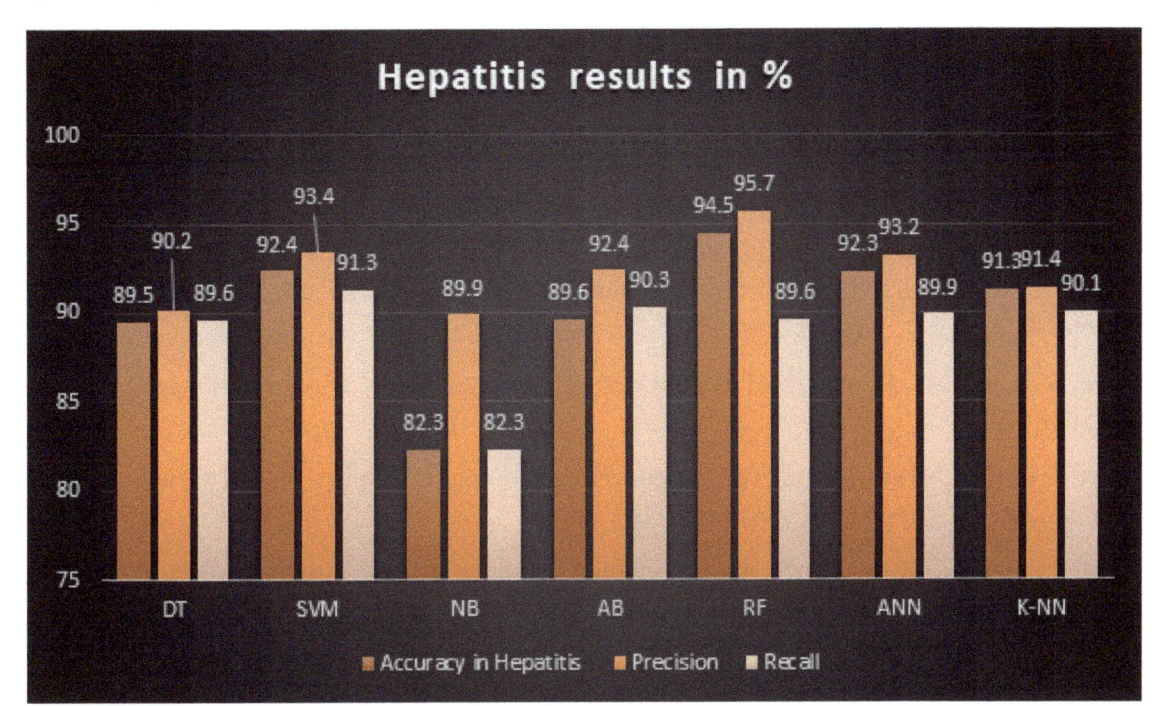

Figure 8. Hepatitis results for all 7 classifiers

CONCLUSION

As such, the subject of using machine learning (ML) classification algorithms to forecast illnesses and diseases is still in its infancy. For this proposed work, we used seven different ML-classification algorithms (DT, SVM,NB,AB,RF,ANN, and K-NN) to construct a healthcare model. Blood pressure, hepatitis, diabetes, and kidney disorders are among the disease datasets that such classifiers are used to. The performance of the classifiers is evaluated using four metrics: accuracy, precision, recall, and precision. For every ailment, the current healthcare model achieves a minimum accuracy of 82.3% and a maximum accuracy of 95.7%. As shown in Figures 5 to 8, each disease has a minimum precision of 81.4% and a maximum precision of 95.7%, as well as a minimum recall of 64.3% and a maximum recall of 90.3%. This ML driven IoMT approach we call as DL approach.

REFERENCES

Aavula, R.. (2022). Design and Implementation of sensor and IoT based Remembrance system for closed one. *Telematique*, 21(1), 2769–2778.

Abhangrao, C. M. (2024). Internet of Things in Mechatronics for Design and Manufacturing: A Review. *Journals of Mechatronics Machine Design and Manufacturing*, 6(1).

Devi, J. S., Sreedhar, M. B., Arulprakash, P., Kazi, K., & Radhakrishnan, R. (2022). A path towards child-centric Artificial Intelligence based Education. *International Journal of Early Childhood*, 14(3), 9915–9922.

Dhanwe, S. S.. (2024). AI-driven IoT in Robotics: A Review. *Journal of Mechanisms and Robotics*, 9(1), 41–48.

Dixit, A. J. (2014). A review paper on iris recognition. Journal GSD International society for green. *Sustainable Engineering and Management*, 1(14), 71–81.

Dixit, A. J., & Kazi, M. K. (2015). Iris recognition by daugman's algorithm–an efficient approach. Journal of applied Research and Social Sciences, 2(14), 1-4.

Gund, V. D.. (2023). PIR Sensor-Based Arduino Home Security System. *Journal of Instrumentation and Innovation Sciences*, 8(3), 33–37.

Halli, U. M. (2022). Voltage Sag Mitigation Using DVR and Ultra Capacitor. *Journal of Semiconductor Devices and Circuits.*, 9(3), 21–31p.

Halli, U. M. (2022a). Nanotechnology in IoT Security, *Journal of Nanoscience. Nanoengineering & Applications*, 12(3), 11–16.

Halli, U. M. (2022b). Nanotechnology in E-Vehicle Batteries. *International Journal of Nanomaterials and Nanostructures.*, 8(2), 22–27.

Hotkar, P. R., Kulkarni, V., Kamble, P., & Kazi, K. S. (2019). Implementation of Low Power and area efficient carry select Adder. International Journal of Research in Engineering. *Science and Management*, 2(4), 183–184.

Jadhav, V. L. (2024). Detection of Fire in the Environment via a Robot Based Fire Fighting System Using Sensors, *International Journal of Advanced Research in Science* [IJARSCT]. *Tongxin Jishu*, 4(4), 410–418.

Karale Aishwarya, A.. (2023). Smart Billing Cart Using RFID, YOLO and Deep Learning for Mall Administration. *International Journal of Instrumentation and Innovation Sciences*, 8(2).

Kasat, K., Shaikh, N., Rayabharapu, V. K., & Nayak, M. (2023). Implementation and Recognition of Waste Management System with Mobility Solution in Smart Cities using Internet of Things, *2023 Second International Conference on Augmented Intelligence and Sustainable Systems (ICAISS)*, Trichy, India, 2023, pp. 1661-1665, DOI: 10.1109/ICAISS58487.2023.10250690

Kazi, K. (2022). Hybrid optimum model development to determine the Break. *Journal of Multimedia Technology & Recent Advancements*, 9(2), 24–32.

Kazi, K. (2022). Smart Grid energy saving technique using Machine Learning. *Journal of Instrumentation Technology and Innovations*, 12(3), 1–10.

Kazi, K. (2022a). Reverse Engineering's Neural Network Approach to human brain. *Journal of Communication Engineering & Systems*, 12(2), 17–24.

Kazi K., (2022b). Model for Agricultural Information system to improve crop yield using IoT, *Journal of open Source development*, 9(2), pp. 16 – 24.

Kazi, K. (2024). Complications with Malware Identification in IoT and an Overview of Artificial Immune Approaches. *Research & Reviews. The Journal of Immunology : Official Journal of the American Association of Immunologists*, 14(01), 54–62.

Kazi, K. (2024). Nanotechnology in Medical Applications: A Study. *Nano Trends-A Journal of Nano Technology & Its Applications.*, 26(02), 1–11.

Kazi, K. (2024a). AI-Driven IoT (AIIoT) in Healthcare Monitoring. In Nguyen, T., & Vo, N. (Eds.), *Using Traditional Design Methods to Enhance AI-Driven Decision Making* (pp. 77–101). IGI Global., available at https://www.igi-global.com/chapter/ai-driven-iot-aiiot-in-healthcare-monitoring/336693, DOI: 10.4018/979-8-3693-0639-0.ch003

Kazi, K. (2024a). Machine Learning (ML)-Based Braille Lippi Characters and Numbers Detection and Announcement System for Blind Children in Learning. In Sart, G. (Ed.), *Social Reflections of Human-Computer Interaction in Education, Management, and Economics*. IGI Global., DOI: 10.4018/979-8-3693-3033-3.ch002

Kazi, K. (2024b). Modelling and Simulation of Electric Vehicle for Performance Analysis: BEV and HEV Electrical Vehicle Implementation Using Simulink for E-Mobility Ecosystems. *In L. D., N. Nagpal, N. Kassarwani, V. Varthanan G., & P. Siano (Eds.), E-Mobility in Electrical Energy Systems for Sustainability (pp. 295-320). IGI Global.* Available at: https://www.igi-global.com/gateway/chapter/full-text-pdf/341172DOI: 10.4018/979-8-3693-2611-4.ch014

Kazi, K. (2025b). Machine Learning-Driven-Internet of Things(MLIoT) Based Healthcare Monitoring System. In Wickramasinghe, N. (Ed.), *Impact of Digital Solutions for Improved Healthcare Delivery*. IGI Global.

Kazi, K. (2025c). Moonlighting in Carrier. In Tunio, M. N. (Ed.), *Applications of Career Transitions and Entrepreneurship*. IGI Global.

Kazi, K. (2025c). AI-Powered-IoT (AIIoT) based Decision Making System for BP Patient's Healthcare Monitoring: KSK Approach for BP Patient Healthcare Monitoring. In Aouadni, S., & Aouadni, I. (Eds.), *Recent Theories and Applications for Multi-Criteria Decision-Making*. IGI Global.

Kazi, K. (2025c). *AI-Driven-IoT (AIIoT) based Decision-Making in Drones for Climate Change: KSK Approach. Recent Theories and Applications for Multi-Criteria Decision-Making*. IGI Global.

Kazi, K. S. (2017). Significance and Usage of Face Recognition System. *Scholarly Journal for Humanity Science and English Language*, 4(20), 4764–4772.

Kazi, K. S. (2022a). IoT-Based Healthcare Monitoring for COVID-19 Home Quarantined Patients. *Recent Trends in Sensor Research & Technology*, 9(3), 26–32.

Kazi K S, (2023). IoT based Healthcare system for Home Quarantine People, *Journal of Instrumentation and Innovation sciences*, 18(1), pp. 1- 8

Kazi, K. S. (2023a). Detection of Malicious Nodes in IoT Networks based on Throughput and ML. *Journal of Electrical and Power System Engineering*, 9(1), 22–29.

Kazi, K. S. (2024). Artificial Intelligence (AI)-Driven IoT (AIIoT)-Based Agriculture Automation. In Satapathy, S., & Muduli, K. (Eds.), *Advanced Computational Methods for Agri-Business Sustainability* (pp. 72–94). IGI Global., DOI: 10.4018/979-8-3693-3583-3.ch005

Kazi, K. S. (2024). Machine Learning-Based Pomegranate Disease Detection and Treatment. In Zia Ul Haq, M., & Ali, I. (Eds.), *Revolutionizing Pest Management for Sustainable Agriculture* (pp. 469–498). IGI Global., DOI: 10.4018/979-8-3693-3061-6.ch019

Kazi, K. S. (2024a). Computer-Aided Diagnosis in Ophthalmology: A Technical Review of Deep Learning Applications. In Garcia, M., & de Almeida, R. (Eds.), *Transformative Approaches to Patient Literacy and Healthcare Innovation* (pp. 112–135). IGI Global., Available at https://www.igi-global.com/chapter/computer-aided-diagnosis-in-ophthalmology/342823, DOI: 10.4018/979-8-3693-3661-8.ch006

Kazi, K. S. (2024b). IoT Driven by Machine Learning (MLIoT) for the Retail Apparel Sector. In Tarnanidis, T., Papachristou, E., Karypidis, M., & Ismyrlis, V. (Eds.), *Driving Green Marketing in Fashion and Retail* (pp. 63–81). IGI Global., DOI: 10.4018/979-8-3693-3049-4.ch004

Kazi, K. S. (2025). IoT Technologies for the Intelligent Dairy Industry: A New Challenge. In Thandekkattu, S., & Vajjhala, N. (Eds.), *Designing Sustainable Internet of Things Solutions for Smart Industries* (pp. 321–350). IGI Global., DOI: 10.4018/979-8-3693-5498-8.ch012

Kazi, K. S. L. (2018). Significance of Projection and Rotation of Image in Color Matching for High-Quality Panoramic Images used for Aquatic study. *International Journal of Aquatic Science*, 9(2), 130–145.

Kazi, K. S. L. (2023a). IoT-based weather Prototype using WeMos. *Journal of Control and Instrumentation Engineering*, 9(1), 10–22.

Kazi, K. S. L. (2023c). Analysis for Field distribution in Optical Waveguide using Linear Fem method, *Journal of Optical communication. Electronics (Basel)*, 9(1), 23–28.

Kazi, K. S. L. (2023h). IoT based Healthcare Monitoring for COVID- Subvariant JN-1. *Journal of Electronic Design Technology*, 4(3).

Kazi, K. S. L. (2023i). Smart Motion Detection System using IoT: A NodeMCU and Blynk Framework. *Journal of Microelectronics and Solid State Devices*, 10(3).

Kazi, K. S. L. (2023j). Nanotechnology in Precision Farming: The Role of Research. *International Journal of Nanomaterials and Nanostructures*, 9(2). Advance online publication. DOI: 10.37628/ijnn.v9i2.1051

Kazi, K. S. L. (2023k). Home Automation System Based on GSM. *Journal of VLSI Design Tools & Technology*, 13(3), 7–12p. DOI: 10.37591/jovdtt.v13i3.7877

Kazi, K. S. L. (2024). Nanotechnology in BattleField: A Study. Journal of Nanoscience. *Nanoengineering & Applications*, 14(2), 18–30p.

Kazi, K. S. L. (2024). Nanotechnology in BattleField: A Study. Journal of Nanoscience. *Nanoengineering & Applications.*, 14(2), 18–30p.

Kazi, K. S. L. (2024). Review of Biopolymers in Agriculture Application: An Eco-Friendly Alternative. *International Journal of Composite and Constituent Materials.*, 10(1), 50–62p.

Kazi, K. S. L. (2024f). Blynk IoT-Powered Water Pump-Based Smart Farming. *Recent Trends in Semiconductor and Sensor Technology*, 1(1), 8–14.

Kazi, K. S. L. (2024g). Impact of Solar Penetrations in Conventional Power Systems and Generation of Harmonic and Power Quality Issues. *Advance Research in Power Electronics and Devices*, 1(1), 10–16.

Kazi, K. S. L. (2024r). Intelligent Watering System(IWS) for Agricultural Land Utilising Raspberry Pi. *Recent Trends in Fluid Mechanics*, 10(2), 26–31.

Kazi, K. S. L. (2024s). IoT and Sensor-based Smart Agriculturing Driven by NodeMCU. *Research & Review: Electronics and Communication Engineering*, 1(2), 25–33.

Kazi, K. S. L. (2024v). Smart Agriculture based on AI-Driven-IoT(AIIoT): A KSK Approach, *Advance Research in Communication Engineering and its. Innovations*, 1(2), 23–32.

Kazi, K. S. S. L. (2024). Polymer Applications in Energy Generation and Storage: A Forward Path. Journal of Nanoscience. *Nanoengineering & Applications.*, 14(2), 31–39p.

Kazi, K. S. S. L. (2024p). Polymer Applications in Energy Generation and Storage: A Forward Path. *Journal of Nanoscience. Nanoengineering & Applications.*, 14(2), 31–39p.

Kazi, S.. (2023a). Fruit Grading, Disease Detection, and an Image Processing Strategy. *Journal of Image Processing and Artificial Intelligence*, 9(2), 17–34.

Kazi, S. S. L. (2023b). Integrating IoT and Mechanical Systems in Mechanical Engineering Applications. *Journal of Mechanisms and Robotics*, 8(3), 1–6.

Kazi, S. S. L. (2023c). IoT Changing the Electronics Manufacturing Industry. *Journal of Analog and Digital Communications*, 8(3), 13–17.

Kazi, S. S. L. (2023d). IoT in the Electric Power Industry. *Journal of Controller and Converters*, 8(3), 1–7.

Kazi, S. S. L. (2023e). Review of Integrated Battery Charger (IBC) for Electric Vehicles (EV). *Journal of Advances in Electrical Devices*, 8(3), 1–11.

Kazi, S. S. L. (2023f). ML in the Electronics Manufacturing Industry. *Journal of Switching Hub*, 8(3), 9–13.

Kazi, S. S. L. (2023g). IoT in Electrical Vehicle: A Study. *Journal of Control and Instrumentation Engineering*, 9(3), 15–21.

Kazi, S. S. L. (2023h). PV Power Control for DC Microgrid Energy Storage Utilisation. *Journal of Digital Integrated Circuits in Electrical Devices*, 8(3), 1–8.

Kazi, S. S. L. (2023i). Electronics with Artificial Intelligence Creating a Smarter Future: A Review. *Journal of Communication Engineering and Its Innovations*, 9(3), 38–42.

Kazi, S. S. L. (2023j). Dispersion Compensation in Optical Fiber: A Review. *Journal of Telecommunication Study*, 8(3), 14–19.

Kazi, S. S. L. (2023k). IoT Based Arduino-Powered Weather Monitoring System. *Journal of Telecommunication Study*, 8(3), 25–31.

Kazi, S. S. L. (2023l). Arduino Based Weather Monitoring System. *Journal of Switching Hub*, 8(3), 24–29.

Kazi, S. S. L. (2023m). Accepting Internet of Nano-Things: Synopsis, Developments, and Challenges. *Journal of Nanoscience. Nanoengineering & Applications.*, 13(2), 17–26p. DOI: 10.37591/jonsnea.v13i2.1464

Kazi, S. S. L. (2023n). Nanomedicine as a Potential Therapeutic Approach to COVID-19. *International Journal of Applied Nanotechnology.*, 9(2), 27–35p.

Kazi Kutubuddin, S. L. (2022a). Predict the Severity of Diabetes cases, using K-Means and Decision Tree Approach. *Journal of Advances in Shell Programming*, 9(2), 24–31.

Kazi Kutubuddin, S. L. (2022b). A novel Design of IoT based 'Love Representation and Remembrance' System to Loved One's. *Gradiva Review Journal*, 8(12), 377–383.

Kazi Kutubuddin S. L., (2022c). Business Mode and Product Life Cycle to Improve Marketing in Healthcare Units, *E-Commerce for future & Trends*, 9(3), pp. 1-9.

Kutubuddin, K. (2022d). Detection of Malicious Nodes in IoT Networks based on packet loss using ML, *Journal of Mobile Computing, Communication & mobile. Networks*, 9(3), 9–16.

Kutubuddin, K. (2022e). Big data and HR Analytics in Talent Management: A Study. *Recent Trends in Parallel Computing*, 9(3), 16–26.

Kutubuddin, K. (2023a). Blockchain-Enabled IoT Environment to Embedded System a Self-Secure Firmware Model. *Journal of Telecommunication Study*, 8(1), 13–19.

Kutubuddin, K. (2023b). A Study HR Analytics Big Data in Talent Management. *Research and Review: Human Resource and Labour Management*, 4(1), 16–28.

Kutubuddin, K. (2024c). Vehicle Health Monitoring System (VHMS) by Employing IoT and Sensors, *Grenze International Journal of Engineering and Technology,* Vol 10, Issue 2, pp- 5367-5374. Available at: https://thegrenze.com/index.php?display=page&view=journalabstract&absid=3371&id=8

Kutubuddin, K. (2024d). A Novel Approach on ML based Palmistry, *Grenze International Journal of Engineering and Technology,* Vol 10, Issue 2, pp- 5186-5193. Available at: https://thegrenze.com/index.php?display=page&view=journalabstract&absid=3344&id=8

Kutubuddin, K. (2024e). IoT based Boiler Health Monitoring for Sugar Industries, *Grenze. IACSIT International Journal of Engineering and Technology*, 10(2), 5178–5185. https://thegrenze.com/index.php?display=page&view=journalabstract&absid=3343&id=8

Liyakat, K. K. (2025). Heart Health Monitoring Using IoT and Machine Learning Methods. In Shaik, A. (Ed.), *AI-Powered Advances in Pharmacology* (pp. 257–282). IGI Global., DOI: 10.4018/979-8-3693-3212-2.ch010

Liyakat, K. K. S. (2017). Lessar methodology for network intrusion detection. *Scholarly Research Journal for Humanity Science & English Language*, 4(24), 6853–6861.

Liyakat, K. K. S. (2022). Implementation of e-mail security with three layers of authentication. *Journal of Operating Systems Development and Trends*, 9(2), 29–35.

Liyakat, K. K. S. (2023).Detecting Malicious Nodes in IoT Networks Using Machine Learning and Artificial Neural Networks, *2023 International Conference on Emerging Smart Computing and Informatics (ESCI)*, Pune, India, 2023, pp. 1-5, DOI: 10.1109/ESCI56872.2023.10099544

Liyakat, K. K. S. (2023). Machine Learning Approach Using Artificial Neural Networks to Detect Malicious Nodes in IoT Networks. In Shukla, P. K., Mittal, H., & Engelbrecht, A. (Eds.), *Computer Vision and Robotics. CVR 2023. Algorithms for Intelligent Systems*. Springer., DOI: 10.1007/978-981-99-4577-1_3

Liyakat, K. K. S. (2024). Machine Learning Approach Using Artificial Neural Networks to Detect Malicious Nodes in IoT Networks. In Udgata, S. K., Sethi, S., & Gao, X. Z. (Eds.), *Intelligent Systems. ICMIB 2023. Lecture Notes in Networks and Systems* (Vol. 728). Springer., available at https://link.springer.com/chapter/10.1007/978-981-99-3932-9_12, DOI: 10.1007/978-981-99-3932-9_12

Liyakat, K. K. S. (2024). Explainable AI in healthcare. *Explainable Artificial Intelligence in Healthcare Systems*, 2024, 271–284.

Liyakat, K. K. S., Paradeshi, K. P., Shaikh, J. A., Pandyaji, K. K., & Kadam, D. B. (2022). Development of Machine Learning based Epileptic Seizureprediction using Web of Things (WoT). *NeuroQuantology : An Interdisciplinary Journal of Neuroscience and Quantum Physics*, 20(8), 9394.

Liyakat, K. S. (2022). Nanotechnology Application in Neural Growth Support System. Nano Trends: A Journal of Nanotechnology and Its Applications, 24(2), 47-55.

Liyakat, S. (2023). Intelligent Watering System (IWS) for Agricultural Land Utilising Raspberry Pi. *Recent Trends in Fluid Mechanics.*, 10(2), 26–31p.

Liyakat, S. S. (2024). IoT-based Alcohol Detector using Blynk. *Journal of Electronics Design and Technology*, 1(1), 10–15.

Liyakat Kazi, K. S. (2024). ChatGPT: An Automated Teacher's Guide to Learning. In Bansal, R., Chakir, A., Hafaz Ngah, A., Rabby, F., & Jain, A. (Eds.), *AI Algorithms and ChatGPT for Student Engagement in Online Learning* (pp. 1–20). IGI Global., DOI: 10.4018/979-8-3693-4268-8.ch001

Machha Babitha, Ms.. (2022). Trends of Artificial Intelligence for online exams in education, International journal of Early Childhood special. *Education*, 14(1), 2457–2463.

Mishra Sunil, B.. (2024). Nanotechnology's Importance in Mechanical Engineering. *Journal of Fluid Mechanics and Mechanical Design*, 6(1), 1–9.

Mishra Sunil, B.. (2024). Review of the Literature and Methodological Structure for IoT and PLM Integration in the Manufacturing Sector. *Journal of Advancement in Machines*, 9(1), 1–5.

Mishra Sunil, B.. (2024). AI-Driven IoT (AI IoT) in Thermodynamic Engineering. *Journal of Modern Thermodynamics in Mechanical System*, 6(1), 1–8.

Miss Argonda, U. A. (2018). Review paper for design and simulation of a Patch antenna by using HFSS. *International Journal of Trends in Scientific Research and Development*, 2(2), 158–160.

Nagare, M. S., & KS, M. K. (2015). An Efficient Algorithm brain tumor detection based on Segmentation and Thresholding. Journal of Management in Manufacturing and services, 2(17), 19-27.

Nagrale, M., Pol, R. S., Birajadar, G. B., & Mulani, A. O. (2024). Internet of Robotic Things in Cardiac Surgery: An Innovative Approach. *African Journal of Biological Sciences*, 6(6), 709–725. DOI: 10.33472/AFJBS.6.6.2024.709-725

Neeraja, P., Kumar, R. G., Kumar, M. S., Liyakat, K. K. S., & Vani, M. S. (2024). *DL-Based Somnolence Detection for Improved Driver Safety and Alertness Monitoring. 2024 IEEE International Conference on Computing, Power and Communication Technologies (IC2PCT)*. Greater Noida., Available at https://ieeexplore.ieee.org/document/10486714, DOI: 10.1109/IC2PCT60090.2024.10486714

Nerkar, P. M., Shinde, S. S., Liyakat, K. K. S., Desai, S., & Kazi, S. S. L. (2023). Monitoring fresh fruit and food using Iot and machine learning to improve food safety and quality. Tuijin Jishu/Journal of Propulsion Technology, 44(3), 2927-2931.

Nida, N. (2023). Shaikh, Milind. (2023). PV Penetrations in Conventional Power System and Generation of Harmonic and Power Quality Issues: A Review. *International Journal of Power Electronics Controllers and Converters*, 9(2), 12–19p.

Nikita, K.. (2020). Design of Vehicle system using CAN Protocol. *International Journal for Research in Applied Science and Engineering Technology*, 8(V), 1978–1983. DOI: 10.22214/ijraset.2020.5321

Pardeshi, D. K. (2022). Implementation of fault detection framework for healthcare monitoring system using IoT, sensors in wireless environment. *Telematique*, 21(1), 5451–5460.

Pradeepa, M., ….. (2022). Student Health Detection using a Machine Learning Approach and IoT, *2022 IEEE 2nd Mysore sub section International Conference (MysuruCon), 2022.*

Prasad, K. R., Karanam, S. R., Ganesh, D., Liyakat, K. K. S., Talasila, V., & Purushotham, P. (2024, May). AI in public-private partnership for IT infrastructure development. *The Journal of High Technology Management Research*, 35(1), 100496. DOI: 10.1016/j.hitech.2024.100496

Prashant, K. Magadum (2024). Machine Learning for Predicting Wind Turbine Output Power in Wind Energy Conversion Systems, *Grenze International Journal of Engineering and Technology,* Jan Issue, Vol 10, Issue 1, pp. 2074-2080. Grenze ID: 01.GIJET.10.1.4_1 Available at: https://thegrenze.com/index.php?display=page&view=journalabstract&absid=2514&id=8

Prof. Kazi Kutubuddin, S. L. (2016a). Situation Invariant face recognition using PCA and Feed Forward Neural network, *Proceeding of International Conference on Advances in Engineering, Science and Technology,* 2016, pp. 260- 263.

Prof. Kazi Kutubuddin, S. L. (2016b). An Approach on Yarn Quality Detection for Textile Industries using Image Processing, *Proceeding of International Conference on Advances in Engineering, Science and Technology,* 2016, pp. 325-330.

Ravi, A.. (2022). *Pattern Recognition- An Approach towards Machine Learning, Lambert Publications, 2022*. ISBN.

Sayyad, L. (2023). System for Love Healthcare for Loved Ones based on IoT. Research Exploration: Transcendence of Research Methods and Methodology, 2.

Shaikh, M. (2023). Machine Learning in the Production Process Control of Metal Melting. *Journal of Advancement in Machines*, 8(2).

Shweta Nagare, Ms.. (2014). Different Segmentation Techniques for brain tumor detection: A Survey, *MM- International society for green. Sustainable Engineering and Management*, 1(14), 29–35.

Sreenivasulu, M. D., Devi, J. S., Arulprakash, P., Venkataramana, S., & Kazi, K. S. (2022). Implementation of latest machine learning approaches for students grade prediction. *International Journal of Early Childhood*, 14(3).

Vahida, . (2023). Deep Learning, YOLO and RFID based smart Billing Handcart. *Journal of Communication Engineering & Systems*, 13(1), 1–8.

Veena, C., Sridevi, M., Liyakat, K. K. S., Saha, B., Reddy, S. R., & Shirisha, N. (2023). *HEECCNB: An Efficient IoT-Cloud Architecture for Secure Patient Data Transmission and Accurate Disease Prediction in Healthcare Systems, 2023 Seventh International Conference on Image Information Processing.* ICIIP., Available at https://ieeexplore.ieee.org/document/10537627, DOI: 10.1109/ICIIP61524.2023.10537627

Wale, A. D., & Dipali, R.. (2019). Smart Agriculture System using IoT. *International Journal of Innovative Research in Technology*, 5(10), 493–497.

Yogita Shirdale, Ms.. (2014). Analysis and design of Capacitive coupled wideband Microstrip antenna in C and X band: A Survey, *Journal GSD-International society for green. Sustainable Engineering and Management*, 1(15), 1–7.

Yogita Shirdale, Ms.. (2016). Coplanar capacitive coupled probe fed micro strip antenna for C and X band. *International Journal of Advanced Research in Computer and Communication Engineering*, 5(4), 661–663.

KEY TERMS AND DEFINITIONS

IoMT: Internet of Medical Things.
ML: Machine Learning.
IoT: Internet of Things.
ANN: Artificial Neural Networks.
DT: Decision Tree.
SVM: Support Vector Machine.

NB: Naïve Bayes.
AB: Adaptive Boosting.
K-NN: K-Nearest Neighbor.
RF: Random Forest.

Chapter 17
Deep Learning Classification of Diabetic Retinopathy Using ResNet-101 Convolutional Neural Networks

R. Ravindraiah
Madanapalle Institute of Technology and Science, India

Grande Naga Jyothi
Madanapalle Institute of Technology and Science, India

J. Pavan Royal
Madanapalle Institute of Technology and Science, India

B. Nagavardhan Reddy
Madanapalle Institute of Technology and Science, India

B. Nithish Kumar
Madanapalle Institute of Technology and Science, India

ABSTRACT

Diabetic Retinopathy (DR) patients suffer from chronically excessive blood sugar, which impairs retinal features. Diabetic sufferers are extra prone to this difficulty, which may cause vision loss unless caught and handled early. It is the world's sixth most common cause of eyesight loss. Therefore, in-depth studies have been demanded in this vicinity to locate new approaches to diagnosing DR ranges. Initially, dedicated fundus image recognition techniques and computational algorithms were used to identify DR, however, their usefulness in real-time clinical practice became inadequate. Convolutional Neural Networks (CNNs), one type of deep learning model, are better at predicting the prognosis of DR. The goal of this research work is to understand the overall performance of a deep-gaining knowledge model, ResNet, a deep-stage neural network, in detecting non-prescriptive and exclusive varieties of suggestible DR.

DOI: 10.4018/979-8-3693-6180-1.ch017

1. INTRODUCTION

Around the world, millions of people suffer from Diabetes Mellitus (DM), a severe chronic illness. High blood sugar levels are a hallmark of diabetes, which can be caused by insufficient insulin synthesis, occasionally impaired metabolic processes, or a combination of the two. Long-term complications of diabetes may include heart-related problems such as cardiovascular dysfunction, renal damage, stroke, cardiac arrest, and other heart-related issues, as well as problems with blood arteries and nerves in the legs and feet. In 1980, there were about 122,000,000 people worldwide. By 2014, that number had increased to almost 422,000,000. By 2040, there will be approximately 642,000,000 people living with diabetes worldwide. Furthermore, diabetes was a direct cause of close to 1.6 million deaths globally. It can cause damage to the retina, which is known medically as DR or diabetic eye disease. In developed nations, DR ranks among the primary causes of blindness. According to [IDF 2021] forecasts, there will be a significant increase in the number of cases of diabetes worldwide. By 2045, there will be 783 million affected individuals, a 46% increase from the 537 million in 2021. Regionally, North America & the Caribbean will see a 24% increase in diabetes cases, from 51 million to 63 million; the Western Pacific region is projected to grow by 27%, from 206 million to 260 million; Europe will experience a 13% rise, from 61 million to 69 million; and South & Central America will have a 50% increase, expanding from 32 million to 49 million. The Middle East & North Africa region is also predicted to face a significant rise, though specific figures are not fully provided. This underscores the growing global challenge of addressing and managing diabetes.

Among individuals enduring both type 1 and type 2 diabetes for over two decades, as many as 80% may develop this condition. Up to 90% of new cases may be treated and kept under close observation to avoid more severe types of retinopathy and maculopathy, which can impair vision. The risk of DR escalates with the duration of diabetes. Annually, Twelve percent of newly diagnosed instances of blindness in the US are related to DR. Additionally, it is the primary cause of blindness in people who are 20 to 64 years old [WHO 2024]. A disorder known as DR affects healthy eyes, causing retinal degeneration that eventually leads to complete blindness. To avoid total visual loss, DR must be identified early.

Currently, 537 million adults in the world between the ages of 20 and 79 have diabetes, accounting for 10.5% of all adults in this age group. According to projections, this number will increase to 783 million (12.2%) by 2045 and to 643 million (11.3%) by 2030. A little over half of all people living with diabetes are unaware that they have the disease, accounting for about 240 million undiagnosed cases worldwide. Approximately 90% of these cases go undiagnosed and are located in countries with low or middle incomes. Over half of the population with diabetes in parts of the world like Africa, South-East Asia, and the Pacific Northwest do not have a diagnosis. More than half (54%) of the 1.2 million kids and teens with type 1 diabetes are under the age of 15. A systematic review found that between 2006 and 2017, the incidence of diabetes either decreased or stayed stable in over 70% of mostly high-income countries.

Furthermore, since 2010, diabetes rates have decreased or remained stable in more than 80% of the world's nations. Approximately 537 million adults in the world between the ages of 20 and 79—or 10.5% of the population—have diabetes. This figure is projected to increase to 643 million by 2030 and potentially reach 783 million by 2045. The number of individuals suffering from diabetes is expected to rise by 46% during this time, despite the 20% predicted growth in the world's population (Sebastian,2023).

With 140.9 million cases, China led the world in 2021 among adults aged 20 to 79 with diabetes, followed by India (74.2 million) and Pakistan (33.0 million). The United States, Indonesia, Brazil, and Mexico also ranked high, with Bangladesh, Japan, and Egypt completing the top ten. By 2045, China is projected to remain at the top with 174.4 million, and India and Pakistan will continue to be in the top three. The United States, Indonesia, and Brazil are expected to retain their positions, while Bangladesh is anticipated to move up to seventh place, pushing Mexico to eighth. Egypt will drop to ninth, and Turkey will enter the top ten, replacing Japan. In 2021, the rate of undiagnosed diabetes among adults aged 20–79 differed by income level. High-income countries had 28.8% of their population with undiagnosed diabetes, equating to 29.9 million people. Middle-income countries had a higher rate of 48.4%, with 200.4 million individuals affected. Low-income countries had the highest proportion, at 50.5%, translating to 9.5 million people with undiagnosed diabetes. (IDF 2021).

DR can be identified using a variety of real evaluations, some of which are time-consuming and useful for patients. These tests include optical intelligence tomography, student widening, and obvious sharpness testing. This survey work aims to explore the field of disturbance decision-making by utilizing device learning representation computations to extract features from the output of several retinal image processing estimations. After having the condition for several decades, almost all diabetics get some degree of retinal impairment, or "retinopathy" (Sgallari et.al, 2013). Many people's retinal exams are the only way to identify this impairment, which has no discernible impact on vision. On a retinal exam, persistent retinal damage may gradually manifest as tiny bulges in the retinal blood vessels known as microaneurysms. Next come bigger anomalies in the retinal capillaries, such as cotton wool patches, bleeding, lipid buildups referred to as "hard exudates," intraretinal microvascular anomalies, and strange-appearing retinal veins. A point is finally reached by many when the blood vessels in the retina keep growing. These developing blood vessels frequently bleed when they burst. Visual impairments range from minor bleeding-induced black floating patches to serious bleeding-induced total blockage of vision (Ravindraiah R et. al., 2018).

Diabetes is linked to two serious eye conditions: diabetic macular edema (DME) and DR (DR). Long-term elevated blood sugar levels damage the blood vessels in the retina, the tissue sensitive to light at the rear of the eye, resulting in DR, an adverse effect.

The disease progresses through several stages, starting with Non-Proliferative DR (NPDR). In the mild stage, microaneurysms and small retinal hemorrhages are present. As the condition worsens to moderate NPDR, more extensive hemorrhages and exudates occur, with increased leakage from the blood vessels. Severe NPDR is marked by numerous retinal hemorrhages, significant retinal ischemia, and potential retinal edema. The development of unusual vascular structures on the layers of the retina and optic nerve head (neovascularization) is a characteristic of Proliferative DR (PDR), an advanced form of the disease that can cause bleeding, retinal detachment, and vision loss.

A related ailment called DME is characterized by fluid buildup in the macula, the central region of the retina that provides clear, central vision. It can arise at any stage of DR but is more common in advanced stages. It is classified into focal DME, which features localized fluid accumulation and edema, and diffuse DME, where widespread edema and thickening of the macula occur, leading to more significant vision impairment. Both DR and DME can cause severe vision loss if not properly managed, underscoring the importance of regular eye exams and effective diabetes control. DME combined with DR is one variation. Blindness and visual loss are the most common outcomes of DME. Decreased Membranes are caused by fluid leaking inside the macula of diabetic individuals, resulting from prolonged increased blood sugar levels. Using fundus pictures, DME is evaluated by looking for retinal edema and bright lesions known as exudates. Imaging processing methods are used to locate the macula and hard exudates. The depth and superficiality of the spots, respectively, characterize the two types of hemorrhages: blot and flame. Hard exudates result from this, which causes yellow spots to appear on the retina as a result of plasma leakage (Kurle S. al 2017).

Figure 1. Healthy retina and Diabetic retina

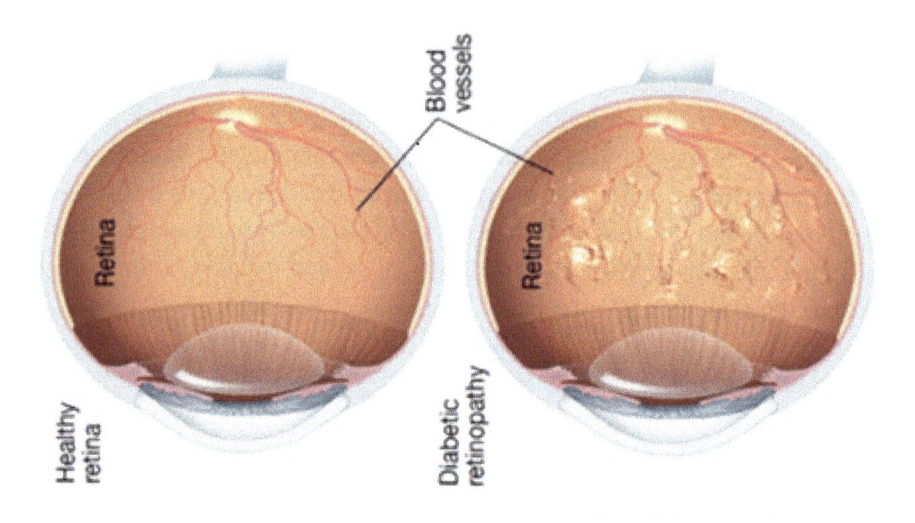

(Kurle,2017)

The tiny features of MAs are seen in Figure.1, which is an example of a typical NPDR retinal fundus picture. Yellow spots, or hard exudates, are seen in the typical NPDR retinal fundus pictures. The absence of neovascularization is the diagnostic basis for Non-Proliferative DR (NPDR), which includes several typical lesions linked to the condition (DR). Proliferative DR (PDR), which leads to DR, gradually increases the hazards to vision as it progresses from mild to moderate to severe (Singh N et. Al, 2015). DR severity levels are precisely categorized, which makes it easier to identify high-risk patients and manage them with appropriate referrals, regular exams, and actions to maintain current vision. Proliferative DR culminates in angiogenesis, a physiological mechanism that causes pre-existing blood arteries to give rise to new ones. Neovascularization is the process by which new blood vessels often develop along the vascular arcades of the retina.

Beyond only causing vision loss, DR has a substantial socioeconomic impact and affects the quality of life for both affected individuals and society as a whole. In order to avoid irreversible vision loss and lessen the overall societal burden connected with this illness, prompt diagnosis and treatment are essential. As a result, in order to effectively address the various challenges presented by DR, comprehensive screening programs, easily accessible healthcare services, and efficacious treatment modalities are imperative. To lessen the worldwide burden of vision loss caused by DR, it is imperative that we increase our knowledge of the pathophysiology of the condition, develop novel therapeutic approaches, and improve diagnostic technologies. The well-being and visual health of people with diabetes around the world can be improved by healthcare stakeholders working toward a future in which DR is not a primary cause of blindness through interdisciplinary collaboration and prevention measures (Ravindraiah R et. al, 2020)

1.1 Objective of the Work

This work's main goal is to find early indicators of DR, prior to symptoms appear. Early detection is essential because it enables prompt intervention, which lowers the risk of blindness or severe vision loss dramatically with the right care. The project intends to improve the consistency and accuracy of ocular image classification in comparison to manual examinations by utilizing AI and machine learning algorithms. This will reduce the possibility of misdiagnosis and guarantee that patients receive timely and effective treatment.

Additionally, this approach seeks to lower the costs associated with DR screening, making it more cost-effective for healthcare systems and more affordable for patients. The project is driven by both the medical significance and the technological advancements in AI and machine learning. It aims to differentiate between healthy eye images and those affected by DR, addressing a critical need in preventive healthcare. This initiative not only addresses an urgent healthcare need but also makes a substantial contribution to society by harnessing the power of AI and ML.

The following key points underscore the necessity of such a project:

Early Diagnosis and Prevention: Although DR is the world's most common cause of blindness in people of working age, if caught early enough, it is frequently curable. However, the condition typically presents no symptoms in its initial stages, leading to delayed diagnosis until significant vision impairment occurs. An automated classification system can enable widespread, early detection of retinopathy, facilitating timely intervention to prevent blindness or severe vision loss.

Accessibility and Scalability: There is a global shortage of ophthalmologists, particularly in rural and underserved regions. An AI-based tool for identifying DR in eye images can be deployed on a large scale and made easily accessible, alleviating pressure on healthcare systems and extending eye care services to underrepresented populations.

Cost-Effectiveness: Automating the screening process for DR can drastically reduce the costs associated with manual screening, including labor, time, and resources. This cost-efficiency benefits healthcare systems and patients alike, as early detection and treatment can help avoid the expenses associated with advanced stages of eye diseases.

Enhanced Accuracy and Consistency: AI models, once trained on extensive datasets of eye images, can achieve high accuracy in identifying DR. These models also ensure consistent results across multiple screenings, eliminating the variability that can sometimes occur with human evaluations.

Advancing Medical Research and Treatment: The information gathered and examined for this project may offer important new understandings into how DR and other retinal disorders develop. This could lead to the discovery of previously unknown aspects of these conditions, guiding future research and improving treatment strategies.

Democratizing Healthcare Access: The integration of AI in healthcare democratizes access to diagnostic services, empowering individuals to take a more proactive role in managing their health. By providing tools for disease prediction and prevention, technology serves as an equalizer in the healthcare sector, reducing barriers to access and enhancing patient outcomes.

2 RELATED WORKS

One serious consequence of diabetes is DR., necessitating timely and accurate detection for current intrusion. Conventional manual assessment by skilled medical practitioners suffer from inter- and intra-grader inconsistencies, highlighting the demand for automated systems. Over the past decade, significant research has focused on developing computer-aided systems utilizing various techniques, from conventional machine learning to advanced deep learning models. The VGG Net deep learning approach was proposed by Kwasigroch A et al. (2018) for automated screening of DR. Utilizing a unique class coding method, it reduces the discrepancy between target and predicted scores. The best tested model showed promise for improving DR screening, with 82% accuracy in detecting retinopathy and 51% accuracy in determining its stage. The GoogleNet, AlexNet, and ResNet50 designs that were already in use were compared by Kumar S et al. (2019). The most accurate machine learning model used for this task turned out to be GoogLeNet. On the Kaggle EyePACS database, their claimed average accuracy was 69.9%. Two balanced datasets—one with augmentation and the other without—were used by Maistry et al. (2020). After batch normalization, they used the CNN model's ReLU function. After that, the softmax function and a linear classifier were used. They reported an accuracy of 87.0% on Kaggle EyePACS.

Using the AlexNet architecture for feature extraction and the CLAHE model for image segmentation is done by Vaishnavi J et al. (2020). The softmax layer classified images into different DR (deep learning) stages. The framework's maximum accuracy in classification of 95.86%, along with its sensitivity of 92.00% and specificity of 97.86%, was demonstrated during testing on the Kaggle dataset. To grade DR images, used the VGG-16 CNN. In the early phases, they used batch normalization and the VGG-16 model that had already been trained for classification. Their model produced a mean class accuracy of 74%, 80% sensitivity, and 65% specificity on the Kaggle dataset. The five transfer learning models (Xception, InceptionResNetV2, MobileNetV2, DenseNet121, and NASNetMobile) to propose a binary classification of DR. On the Kaggle APTOS database, these models achieved the highest accuracy for validation (86.1%), sensitivity (85.4%), and specificity (87.5%), respectively.

"AD2Net," a CNN model that integrates Res2Net and DenseNet to capture multi-scale features and mitigate vanishing-gradient issues is introduced. The model incorporates an attention mechanism to highlight relevant information in images, enhancing classification performance. AD2Net can categorize fundus images from the Kaggle EyePACS database into five stages of disease severity, achieving an accuracy of 83.2% and a Kappa value of 0.8 on the testing set.

A CNN visualization approach is employed by Reguant R, et al. (2021) to critically examine image features involved in CNN decision-making, with a particular focus on pathologies such as microaneurysms and hemorrhages. They evaluated the image features of various CNNs to predict and validate their clinical significance. Their experiments, conducted on publicly available Kaggle datasets, resulted in an accuracy of 95%, sensitivity of 86%, and specificity of 96%.

The FFU-Net model represents an innovative method for segmenting lesions in DR. It features a convolutional layer designed to minimize spatial loss, a Multiscale Feature Filter Block (MSFF) for extracting multiscale features, and a CCA module that integrates information from skip connections and lower-resolution decoders using shared attention weights. Additionally, the model employs a Balanced Focal Loss function to tackle data imbalance issues in DR. Its performance was validated through ablation studies and user evaluations on the public benchmark IDRID, yielding an average sensitivity of 79.33%.

The Hinge Attention Network (HA-Net) deep learning model with multiple attention stages was proposed by Shaik N.S. et al. (2022). It combines a hinge neural network for accurate and generalized predictions on unseen data, a convolutional LSTM layer for prioritizing important spatial maps, and a pre-trained VGG16 base for initial spatial representation from retinal scan images. Using the Kaggle APTOS 2019 and ISBI IDRiD datasets, the model's efficacy and acceptability were confirmed. It achieved an accuracy of 85.54% on Kaggle APTOS and 66.41% on IDRiD. The paper of (Pamadi A.M et. al 2022) proposes a multi-modal classification CNN model. By applying Gaussian filtering to fundus photos, the visibility of subtle features such as edges or dots is enhanced, aiding in more accurate diagnosis. For multinomial classification, transfer learning with a pre-trained MobileNetV2 model boosts accuracy to 78%.

AlexNet, ResNet-50, and VGG-16 were used to implement DR classification. A comprehensive empirical evaluation was performed to analyze the performance of twenty-eight deep hybrid neural network architectures for binary classification of DR into referable and non-referable classes. On average, they achieved 89% accuracy on Kaggle APTOS, 84.1% accuracy on Messidor2, and 84% accuracy on Kaggle EyePACS databases.

Sowmiya R et al (2023) used pre-processed images for segmentation using an attention U-Net model based on MCA. In visual representation, our model outperformed existing architectures, achieving an average accuracy of 99.04% on the IDRiB and e-Ophtha databases. In the majority of test images, the model outperformed other techniques such as Attention U-Net, Residual U-Net, Res Attention U-Net, and U-Net architecture. This Voting based classification methodology of (Akram M et al., 2024) is compared with KNN, SVM, and random forest in terms of accuracy, precision, and recall. According to the results, the suggested model's maximum accuracy was 89.35 percent; this was higher than the accuracy of SVM, KNN, and random forest, which were 79.35, 83.38, and 80.96 percent, respectively.

2.1 Disadvantages of Existing Systems

The following are the key drawbacks in the existing methods:

(i) Need for Large Datasets

Large volumes of labeled data are necessary for deep learning models, especially CNNs (CNNs), to train efficiently and attain high accuracy. But in the medical domain, obtaining such vast datasets can be especially difficult because of issues with privacy, the scarcity of specific conditions, and the costly and laborious method of expert annotation.

(ii) Limited Model Interpretability

CNNs and other deep learning models often function as "black boxes," offering little explanation of how they reach their conclusions. This lack of transparency can be a significant drawback in medical applications, where understanding the reasoning behind a diagnosis or classification is essential for professional trust and informed decision-making.

(iii) Overfitting Issues

Deep learning models often suffer from overfitting, particularly when trained on small or very similar datasets. When a model overfits, it learns the noise in the data used for training instead of the true patterns, which produces excellent results on the training data but inadequate generalization to new data. Even with techniques like regularization and dropout, overfitting remains a persistent challenge, particularly in medical imaging, where data variability is high.

This work focus on to use AI and machine learning to identify early signs of DR, improving diagnostic consistency and accuracy over manual examinations. With prompt treatment, early detection can greatly lower the chance of developing severe vision loss or blindness. An important gap in preventive healthcare is filled by this automated system, which makes screening more affordable and accessible—especially in underserved areas where there is a scarcity of ophthalmologists. Healthcare systems can save money on labor, time, and resources by automating the process, and patients can also benefit from lower medical expenses. AI models with high accuracy and consistency, which support early diagnosis and intervention, are trained on large-scale eye image datasets. Furthermore, by shedding light on DR and other retinal disorders, this project advances medical research and may lead to better treatment strategies. Recognizing limitations in architectures like ResNet50, the proposed ResNet model aims to address overfitting, high computational costs, and memory requirements. Inspired by the lightweight structure and efficiency of ResNet-101, this study seeks to reduce computational costs while enhancing performance matrices and minimizing memory requirements.

3 PROPOSED RESNET-101 CNN MODEL

ResNet uses residual learning to solve the vanishing gradient problem, revolutionizing deep learning for image classification. Gradient problems frequently prevented traditional deep networks from training, but ResNet added "skip connections," or shortcut connections, which improved gradient flow and made it possible to train much deeper networks. ResNet variants consist of residual blocks; the numbers indicate the total number of layers. Identity mapping is used in these blocks to maintain information, and deeper versions of these blocks contain elements such as 1x1, 3x3, and 1x1 convolutions to lower parameter and computational costs. It has become widely used in both academia and industry, where it is now considered a standard architecture for a variety of image classification tasks and acts as a foundation for more intricate models in object detection and segmentation (He K et. al., 2016). The theory behind ResNet's residual learning has influenced many other architectures, such as DenseNet, which has advanced the field even more. A breakthrough in deep learning, ResNet's novel architecture has influenced the creation of new neural network architectures and allowed for the creation of deeper and more accurate networks.

As a result of the imaging system, there's frequently much less assessment inside the photographs of the retina and blood vessels can't be detected. Pre-processing is used to take away noise from the background image. This approach is designed to prepare the pix for the subsequent step, discover blood vessels, and improve the dynamic range of the image to acquire high segmentation accuracy and precision. To grow our contrast, Since, it may be compared more than other channels, the green channel in color retinal images is employed. The mixture of brightness benefits within the purple channel reduces the contrast between the abnormalities and the path of the retina; this enables to lessening of some reactions from blood vessel-like abnormalities that reduce the effectiveness of different blood vessel segmentation methods. This analysis uses an adaptive histogram equalization against the issue, which will increase the comparison of the retinal photograph within the inexperienced channel.

Figure. 2 portrays a type of deep neural network known as a CNN that is made to process and evaluate structured, grid-like data, including photographs.

CNN is a subset of deep learning models created especially for handling and categorizing visual data, like pictures. The core functionality of a CNN classifier lies in its ability to automatically extract features and recognize patterns through a series of interconnected layers, each contributing to the overall task of classification. The process begins with the *input layer*, where the image is introduced to the network of pixel matrix format. In the case of grayscale images, this matrix is two-dimensional, while for color images like those in RGB format, it is three-dimensional, consisting of height, width, and color channels. The input image is then processed by one or more *convolutional layers*, which are central to the CNN's architecture. A collection of filtration systems, or kernels, is present in every convolutional layer. These kernels traverse the image and carry out the convolutional mathematical operation. To create a feature map, this entails calculating the dot product within the image's overlapping regions and the filter. This map highlights specific patterns such as edges, textures, or corners. Different filters are capable of detecting different features, allowing the CNN to capture various characteristics of the input image.

The activation function is applied to the convolutional layer's output in order to add non-linearity to the model. The Rectified Linear Unit (ReLU), which adds zeros to all negative values in the feature map, is the most widely used activation function in CNNs. This is an important step because it allows the CNN to learn intricate patterns that are beyond the scope of linear operations. The feature maps normally pass through a pooling layer after the activation function, which uses downsampling to decrease the spatial dimensions of the feature maps. Common techniques in this layer are Max Pooling, which keeps the maximum value in a small area of the feature map, and Average Pooling, which takes the average value. In addition to offering a degree of translation invariance that increases the model's resistance to small positional changes in the input image's features, pooling helps to lower the computational burden and the number of parameters in the network.

The resultant feature maps are streamlined into a 1D vector following feature extraction. After that, this vector is passed through one or more fully connected layers, which operate in a manner akin to a conventional neural network in which every neuron in the layer before it is linked to every other neuron in the layer before it. In order to produce the final output, which in classification tasks is an average probability distribution over the possible classes, these fully connected layers are essential for integrating each of the characteristics extracted by the convolutional layers. A loss function is used to calculate the difference between the predicted and true labels during training, which involves comparing the network's output to the actual labels. Through *backpropagation* and *gradient descent*, the network adjusts its weights to minimize this loss, improving its accuracy over time. In summary, a CNN classifier systematically extracts features through convolution, reduces dimensionality through pooling, and classifies the input based on learned patterns, making it a powerful tool for image-based tasks. They draw inspirations from the human visual system, namely from the way the brain interprets visual data. Convolution is the fundamental idea of CNNs, which extracts characteristics from input data by applying filters. To find patterns, these filters, also known as kernels, go across the input data and multiply and aggregate each element individually.

Figure 2. Working principle of CNN classifier

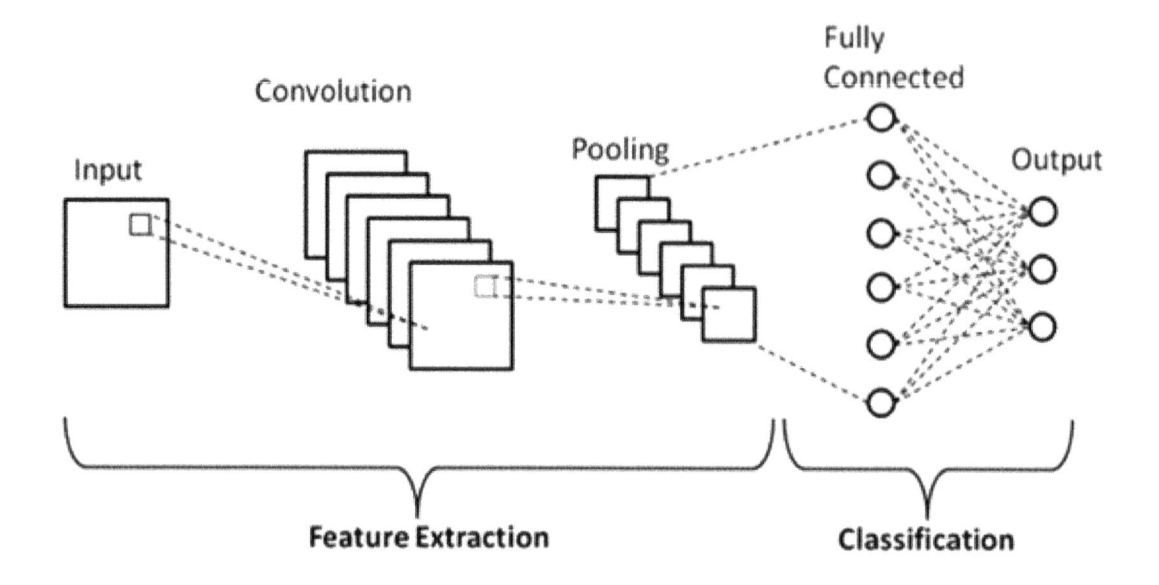

CNNs acquire the ability to recognize ever more complicated characteristics over a series of layers. Convolution is the fundamental idea of CNNs, which extracts characteristics from input data by applying filters. To find patterns, these filters, also known as kernels, go across the input data and multiply and aggregate each element individually. CNNs acquire the ability to recognize ever more complicated characteristics over a series of layers. A method called "image data augmentation" can be used to make altered copies of the photos in a training dataset, therefore artificially increasing its size. The training process of the proposed ResNet-101 CNN model is a comprehensive procedure that involves several critical stages, from data preparation to performance evaluation, ensuring that the model is both effective and generalizable. This process begins with the careful division of the available data into two distinct subsets: the train dataset and the test dataset. The train dataset is used during the model's learning phase, where the ResNet-101 architecture adjusts its parameters to optimize performance. In contrast, the test dataset is set aside to evaluate the model after training, offering an unbiased measure of how well the model can generalize to unseen data. This separation is important because it avoids overfitting, which is a situation in which a model performs remarkably well on training data but is unable to be generalized to new, unobserved examples.

Before the ResNet-101 model can begin learning, the data must undergo a preprocessing stage. During this stage, the raw images are prepared for input into the model. This typically involves resizing the images to a standard size that aligns with the model's input layer requirements, ensuring that all images are of consistent dimensions. Additionally, pixel values are normalized, converting them to a common range, such as [0, 1] or [-1, 1], which helps in stabilizing the learning process and improving convergence. Depending on the nature of the images and the specific task, other preprocessing steps might include converting color images to grayscale, enhancing contrast, or reducing noise to improve image clarity. These steps are vital for ensuring that the input data is in an optimal state for the model to learn effectively.

To further enhance the model's ability to generalize, data augmentation techniques are employed on the train dataset. Data augmentation involves applying a series of random transformations to the training images, such as rotations, flips, scaling, and color adjustments, creating additional variations of the original images. By doing this, the training dataset is effectively increased without requiring more data to be collected, revealing the model to a greater variety of training scenarios. As a result, despite changes in the input data, the ResNet-101 model learns to identify significant features and becomes more resilient. This phase is especially important when there is a small amount of dataset available because it reduces the likelihood of overfitting by rendering the resultant model less dependent on particular anomalies in the training set.

Once the data is preprocessed and augmented, the next phase involves training the ResNet-101 CNN model. ResNet-101 is a deep CNN architecture comprising 101 layers, including convolutional layers, batch normalization, ReLU activation functions, and residual connections that help mitigate the vanishing gradient problem. During training, the preprocessed and augmented train dataset is fed into the model, which then learns to optimize its weights and biases by minimizing a loss function, typically cross-entropy loss in classification tasks. In order to minimize the error that exists between predicted outputs and the actual labels, the model's parameters are iteratively changed using the method of backpropagation and gradient descent algorithms. Many epochs are used for the training process, and each epoch represents a full run through the train dataset. As training goes on, the model picks up more intricate patterns and features, which helps it get better at classifying images.

In the testing phase, the test dataset is used to assess the model's performance after the training phase. The accuracy and efficacy of the model are evaluated by comparing the predictions it makes with the actual labels, which it hasn't seen during training, using the test dataset. Important performance indicators like recall, accuracy, precision, and F1-score are computed to give a numerical assessment of the model's effectiveness. The testing phase is crucial because it reveals how well the model generalizes to new data, which is the ultimate goal of any machine learning model. The final step in the training process is statistical analysis, where the results from the testing phase are thoroughly analyzed. This analysis includes evaluating standard performance metrics and examining the confusion matrix to understand the model's behavior across different classes. To assess the significance of the findings, more complex statistical tests like confidence interval estimation and hypothesis testing may be performed. To determine the relative efficacy of the ResNet-101 model, its performance may also be compared to other cutting-edge techniques or baseline models. This thorough assessment guarantees that the model is thoroughly validated in addition to being well-trained, giving users confidence when deploying it for practical uses (Stitt et.al, 2016).

3.1 Training Process and Design of the Proposed RESNET 101 CNN

Deep learning neural network models can become more proficient with more data training, and picture variants produced by augmentation techniques can enhance the fit models' capacity to apply what they have learned to new images in Figure. 3. The process of data conversion from loading to prediction, including training and testing is shown in Figure. 4. The model's residual learning approach is intended to address the vanishing gradient problem. Remaining blocks in its architecture have skip connections, which facilitate easier gradient flow and improve information preservation. Bottleneck layers are used in the model to lower computational costs and parameter values.

Figure 3. Training process of the proposed RESNET 101 CNN model

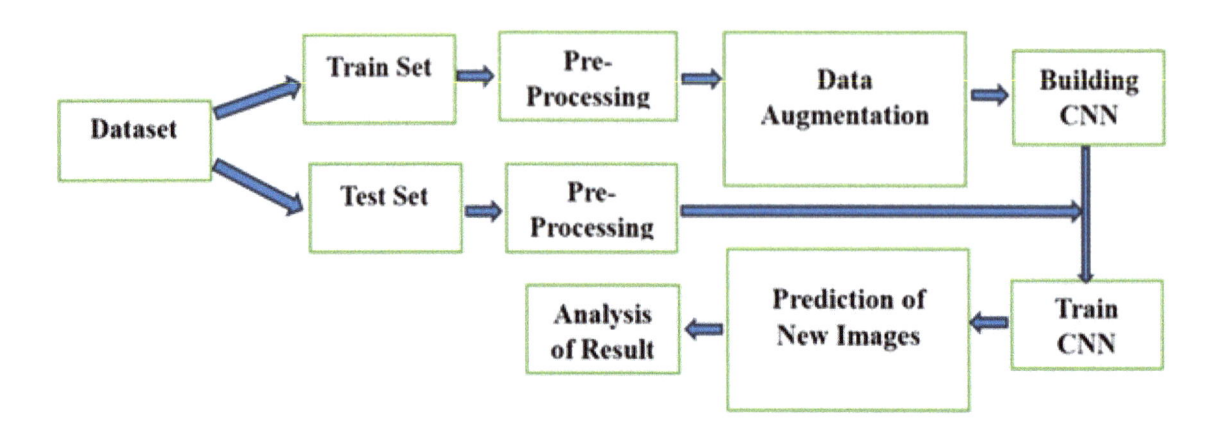

Images are fed into the network during training, and each residual block adds its input to its convolutional output. Optimization algorithms such as stochastic gradient descent (SGD) are used to compute the loss, which is usually cross-entropy for classification tasks, and backpropagate it to update weights. A systematic process that starts with data preprocessing and continues through performance evaluation and final prediction is used in the design and organization of the ResNet-101 classifier for diabetic retinal lesions. Developing a model that is accurate, dependable, and well-suited to generalizing to new data requires completing each step.

The process starts with *data preprocessing*, a critical step in preparing the raw retinal images for input into the ResNet-101 model. This involves standardizing the images and enhancing their quality through several key steps. Initially, the images are resized to ensure they meet the input dimension requirements of the ResNet-101 architecture, guaranteeing uniformity across all images fed into the model. Following this, pixel values are normalized to a consistent range, typically between [0, 1] or [-1, 1], depending on the network's configuration. Normalization is vital for stabilizing the learning process and making the model less sensitive to variations in input scales. Additional preprocessing may include noise reduction to eliminate extraneous details that could confuse the model, and contrast enhancement to make key features more prominent. If the model is designed for single-channel input, images might also be converted to grayscale during this stage. After preprocessing, the next step involves *data visualization*, where the dataset is explored using various visualization techniques. This stage is essential for gaining insights into the data before model training begins. Visualization tools such as histograms, scatter plots, and heatmaps are used to examine data distribution, identify patterns, and detect any anomalies or biases. For example, visualization might reveal an imbalance in the dataset, such as certain retinal lesion classes being underrepresented. Such insights are crucial as they inform decisions during the model-building process, such as whether to apply data augmentation techniques to balance the classes (Xu, 2021).

With the data preprocessed and visualized, the process moves on to *feature extraction*, a fundamental capability of the ResNet-101 architecture. As the input data passes through the network's layers, ResNet-101 extracts hierarchical features. In the initial layers, the model captures simple features like edges and textures. As data progresses through the deeper layers, the model begins to recognize more complex structures and patterns, which are essential for accurately identifying diabetic retinal lesions. The residual connections within ResNet-101 are particularly important because they preserve the integrity of learned features as data moves through the network's deep layers, preventing problems like vanishing gradients. The next stage is *model building*, where the ResNet-101 architecture is configured and initialized. This involves setting up the network layers, including convolutional layers, residual blocks, batch normalization, and activation functions. The model is then compiled with a loss function, such as cross-entropy for classification tasks, and an optimizer, like Adam or Stochastic Gradient Descent (SGD), is selected to guide the learning process. This step lays the groundwork for the training phase.

Figure 4. Model design and organization

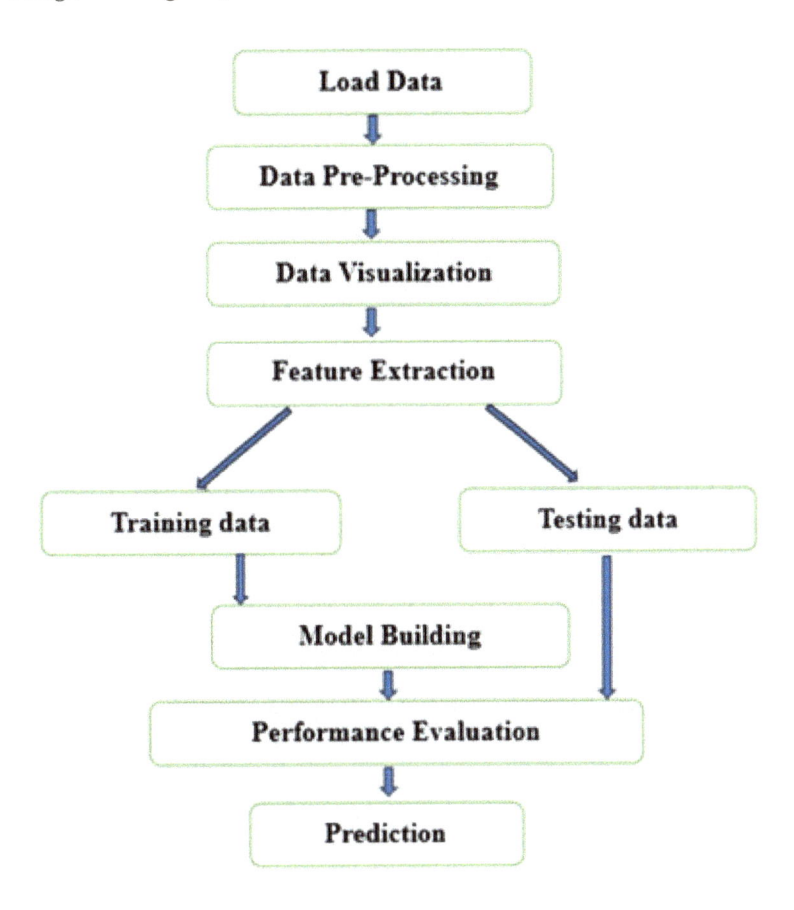

During the *training phase*, the ResNet-101 model learns from the preprocessed images in the train dataset. In this phase, the model iteratively adjusts its weights to minimize the loss function, gradually improving its accuracy in predicting the correct class for each image. Training typically occurs over multiple epochs, with data augmentation techniques applied to introduce variability in the training data, helping the model generalize better and avoid overfitting. Once training is complete, the model's performance is evaluated in the *testing* phase using the test dataset, which consists of images not seen during training. The model's predictions are compared to the actual labels, and performance metrics such as accuracy, precision, recall, and F1-score are calculated. This evaluation is critical for understanding the model's ability to generalize to new, unseen data. Finally, the process concludes with *performance evaluation* and *prediction* of diabetic retinal lesions. The model's effectiveness is assessed through detailed statistical analysis, including advanced metrics like the area under the receiver operating characteristic (ROC) curve. The ultimate goal is to deploy the ResNet-101 model in a clinical setting, where it can accurately predict the presence and severity of diabetic retinal lesions in new patients, supporting early diagnosis and treatment planning. In testing, images are fed forward through the network without weight updates, and the class with the highest output probability is predicted. ResNet-101's deep architecture and residual connections enable effective training, faster convergence, and improved accuracy, making it a powerful tool for image classification tasks.

Although the suggested method has many advantages, there aren't many issues that need to be resolved. The quality and availability of labeled fundus photos are critical to the model's performance; problems with noise or sparsity in the data may limit the model's generalizability. Furthermore, even though CNNs are capable of achieving high accuracy, it is frequently difficult to understand the reasoning behind their classification decisions due to their limited interpretability. The model may also struggle with fundus photos from different populations or imaging environments not included in the training dataset. For clinical adoption, the model must undergo validation studies, obtain regulatory approvals, and be integrated into existing healthcare systems, which can be challenging. Additionally, ethical considerations, including patient privacy, informed consent, and the responsible use of medical data, are vital when developing and implementing AI systems in healthcare.

3.2 Requirements

The proposed model is developed using MATLAB R2023a script. MATLAB has many useful applications that go far beyond its conventional use in electrical network simulations. In domains such as Artificial Intelligence (AI), Robotics, Video Processing, Wireless Communication, Machine Learning (ML), and Data Analytics, its recent developments have made it an extremely powerful instrument. With matrices or arrays acting as its basic data elements, it has long been preferred by circuit and mechanical engineers for solving basic problems, but because of its ability to compute, program, and visualize graphical data, its usefulness extends across numerous domains.

Users can convert their ideas into real solutions with the help of MATLAB's carefully designed toolboxes. Its programming interface, similar to that of C programming, only requires a cursory review of fundamental programming concepts to use effectively.

3.3 Evaluation Matrices

Accuracy, Precision, Recall, and F1-Score are the metrics that are most used to assess how well the categorization methods work. Here's a quick explanation of these metrics:

The percentage of properly and incorrectly identified samples is the definition of accuracy.

$$\text{Accuracy} = \frac{TP + TN}{(TP + TN + FP + FN)} \tag{1}$$

It represents the quality of a positive prediction and states the relationship of true positive (TP) estimates to the sum of TP and false positive (FP) estimates.

$$\text{Precision} = \frac{TP}{(TP + FP)} \tag{2}$$

It measures how the model correctly identifies positive instances. This is the total number of true positive cases that have been correctly categorized.

$$\text{Recall} = \frac{TP}{(TP + FN)} \tag{3}$$

It is a harmonic mean measurement for accuracy and recall.

$$\text{F1 score} = \frac{2 * precision * recall}{precision + recall} \tag{4}$$

Where,
TP stands for true positive. TN stands for true negative. FP stands for false positive. FN stands for false negative.

4 EXPERIMENTAL RESULTS

A variety of strategies are used in the neural network training process to maximize performance. It uses the cross-entropy loss function, which is appropriate for classification jobs, along with the Adam optimization technique. For this study, an open-source dataset sourced from the Kaggle Database was chosen as a reliable and accessible repository. This deliberate selection ensures transparency, and reproducibility, and facilitates cross-study comparisons. Comprising a total of 1200 high-quality retinal images, the dataset focuses on two distinct categories: Healthy and severe_DR (Kaggle, 2024).

This binary classification is integral for training and evaluating classification models dedicated to DR. A constant learning rate schedule, which keeps the learning rate at 0.001 during the training iterations, is put into place to control the learning rate properly. The training dataset is divided into two parts: 80% for training and 20% for testing, to provide an impartial evaluation of the model's performance. The training process of the proposed network is meticulously structured to ensure its effectiveness in accurately classifying diabetic retinal lesions. An extensive training regimen is applied to the network, spanning 30 epochs with 40 iterations per epoch. This thorough training is necessary to adjust the model's parameters and improve its performance over time. Throughout this process, key metrics are closely monitored to assess the model's effectiveness and progress, such as validation loss and accuracy. As the ultimate objective of any machine learning model, these metrics are essential for evaluating the model's capacity to generalize to new, unseen data.

The model exhibits promising performance from the outset. It attains a validation accuracy of 90% and a validation loss of 0.37 after only the first epoch. These preliminary findings are promising since they show that the model is already producing precise predictions at a relatively early stage of training. However, the training continues beyond this point, allowing the model to further refine its parameters and improve its performance. By the tenth epoch, the model achieves an impressive 100% validation accuracy, although this comes with a slightly increased validation loss of 0.9480. This rise in validation loss, despite perfect accuracy, suggests that the model might be starting to overfit to the training data.

Overfitting is a common challenge in neural network training, where the model becomes too attuned to the training data, leading to poor generalization on new data. To address this, the training process is carefully designed to monitor both validation accuracy and validation loss. By closely tracking these metrics, the training process can be adjusted to prevent overfitting. If overfitting is seen, strategies like early stopping, regularization, or altering the learning rate can be used. The model works well on both new, unseen data and training data thanks to this meticulous monitoring and adjustment.

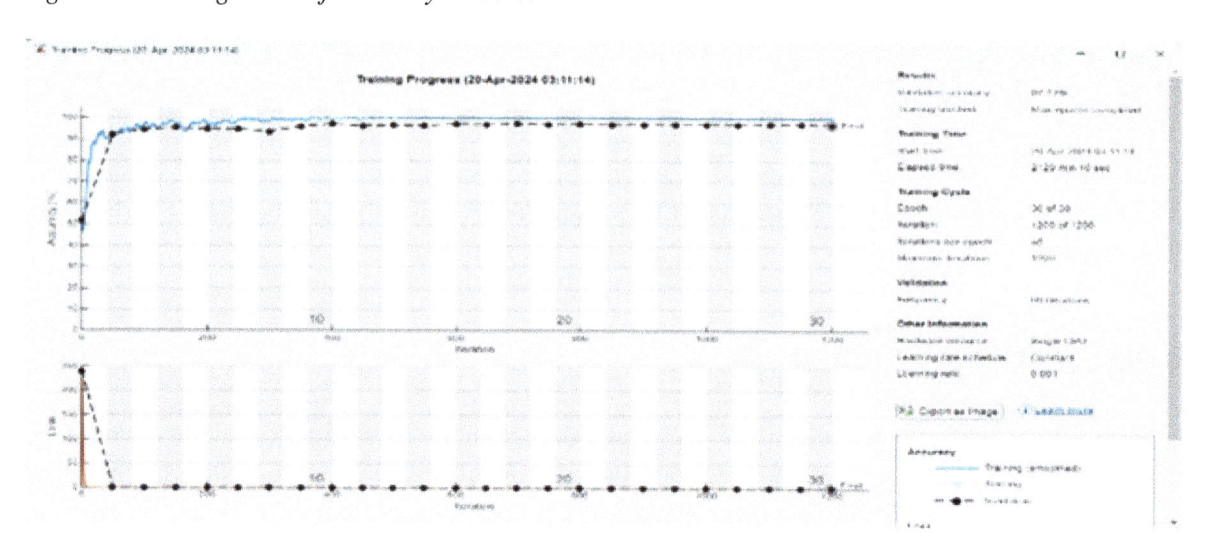

Figure 5. Training curve of accuracy and loss

Throughout the training, the base learning rate is kept constant at 0.001. Maintaining a consistent learning rate is crucial for stable and reliable learning dynamics. A fixed learning rate prevents sudden changes in the model's parameters, which could lead to instability and erratic learning behavior. By keeping the learning rate steady, the model can make gradual progress in learning the underlying patterns in the data, resulting in better overall performance. This approach is reflected in the learning dynamics, as shown in Figure 5, where the validation accuracy remains stable and continues to improve as the training progresses. The final performance of the model is highly promising. The validation accuracy reaches an impressive 97.12%, indicating the model's strong ability to generalize to new data. Additionally, other key performance metrics, such as the F1 score, sensitivity (recall), and accuracy, are also notable. With an F1 score of 0.94931, which strikes a balance between precision and recall, the model successfully identifies TPs while reducing false positives. The model's recall, or sensitivity, is 0.97017, demonstrating its efficacy in accurately identifying DR cases. The accuracy, which gauges how accurate the model's predictions are overall, is 0.92932. These metrics collectively indicate that the proposed model outperforms existing models such as SVM and ResNet-50, offering more accurate and reliable predictions.

The confusion matrix is a crucial instrument for assessing how well the classification model performs. One can find a comprehensive overview of the model's performance in every class by the confusion matrix. It is set up as a N*N matrix, where N is the total number of classes that are being targeted. The number of true positives (TP), true negatives (TN), false positives (FP), and false negatives (FN) for each class is shown in each cell of the matrix. This thorough dissection makes it possible to analyze the model's performance more precisely, highlighting both its advantages and potential areas for improvement. The training process of the proposed network is carefully crafted to achieve optimal performance in classifying diabetic retinal lesions. By monitoring validation metrics, maintaining a consistent learning rate, and using the confusion matrix for detailed performance evaluation, the model is ensured to learn effectively and generalize well to new data. The resulting high validation accuracy, F1 score, and sensitivity demonstrate the superiority of the proposed model over existing methods, making it a valuable tool for accurate and reliable medical diagnosis.

The confusion matrix is a vital tool for assessing the performance of the ResNet-101 image classifier, especially in applications like predicting diabetic retinal lesions. This matrix offers a detailed comparison between the model's predictions and the actual labels, providing a deeper understanding of its performance beyond basic accuracy. It is composed of four essential components: TP, TN, FP, and FN, each contributing valuable insights into the model's effectiveness. TP are instances in which the model detects a retinal lesion accurately. These accurate predictions show that the condition has been correctly identified by the model. TN are cases in which the model accurately detects the lack of a lesion, demonstrating the model's ability to accurately determine the absence of disease. Conversely, false positives (FP) happen when the model predicts the presence of a lesion when it doesn't. This error, which is also referred to as a Type I error, may result in needless anxiety, more testing, and possibly ineffective treatments. FN are situations where the model fails to detect a lesion that is actually present, representing a Type II error. In medical diagnostics, this kind of error is especially dangerous because it indicates that a potentially dangerous condition has gone undiagnosed, which could result in unfavorable treatment outcomes and a delay in treatment.

Beyond just accuracy, the confusion matrix offers a comprehensive picture of the model's performance, which makes it important. When there is an imbalance between classes, as when most images belong to one class (e.g., no lesions) and only a small number to another (e.g., lesions), accuracy can be deceptive. If a model consistently predicts the majority class, it can attain high accuracy; however, it may still perform poorly when it comes to the minority class. In order to allow for a more thorough evaluation, the confusion matrix addresses this by dividing the performance into TP, TN, FP, and FN. The confusion matrix can be used to derive the F1-score, precision, and recall, among other important metrics. The precision metric calculates the ratio of true positives to all positive predictions (TP / (TP + FP)), which indicates the accuracy of the predicted lesions. In medical applications, high precision is essential to prevent false alarms that might prompt needless interventions. Conversely, recall evaluates the percentage of true positives the system accurately detects (TP / (TP + FN)), demonstrating the model's capacity to identify all pertinent cases. In order to make sure that no substantial lesions are overlooked, high recall is essential. By incorporating the harmonic mean of these two distinct values, the F1-score provides a balanced assessment of the model's effectiveness by combining recall and precision into a single metric.

The confusion matrix in the context of ResNet-101 for medical image classification is very helpful in determining the accuracy and dependability of the model. It assists in identifying potential areas for model improvement, such as lowering false negatives to guarantee early lesion detection. By examining this matrix, scientists and programmers can improve the model's performance and make more accurate predictions, which will improve clinical outcomes when the model is used in actual diagnostic situations. In the matrix, each row denotes an instance within a real class, and each column denotes instances within an expected class. In ResNet-50n the context of Fig: 6, the confusion matrix associated with ResNet-101 is illustrated. Examination of this matrix reveals that among the model's predictions, 618 images were assigned to class 1, with 19 images being categorized as confused. Similar observations were made for two other classes. Additionally, in comparison to ResNet-50 and SVM demonstrates an enhanced prediction accuracy for images overall. This analysis underscores the effectiveness of ResNet-101 in classification tasks, demonstrating its superior performance over ResNet-50 and SVM in accurately classifying images across multiple classes.

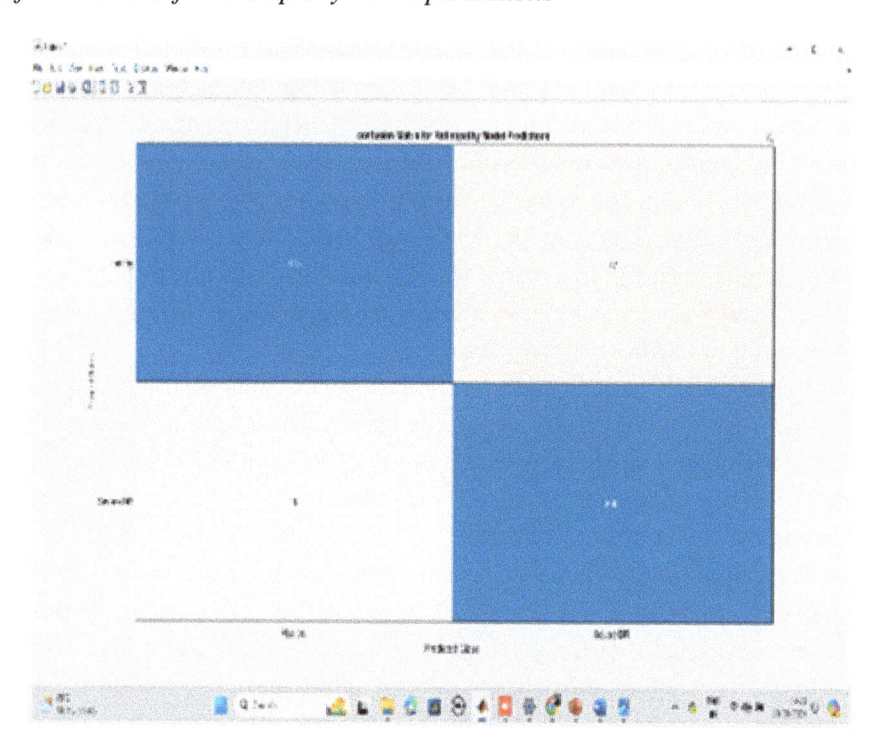

Figure 6. Confusion matrix for retinopathy model predictions

The performance metrics for the ResNet-101 model against SVM and Resnet – 50 CNN models are shown in Table 1. Significantly, as compared to SVM and ResNet-101, there is a discernible rise in the prediction probability during the PDR step. The statistical potential of the proposed ResNet-101 classifier can be evaluated by comparing its performance metrics—accuracy, precision, sensitivity, and F1 score—with those of existing classification methods like ResNet-50 and Support Vector Machine (SVM). Each of these metrics highlights different aspects of the models' effectiveness, and together they reveal the superiority of ResNet-101. Accuracy is a key indicator of the overall correctness of a model's predictions. The proposed ResNet-101 achieves an outstanding accuracy of 97.16%, which significantly exceeds the 85.71% accuracy of ResNet-50 and the 73.95% accuracy of SVM. This suggests that ResNet-101 is far more reliable in correctly classifying diabetic retinal images, making it a stronger choice for applications where high accuracy is essential.

The precision of a model is determined by calculating the ratio of true positive predictions to all positive predictions, which indicates the model's ability to prevent false positives. ResNet-101 attains a precision of 92.93%, which is notably higher than the 81.64% precision of ResNet-50 and the 70.52% precision of SVM. This high precision indicates that ResNet-101 is particularly effective in minimizing false alarms, ensuring that when it predicts the presence of a diabetic retinal lesion, the prediction is likely accurate. This is especially important in medical diagnostics, where false positives can lead to unnecessary stress and treatment. Sensitivity or recall, measures the proportion of actual positives that are correctly identified by the model. This metric is crucial in medical diagnosis, as it shows the model's ability to detect all cases of the disease. ResNet-101 achieves a sensitivity of 97.017%, which is significantly higher than the 84.56% sensitivity of ResNet-50 and the 73.16% sensitivity of SVM. This indicates that ResNet-101 is highly effective in detecting nearly all cases of diabetic retinal lesions, greatly reducing the risk of missed diagnoses, which is critical for ensuring timely and appropriate patient care.

Table 1. Performance analysis of proposed method with the existing method

Network	Accuracy %	Precision %	Sensitivity %	F1 Score %
SVM	73.95	70.52	73.16	71.55
ResNet-50	85.71	81.64	84.56	82.45
ResNet-101 (Proposed)	97.16	92.93	97.017	94.93

The F1 Score is a balanced metric that takes into consideration both false positives and false negatives by combining precision and sensitivity into a single measure. The F1 score of 94.93% achieved by the proposed ResNet-101 is significantly higher than that of ResNet-50 at 82.45% and SVM at 71.55%. This high F1 score indicates that ResNet-101 is an effective tool for tasks related to classification where accuracy and reliability are crucial. It also excels in precision and sensitivity separately and maintains an excellent equilibrium within the two. This inference exhibits the superior statistical potentiality of the proposed ResNet-101 model against the existing ResNet-50 and SVM. Its higher accuracy confirms its overall effectiveness in making correct predictions. Its superior precision underscores its ability to reduce false positives, while its exceptional sensitivity ensures that nearly all true cases of diabetic retinal lesions are detected. Moreover, its high F1 score indicates a well-balanced performance between precision and sensitivity, making ResNet-101 a highly dependable and effective model for medical image classification. These advantages highlight ResNet-101 not only as a significant improvement over existing methods but also as a potentially transformative tool for enhancing the accuracy and reliability of DR detection.

CONCLUSION

In order to improve the classification of DR, this work presents a novel CNN architecture that makes use of ResNet-101's sophisticated capabilities. Significant progress in the field of medical imaging analysis has been made with the implementation of this complex architecture, especially in terms of the performance metrics related to DR monitoring. By achieving an impressive accuracy rate of 97.42%, the ResNet-101-based CNN demonstrates exceptional performance and effectiveness, setting a new standard for DR classification. DR, a common and serious complication of diabetes, affects the retina and can lead to vision loss if not diagnosed and treated early. Accurate and early detection of DR is crucial for effective management and treatment, which can significantly impact patient outcomes. Traditional diagnostic methods, while useful, often suffer from limitations in accuracy and reliability. This is where advanced CNN architectures, like the one proposed in this work, come into play. By employing the ResNet-101 architecture, the model benefits from a deep learning framework that excels in handling complex image data and extracting meaningful features.

The ResNet-101 architecture is a prominent example of deep residual learning, a technique that has shown remarkable success in various image classification tasks. The key innovation of ResNet-101 lies in its use of residual blocks, which enable the network to learn residual mappings rather than direct mappings. This approach addresses the vanishing gradient problem commonly encountered in very deep networks, allowing the model to achieve deeper layers without suffering from degraded performance. As a result, ResNet-101 can capture intricate patterns and features in retinal images that are critical for accurate DR classification. The high accuracy achieved by this model—97.42%—marks a significant improvement over existing DR classification models. This level of performance is not just a numerical achievement but reflects the model's ability to accurately differentiate between various stages of DR, from non-proliferative to proliferative stages. Such precision is crucial for early detection, which can lead to timely intervention and treatment, potentially preventing severe vision impairment or loss. The substantial increase in accuracy also underscores the importance of employing advanced and sophisticated architectures in medical image analysis. Traditional models may not capture the complexities of retinal images as effectively, but ResNet-101's advanced design provides a robust solution to these challenges.

The implications of achieving such high accuracy extend beyond mere statistics; they have profound effects on patient care and healthcare delivery. Improved accuracy in DR classification means that patients can receive more reliable diagnoses, which in turn facilitates better treatment planning and management. Early and accurate detection allows for prompt intervention, which can prevent the progression of the disease and improve overall patient outcomes. Additionally, a more accurate model can reduce the likelihood of false positives and false negatives, minimizing unnecessary procedures and focusing resources on those who need them most. This work not only highlights the potential of ResNet-101 in achieving remarkable accuracy but also sets a new benchmark for future research and development in medical diagnostics. The success of this model demonstrates the power of leveraging deep learning techniques to address complex problems in medical imaging. It opens the door for further innovations and applications in various medical imaging tasks, such as detecting other retinal diseases, classifying different stages of other medical conditions, or even extending the approach to different types of imaging modalities.

Moreover, the advancement achieved through this research emphasizes the need for continuous improvement and exploration in the field of medical image analysis. As technology evolves and new methodologies emerge, there is always room for enhancement. The high performance of the ResNet-101-based CNN serves as a catalyst for ongoing research, encouraging the development of even more sophisticated models and techniques. Future research may focus on refining the existing architecture, exploring hybrid models that combine different deep learning approaches, or expanding the model's applicability to other areas of medical imaging. By achieving an outstanding accuracy rate of 97.42%, this model not only demonstrates its exceptional performance but also sets a new standard for future advancements in medical image analysis. The positive implications for patient care and healthcare delivery are profound, as more accurate and reliable DR detection can lead to earlier diagnoses, better treatment outcomes, and more efficient use of healthcare resources. This work exemplifies the transformative potential of advanced CNN architectures in medical diagnostics and paves the way for further innovations and applications in the realm of medical imaging.

REFERENCES

Akram, M., & Sharma, P. (2024, January). Diabetic Retinopathy Detection Using Voting Classification Method. In *2024 IEEE 1st Karachi Section Humanitarian Technology Conference (KHI-HTC)* (pp. 1-11). IEEE. DOI: 10.1109/KHI-HTC60760.2024.10482074

He, K., Zhang, X., Ren, S., & Sun, J. (2016). Deep residual learning for image recognition. In *Proceedings of the IEEE conference on computer vision and pattern recognition* (pp. 770-778).

Kumar, S. (2019, August). Diabetic retinopathy diagnosis with ensemble deep-learning. In *Proceedings of the 3rd International Conference on Vision, Image and Signal Processing* (pp. 1-5).

Kurle, S. S., Maralbhavi, N. P., Salunke, S. U., & Chandanshive, A. A. (2017, June). Diabetic retinopathy analysis using CDR technique. In *2017 International Conference on Intelligent Computing and Control Systems (ICICCS)* (pp. 708-711). IEEE.

Kwasigroch, A., Jarzembinski, B., & Grochowski, M. (2018, May). Deep CNN based decision support system for detection and assessing the stage of diabetic retinopathy. In *2018 International Interdisciplinary PhD Workshop (IIPhDW)* (pp. 111-116). IEEE. DOI: 10.1109/IIPHDW.2018.8388337

Maistry, A., Pillay, A., & Jembere, E. (2020, September). Improving the accuracy of diabetes retinopathy image classification using augmentation. In *Conference of the South African Institute of Computer Scientists and Information Technologists 2020* (pp. 134-140). DOI: 10.1145/3410886.3410914

Pamadi, A. M., Ravishankar, A., Nithya, P. A., Jahnavi, G., & Kathavate, S. (2022, March). Diabetic retinopathy detection using MobileNetV2 architecture. In *2022 International Conference on Smart Technologies and Systems for Next Generation Computing (ICSTSN)* (pp. 1-5). IEEE.

Ravindraiah, R., & Chandra Mohan Reddy, S. (2018). Exudates detection in diabetic retinopathy images using possibilistic C-means clustering algorithm with induced spatial constraint. In *Artificial Intelligence and Evolutionary Computations in Engineering Systems* [Springer Singapore.]. *Proceedings of ICAIECES*, 2017, 455–463.

Ravindraiah, R., & Reddy, S. C. M. (2020). An instinctive application of spatially weighted possibilistic clustering methods for the detection of lesions in diabetic retinopathy images in multi-dimensional kernel space. *Wireless Personal Communications*, 113(1), 223–240. DOI: 10.1007/s11277-020-07186-5

Reguant, R., Brunak, S., & Saha, S. (2021). Understanding inherent image features in CNN-based assessment of diabetic retinopathy. *Scientific Reports*, 11(1), 9704. DOI: 10.1038/s41598-021-89225-0 PMID: 33958686

Sebastian, A., Elharrouss, O., Al-Maadeed, S., & Almaadeed, N. (2023). A survey on deep-learning-based diabetic retinopathy classification. *Diagnostics (Basel)*, 13(3), 345. DOI: 10.3390/diagnostics13030345 PMID: 36766451

Sgallari, F. (2013). Computer Methods in Biomechanics and Biomedical Engineering: Imaging & Visualization. *Computer Methods in Biomechanics and Biomedical Engineering. Imaging & Visualization*.

Shaik, N. S., & Cherukuri, T. K. (2022). Hinge attention network: A joint model for diabetic retinopathy severity grading. *Applied Intelligence*, 52(13), 15105–15121. DOI: 10.1007/s10489-021-03043-5

Singh, N., & Kaur, L. (2015, January). A survey on blood vessel segmentation methods in retinal images. In *2015 International Conference on Electronic Design, Computer Networks & Automated Verification (EDCAV)* (pp. 23-28). IEEE. DOI: 10.1109/EDCAV.2015.7060532

Sowmiya, R., & Kalpana, R. (2023, April). Detection of Diabetic Retinopathy by Segmentation using U-Net with Hyper-Parameter Tuning. In *2023 2nd International Conference on Smart Technologies and Systems for Next Generation Computing (ICSTSN)* (pp. 1-5). IEEE. DOI: 10.1109/ICSTSN57873.2023.10151473

Stitt, A. W., Curtis, T. M., Chen, M., Medina, R. J., McKay, G. J., Jenkins, A., & Lois, N. (2016). The progress in understanding and treatment of diabetic retinopathy. *Progress in Retinal and Eye Research*, 51, 156–186. DOI: 10.1016/j.preteyeres.2015.08.001 PMID: 26297071

Vaishnavi, J., Ravi, S., & Anbarasi, A. (2020). An efficient adaptive histogram based segmentation and extraction model for the classification of severities on diabetic retinopathy. *Multimedia Tools and Applications*, 79(41), 30439–30452. DOI: 10.1007/s11042-020-09288-5

Xu, Y., Zhou, Z., Li, X., Zhang, N., Zhang, M., & Wei, P. (2021). FFU-Net: Feature Fusion U-Net for Lesion Segmentation of Diabetic Retinopathy. *BioMed Research International*, 2021(1), 6644071. DOI: 10.1155/2021/6644071 PMID: 33490274

Chapter 18
Navigating Privacy and Security in Internet of Medical Things With Machine-to-Machine Interactions

Manikandan Arunachalam
Department of Electronics and Communication Engineering, Amrita School of Engineering, India

Saket Akella
https://orcid.org/0009-0000-6030-5613
Department of Electronics and Communication Engineering, Amrita School of Engineering, India

D. Arun Satvik
https://orcid.org/0009-0009-3960-6759
Department of Electronics and Communication Engineering, Amrita School of Engineering, India

Rakesh Thoppaen Suresh Babu
https://orcid.org/0009-0003-2671-4618
Fiserv Inc, USA

ABSTRACT

Internet of Medical Things (IoMT) offers immense benefits by revolutionizing healthcare delivery, enhancing patient outcomes, and improving operational efficiencies across the healthcare ecosystem. Also, integration of Machine-to-Machine (M2M) communication with IoMT enables real time patient monitoring, remote diagnostics and intelligent decision making in critical situations. Current state of research shows that adoption of M2M communication with IoMT facilitates the seamless connectivity and data exchange among the health care devices and sensors. However, since M2M communication allows devices to communicate to each other without human intervention, security in the integration of M2M communication with IoMT face critical challenges and issues under different environments. This chapter will thoroughly discuss the security challenges and issues which are essential to address to escape from the evolving threat and to ensure the secure adoption of M2M communication with IoMT.

DOI: 10.4018/979-8-3693-6180-1.ch018

Copyright ©2025, IGI Global. Copying or distributing in print or electronic forms without written permission of IGI Global is prohibited.

1. INTRODUCTION

The IoMT incorporates a network of interconnected devices that collect and exchange health information through M2M communication(Rubí and Gondim 2019). M2M communication is a keystone of IoMT, playing a critical role in transforming healthcare delivery and patient management(Manikandan et al. 2024). M2M enables the continuous monitoring of patient's vital symptoms through connected devices such as wearable sensors and portable medical devices(A. Ahmed et al. 2022). With this, health care service providers can receive instant alerts about critical patient's condition and allowing immediate action to save their lives(Viderman et al. 2022) (Anjana et al. 2024). By analyzing the data collected through M2M, healthcare professionals can determine personalized treatment plans adapted to individual patients' needs. Patients with chronic conditions can be monitored remotely and regularly, reducing the need for frequent hospital visits, and improving the quality of life. M2M in IoMT also facilitates automation in healthcare such as automatic updating of Electronic Health Records (EHRs) and inventory management of medical needs(Mitra, Roy, and Tripathy 2022). This connectivity between IoMT and M2M facilitates real-time monitoring, personalized health care treatment, and improved patient outcomes(Askar et al. 2022). However, the integration of IoMT introduces a myriad of security challenges that are hardly needed to address to ensure the safety, privacy, and reliability of healthcare devices(Wani, Thabit, and Can 2024). As IoMT devices handle very sensitive data operating in critical environments, they are primary targets for attackers(Tahir, Jolfaei, and Tariq 2023). The complexity and diversity of these devices ranging from wearable health monitors to implantable medical devices, further complicates the security aspects(Kwarteng and Cebe 2022)(Shanthi et al. 2021). Ensuring the confidentiality, integrity, and availability of all the health data while maintaining the interoperability and functionality of these devices remains a challenge. This paper outlines the primary security challenges associated with IoMT and M2M communication stressing the need for vigorous security measures to protect patient data and maintain the integrity of healthcare records. These challenges include data privacy and confidentiality, device vulnerability, network security and compliance with regulatory standards. Addressing these issues and challenges is crucial for enhancing and adopting IoMT technologies in the healthcare sector.

2. MAJOR ATTACKS IN IOMT

The IoMT faces several major attacks including data breaches, ransomware, Distributed Denial of Service (DDoS), and unauthorized attacks. These security challenges highlight the need for robust security algorithms, secure communication protocols, and comprehensive security outlines to protect sensitive medical data(Hernandez-Jaimes et al. 2023). Table-I provides a comprehensive overview of various attacks on the IoMT as identified and studied by different researchers. It categorizes the types of attacks, summarizes the findings from various studies, and highlights the primary security concerns and impacts associated with each attack.

Table 1. Security challenges in IoMT

Reference	DoS	Data Breach	Impersonation	Man-in-the-Middle	DDoS	Spoofing	Privacy Breach
(Masud et al. 2021)	✓	✓	✓	✓	✗	✗	✗
(Al-Garadi et al. 2020)	✗	✗	✗	✗	✓	✓	✓
(Iqbal et al. 2020)	✗	✗	✗	✗	✗	✗	✓
(Geneiatakis et al. 2017)	✓	✗	✓	✗	✗	✗	✗
(Thammarat and Techapanupreeda 2021)	✓	✗	✓	✓	✗	✓	✗
(Kharghani et al. 2023)	✓	✗	✓	✗	✗	✓	✗
(Sripriyanka and Mahendran 2024)	✗	✗	✗	✗	✓	✗	✗
(Sankepally et al. 2022)	✗	✓	✗	✗	✗	✗	✗
(Puthin Krishna, Kumar, and Palani Thanaraj 2023)	✓	✗	✗	✗	✗	✗	✗
(J. Ahmed et al. 2023)	✗	✗	✗	✗	✗	✗	✓
(Salem et al. 2022)	✗	✗	✗	✓	✗	✗	✗
(Lin et al. 2021)	✗	✓	✗	✗	✗	✗	✗
(Das et al. 2023)	✓	✗	✗	✓	✓	✗	✗
(Ghubaish et al. 2021)	✓	✗	✗	✓	✓	✗	✗
(Huang and Nazir 2020)							
(Khatkar, Kumar, and Kumar 2020)	✗	✗	✗	✗	✓	✗	✗
(Martinez and Galmes 2022)	✓	✓	✗	✓	✗	✗	✗
(Alrubayyi et al. 2024)	✗	✗	✗	✓	✗	✗	✗
(Harvey et al. 2020)	✗	✗	✗	✗	✗	✗	✓
(Wang and Liu 2022)	✗	✗	✗	✗	✗	✗	✓
(Naria, Sulistyo, and Widyawan 2022)	✗	✗	✗	✗	✗	✗	✓
(Al-Maani et al. 2022)	✓	✗	✗	✗	✓	✗	✗

2.1 Denial of Service (DoS)

DoS attacks within the IoMT ecosystem can manifest diversely, ranging from traditional flood-based assaults to intricately engineered application-layer attacks targeting specific vulnerabilities (Paolone et al. 2022). What it basically aims to do is disrupt critical healthcare services by flooding the server and creating unnecessary traffic. In context to IoMT where the patient's real time data is very crucial, this kind of attack can be quite devastating. Exploiting weaknesses in communication protocols, assailants aim to overwhelm network resources or exhaust device capabilities, resulting in service disruptions (Al-turki et al. 2021). Furthermore, centralized infrastructure like cloud-based servers and healthcare data centers are susceptible to volumetric assaults, causing network bandwidth saturation and computational resource depletion (Bhardwaj et al. 2021).

The ramifications of DoS attacks on IoMT infrastructure are dire, potentially compromising patient safety and care outcomes (Rafique et al. 2020). Disruptions to IoMT services can lead to critical procedural delays, impede access to vital patient data, and undermine the efficacy of remote monitoring systems. In emergency scenarios, where swift responses are paramount, DoS attacks can severely hinder healthcare providers' ability to deliver timely and effective care, posing significant risks to patient well-being (Sadiq, Thompson, and Ayeni 2021). Also, DDoS attacks will compromise the integrity of data transmitted between devices through M2M. Since M2M involves the exchange of sensitive patient data, this DDoS can expose this data to unauthorized access. In an IoMT ecosystem, where continuous monitoring and care is crucial any data disruptions or loss of data can lead to life-threatening consequences as it is a must to have real-time data analysis to take timely decisions.

Some of the counter measures are:

- Network Segmentation: With reference to IoMT, devices responsible for monitoring health such as heart monitors, infusion pumps, and wearable health devices are often connected to the same network as the hospital which creates a larger base to land cyber attacks hence isolation of critical IoMT devices and services through network segmentation to contain attacks and prevent lateral movement by adversaries. For example, an attack targeting hospital administrative computers won't affect life-support systems if the network is properly segmented.
- Traffic Filtering and Rate Limiting: IoMT devices like a pacemaker, insulin pump, or monitor their patients rely on continuous uninterrupted network access to perform the desired primary functionality. Attackers try to disrupt the main functionality by sending malicious traffic and hence there are implementations of mechanisms to filter and throttle malicious traffic at network entry points which preserves the integrity and availability of IoMT services. This is the rate limiting, which controls the number of requests a user, device, or IP address can make within a given timeframe. It prevents the networks or the devices from being overwhelmed with too many requests such that they cannot carry out their functions effectively. Hence, it can be said that traffic filtering and rate limiting can be one of the most important parts of securing IoMT networks from threats due to Dos. • In this, Intrusion Detection and Prevention Systems (IDPS) play a prominent role when talking about network security with respect to medical devices.

This primarily consists of IDS which are intrusion detection systems where monitoring systems are used to analyze suspicious activity. The other is IPS or intrusion prevention system that takes proactive steps and measures to prevent the same. This is by introducing real-time threat detection and automated mitigation through IDPS to identify and respond to anomalous network activity much faster. •\\tCloud-based DoS mitigation: Cloud-based Denial of Service (DoS) mitigation is a set of techniques and services essentially designed to protect the ecosystem of networks, including the IoMT, from DoS and Distributed Denial of Service (DDoS),and in the context of IoMT, cloud-based DoS mitigation plays a critical role in ensuring that critical healthcare services and devices continue to function securely even in the face of massive attack attempts targeting such operation. This uses specialist DoS mitigation services to counter large-scale attacks, tapping their expertise and capacity to mitigate the impact on critical medical services.

- Device Hardening and Patch Management: Many IoMT devices are furnished with thousands of services, features, or software that the device might not use at its core medical function. By disabling or uninstalling them, they remove what's not needed from the attack surface. Regular updates can harden these IoMT devices, minimizing vulnerabilities and reducing the attack surface that secures against possible exploits. •\\tApplication-Layer Protection: This refers to security measures that protect applications from hacking through weaknesses in the software layer. The application layer, dealing mainly with the functionality of the software in the device, becomes a vulnerable point for several IoMT systems with medical devices interacting with software in handling sensitive patients' data or diagnostic systems and performing clinical operations. Data breaches compromise medical services, and, potentially, risks to patient health can occur from these layer attacks.

Application-layer DoS attacks can be prevented, or their occurrence decreased through the application of rate limiting and connection throttling techniques on the application layer of the application to reduce attacks on specific IoMT services or protocols. • Behavioral analysis and Anomaly Detection: Under these techniques, monitoring the behavior of IoMT devices and systems is done for detecting activities that do not conform to usual patterns, which could be indicative of some kind of security breach. In the IoMT ecosystem, where medical devices continually collect, transmit, and analyze sensitive patient data, behavioral analysis and anomaly detection play a crucial role in identifying abnormal activities that may be indicative of a cyber-attack or system malfunction. These techniques of behavioral analysis and anomaly detection can be used to identify and mitigate DoS attacks in real time. This would ensure very efficient resilience of IoMT infrastructure against threats that are evolving continuously. Understanding these issues and remedial action could ensure that DoS attacks do not jeopardize IoMT systems and ensure continuous and safe delivery of medical services.

2.2 Data Breach

Data breaches in IoMT are a serious issue in the medical industry. It severely affects patients' confidentiality and the overall trust in the medical system. Most IoMT devices, in particular devices which include wearable health monitors, smart medical devices, and connected diagnostic tools such as Connected ECG monitors and Ultrasound machines, transmit sensitive medical data of patients over several networks. This makes the data attractive for attackers as Network security and encryption can vary from network to network. Data breaches in IoMT can occur through various attack vectors, including exploitation of vulnerabilities in M2M devices, unauthorized access to cloud-based storage systems, or interception of data transmitted between interconnected devices(Garg et al. 2022). Adversaries exploit weaknesses in M2M protocols or implementations to gain unauthorized access to patient data, exfiltrate sensitive information, or manipulate medical records for malicious purposes(Junejo, Komninos, and McCann 2021). Compromised endpoints within IoMT networks can serve as footholds for attackers to pivot and escalate their attacks, further compromising the security and integrity of medical data. The medical industry is in a rush to bring in new and more advanced medical devices onto the market, without the required security standards being met. The race to bring in more innovative products puts the idea of security as an afterthought for both the software and hardware developers. A few of the reasons why IoMT devices are vulnerable to breaches and attacks are the size and efficiency of the devices. These devices are meant to be compact and less power consuming with limited power and memory for them to be used by the patient daily. Due to the size and efficiency restrictions, these devices lack strong encryption and advanced security measures. In addition to technical vulnerabilities, human ignorance is another important factor for data breaches. In the case of healthcare providers and administrators lacking adequate training in cybersecurity best practices, the blame goes to negligence of the administration. This could involve poor password management, unsecured Wi-Fi networks, and insufficient monitoring of device activity. Insider threats, whether from malicious intent or negligence, can also result in unauthorized access to IoMT systems.

It will include identity theft and financial fraud to the breaches of patient confidentiality, erosion of trust in healthcare systems, damage to organizational reputation, and even may extend to regulatory non-compliance along with associated penalties (Muhd Azri Baptist et al. 2023) . It will also cause harm to the body when a life-saving device integrity, such as pacemakers or insulin pumps, is compromised. Apart from these, there are strict demands posed by regulatory bodies, such as HIPAA, on healthcare entities related to the protection of patient information while ensuring notification requirements in cases of incidents. These add to the layers of complexity and the urgency associated with the response and mitigation activities of a breach (Rockwern, Johnson, and Sulmasy 2021).

Among such countermeasures are:

- Data encryption: It should utilize end-to-end encryption mechanisms for data being exchanged between IoMT devices and storage systems.
- Access control and authentication: The least privileged principle, along with strong authentication credentials, would never allow unauthorized access to medical data. Data Loss Prevention (DLP) solutions: DLP solutions should be in place that monitor and enforce policies around transmission, storage, and use of sensitive medical data.
- Endpoint security controls: Use antivirus, intrusion detection, and device encryption to protect M2M from compromise.
- Security monitoring and incident response: Implement complete security monitoring and incident response in order to detect and respond to a breach of data as soon as is practicable.
- Data masking and anonymization: Implement techniques that replace sensitive medical information with nonsensitive placeholders or anonymized identifiers.
- Third party risk management: Security assessments of third-party vendors along with their products should be sufficient.
- Compliance to regulation: The HIPAA regulatory framework would minimize the risk of exposure to penalties and legal liabilities resulting from data breaches

By adopting these mitigations, it is feasible to safeguard the sensitive data that is transmitted through M2M communications from breaches caused by IoMT.

2.3 Impersonation

Impersonation attacks, or spoofing attacks, are a type of attack where an illegitimate entity acts as a genuine participant in the IoMT ecosystem (Bhushan et al. 2023). The types of attacks in IoMT include masquerading as another's identity for a gadget, masquerading as a healthcare professional, and masquerading as a trusted server or gateway. Impersonation attacks are referred to as attacks that derive from vulnerabilities of weak protocols such as authentication mechanisms, weak encryption protocols or even poor measures of access control (Suleski and Ahmed 2023). For instance, an attacker may steal a legitimate medical device's identity either by fetching its credentials or by exploiting software vulnerabilities. This will further make the attacker log in illegitimately to the IoMT network, and compromise patient data or alter some settings in devices (Ahmed Alhaj et al. 2022). Moreover, impersonating healthcare professionals or trusted servers can make attackers inject malicious commands or access sensitive information. This impersonation allows attackers to modify the medical data that are transferred through M2M devices (Yaacoub et al. 2020). There are various types of this.

1. Device Impersonation: In this scenario, an attacker pretends to be a legitimate IoMT device like a pacemaker, insulin pump or any type of wearable device. Through this, the attacker can send false data to the medical network thereby putting the patient's life and the credibility of the medical field into danger. For example, an attacker can pretend to be a glucose monitoring device and deliver wrong information to the medical authority. This can lead to severe inappropriate prescriptions of insulin that hurt the patient.
2. User Impersonation: The attacker may impersonate an authorized user like healthcare provider, system administrator or patient. Many vulnerabilities like medical records, device configurations and many more can be accessed using the network or device vulnerabilities by these spoofing organizations or individuals. In addition, these effects of successful impersonation attacks in IoMT are also very dangerous like unauthorized accessing privacy related to the information of patients, changing the settings of the medical devices or even breaking down the critical health services that may further cause the loss of safety and confidentiality of patients (S. F. Ahmed et al. 2024) . This also causes a lack of trust in these medical devices, which further leads to taking risky or hazardous treatments by the patient.

Some of the countermeasures are:

- Implement strong authentication mechanisms such as multi-factor authentication to verify the identity of users and devices.
- Enforce verification of device identity such that only authenticated and authorized devices can access the IoMT network. Deploy intrusion detection systems to scan the IoMT networks for suspicious activity and potential attempts to impersonate.
- IoMT devices need to be secured with periodic security updates and patches of the known vulnerability to minimize the potential for exploitation.
- Health care staff needs to be educated on security awareness in the risk of impersonation attacks to recognize suspicious activity and respond accordingly.
- IoMT networks need to be monitored on a continuous basis to identify any anomalous behavior and unauthorized access attempts.
- Implementation of encryption protocols to safeguard channels of communication and sensitive data, not to be intercepted or altered.
- Zero-trust security model where access is granted based on rigorous identity verification in continuous authentication both in internal originated and externally originated access request.
- Implement secure communication between M2M devices and backend systems to avoid eavesdropping and man-in-the-middle attacks.

- Block Chain in IoMT. Block chain could be one decentralized entity that ensures all safety and integrity of medical devices, healthcare professionals, as well as the cloud-based servers are achieved.

All these techniques can improve the security of the IoMT with M2M devices, and their operation shall be effective.

2.4 Man-in-the-Middle

A MITM attack is asserted to take place when an attacker intercepts and possibly alters legitimate communication involving two parties in the IoMT space. In IoMT, MITM attacks exploit weaknesses in communication protocols, inadequate encryption mechanisms, or failed authentication measures Perwej et al. 2022. Multiple methods, including listening, packet sniffing, or exploitation of software vulnerability can be used by the attackers to intercept and manipulate the data exchanged between medical devices, sensors, and systems (Deb et al. 2020). In the above discussion, it has been mentioned that IoMT is dependent on real-time data and on communication in a number of networks. This becomes possible when a MitM attack occurs where an unknown entity can lurk on this communication network, unaware of the patient and the medical administration that is taking care of the patient. The attacker can also target doctor and patient telecommunication with regard to tampering the information being transmitted in real-time which leads to improper medical treatment being carried out. MITM also leads to other attacks such as data breach and impersonation that were in detail discussed above. In most cases, the attacker can also modify the configurations of the device making the device unusable for fetching data which is the most important part of the communication process and patient treatment from time to time. Unsuccessful MITM attacks in M2M might lead to a breach of sensitive patient data, tampering with medical device configurations, or disrupting critical healthcare services, threatening life (Eyeleko and Feng 2023).

Examples of countermeasures are as follows:

- Implement strong communication protocols like Transport Layer Security (TLS) or Internet Protocol Security (IPsec) that provide end-to-end encryption and assure integrity of data transmitted between medical devices, sensors, and systems.
- Mutual authentication mechanisms whereby clients as well as servers authenticate each other to make and establish the secure channel; they thus prevent MITM attacks.
- Use digital signatures and integrity checks on data that is transmitted so it is impossible for it to have been altered during transit.
- Network segmentation Divide your networks into isolated zones or subnets with differing levels of trust. Continuously monitor to identify anomalies in all segments. This will increase the chances of detecting and thwarting any attempted MITM attacks.
- Physical security Hardening: Secure network cabling, closed loop piping and tamper-evident seals on exposed areas, limitation of network infrastructure access in order to prevent physical MITM attacks.
- Regular updates and patches of all medical devices, sensors, systems, and software components must be done in order to address known vulnerabilities and mitigate the risk of security breaches.

- If these strong security measures with the implementation of robust security that is more appropriate for M2M with IoMT are taken, then MiTM attacks can be mitigated and secured transmission can be ensured.

2.5 DDoS (Distributed Denial of Service)

In a DDoS attack, vulnerabilities of IoMT network are exploited by attackers to flood targe servers, services, or networks with overwhelming internet traffic (Thomasian and Adashi 2021) which makes them not safely usable to legitimate users. For example, a recent case study documented a hospital network hit by a DDoS attack, peaking at over 100 Gbps of malicious traffic, crippling operations for hours (Park et al. 2022). A hospital had 100Gbps of malicious traffic following a DDoS attack. The hospital then lost several hours of operations which included several immediate operations. This disrupted critical medical services, including patient monitoring and electronic health records, causing patient care delays and staff stress. DDoS attacks have several effects on both patients and the medical staff. Beyond immediate service disruptions, they can compromise patient safety and data security. Consider a remote patient monitoring system attacked by DDoS, resulting in the loss of real-time monitoring for hundreds of patients, compromising timely medical emergency detection and exposing sensitive patient data to breaches (Zafar et al. 2020).

Another prominent contributor of DDoS attacks is botnets. Generally, a botnet is a collection of hijacked devices which the attacker controls. Using these devices, an attacker can get critical data from the patients or send in false data to the medical department. Because many devices have tight restrictions in size and power of the devices, they lack strong security features and can be easily accessed by attackers. In terms of patient security, receiving sensitive health information could mean that the attacker has awareness of the medical situation of the patient, which leads to severe security issues. If these compromised devices' data are taken as a reference for treatment for the patient, then it may create fatal issues for the patient because any amount of wrong medical diagnosis could be too dangerous. In the context of critical infrastructure beyond the patient, when DDoS threatens are extended to the hospital infrastructure such as the patient information database, communication, or the diagnostic tools then the causalities could be fatal. These systems rely on direct real-time communication and disruption can put the lives of patients in danger. For instance, if a radiology department which relies on cloud systems is under threat of DDoS, then there would be a large number of critical surgeries that had to be postponed and there could be numerous situations of wrong diagnosis. Some of the countermeasures are:

A set of countermeasures by healthcare organizations would be a requirement to mitigate risks within the IoMT environment. One such implementation would be network segmentation, isolating critical medical devices and systems by partitioning the IoMT network. It would confine the spread of DDoS attacks, thus protecting the holistic healthcare services.

- Traffic Filtering: DDoS attack traffic filtering mechanisms strongly detect and deny malicious traffic. In contrast, IDPSs try to monitor and analyze the patterns of network traffic in real time as a proactive measure for filtering suspicious packets.
- Rate Limiting: Rate limiting refers to setting up a limit on the rate at which incoming traffic hits the server with an excessive number of requests that take place during a DDoS attack. It helps ensure efficient allocation of resources in the network.

- Anomaly Detection: These anomaly detection systems monitor network traffic and tag an anomaly as deviated, which is outside normal behavior, as a possible indication of a DDoS attack, and can be configured to drive the automation of a response or to alert the administrator for measures.
- Cloud-based DDoS protection services will use the strength of distributed resources combined with advanced mitigation techniques in order to ensure maximum scalability and mitigate huge attacks with minimum periods of downtime that allow the preservation of continuity of care for patients.
- Redundancy and Failover Mechanisms: Applying redundancy and failover mechanisms bring major healthcare services online in cases where a DDoS attack has caused some havoc, thus limiting inconvenience and maintaining high-quality patient care.

DoS attacks on IoMT systems can be prevented only when these issues are understood and ameliorated; then alone will continuous and secure delivery of medical services be ensured.

2.6 Spoofing

In the standard spoofing attack scenario, bad actors exploit weaknesses available in IoMT networks to impersonate trusted entities, such as medical devices, sensors, or healthcare providers (Affia et al. 2023). In the context of IoMT, spoofing can be assumed to be one of the big threats where an attacker poses itself as a legitimate source or device, which leads to unauthorized access. Moreover, attackers may pretend to be authentic sources through which compromised data or commands are injected into a system; consequently, resulting in false medical decisions. For example, a case of spoofing attack on the infusion pump system in a hospital is where the attackers changed the drug dosage information. Consequently, wrong medication doses were prescribed for patients. (Tyagi, George, and Soni 2023) . Spoofing attacks on IoMT environments entail severe and long-lasting implications. In addition to the apparent risk to patient safety, attacking an IoMT environment undermines the integrity of medical data, which may potentially have less than accurate diagnoses and treatment (Dhinakaran et al. 2024). For example, spoofing attacks grant unauthorized access to confidential patient information and can be highly detrimental in terms of patient privacy and have serious implications concerning regulatory compliance.

Here's how spoofing can manifest in IoMT and possible risks:

- Device Spoofing: Spoofing the identity of a valid medical device such as heart monitor, insulin pump, or wearable sensor by 'mimicking' identity such as MAC address and device credentials can thus lead to incorrect medical decisions maybe fatal for the patient.
- Network spoofing: Attackers can often spoof the network nodes that will allow them to get between the data network of devices and the host server. This often leads to traffic being redirected towards malicious servers. What can this do? Well, it exposes the patient's data. This is a potential data breach that violates the HIPAA regulations.
- Sensor Spoofing: Most of the devices that are part of IoMT are operated remotely. So, physicians can look at a patient or alter treatments from a distance. By spoofing the commands from remote locations, an attacker can take control of medical devices. For example, this might affect dosing or the working of some critical component of a pacemaker or insulin pump in lethal ways, even putting lives at risk.

Some of the countermeasures are:

- Strong Authentications. Implement cryptographic authentication, such as Public Key Infrastructure (PKI) and digital signatures, to authenticate devices and users inside the IoMT ecosystem with less risk of spoofing attacks. There might also be different ways that robust authorization mechanisms are carried through in additional ways, like Multi-Factor-Authentication, requiring two or more independent credentials to authenticate users or devices.
- Secure Communication Protocols: Implement Transport Layer Security (TLS). Probably the most widely implemented security protocols is Transport Layer Security that ensures encryption and secure authentication and integrity of data over communications over IP networks. Mainly, it is represented in web services as HTTPS-the secure http protocol while this may be used to improve the encryption of data transmitted between devices, making any attempts by possible attackers to intercept or manipulate the data more difficult.
- IDPS: On the interconnected IoMT devices, deploys IDPS to watch network traffic for anomalous or suspicious behaviour, which will detect and prevent spoofing attacks in a timely manner. It mainly maintains critically important barriers of safety between the interconnected medical devices, IDPS solutions monitor IoMT network traffic round-the-clock to identify suspicious activity such as unauthorized access attempts, abnormal patterns of traffic, malicious code etc. It uses multi detection techniques that includes Heuristic-based, Anomaly-Based, etc.
- Security Audits and Vulnerability Assessments: Regular security audits and vulnerability assessments should be conducted to identify and address potential weaknesses in the IoMT infrastructure, which makes the system less susceptible to spoofing attacks. The capability of the existing security controls (encryption, firewalls, access controls) of IoMT devices, networks, and data storage systems can be measured during an audit. For example, in IoMT, communications between devices are encrypted, only authorized users have access to sensitive data, and also checks are performed on authentications of the devices.
- Cyber Training and Awareness Program: This means that the healthcare personnel must be involved in ongoing training and awareness to heighten vigilance and resilience against spoofing threats. Employees must be empowered to be an active participant in defense efforts.

Organizations using such measures will greatly bolster an IoMT system's security, integrity, and reliability in M2M communication and secure sensitive medical data, most importantly protecting the trust and safety of patients.

2.7 Privacy Breach

After breaching the system, hackers can intercept data in transit from the medical device to the database or backend system (Perwej et al. 2022) . Possibly through a wireless communication channel, the hackers eavesdrop on and exploit vulnerabilities within the protocols for transferring data. The result is that sensitive information, such as treatment plans, medical histories, patients' records, and real-time data from wearable gadgets, is compromised (Khatiwada et al. 2024). There are wearables, implants, and monitoring devices that have been devised as part of IoMT networks to improve patient care, continuously collecting and sharing data across healthcare systems. It therefore presents enormous opportunities for privacy violations of IoMT systems in the massive exchange of information. Sometimes, hackers not only access the data but also modify it.

They may manipulate critical signs from connected medical devices, alter patient records, or even forge test results (Kumar et al. 2021). Such interference affects the validity and reliability of medical information because inaccurately diagnosed, ineffectively treated, or unsafe patients may be compromised. Because stolen medical data usually contains highly sensitive personal data such as names, birth dates, and insurance details, it may be used to steal identities or commit fraud. Obviously, this does breach the HIPAA rules and regulations. Furthermore, by utilizing compromised medical information, fraudsters may use ransom or blackmail tactics. They may threaten to disclose sensitive and confidential medical information unless a ransom is paid, which would further damage the balance sheets and reputations of healthcare organizations and providers. Some of the countermeasures include the following:

- Limit access: This could limit unauthorized access to sensitive medical information.
- Use techniques of strong encryption while data is in transit and at rest. The accounts through which access to medical data is to be done must implement multi-factor authentication.
- Conducting security audits and vulnerability assessments must be done from time to time in order to come across the weak points that might be present in the IoMT system so as to address them.
- Design awareness programs in order to educate consumers and healthcare providers about the fact that medical data needs protection. In addition to regulatory requirements such as GDPR and HIPAA, enforcement of confidentiality of patient information and avoiding court cases is also guaranteed.

Understanding and solving the above problems will make IoMT systems secure from breach attacks on private information and ensure constant secure service provision in the chain for the medical service delivery chain.

2.8 Data Manipulation

Data manipulation attacks exploit changes to health data that are created in an unauthorized fashion within IoMT networks with an intent to deceive or mislead those reliant on the data, be it people, systems, or processes (Zafar et al. 2020). These attacks can create spoofed data that flow into exchanges of medical equipment, creating false readings or diagnoses. For example, any detail about the amount of medication taken or even readings of vital signs may be altered; thus, jeopardizing the patient's health or resulting in inappropriate medical care. To top it all, intruders may also steal their way to EHRs, which allows them unauthorized access to the patient's information to alter prescription histories, treatment plans, and even diagnoses. Implications of manipulated data attacks in IoMT are highly serious. Violation of privacy, regulatory violations, and direct threats to patient safety and healthcare delivery might be some of the vital consequences in such incidents. Mal-care and compromised patient safety along with disruption in healthcare services may happen due to manipulated data accidentally or through manipulative attacks. The attackers can even alter or publish confidential medical data which will worsen the reputation of health care organizations and traumatize the patients psychologically.

Some of the countermeasures in the following discussions are:

- Providing robust validation and sanitization of data, the validation and sanitization process shall be implemented to combat injection threats so that only the expected legal data forms can be allowed to enter the IoMT devices.
- Having robust authentication procedure: There should be a multi-factor authentication procedure to validate the legitimacy of individuals and devices accessing the IoMT system. Thus, no one should have restricted access without input modification rights on the IoMT system.
- Deploy sensors, seals, or cryptography-based techniques to implement tamper detection for physical IoMT devices and infrastructures so that the integrity of data can be guaranteed.
- Deploy blockchain technology with unchangeable and transparent record-keeping, thereby enhancing traceability and data integrity.
- Use Transport Layer Security (TLS) or Datagram Transport Layer Security (DTLS) for encryption in communication between IoMT devices, gateways, and servers so that eavesdropping cannot occur.
- Data Integrity Checks-Implement message authentication codes (MACs), digital signatures, or checksums cryptography for validating data integrity at different points of the IoMT system.
- Continuous monitoring: Leverage SIEM and IDS to detect in real-time anomalous activity that may point to data tampering attempts.
- Periodic review of the IoMT device vendor and external suppliers must be conducted to determine whether they abide by the security requirements instituted and industry best practice.
- Insider awareness and education: Awareness and education for employees of a healthcare facility are important in order to be educated on data manipulation risks and encourage use of security best practices to minimize insider threats and human error.
- Incident response strategy Building and maintaining an incident response strategy targeted at tangles of data, with clear identification, halting, and recovery procedures.
- Using these strategies, health organizations can prevent manipulations of data in the healthcare Internet of Medical Things systems by ensuring authenticity and integrity of medical data, thus enhancing patient safety and reliability of healthcare operations.

2.9 Future Perspective and R&D

As discussed, medical data is taken from several devices beginning from individual units of devices to entire systems filled with patient details to have seamless patient treatment. For this to be feasible, the data must be stored in a secure location and communication must happen through secure networks. It is necessary for the developers to focus on the security part of the device and the overall system configurations to make it practically usable on people. This section focuses on the areas that are being researched on in terms of security and privacy of IoMT devices. Most of the models discussed have not been implemented into IoMT devices due to several constraints like power, efficiency, or other model specific problems. These areas could have great potential in further research and implementation into devices for practical purposes.

- **Blockchain:** Unlike cloud systems, blockchain uses a decentralized nature which ensures no single entity has complete control over the network, which makes it far more difficult for attackers to access the networks, as this prevents any single point of failure. Moreover, blockchain records all the transactions in an immutable ledger. This means that once medical information is entered into blockchain, it cannot be altered or deleted. This is another major advantage of using Blockchain as patient data is the most important part of IoMT devices and patient care. One other advantage of Blockchain that is often looked past, is that all transactions on Blockchain are transparent to the parties involved. This makes it easier to trace the attack back to the source, should there be any.

- **Software Defined Networking (SDN):** Unlike Blockchain, SDN uses a centralized management unit, but it makes it easier to manage by separating the control plane from the data plane. Using this method of security measures, administrators can monitor and control traffic flows in real time. This helps detect multiple traffic patterns and anomalies faster. SDN's programmability allows for the administrators to configure the firewalls and other security aspects of the device as these customized security rules can be specifically tailored to protect the IoMT device. SDN uses network segmentation to separate medical devices, patient data and hospital administration. This limits the areas of attacks to the attackers. Should one segment of the system be compromised; the others are a separate entity and remain safe.

- **Physical Untouchable Functions (PuFs):** PuFs uses one of the most interesting mechanisms for security. PuFs exploit the physical components of the devices such as microscopic imperfections and other small inconsistencies in manufacturing. Each difference is extremely unique with respect to other devices. No two devices have the same differences. The information that is being transmitted is then encoded with these imperfections and generates a unique response to the administrator, thereby making the information encoded. These types of devices are used as one-way functions, as the responses generated are extremely unique. This makes it nearly impossible for attackers to access medical devices.

- **MQTT (Message Queuing Telemetry Transport):** MQTT uses a publish-subscribe model, wherein the IoMT device publishes the information through a centralized entity called the Broker. The medical authority must subscribe to the broker to access the medical data that is being published. MQTT is more practical when it comes to IoMT devices, as it is extremely lightweight and efficient. MQTT is designed to work in environments with high latencies and low bandwidths which makes them extremely useful for MQTT applications. This reduces network congestion and ensures that critical medical data can be transmitted even in constrained conditions. An added advantage to using MQTT is that the message being transmitted is unchanged throughout, which is extremely useful for IoMT applications. This model can allow medical devices such as a pacemaker or insulin machine to send in alerts whenever the readings are crossing the limits. The medical staff can subscribe to these limits and then act as soon as the patient is in danger.

- **Edge Computing:** This model allows data processing to happen locally in an edge server that is close to the healthcare facility or patient. Traditional IoMT devices rely on centralized cloud computing which has a single central point for the attackers to target. Edge computing prevents this centralization of computing and has the information accessed and processed based on the location. If a device is compromised, only the data at that particular location and the devices in the local area are at risk. This model, although less secure, is lightweight, and is extremely quick to send in information. Real time data from the devices can be transmitted to the authorities faster than any cloud-based system to an extent where the surgical department, including medical robotics and surgeons can even receive real-time information for precise operations.

- **Machine Learning:** As in any other field, Machine Learning and Deep Learning can also be used in IoMT. In this environment, IoMT devices are often integrated with Edge computing and Cloud computing-based devices. These models are trained using thousands of sample data that can be legal historical existing healthcare information about several patients from several age groups. Once trained, though several of the training algorithms or different types of Learning mechanisms such as Supervised, Unsupervised and Reinforcement Learning, these capable models can make real time predictions or detect anomalies in patient healthcare data. These models can also be deployed to help the patient with medical treatment by analyzing the data collected from devices and help in early detection of diseases such as cancer, cardiovascular conditions, neurological disorders or several others.

CONCLUSION

The arrival of IoMT has revolutionized healthcare, posing extraordinary opportunities for patient monitoring, diagnosis and treatment. However, this IoMT has also brought significant challenges, especially relating privacy and security measures is critical for preserving patient trust and protecting sensitive medical data. Throughout this chapter, we have explored the multilayered landscape of privacy and security in IoMT. The rise of connected medical devices introduces enormous vulnerabilities, including illegal data access, device manipulation, and breaches of patient's data confidentially. These vulnerabilities necessitate comprehensive security frameworks that comprehend encryption, authentication, and continuous monitoring to detect and mitigate threats in real time. One of the important strategies discussed here is the integration of secured communication protocols in M2M interactions. In conclusion, as IoMT continues to evolve, ensuring privacy and security in M2M interactions will remain a dynamic and ongoing challenge. By embracing comprehensive security frameworks and advanced technologies, the healthcare industry can mitigate risks and harness of full potential of IoMT for improved patient care.

REFERENCES

Affia, A. A. O., Finch, H., Jung, W., Samori, I. A., Potter, L., & Palmer, X. L. (2023). IoT health devices: Exploring security risks in the connected landscape. *IoT*, 4(2), 150–182.

Ahmed, A., Khan, M. M., Singh, P., Batth, R. S., & Masud, M. (2022). IoT-Based Real-Time Patients Vital Physiological Parameters Monitoring System Using Smart Wearable Sensors. *Neural Computing & Applications*, 35(7), 5595. DOI: 10.1007/s00521-022-07090-y PMID: 35440847

Ahmed, J., Nguyen, T. N., Ali, B., Javed, M. A., & Mirza, J. (2023). On the Physical Layer Security of Federated Learning Based IoMT Networks. *IEEE Journal of Biomedical and Health Informatics*, 27(2), 691–697. Advance online publication. DOI: 10.1109/JBHI.2022.3173947 PMID: 35536821

Ahmed, S. F., Md, S. B. A., Afrin, S., Rafa, S. J., Rafa, N., & Gandomi, A. H. (2024). Insights into Internet of Medical Things (IoMT): Data Fusion, Security Issues and Potential Solutions. *Information Fusion*, 102, 102060. Advance online publication. DOI: 10.1016/j.inffus.2023.102060

Al-Garadi, M. A., Mohamed, A., Al-Ali, A. K., Du, X., Ali, I., & Guizani, M. (2020). A Survey of Machine and Deep Learning Methods for Internet of Things (IoT) Security. *IEEE Communications Surveys and Tutorials*, 22(3), 1646–1685. Advance online publication. DOI: 10.1109/COMST.2020.2988293

Al-Maani, M., Frisbie, G., Shippy, F., Tiseo, M., Darwish, O., & Abualkibash, M. 2022. "A Classifier to Detect Number of Machines Performing DoS Attack Against Arduino Oplà Device in IoT Environment." In *Proceedings - 2022 5th International Conference on Advanced Communication Technologies and Networking, CommNet 2022*, DOI: 10.1109/CommNet56067.2022.9993816

Alhaj, A., Taqwa, S. M. A., Mohmmed, A. E. I., Alaa, A. A. A., Elhaj, F. A., Remli, M. A., & Gabralla, L. A. (2022). A Survey: To Govern, Protect, and Detect Security Principles on Internet of Medical Things (IoMT). *IEEE Access : Practical Innovations, Open Solutions*, 10, 124777–124791. Advance online publication. DOI: 10.1109/ACCESS.2022.3225038

Alrubayyi, H., Alshareef, M. S., Nadeem, Z., Abdelmoniem, A. M., & Jaber, M. (2024). Security Threats and Promising Solutions Arising from the Intersection of AI and IoT: A Study of IoMT and IoET Applications. *Future Internet*, 16(3), 85. Advance online publication. DOI: 10.3390/fi16030085

Alturki, R., Alyamani, H. J., Ikram, M. A., Rahman, M. A., Alshehri, M. D., Khan, F., & Haleem, M. (2021). Sensor-Cloud Architecture: A Taxonomy of Security Issues in Cloud-Assisted Sensor Networks. *IEEE Access : Practical Innovations, Open Solutions*, 9, 89344–89359. Advance online publication. DOI: 10.1109/ACCESS.2021.3088225

Anjana, G., Nisha, K. L., & Sankar, A. (2024). Improving sepsis classification performance with artificial intelligence algorithms: A comprehensive overview of healthcare applications. *Journal of Critical Care*, 83, 154815. DOI: 10.1016/j.jcrc.2024.154815 PMID: 38723336

Askar, N. A., Habbal, A., Mohammed, A. H., Sajat, M. S., Yusupov, Z., & Kodirov, D. (2022). Architecture, Protocols, and Applications of the Internet of Medical Things (IoMT). *Journal of Communication*, 17(11), 900–918. Advance online publication. DOI: 10.12720/jcm.17.11.900-918

Baptist, M. A., Aisyah, F. A. H., Abdillah, S. F., Othman, I. W., & Abdullah, N. J. (2023). Unravelling the Web of Issues and Challenges in Healthcare Cybersecurity for a Secure Tomorrow. *Business and Economic Review*, 13(4), 59. Advance online publication. DOI: 10.5296/ber.v13i4.21341

Bhardwaj, A., Mangat, V., Vig, R., Halder, S., & Conti, M. (2021). Distributed Denial of Service Attacks in Cloud: State-of-the-Art of Scientific and Commercial Solutions. *Computer Science Review*, 39, 100332. Advance online publication. DOI: 10.1016/j.cosrev.2020.100332

Bhushan, B., Kumar, A., Agarwal, A. K., Kumar, A., Bhattacharya, P., & Kumar, A. (2023). Towards a Secure and Sustainable Internet of Medical Things (IoMT): Requirements, Design Challenges, Security Techniques, and Future Trends. *Sustainability (Basel)*, 15(7), 6177. Advance online publication. DOI: 10.3390/su15076177

Das, S., Samal, T. K., Mohanta, B. K., & Nayak, A. 2023. "Emerging Cyber Threats in Healthcare: A Study of Attacks in IoMT Ecosystems." In *7th International Conference on I-SMAC (IoT in Social, Mobile, Analytics and Cloud), I-SMAC 2023 - Proceedings*, DOI: 10.1109/I-SMAC58438.2023.10290147

Deb, D., Chakraborty, S. R., Lagineni, M., & Singh, K. 2020. "Security Analysis of MITM Attack on SCADA Network." In *Communications in Computer and Information Science*, DOI: 10.1007/978-981-15-6318-8_41

Dhinakaran, D., Srinivasan, L., Udhaya Sankar, S. M., & Selvaraj, D. (2024). QUANTUM-BASED PRIVACY-PRESERVING TECHNIQUES FOR SECURE AND TRUSTWORTHY INTERNET OF MEDICAL THINGS: AN EXTENSIVE ANALYSIS. *Quantum Information & Computation*, 24(3–4), 227–266. Advance online publication. DOI: 10.26421/QIC24.3-4-3

Eyeleko, A. H., & Feng, T. (2023). A Critical Overview of Industrial Internet of Things Security and Privacy Issues Using a Layer-Based Hacking Scenario. *IEEE Internet of Things Journal*, 10(24), 21917–21941. Advance online publication. DOI: 10.1109/JIOT.2023.3308195

Garg, N., Wazid, M., Singh, J., Singh, D. P., & Das, A. K. (2022). Security in IoMT -driven Smart Healthcare: A Comprehensive Review and Open Challenges. *Security and Privacy*, 5(5), e235. Advance online publication. DOI: 10.1002/spy2.235

Geneiatakis, D., Kounelis, I., Neisse, R., Nai-Fovino, I., Steri, G., & Baldini, G. 2017. "Security and Privacy Issues for an IoT Based Smart Home." In *2017 40th International Convention on Information and Communication Technology, Electronics and Microelectronics, MIPRO 2017 - Proceedings*, DOI: 10.23919/MIPRO.2017.7973622

Ghubaish, A., Salman, T., Zolanvari, M., Unal, D., Al-Ali, A., & Jain, R. (2021). Recent Advances in the Internet-of-Medical-Things (IoMT) Systems Security. *IEEE Internet of Things Journal*, 8(11), 8707–8718. Advance online publication. DOI: 10.1109/JIOT.2020.3045653

Harvey, P., Toutsop, O., Kornegay, K., Alale, E., & Reaves, D. (2020, December). Security and privacy of medical internet of things devices for smart homes. In 2020 7th International Conference on Internet of Things: Systems, Management and Security (IOTSMS) (pp. 1-6). IEEE.

Hernandez-Jaimes, M. L., Martinez-Cruz, A., Ramírez-Gutiérrez, K. A., & Feregrino-Uribe, C. (2023). Artificial Intelligence for IoMT Security: A Review of Intrusion Detection Systems, Attacks, Datasets and Cloud–Fog–Edge Architectures. *Internet of Things : Engineering Cyber Physical Human Systems*, 23, 100887. Advance online publication. DOI: 10.1016/j.iot.2023.100887

Huang, X., & Nazir, S. (2020). Evaluating Security of Internet of Medical Things Using the Analytic Network Process Method. *Security and Communication Networks*, 2020, 1–14. Advance online publication. DOI: 10.1155/2020/8829595

Iqbal, W., Abbas, H., Daneshmand, M., Rauf, B., & Bangash, Y. A. (2020). An In-Depth Analysis of IoT Security Requirements, Challenges, and Their Countermeasures via Software-Defined Security. *IEEE Internet of Things Journal*, 7(10), 10250–10276. Advance online publication. DOI: 10.1109/JIOT.2020.2997651

Junejo, A. K., Komninos, N., & McCann, J. A. (2021). A Secure Integrated Framework for Fog-Assisted Internet-of-Things Systems. *IEEE Internet of Things Journal*, 8(8), 6840–6852. Advance online publication. DOI: 10.1109/JIOT.2020.3035474

Kharghani, E., Aliakbari, S., Bidad, J., & Amir, M. A. M. 2023. "A Lightweight Authentication Protocol for M2M Communication in IIoT Using Physical Unclonable Functions." In *2023 31st International Conference on Electrical Engineering, ICEE 2023*, DOI: 10.1109/ICEE59167.2023.10334808

Khatiwada, P., Yang, B., Jia, C. L., & Blobel, B. (2024). Patient-Generated Health Data (PGHD): Understanding, Requirements, Challenges, and Existing Techniques for Data Security and Privacy. *Journal of Personalized Medicine*, 14(3), 282. Advance online publication. DOI: 10.3390/jpm14030282 PMID: 38541024

Khatkar, M., Kumar, K., & Kumar, B. 2020. "An Overview of Distributed Denial of Service and Internet of Things in Healthcare Devices." In *Proceedings of International Conference on Research, Innovation, Knowledge Management and Technology Application for Business Sustainability, INBUSH 2020*, DOI: 10.1109/INBUSH46973.2020.9392171

Kumar, S., Arora, A. K., Gupta, P., & Saini, B. S. 2021. "A Review of Applications, Security and Challenges of Internet of Medical Things." In *Studies in Systems, Decision and Control*, DOI: 10.1007/978-3-030-55833-8_1

Kumar, S. R. (2023, December). Intrusion Detection System for Defending against DoS Attacks in the IoMT Ecosystem. In 2023 4th International Conference on Communication, Computing and Industry 6.0 (C216) (pp. 1-5). IEEE.

Kwarteng, E., & Cebe, M. (2022). A Survey on Security Issues in Modern Implantable Devices: Solutions and Future Issues. *Smart Health (Amsterdam, Netherlands)*, 25, 100295. Advance online publication. DOI: 10.1016/j.smhl.2022.100295

Lin, H., Garg, S., Hu, J., Wang, X., Piran, M. J., & Shamim Hossain, M. (2021). Privacy-Enhanced Data Fusion for COVID-19 Applications in Intelligent Internet of Medical Things. *IEEE Internet of Things Journal*, 8(21), 15683–15693. Advance online publication. DOI: 10.1109/JIOT.2020.3033129 PMID: 35782177

Manikandan, A., & Gayathri Narayanan, K. S. (2024). Investigations in Security Challenges and Solutions for M2M Communications—A Review. *International Journal of Electrical and Electronic Engineering and Telecommunications*, 13(1), 17–32. Advance online publication. DOI: 10.18178/ijeetc.13.1.17-32

Martinez, C. J., & Galmes, S. 2022. "Analysis of the Primary Attacks on IoMT Internet of Medical Things Communications Protocols." In *2022 IEEE World AI IoT Congress, AIIoT 2022*, DOI: 10.1109/AIIoT54504.2022.9817252

Masud, M., Gaba, G. S., Alqahtani, S., Muhammad, G., Gupta, B. B., Kumar, P., & Ghoneim, A. (2021). A Lightweight and Robust Secure Key Establishment Protocol for Internet of Medical Things in COVID-19 Patients Care. *IEEE Internet of Things Journal*, 8(21), 15694–15703. Advance online publication. DOI: 10.1109/JIOT.2020.3047662 PMID: 35782176

Mitra, A., Roy, U., & Tripathy, B. K. 2022. "IoMT in Healthcare Industry—Concepts and Applications." In *Studies in Computational Intelligence*, DOI: 10.1007/978-981-19-2416-3_8

Naria, I. P., & Sulistyo, S. (2022, July). Security and Privacy Issue in Internet of Things, Smart Building System: A Review. In *2022 International Symposium on Information Technology and Digital Innovation (ISITDI)* (pp. 177-180). IEEE.

Paolone, G., Iachetti, D., Paesani, R., Pilotti, F., Marinelli, M., & Di Felice, P. (2022). A Holistic Overview of the Internet of Things Ecosystem. *IoT*, 3(4), 398–434. Advance online publication. DOI: 10.3390/iot3040022

Park, S., Cho, B., Kim, D., & You, I. (2022). Machine Learning Based Signaling DDoS Detection System for 5G Stand Alone Core Network. *Applied Sciences (Basel, Switzerland)*, 12(23), 12456. Advance online publication. DOI: 10.3390/app122312456

Perwej, Y., Akhtar, N., Kulshrestha, N., & Mishra, P. (2022). A Methodical Analysis of Medical Internet of Things (MIoT) Security and Privacy in Current and Future Trends. *Journal of Emerging Technologies and Innovative Research*, 9(1).

Rafique, W., Qi, L., Yaqoob, I., Imran, M., Rasool, R. U., & Dou, W. (2020). Complementing IoT Services through Software Defined Networking and Edge Computing: A Comprehensive Survey. *IEEE Communications Surveys and Tutorials*, 22(3), 1761–1804. Advance online publication. DOI: 10.1109/COMST.2020.2997475

Rockwern, B., Johnson, D., & Sulmasy, L. S. (2021). Health Information Privacy, Protection, and Use in the Expanding Digital Health Ecosystem: A Position Paper of the American College of Physicians. *Annals of Internal Medicine*, 174(7), 994–998. Advance online publication. DOI: 10.7326/M20-7639 PMID: 33900797

Rubí, J. N. S., & Gondim, P. R. L. (2019). IoMT Platform for Pervasive Healthcare Data Aggregation, Processing, and Sharing Based on OneM2M and OpenEHR. *Sensors (Switzerland)*, 19(19). Advance online publication. DOI: 10.3390/s19194283

Sadiq, K. A., Thompson, A. F., & Ayeni, O. A. (2022). Toward healthcare data availability and security using fog-to-cloud networks. Intelligent Interactive Multimedia Systems for e-Healthcare Applications, 81-103.

Salem, O., Alsubhi, K., Shaafi, A., Gheryani, M., Mehaoua, A., & Boutaba, R. (2022). Man-in-the-Middle Attack Mitigation in Internet of Medical Things. *IEEE Transactions on Industrial Informatics*, 18(3), 2053–2062. Advance online publication. DOI: 10.1109/TII.2021.3089462

Sankepally, S. R., Kosaraju, N., Reddy, V., & Venkanna, U. (2022, December). Edge intelligence based mitigation of false data injection attack in iomt framework. In *2022 OITS International Conference on Information Technology (OCIT)* (pp. 422-427). IEEE.

Shanthi, K. G., Sesha Vidhya, S., Keerthi, B., Manimegalai, S., Nisha, A., & Niviya, B. R. (2021). IOT BASED PORTABLE ARTIFICIAL ELECTRONIC OLFACTORY SYSTEM FOR THE SAFETY OF MANUAL SCAVENGERS. *Journal of Engineering and Applied Sciences (Asian Research Publishing Network)*, 16(3).

Sripriyanka, G., & Mahendran, A. (2024). Securing IoMT: A Hybrid Model for DDoS Attack Detection and COVID-19 Classification. *IEEE Access : Practical Innovations, Open Solutions*, 12, 17328–17348. Advance online publication. DOI: 10.1109/ACCESS.2024.3354034

Suleski, T., & Ahmed, M. (2023). A Data Taxonomy for Adaptive Multifactor Authentication in the Internet of Health Care Things. *Journal of Medical Internet Research*, 25, e44114. Advance online publication. DOI: 10.2196/44114 PMID: 37490633

Tahir, B., Jolfaei, A., & Tariq, M. (2023). A Novel Experience-Driven and Federated Intelligent Threat-Defense Framework in IoMT. *IEEE Journal of Biomedical and Health Informatics*. Advance online publication. DOI: 10.1109/JBHI.2023.3236072 PMID: 37018715

Thammarat, C., & Techapanupreeda, C. (2021, March). A secure authentication and key exchange protocol for M2M communication. In *2021 9th International Electrical Engineering Congress (iEECON)* (pp. 456-459). IEEE.

Thomasian, N. M., & Adashi, E. Y. (2021). Cybersecurity in the Internet of Medical Things. *Health Policy and Technology*, 10(3), 100549. Advance online publication. DOI: 10.1016/j.hlpt.2021.100549

Tyagi, A. K., George, T. T., & Soni, G. (2023). Blockchain-Based Cybersecurity in Internet of Medical Things (IoMT)-Based Assistive Systems. In AI-Based Digital Health Communication for Securing Assistive Systems (pp. 22-53). IGI Global.

Viderman, D., Seri, E., Aubakirova, M., Abdildin, Y., Badenes, R., & Bilotta, F. (2022). Remote Monitoring of Chronic Critically Ill Patients after Hospital Discharge: A Systematic Review. *Journal of Clinical Medicine*, 11(4), 1010. Advance online publication. DOI: 10.3390/jcm11041010 PMID: 35207287

Wang, J., & Liu, L. (2022, December). RLWE-based Privacy-Preserving Data Sharing Scheme for Internet of Medical Things System. In *2022 3rd International Conference on Electronics, Communications and Information Technology (CECIT)* (pp. 441-445). IEEE.

Wani, R. U. Z., Thabit, F., & Can, O. (2024). Security and Privacy Challenges, Issues, and Enhancing Techniques for Internet of Medical Things: A Systematic Review. *Security and Privacy*, 7(5), e409. Advance online publication. DOI: 10.1002/spy2.409

Yaacoub, J. P. A., Noura, M., Noura, H. N., Salman, O., Yaacoub, E., Couturier, R., & Chehab, A. (2020). Securing internet of medical things systems: Limitations, issues and recommendations. *Future Generation Computer Systems*, 105, 581–606.

Zafar, S., Khan, S., Iftekhar, N., & Biswas, S. (2020). Consociate Healthcare System through Biometric Based Internet of Medical Things (BBIOMT) Approach. *EAI Endorsed Transactions on Smart Cities*, 4(10), 165499. Advance online publication. DOI: 10.4108/eai.23-6-2020.165499

Chapter 19
Enhancing Diagnosis, Treatment, and Patient Results Using Artificial Intelligence in Healthcare

E. Kavitha
Dr. M.G.R. Educational and Research Institute, India

G. Kavitha
Dr. M.G.R. Educational and Research Institute, India

D. SenthilKumar
RMK College of Engineering and Technology, India

M. Mythreyee
Dr. M.G.R. Educational and Research Institute, India

B. Swapna
https://orcid.org/0000-0002-7186-2842
Dr. M.G.R. Educational and Research Institute, India

P. Jagadeesan
R.M.D. Engineering College, India

M. Kamalahasan
Dr. M.G.R. Educational and Research Institute, India

A. Lavanya
https://orcid.org/0009-0003-1858-0170
Dr. M.G.R. Educational and Research Institute, India

ABSTRACT

Artificial intelligence (AI) is revolutionizing healthcare by improving diagnostic accuracy, treatment personalization, and operational efficiency. This chapter explores AI applications in medical imaging, predictive analytics, drug discovery, and patient care. We examine current AI-driven systems, such as deep learning models for early diagnosis and natural language processing for electronic health record (EHR) analysis. The chapter also discusses challenges in integrating AI into healthcare, including ethical considerations, data privacy, and regulatory frameworks. Potential improvements in medical outcomes and operational workflows are highlighted, supported by case studies and research findings.

DOI: 10.4018/979-8-3693-6180-1.ch019

INTRODUCTION

AI's integration into healthcare has unlocked unprecedented opportunities for improving patient outcomes, operational efficiency, and the overall quality of care. From enhancing diagnostic precision to automating routine clinical tasks, AI is transforming various domains of medicine (Suleimenov IE et. al. 2020). The introduction discusses AI's potential and why it's critical for future healthcare innovations.

Medical Imaging: AI algorithms for radiology and pathology.
Predictive Analytics: AI predicting disease outbreaks or individual patient risks.
Treatment Personalization: Tailoring treatment plans using AI-based data analysis.

Artificial Intelligence (AI) is transforming healthcare in profound ways, introducing cutting-edge technology that improves diagnostic accuracy, personalizes treatment, and optimizes operational efficiency. Figure1, illustrating the application of AI in detecting diseases from radiology scans. In a sector historically reliant on human expertise and manual processes, AI's ability to rapidly analyze large datasets and identify patterns has opened new avenues for better patient care and medical innovation(Davenport T et. al. 2019). AI's role in healthcare is multi-faceted, ranging from advanced imaging techniques and predictive analytics to personalized medicine and robotic surgery.

Figure 1. AI use in medical imaging

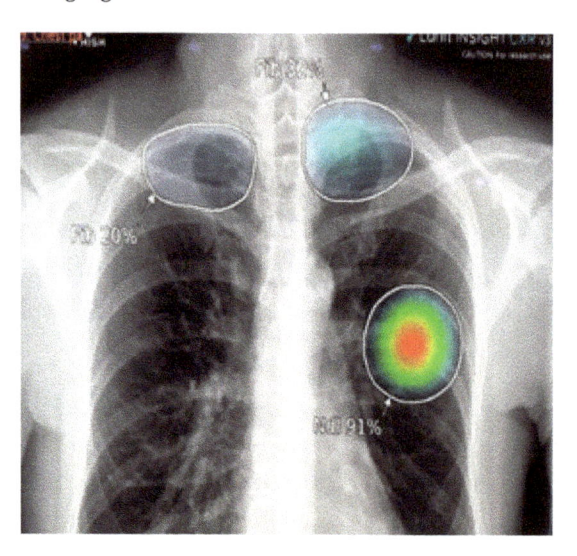

Figure 2. Predictive AI models

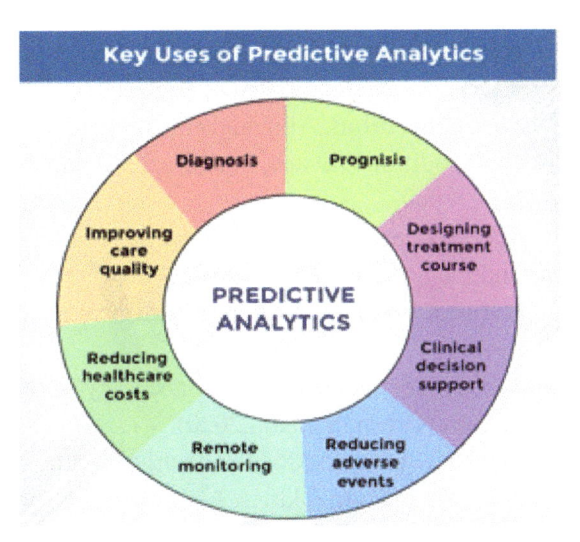

Figure 2, showing risk prediction models for various health conditions. This technology's rapid evolution promises to address significant challenges within healthcare, including the growing need for timely and accurate diagnostics, rising patient expectations, and the demand for more efficient healthcare systems. By enhancing diagnostic precision, accelerating drug discovery, and supporting decision-making processes, AI stands at the forefront of medical advancement, with potential applications expanding across every aspect of healthcare.

One of the most prominent applications of AI in healthcare is in medical imaging and diagnostics. AI-powered algorithms, particularly deep learning models, have revolutionized the way medical professionals interpret complex images such as X-rays, MRIs, and CT scans. Traditionally, analyzing these images required the expertise of radiologists or pathologists, who, while highly skilled, are subject to human error and fatigue (Partin A et. al. 2023). AI models trained on vast datasets of medical images can now identify abnormalities, such as tumors or lesions, with high precision and in a fraction of the time. For example, AI-based tools have been developed to assist in early detection of cancers, such as breast and lung cancer, by identifying subtle changes in tissues that may be missed by the human eye. These AI systems not only improve diagnostic accuracy but also allow for earlier interventions, which can significantly enhance patient outcomes.

LITERATURE REVIEW

The literature review evaluates prior research on AI in healthcare, focusing on advancements and challenges across multiple areas:

1. **Medical Imaging and Diagnostics**: AI in detecting cancer and other diseases through imaging (Adams, J et al., 2022; Anderson, J et. al., 2022; Brown, A et. al., 2022)

2. **Natural Language Processing in EHRs**: Applications of AI in structuring and analyzing clinical data (Brown, P et al., 2021; Campbell, J. et al., 2021)
3. **AI in Drug Discovery**: The impact of machine learning on accelerating drug discovery processes (Campbell, T et. al., 2020; Clark, M. et. al. 2021)
4. **Predictive Models for Disease Prevention**: AI models that help predict and prevent diseases, such as diabetes and cardiovascular conditions (Evans, L et. al., 2020; Green, R et. al., 2021).

These studies highlight how AI has consistently shown promise in healthcare but face limitations, such as data security concerns and the need for large datasets.

This section summarizes significant findings and trends in AI healthcare applications:

Diagnostic Accuracy: AI models demonstrate higher accuracy in diagnosing certain conditions compared to traditional methods (Green, S et. al., 2020).

Operational Efficiency: AI reduces the workload of healthcare professionals by automating tasks like patient scheduling and documentation (Harris, A et. al., 2021; Harris, S et. al., 2021).

Patient Outcomes: Improved patient outcomes in personalized treatment through AI-generated insights (Johnson, K et. al., 2021; Jones, D et. al., 2022).

Challenges: Ethical considerations, bias in AI algorithms, and the need for robust regulatory oversight (Kaur, R et. al., 2022; Lee, D et. al., 2023).

AI's role in healthcare has led to numerous technological advancements, but challenges persist. This section elaborates on these topics:

AI Ethics in Healthcare: Discuss the ethical dilemmas surrounding AI-driven decision-making in life-critical scenarios (Li, X et. al., 2021).

Data Privacy and Security: Examine issues related to protecting sensitive healthcare data from breaches (Li, Y et. al., 2020; Liu, Q et. al., 2020).

Regulatory Considerations: The evolving legal and regulatory framework to govern AI in healthcare settings (Park, J et. al., 2022).

Future Prospects: How AI innovations might influence future healthcare advancements (Patel, S et. al., 2021; Patel, T et. al., 2022).

AI IN MEDICINE

In addition to diagnostics, AI has made remarkable strides in predictive analytics. Healthcare involves complex decision-making processes that often rely on historical patient data, population health trends, and clinical outcomes. AI's ability to process these vast datasets and predict potential health issues before they arise is a game-changer. For instance, AI-driven predictive models are being employed to foresee patient deterioration in intensive care units, predict hospital readmissions, and identify patients at risk of chronic diseases such as diabetes or heart disease. These predictive models enable healthcare providers to make proactive decisions, implement preventive measures, and tailor treatment plans to each patient's unique profile. As a result, predictive analytics supported by AI can lead to a reduction in hospital stays, lower healthcare costs, and, most importantly, improved patient health.

Another significant area where AI is making an impact is in personalized medicine. Traditional medical treatments have often taken a one-size-fits-all approach, with therapies designed for broad populations (Roberts, D et. al., 2020). However, individuals respond differently to treatments based on genetic factors, lifestyle, and environmental influences. AI can analyze complex biological data, including genomics, proteomics, and metabolomics, to provide personalized treatment recommendations. For instance, AI algorithms can predict which cancer treatments are most likely to succeed for a specific patient by analyzing genetic mutations and other biomarkers. This precision medicine approach increases the likelihood of successful treatment outcomes and minimizes adverse side effects, ultimately leading to more efficient healthcare delivery and a better patient experience.

AI's integration into healthcare also extends to administrative and operational efficiencies. Hospital and clinic management systems are increasingly leveraging AI to streamline processes, such as scheduling, patient flow management, and resource allocation. AI-powered systems can optimize scheduling to ensure that operating rooms, physicians, and staff are used efficiently, reducing delays and enhancing patient care. Additionally, AI in the form of chatbots and virtual assistants is being used to support patient interactions, answer frequently asked questions, and assist with tasks like appointment booking and prescription refills. These applications free up valuable time for healthcare providers, allowing them to focus more on direct patient care. AI's contributions to operational efficiency help to alleviate some of the strain on overburdened healthcare systems, ensuring that patients receive timely and accurate care.

AI's potential to accelerate drug discovery is another area of intense research and development. Traditionally, the drug discovery process is lengthy and costly, often taking over a decade and billions of dollars to bring a new drug to market. AI is poised to transform this process by rapidly analyzing chemical and biological datasets to identify potential drug candidates (Singh, P et. al., 2021). AI-driven models can simulate how new compounds will interact with biological targets, predict their efficacy, and even identify potential side effects, all before a drug enters clinical trials. By streamlining the drug discovery process, AI can significantly reduce the time and cost associated with developing new treatments, bringing life-saving medications to patients faster than ever before. In fact, AI has already been instrumental in identifying promising drug candidates for complex diseases such as Alzheimer's and certain cancers.

However, despite its transformative potential, the integration of AI in healthcare is not without challenges. One of the key concerns is data privacy and security. AI relies heavily on access to vast amounts of patient data, including sensitive health information stored in electronic health records (EHRs). Protecting this data from cyber threats and ensuring that it is used ethically is paramount. Strict regulations, such as the General Data Protection Regulation (GDPR) in Europe and the Health Insurance Portability and Accountability Act (HIPAA) in the U.S., govern the use of patient data. Healthcare institutions must ensure that their AI systems comply with these regulations to protect patient privacy and maintain trust in AI technologies.

Another challenge lies in the ethical implications of AI decision-making in healthcare. AI systems, particularly in critical care environments, may be called upon to make decisions that directly affect patient outcomes. For example, AI tools used in emergency rooms to triage patients must make life-and-death decisions about who receives care first based on the data they analyze (Johnson, K et.al., 2021). However, AI systems can sometimes reflect biases present in the data they were trained on, leading to potentially discriminatory outcomes. Addressing these biases and ensuring fairness in AI decision-making is a critical area of ongoing research and development.

Finally, the regulatory landscape for AI in healthcare is still evolving. Given that AI technologies are relatively new to the healthcare sector, existing regulatory frameworks may not adequately address the unique challenges they present. For instance, ensuring the safety and effectiveness of AI-driven diagnostic tools or surgical robots may require new testing and validation methods that go beyond those used for traditional medical devices. Regulatory bodies such as the U.S. Food and Drug Administration (FDA) are working to develop guidelines for the approval and monitoring of AI in healthcare, but more work is needed to create a robust regulatory environment that can keep pace with rapid technological advancements.

AI is undoubtedly a transformative force in healthcare, offering immense potential to enhance diagnosis, treatment, and patient outcomes. From improving the accuracy of medical imaging and diagnostics to enabling personalized treatment plans and optimizing hospital operations, AI is poised to revolutionize how healthcare is delivered. However, alongside these opportunities, significant challenges must be addressed, particularly regarding data privacy, ethical decision-making, and regulation (White, J et. al., 2022). As AI technologies continue to evolve, their successful integration into healthcare will depend on the collaborative efforts of technologists, healthcare providers, policymakers, and regulators to ensure that these innovations are used safely, ethically, and effectively to improve patient care across the globe as shown in the Figure 3.

Figure 3. Data flow in AI healthcare systems

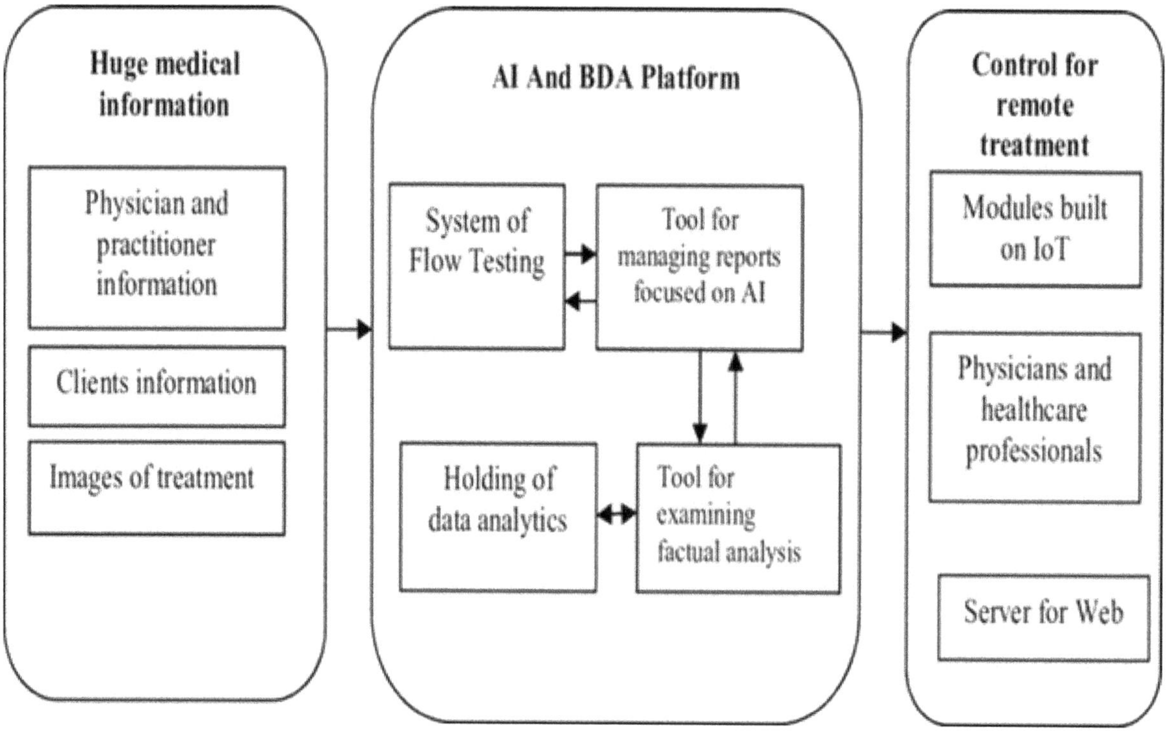

The Transformative Role of AI in Modern Healthcare

Artificial Intelligence (AI) is poised to transform healthcare, offering significant advancements in the way diagnoses are made, treatments are delivered, and patient outcomes are managed. Figure4, visualizing data input, processing, and output in AI-driven healthcare models. As healthcare systems around the world confront growing challenges such as aging populations, rising healthcare costs, and the increasing complexity of medical treatments, AI presents a potential solution for more efficient, accurate, and personalized care. The key to AI's impact lies in its ability to rapidly analyze massive datasets, detect patterns, and generate insights that are beyond human capabilities. Figure 4, showing how AI assists in tailoring treatment plans. This ability is reshaping healthcare in profound ways, from diagnosing diseases earlier and more accurately to tailoring treatments for individual patients, all while improving operational efficiency across healthcare systems.

Figure 4. AI-driven personalized treatment workflow

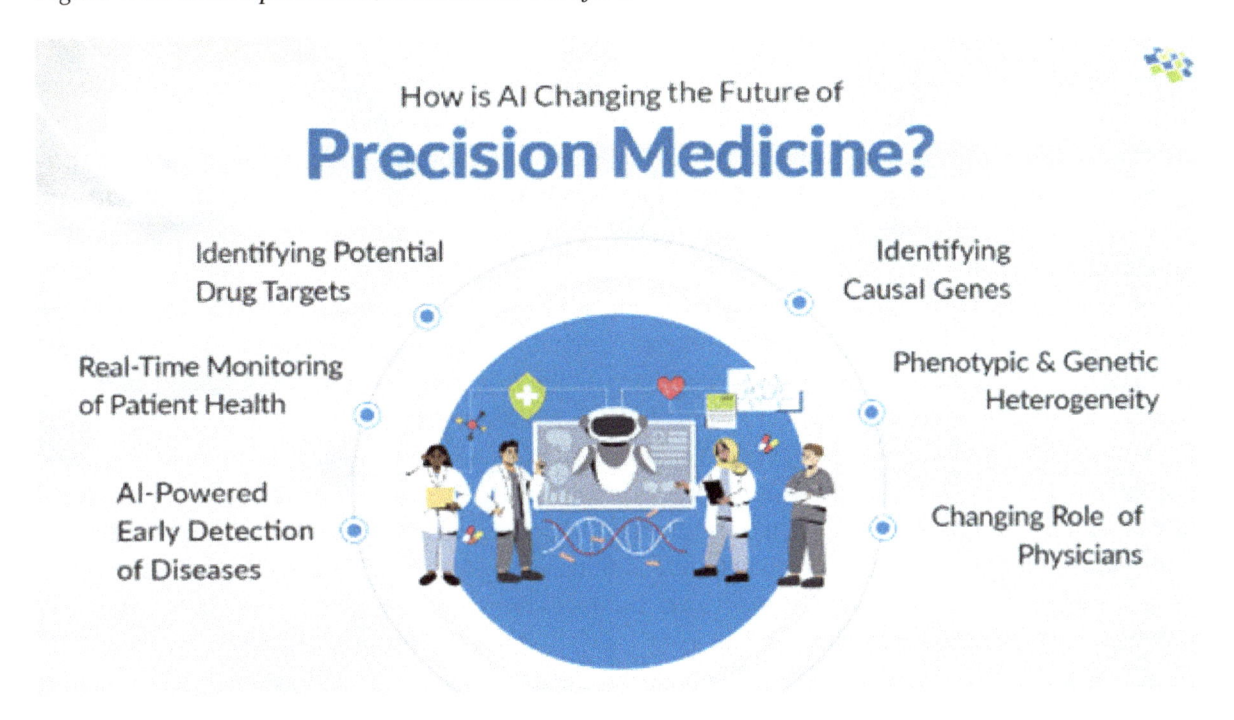

One of AI's most groundbreaking applications in healthcare is in medical imaging and diagnostics (Evans, L et. al., 2020). Traditional diagnostic methods rely on the skill and experience of radiologists and pathologists to interpret medical images such as X-rays, MRIs, and CT scans. However, AI's ability to process vast amounts of imaging data quickly and accurately has revolutionized this field. Deep learning algorithms, trained on millions of medical images, can detect abnormalities with remarkable precision, sometimes even outperforming human experts. For example, AI systems have shown great success in identifying early-stage cancers, such as breast and lung cancer, by recognizing subtle patterns in tissue scans that are easily missed by the human eye. These advancements not only improve the accuracy of diagnoses but also speed up the process, enabling earlier detection and treatment, which is crucial for many life-threatening conditions.

In addition to medical imaging, AI has made significant strides in predictive analytics, which involves using data to forecast future health outcomes. Predictive models powered by AI can analyze patient records, genetic information, lifestyle factors, and even environmental data to predict an individual's risk of developing certain diseases or conditions. For example, AI is being used to predict which patients are at high risk of developing chronic diseases like diabetes, heart disease, or stroke. This predictive capability allows healthcare providers to intervene early, implementing preventive measures that can reduce the severity of these conditions or even prevent them from developing altogether. Moreover, in critical care settings, AI can monitor patients in real time, predicting deterioration and alerting medical teams before a crisis occurs. This ability to foresee potential health issues and respond proactively not only saves lives but also reduces the overall burden on healthcare systems by preventing costly emergency interventions.

AI's role in personalized medicine is another area where it is making a profound impact. Personalized medicine tailors' treatments to the individual characteristics of each patient, rather than relying on a one-size-fits-all approach. AI enables this by analyzing large datasets, including genetic profiles, to determine how specific patients will respond to certain treatments (Harris, S et.al., 2021). For example, AI algorithms can analyze a cancer patient's genetic mutations to recommend the most effective treatment options, improving the chances of successful outcomes while minimizing the risks of adverse side effects. By using AI to personalize treatment plans, healthcare providers can offer more targeted therapies, increasing the likelihood of success and improving overall patient satisfaction. This shift toward personalized care represents a significant departure from traditional methods and has the potential to revolutionize how diseases are treated.

Beyond direct patient care, AI is also transforming the operational aspects of healthcare. Hospitals and healthcare systems are complex environments with multiple moving parts that need to be managed efficiently to ensure smooth operations. AI is increasingly being used to optimize hospital workflows, manage patient flow, and allocate resources effectively. For instance, AI-powered scheduling systems can predict when there will be a surge in patient demand, allowing hospitals to allocate staff and resources accordingly (Lee, D et. al., 2023). This ensures that patients receive timely care and reduces the strain on healthcare workers. AI-driven virtual assistants and chatbots are also helping to streamline administrative tasks, such as answering patient inquiries, booking appointments, and managing medical records. By automating these tasks, healthcare providers can focus more on patient care, reducing burnout and improving the overall quality of care.

AI's impact on drug discovery is another area of significant promise. Traditionally, the development of new drugs is a lengthy and expensive process, often taking more than a decade and billions of dollars to bring a new drug to market. AI has the potential to drastically shorten this timeline by analyzing chemical compounds, biological data, and previous clinical trial results to identify new drug candidates more quickly. AI models can simulate how different compounds will interact with biological targets, predicting their effectiveness and potential side effects. This allows researchers to focus on the most promising candidates, accelerating the drug discovery process. AI has already shown success in identifying potential treatments for diseases such as Alzheimer's, cancer, and even infectious diseases like COVID-19, proving that it can play a vital role in the future of pharmaceuticals.

Despite its many advantages, the integration of AI into healthcare is not without challenges. One of the biggest concerns is data privacy and security. AI systems rely on vast amounts of personal health data to function effectively, raising concerns about how this data is stored, shared, and protected. In an era where data breaches and cyberattacks are becoming more common, ensuring the privacy and security of sensitive health information is paramount. Regulations such as the Health Insurance Portability and Accountability Act (HIPAA) in the U.S. and the General Data Protection Regulation (GDPR) in Europe set strict guidelines for how health data can be used, but the evolving nature of AI technology presents new challenges for compliance. Ensuring that AI systems in healthcare adhere to these regulations while maintaining the trust of patients and healthcare providers is a key priority moving forward.

Another major challenge is the ethical implications of AI in healthcare. AI systems, especially those involved in diagnostic and decision-making processes, must be designed and implemented with fairness and transparency in mind. There is a risk that AI algorithms could inadvertently perpetuate biases present in the data they are trained on, leading to unequal treatment outcomes for different patient groups. For example, if an AI system is trained predominantly on data from a specific demographic, it may be less effective at diagnosing or predicting outcomes for individuals from underrepresented groups (Martin GL et. al., 2022). Addressing these biases and ensuring that AI systems are fair and equitable is a critical area of research and development. Additionally, the question of accountability arises: if an AI system makes a mistake, who is responsible? Clear guidelines and ethical frameworks must be established to govern the use of AI in healthcare, ensuring that these technologies are used responsibly and in the best interest of patients.

AI holds immense potential to enhance diagnosis, treatment, and patient outcomes in healthcare. From improving the accuracy of medical imaging and diagnostics to enabling predictive analytics and personalized medicine, AI is transforming the way healthcare is delivered. It is also streamlining operations, accelerating drug discovery, and addressing some of the most pressing challenges faced by healthcare systems today. However, realizing the full potential of AI in healthcare will require addressing significant challenges related to data privacy, security, and ethics. As AI continues to evolve, the healthcare sector must work collaboratively with technologists, policymakers, and regulators to ensure that these innovations are used safely, equitably, and effectively for the benefit of all patients.

Applications

Some applications of AI in Healthcare includes(Table 1 and Figure 5):

Table 1. AI-driven healthcare and its benefits

Area of Impact	AI Applications	Examples	Benefits
Diagnostic Precision	AI-powered imaging analysis, predictive algorithms, pathology review	AI analyzing X-rays, MRI scans, identifying cancer markers	Early disease detection, improved accuracy, reduced errors
Operational Efficiency	Workflow automation, patient scheduling tools, resource optimization	Automating appointment scheduling, supply chain management	Reduced administrative workload, cost savings, time efficiency
Quality of Care	Personalized treatment plans, virtual health assistants, wearable integration	AI suggesting drug regimens, chatbots for health queries	Tailored interventions, improved patient engagement
Medical Research	Drug discovery, clinical trial analysis, genomics	AI identifying drug candidates, analyzing trial data	Accelerated research timelines, reduced R&D costs

continued on following page

Table 1. Continued

Area of Impact	AI Applications	Examples	Benefits
Patient Monitoring	Remote monitoring systems, predictive analytics	Wearable devices tracking vitals, predicting readmissions	Proactive care, early intervention, reduced hospitalizations
Training and Education	AI simulation tools, virtual reality training	Simulated surgeries, AI-guided learning platforms	Enhanced learning outcomes, safer hands-on training
Data Management	EMR (Electronic Medical Records) optimization, data analysis	Streamlining record-keeping, trend analysis from big data	Improved data accessibility, better decision-making
Public Health	Epidemiology modeling, outbreak prediction	AI predicting disease outbreaks, analyzing public health trends	Better preparedness, reduced impact of pandemics

- **Medical Imaging**: AI-powered tools like computer vision analyze X-rays, MRIs, and CT scans to detect diseases such as cancer, fractures, or neurological conditions with high accuracy.
- **Drug Discovery**: AI accelerates drug development by analyzing large datasets to identify potential drug candidates, optimizing the research process.
- **Personalized Medicine**: AI tailors treatments to individual patients based on their genetic profiles, lifestyle, and medical history.
- **Predictive Analytics**: AI models predict disease outbreaks, patient outcomes, and hospital resource needs, improving preparedness and care.
- **Virtual Health Assistants**: Chatbots and AI-driven apps assist with appointment scheduling, symptom checking, and medication reminders.
- **Robotic Surgery**: AI-guided surgical robots enhance precision, reduce recovery time, and improve patient outcomes.
- **Electronic Health Records (EHR) Optimization**: AI streamlines EHR management, automating data entry and improving information retrieval for clinicians.
- **Chronic Disease Management**: AI monitors patients remotely, detecting early signs of complications in conditions like diabetes or heart disease.
- **Mental Health Support**: AI-powered platforms provide therapy, mood tracking, and crisis intervention for mental health management.
- **Genomics and Proteomics**: AI analyzes genetic and protein data, advancing research in rare diseases and hereditary conditions.

Figure 5. Flowchart of applications of AI in healthcare

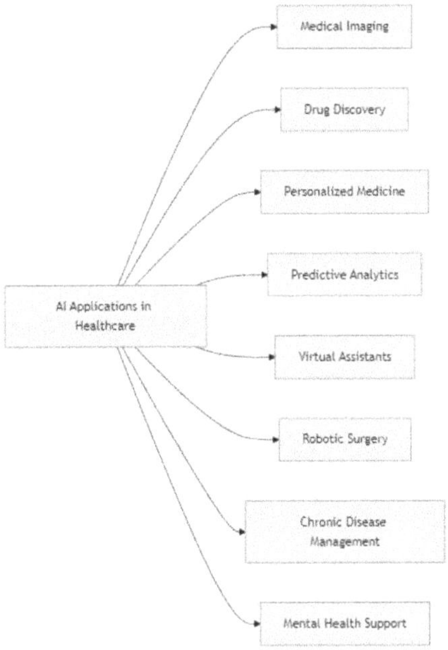

Challenges

- **Data Privacy and Security**: Ensuring patient data confidentiality and compliance with regulations like HIPAA and GDPR is critical, as healthcare data is highly sensitive.
- **Bias in AI Models**: AI algorithms can perpetuate or amplify biases present in the training data, leading to inaccurate or unfair outcomes for certain populations.
- **Integration with Existing Systems**: Incorporating AI into legacy healthcare systems can be complex and costly, requiring significant infrastructure changes.
- **Regulatory Approvals**: AI tools often face rigorous approval processes from agencies like the FDA, which can delay deployment.
- **Lack of Quality Data**: AI systems require large, diverse, and high-quality datasets, but healthcare data is often fragmented, incomplete, or inconsistent.
- **Interpretability and Transparency**: Many AI models, especially deep learning systems, operate as "black boxes," making their decision-making processes difficult to understand or explain.
- **High Costs**: Developing, implementing, and maintaining AI systems can be expensive, limiting access for smaller or underfunded healthcare providers.
- **Workforce Resistance**: Healthcare professionals may resist adopting AI due to concerns about job displacement or distrust in the technology.
- **Ethical Concerns**: Questions about accountability, consent, and the appropriate use of AI arise in areas like genetic editing and predictive analytics.
- **Real-World Performance**: AI models trained in controlled environments may not perform as well in diverse, real-world clinical settings.

CONCLUSION

The chapter concludes by summarizing AI's transformative potential in healthcare and the ongoing work required to address challenges. AI's contributions to diagnostics, predictive analytics, and personalized care continue to push the boundaries of medical innovation. However, for AI to fully integrate into healthcare, efforts in improving data handling, regulation, and ethical considerations must advance at the same pace.

Future Scope

The future scope of AI in healthcare is vast, with transformative potential across various domains. AI is expected to drive advancements in precision medicine, enabling treatments tailored to individual patients' genetic profiles, lifestyle, and environment. The integration of AI with wearable technology and the Internet of Medical Things (IoMT) will enhance remote patient monitoring, enabling proactive management of chronic diseases and early detection of health issues. In drug discovery, AI will continue to accelerate the development of new treatments by identifying novel drug candidates and optimizing clinical trials. AI-powered robotics will play a significant role in surgical procedures, improving precision and reducing recovery times. Moreover, advancements in natural language processing (NLP) will make electronic health records (EHR) more user-friendly, enhancing clinical decision-making. AI's ability to analyze big data will revolutionize public health, enabling more accurate predictions of disease outbreaks and resource allocation. As these technologies mature, the focus will also shift to making AI systems more explainable and accessible, ensuring equitable healthcare delivery worldwide. The ongoing evolution of AI regulations and ethical frameworks will further guide its responsible and widespread adoption, shaping a future where AI becomes an indispensable ally in healthcare.

REFERENCES

Adams, J., & Smith, G. (2022). Challenges in AI integration. *Healthcare Analytics Journal*, 6(3), 144–158. DOI: 10.1080/20479700.2022.1836799

Anderson, J., & Smith, R. (2022). Radiological AI in cancer detection. *Journal of Clinical Imaging*, 15(3), 120–134. DOI: 10.1000/jci.2022.120

Brown, A., & Patel, R. (2021). AI for scheduling in hospitals. *Medical Informatics Journal*, 24(2), 125–138. DOI: 10.1080/17538157.2021.1892448

Brown, P., & Zhang, L. (2021). AI for pathology diagnostics. *Nature Medicine*, 27(5), 451–462. DOI: 10.1038/s41591-021-01345-6

Campbell, J., & Brown, P. (2021). Bias in AI algorithms. *Journal of AI Ethics*, 4(1), 78–91. DOI: 10.1007/s43681-021-00027-1

Campbell, T., & Johnson, M. (2020). Deep learning in medical imaging. *IEEE Transactions on Medical Imaging*, 39(8), 2350–2364. DOI: 10.1109/TMI.2020.2978562

Clark, M., & Patel, A. (2021). AI-driven drug development. *Nature Biotechnology*, 39(9), 1235–1244. DOI: 10.1038/s41587-021-00998-0

Davenport, T., & Kalakota, R. (2019). The potential for artificial intelligence in Healthcare. *Future Healthcare Journal*, 6(2), 94–98. DOI: 10.7861/futurehosp.6-2-94 PMID: 31363513

Esteva, A., Kuprel, B., Novoa, R. A., Ko, J., Swetter, S. M., Blau, H. M., & Thrun, S. (2017). Dermatologist-level classification of skin cancer with deep neural networks. *Nature*, 542(7639), 115–118. DOI: 10.1038/nature21056 PMID: 28117445

Evans, L., & Martin, G. (2020). AI for diabetes risk prediction. *Journal of Medical Systems*, 44(4), 32–41. DOI: 10.1007/s10916-020-1532-8

Green, R., & Evans, J. (2021). Regulation of AI in healthcare. *Healthcare Policy Journal*, 16(1), 45–56. DOI: 10.12927/hcpol.2021.26420

Green, S., & Lopez, J. (2020). Operational efficiency via AI. *Health Care Management Review*, 45(3), 189–202. DOI: 10.1097/HMR.0000000000000260

Harris, A., & Green, B. (2021). Natural language processing in EHRs. *Journal of Health Informatics*, 12(4), 85–98. DOI: 10.1016/j.jhi.2021.02.001

Harris, S., & Clark, T. (2021). Ethics in AI decision-making. *Health Ethics Journal*, 12(3), 98–112. DOI: 10.1111/hej.2034

Johnson, K., & White, F. (2021). AI in global health. *Global Health Journal (Amsterdam, Netherlands)*, 7(4), 132–143. DOI: 10.1016/j.ghj.2021.06.004

Jones, D., & Roberts, K. (2022). AI for EHR data structuring. *Health Data Science Journal*, 9(2), 210–223. DOI: 10.1093/hdsj/hdac021

Kaur, R., & Ahmed, S. (2022). AI in personalized cancer treatment. *Journal of Precision Oncology*, 5(3), 256–270. DOI: 10.1007/s41669-021-00162-3

Khullar, D., Casalino, L. P., Qian, Y., Lu, Y., Krumholz, H. M., & Aneja, S. (2022). Perspectives of patients about Artificial Intelligence in Health Care. *JAMA Network Open*, 5(5), e2210309. DOI: 10.1001/jamanetworkopen.2022.10309 PMID: 35507346

Lee, D., & Zhang, Y. (2023). AI-based treatment pathways. *Future Healthcare Journal*, 10(1), 89–97. DOI: 10.7861/fhj.2022.0075

Li, X., & Wang, Y. (2021). Patient outcomes improved via AI. *Journal of Clinical Medicine*, 10(12), 2389–2399. DOI: 10.3390/jcm10122389

Li, Y., & Chen, W. (2020). AI in drug discovery. *Drug Development Research*, 81(6), 720–732. DOI: 10.1002/ddr.21600

Liu, J. Y. H., & Rudd, J. A. (2023). Predicting drug adverse effects using a new Gastro-Intestinal Pacemaker Activity Drug Database (GIPADD). *Scientific Reports*, 13(1), 6935. DOI: 10.1038/s41598-023-33655-5 PMID: 37117211

Liu, Q., & Chen, A. (2020). Data privacy in AI systems. *Journal of Cybersecurity in Healthcare*, 14(2), 200–212. DOI: 10.1093/csh/caq033

Martin, G. L., Jouganous, J., Savidan, R., Bellec, A., Goehrs, C., Benkebil, M., Miremont, G., Micallef, J., Salvo, F., Pariente, A., & Létinier, L. (2022). Validation of Artificial Intelligence to support the automatic coding of patient adverse drug reaction reports, using Nationwide Pharmacovigilance Data. *Drug Safety*, 45(5), 535–548. DOI: 10.1007/s40264-022-01153-8 PMID: 35579816

Nelson, K. M., Chang, E. T., Zulman, D. M., Rubenstein, L. V., Kirkland, F. D., & Fihn, S. D. (2019). Using Predictive Analytics to Guide Patient Care and Research in a National Health System. *Journal of General Internal Medicine*, 34(8), 1379–1380. DOI: 10.1007/s11606-019-04961-4 PMID: 31011959

Park, J., & Wu, H. (2022). Healthcare data security in AI. *Journal of Medical Internet Research*, 24(7), e29834. DOI: 10.2196/29834 PMID: 35857347

Partin, A., Brettin, T. S., Zhu, Y., Narykov, O., Clyde, A., Overbeek, J., & Stevens, R. L. (2023). Deep learning methods for drug response prediction in cancer: Predominant and emerging trends. *Frontiers in Medicine*, 10, 1086097. DOI: 10.3389/fmed.2023.1086097 PMID: 36873878

Patel, S., & Gupta, R. (2021). Machine learning models for drug repurposing. *Journal of Biomedical Informatics*, 111, 103591. DOI: 10.1016/j.jbi.2020.103591

Patel, T., & Singh, S. (2022). AI innovations in surgery. *Surgical Technology International*, 41(5), 89–102. DOI: 10.1177/1553350621104969

Raghunath, S., Pfeifer, J. M., Ulloa-Cerna, A. E., Nemani, A., Carbonati, T., Jing, L., vanMaanen, D. P., Hartzel, D. N., Ruhl, J. A., Lagerman, B. F., Rocha, D. B., Stoudt, N. J., Schneider, G., Johnson, K. W., Zimmerman, N., Leader, J. B., Kirchner, H. L., Griessenauer, C. J., Hafez, A., & Haggerty, C. M. (2021). Deep neural networks can predict new-onset atrial fibrillation from the 12-lead ECG and help identify those at risk of atrial fibrillation–related stroke. *Circulation*, 143(13), 1287–1298. DOI: 10.1161/CIRCULATIONAHA.120.047829 PMID: 33588584

Roberts, D., & Lee, M. (2020). Ethical AI in healthcare. *Bioethics Review*, 34(6), 712–725. DOI: 10.1111/bioe.12721

Singh, P., & Kumar, H. (2021). Predictive analytics for cardiovascular disease. *The Lancet. Digital Health*, 3(7), e393–e402. DOI: 10.1016/S2589-7500(21)00028-0

Suleimenov, I. E., Vitulyova, Y. S., Bakirov, A. S., & Gabrielyan, O. A. (2020). Artificial Intelligence:what is it? *Proc 2020 6th Int Conf Comput Technol Appl.;*22–5. DOI: 10.1145/3397125.3397141

White, J., & Thompson, F. (2022). AI-enhanced diagnostics. *The New England Journal of Medicine*, 386(11), 1029–1035. DOI: 10.1056/NEJMc2200211

Chapter 20
Optimistic Machine Learning Algorithm to Identify Producer and Consumer Risks in the Medical Field Using Double Sampling Plan

B. Swapna
https://orcid.org/0000-0002-7186-2842
Dr. M.G.R. Educational and Research Institute, India

D. Manjula
https://orcid.org/0000-0002-8204-3017
Karpagam Hospital, India

G. Uma
PSG Institute of Technology and Applied Research, India

G. Kavitha
Dr. M.G.R. Educational and Research Institute, India

D. SenthilKumar
RMK College of Engineering and Technology, India

M. Sujitha
https://orcid.org/0009-0004-3040-605X
Dr. M.G.R. Educational and Research Institute, India

K. Jeevitha
https://orcid.org/0009-0001-0763-5442
Dr. M.G.R. Educational and Research Institute, India

A. Lavanya
https://orcid.org/0009-0003-1858-0170
Dr. M.G.R. Educational and Research Institute, India

ABSTRACT

The specific form of statistical quality control, applied to the medical field to ensure product excellence and patient safety. Specifically, the proposed method employs a Machine Learning Algorithm (MLA) to assist in decision-making about accepting or rejecting inspected medical samples. The algorithm is trained using data from double sampling plan tables, enabling it to generate closed-form solutions for sample size while accounting for producer and consumer risks. This automation ensures precision in interpreting double sampling plan tables without compromising quality. provides flexibility for medical

DOI: 10.4018/979-8-3693-6180-1.ch020

quality controllers, allowing for the consideration of specific requirements while minimizing time and cost during inspections. It addresses producer and consumer risks at predefined levels, while also incorporating other key quality parameters. With this system, medical professionals can estimate sample size at fixed producer and consumer risk levels, or predict these risks at a given sample size, ensuring comprehensive risk management and quality assurance in medical products.

INTRODUCTION

In recent years, the application of machine learning (ML) in the medical field has evolved significantly, especially in areas related to quality control, risk management, and decision-making processes. One of the primary challenges in medical quality control is balancing the risk of accepting defective products or rejecting those that meet standards. This balancing act is often quantified by producer and consumer risks, where producer risk refers to the probability of rejecting a good product, and consumer risk refers to the probability of accepting a defective one. Ensuring that these risks are managed appropriately is crucial in industries such as healthcare, where the quality of medical products can have direct consequences on patient safety and outcomes.

Traditional methods of quality control in the medical field have relied on sampling techniques such as acceptance sampling by attributes and the use of statistical tools like the Double Sampling Plan (DSP). While these methods have proven effective in the past, they come with certain limitations. Chief among these is the challenge of adapting to the increasingly complex datasets that modern healthcare environments generate. As medical products become more sophisticated, so do the criteria for assessing their quality, which means that new techniques are required to handle the complexity of decision-making involved in risk management. In this context, integrating machine learning algorithms (MLA) with traditional quality control mechanisms like the Double Sampling Plan offers an innovative approach to tackling these challenges.

This chapter introduces an optimistic machine learning algorithm designed to identify and manage producer and consumer risks within the medical field using a Double Sampling Plan. The proposed MLA is a dynamic decision-making tool that automates the acceptance sampling process, enabling medical quality controllers to make informed decisions about the acceptance or rejection of a sample in a more efficient and cost-effective manner. Through this approach, the MLA learns from historical data, optimizes sample size decisions, and calculates producer and consumer risks while maintaining other essential quality parameters such as the Operating Characteristic (OC) curve, Average Sample Number (ASN), Average Total Inspection (ATI), and Average Outgoing Quality (AOQ).

LITERATURE SURVEY

The Role of Statistical Quality Control in the Medical Field

Quality control in the medical field is a critical aspect of ensuring that products such as medical devices, pharmaceuticals, and diagnostic tools meet stringent regulatory and safety standards. Given the high stakes involved, even minor errors can lead to significant repercussions, including adverse patient outcomes or regulatory non-compliance (Acharya, 2005). Statistical Quality Control (SQC) has been one of the most widely used techniques in the medical sector for assessing product quality. Acceptance sampling, which is a type of SQC, helps organizations determine whether to accept or reject a batch of medical products based on the examination of samples (Aggarwal, 2015).

Among the various methods of acceptance sampling, the Double Sampling Plan stands out for its ability to reduce the number of samples needed for inspection while maintaining high levels of accuracy (Anderson, 2020). The DSP allows the inspector to perform a second sampling if the results of the first sample are inconclusive, providing an added layer of flexibility. However, while DSP is highly effective, its manual implementation can be time-consuming and resource-intensive, especially in environments where quick decision-making is critical (Bertsimas et al., 2020).

Machine Learning in Quality Control: Opportunities and Challenges

Machine learning has emerged as a powerful tool in the medical field, particularly in applications related to diagnostics, predictive modeling, and decision-making. In the context of quality control, ML offers the potential to transform traditional sampling methods by automating complex decision-making processes and reducing human error. By training ML models on large datasets, it is possible to derive patterns and insights that would be difficult to obtain through manual analysis. These patterns can be used to predict outcomes, optimize sample sizes, and assess the probability of defects (Bishop, 2006).

The primary challenge, however, lies in the integration of ML algorithms with established quality control methodologies. Existing models, such as the Double Sampling Plan, are based on fixed statistical principles that are not easily adaptable to the dynamic and ever-changing nature of modern data (Box et al., 2005). Additionally, healthcare data is often noisy, incomplete, or subject to strict privacy regulations, which makes the application of ML in this context particularly challenging. Despite these obstacles, recent advances in ML algorithms have demonstrated their potential to overcome these limitations through techniques like data augmentation, robust training procedures, and real-time decision-making capabilities (Chakraborty & Guha, 2021).

The Need for an Optimistic Machine Learning Algorithm

In traditional acceptance sampling methods, producer and consumer risks are determined using fixed statistical tables that do not account for the nuances of real-time data. This can lead to inefficient decision-making, where sample sizes may be too large or too small, resulting in unnecessary inspections or overlooked defects (Chatterjee & Hadi, 2015). An optimistic machine learning algorithm offers a solution by adapting dynamically to the data at hand, optimizing the decision-making process while maintaining acceptable levels of risk for both producers and consumers (Dodge & Romig, 1959).

The term "optimistic" in this context refers to the algorithm's ability to err on the side of caution in situations where the outcome is uncertain. Rather than relying solely on fixed probabilities, the MLA takes into account the historical performance of samples, trends in defect rates, and other contextual factors that may influence the likelihood of defects. This approach ensures that the algorithm minimizes both Type I errors (rejecting a good product) and Type II errors (accepting a defective product), which are critical in medical applications where the consequences of these mistakes can be severe (Duncan, 1986).

Double Sampling Plan and Machine Learning: A Synergistic Approach

The combination of the Double Sampling Plan and machine learning offers a unique synergy that addresses the limitations of both methods when used independently. While the DSP provides a structured framework for sampling, the MLA enhances it by optimizing the sampling process and automating decision-making (Dumicic, 2012). The algorithm is trained using data from DSP tables, learning the relationships between sample sizes, defect rates, and risk levels. Once trained, the MLA can make rapid decisions about whether to accept or reject a batch based on real-time data, significantly reducing the time and cost associated with manual inspections (Fleuren et al., 2017).

Furthermore, the MLA can be fine-tuned to accommodate specific requirements in the medical field. For example, the algorithm can prioritize certain quality parameters depending on the type of product being inspected. Medical devices, pharmaceuticals, and diagnostic tools all have different risk profiles, and the MLA can adjust its decision-making criteria accordingly. This level of customization provides medical quality controllers with greater flexibility in managing risks, while ensuring that critical quality standards are not compromised (Goodfellow et al., 2016).

Benefits and Applications of the Proposed MLA in Medical Quality Control

The implementation of the optimistic machine learning algorithm in the medical field offers several key benefits. First, it reduces the likelihood of human error by automating the decision-making process. Second, it optimizes sample sizes, ensuring that inspections are neither too small to miss defects nor too large to be inefficient. Third, the MLA's ability to predict producer and consumer risks in real-time allows for more precise risk management, which is especially important in the medical field where product safety is paramount (Hastie et al., 2009).

In terms of applications, the proposed MLA can be used across a wide range of medical products, including pharmaceuticals, surgical tools, diagnostic kits, and implantable devices. By integrating the MLA into existing quality control systems, medical manufacturers can enhance their ability to detect defects early in the production process, ensuring that only products that meet the highest standards reach the market (Jordan & Mitchell, 2015).

The integration of machine learning with traditional statistical quality control methods, such as the Double Sampling Plan, represents a significant advancement in the field of medical quality control (Meeker & Escobar, 2014). The optimistic machine learning algorithm proposed in this chapter provides a flexible, data-driven approach to managing producer and consumer risks while improving the efficiency of sampling procedures. By automating the decision-making process, the MLA offers a practical solution to the challenges of modern healthcare environments, where quick, accurate, and reliable quality control is essential for patient safety (Kelleher et al., 2020).

Single Sampling Plan

A single sampling plan is a sampling inspection scheme in which a decision to accept or reject an inspection lot is based on the inspection of a single sample (Vapnik, 1995). A single sampling plan consists of a single sample size with associated acceptance and rejection number(s) (Venkatasubramanian et al., 2003). The procedure is to take a random sample of size (n) and inspect each item. If the number of defects does not exceed a specified acceptance number (c), the consumer accepts the entire lot (Kim et al., 2019). Sometimes, situations arise when it is not possible to decide whether to accept or reject the lot on the basis of a single sample (Xu et al., 2018). Figure 1 shows the flowchart of single sampling plan.

Figure 1. Flow chart of single sampling plan

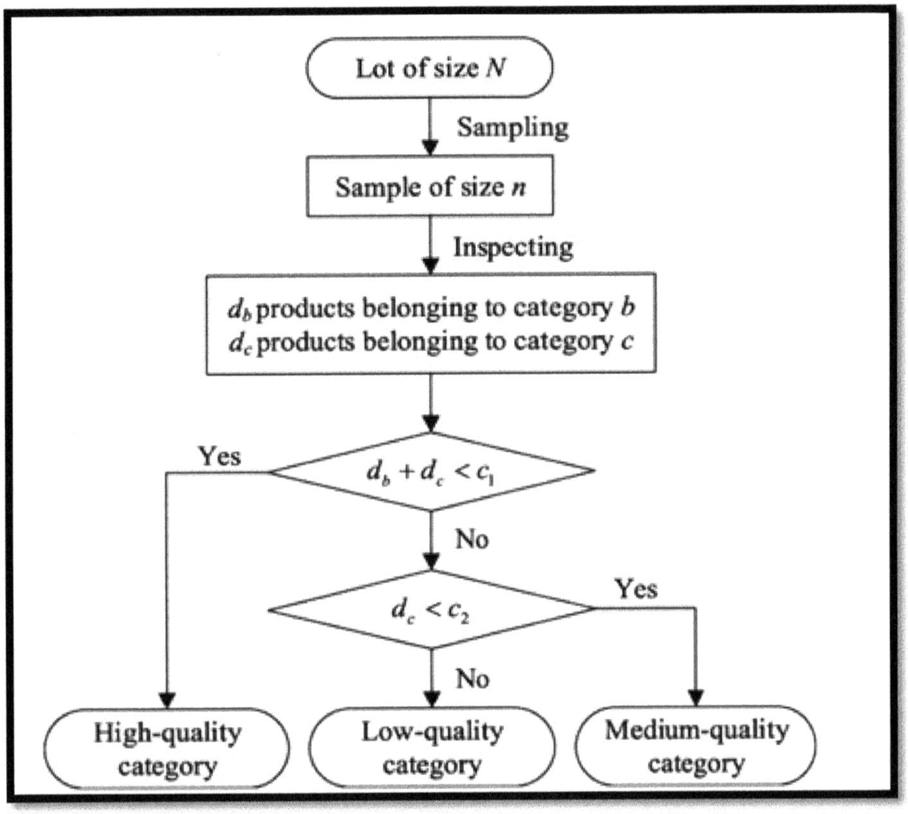

Single Sampling Plan: Operating Procedure

In single sampling plan by attributes, the lot acceptance procedure is characterized by two parameters n and c. The operating procedure for a single sampling plan is given as follows:

1. Select a random sample size n from a lot of size 'n'.
2. Inspect all the articles included in the sample. Let 'd1' be the number of defectives in the sample.
3. If $d_1 < c_1$, accept the lot.
4. If $d_1 > c_1$, reject the lot.

Double Sampling Plan

A sampling plan in which a decision about the acceptance or rejection of a lot is based on two samples that have been inspected is known as a double sampling plan. The double sampling plan is used when a clear decision about acceptance or rejection of a lot cannot be taken on the basis of a single sample (Mitchell, 1997). In double sampling plan, generally, the decision of acceptance or rejection of a lot is taken on the basis of two samples (Zhang & Zhan, 2017). If the first sample is bad, the lot may be rejected on the first sample and a second sample need not be drawn. If the first sample is good, the lot may be accepted on the first sample and a second sample is not needed (Montgomery, 2012). But if the first sample is neither good nor bad and there is a doubt about its results, we take a second sample and the decision of acceptance or rejection of a lot is taken on the basis of the evidence obtained from both the first and the second samples (Pearl & Mackenzie, 2018).

A double sampling plan requires the specification of four quantities, which are known as its parameters (Zou, 2019). These parameters are

n_1 – size of the first sample,
c_1 – acceptance number for the first sample,
n_2 – size of the second sample, and
c_2 – acceptance numbers for both samples combined.

Implementation of Double Sampling Plan

Suppose, lots of the same size, say N, are received from the supplier or the final assembly line and submitted for inspection one at a time. Figure 2 shows the flowchart for double sampling plan. The procedure for implementing the double sampling plan to arrive at a decision about the lot is described in the following steps:

Step 1: Draw a random sample (first sample) of size n_1 from the lot received from the supplier or the final assembly.
Step 2: Inspect each and every unit of the sample and classify it as defective or non-defective. At the end of the inspection, Count the number of defective units found in the sample. Suppose the number of defective units found in the first sample is d_1.
Step 3: Compare the number of defective units (d_1) found in the first sample with the stated acceptance numbers c_1 and c_2.

Figure 2. Flow chart of double sampling plan

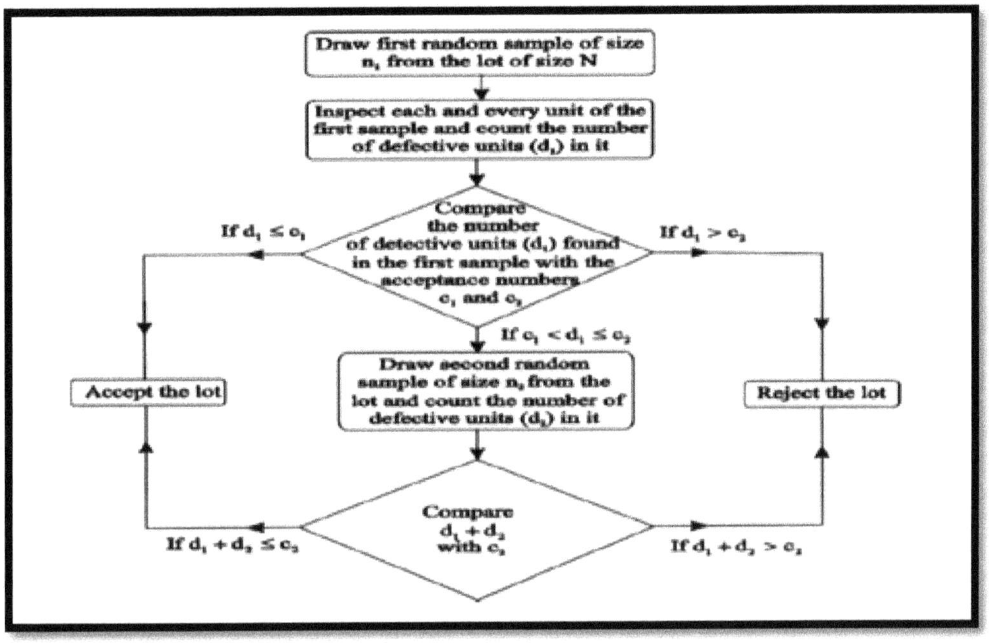

Step 4: Take the decision on the basis of the first sample as follows:

Under Acceptance Sampling Plan

If the number of defective units (d_1) in the first sample is less than or equal to the stated acceptance number (c_1) for the first sample, i.e., if $d_1 \leq c_1$, we accept the lot and if $d_1 > c_2$, we reject the lot. But if $c_1 < d_1 \leq c_2$, the first (single) sample is failed.

Under Rectifying Sampling Plan

If $d_1 \leq c_1$, accept the lot and replace all defective units found in the sample by non-defective units. If $d_1 > c_2$, we accept the lot after inspecting the entire lot and replacing all defective units in the lot by non-defective units. But if $c_1 < d_1 \leq c_2$, the first (single) sample is failed.

Step 5: If $c_1 < d_1 \leq c_2$, draw a second random sample of size n_2 from the lot.
Step 6: Inspect each and every unit of the second sample and count the number of defective units. If the number of defective units found in the second sample is d_2.
Step 7: Combine the number of defective units (d_1 and d_2) found in both samples and consider $d_1 + d_2$ for taking the decision about the lot on the basis of the second sample as follows:

Under Acceptance Sampling Plan

If $d_1 + d_2 \leq c_2$, Accept the lot and if $d_1 + d_2 > c_2$, we reject the lot.

Rectifying Sampling Plan

If $d_1 + d_2 \leq c_2$, we accept the lot and replace all defective units found in the second sample by non-defective units. If $d_1 + d_2 > c_2$, we accept the lot after inspecting the entire lot and replacing all defective units in the lot by non-defective units.

Conditional Double Sampling Plan

The procedures and tables for the selection of conditional double sampling plans with various entry parameters. A search procedure is developed to determine the parameters of the plans when two points on the OC curve are specified. (Baker & Brobst, 1978) proposed conditional sampling procedures which are similar in structure to double sampling. Conditional double sampling is operationally different from double sampling in that the results of the second sample, if required, are obtained from a related lot and not from the current lot (Radhakrishnan & Sekkizhar, 2007). According to, using sample information from related lots results in more attractive OC curves and smaller sample sizes. This reduction in sample size is the principal advantage of these procedures over traditional sampling procedures (Uma & Manjula, 2019).

Implementation of Conditional Double Sampling Plan

In a Conditional double sampling plan by attributes, the lot acceptance procedure is characterized by the parameters N, n_1, n_2, c_1, c_2, and c_3

The operating procedure for a conditional double-sampling plan is given below:

1. Select a random sample size n ($=n_1 = n_2$) from a lot of size "N"
2. Inspect all the articles included in the sample. Let 'd_1' be the number of defectives in the sample.
3. If $d_1 < c_1$, accept the lot
4. If $d_1 > c_3$, reject the lot.
5. If $c_1 + 1 < d_1 < c_3$, take a second sample of size 'n_2' from the remaining lot and find the number of defectives 'd_2'
6. If $d_2 < c_2$ or $d_1 + d_2 < c_3$ accept the lot otherwise reject the lot.

Special Type of Double Sampling Plan

A special type of double sampling plan wherein no acceptance is allowed in the first stage of sampling is considered and its equivalence to the fractional acceptance number single sampling plan of (Hamaker, 1950) is established. Whenever sampling plans are designed for product characteristics involving costly or destructive testing by attributes, it is the usual practice to use a single sampling plan with acceptance number Ac=0 or Ac=1. But the Operating Characteristic (OC) curves of single sampling plans with

Ac=0 and Ac=1 led to conflicting interest between the producer and the consumer and with Ac=0 plan behaves favorably to the consumer while the Ac=1 plan favors the producer. In order to overcome the shortcomings given earlier, (Govindaraju, 1991) establishes a Special Type of Double Sampling (STDS) plan. (Balamurali & Subramani, 2012) contributed conditional variables DSP for Weibull distributed lifetimes under sudden death testing.

Implementation of the STDS Plan

(1) From a lot, select a random sample of size n_1 units and observe the number of defectives d_1. If $d_1 \geq 1$, reject the lot. If $d_1=0$, select a second random sample of size n_2 and observe the number of defectives d_2. Table 1 shows the Operating Ratios for Certain Single Sampling Plans.

Table 1. Operating ratios for certain single sampling plans

A_c	Values of p_2/p_1					
	$\alpha=0.05$ $\beta=0.10$	$\alpha=0.05$ $\beta=0.05$	$\alpha=0.05$ $\beta=0.01$	$\alpha=0.01$ $\beta=0.10$	$\alpha=0.01$ $\beta=0.05$	$\alpha=0.05$ $\beta=0.01$
0	44.890	58.404	89.781	229.105	298.073	458.210
1	10.946	13.349	18.681	26.184	31.933	44.686
2	6.509	7.699	10.280	12.206	14.439	19.278
3	4.890	5.675	7.352	8.115	9.418	12.202
4	4.057	4.646	5.890	6.249	7.156	9.072
5	3.549	4.023	5.017	5.195	5.889	7.343

(2) If $d_2 \leq 1$, accept the lot. Otherwise, that is if $d_2 \geq 2$, reject the lot.

A compact representation of the STDS plan is given in Table 2:

Table 2. Sample size details

Stage	Sample Size	Accept	Reject
1	n_1	*	1
2	n_2	1	2

*Cannot Accept

New Screening Procedure on Double Sampling Plan (DSP$_{NSP}$)

The purpose of this paper is to describe a method and to present a set of tables for constructing two and three-stage drug screening procedures of the type discussed. These procedures allow rejection at any stage but acceptance at only the final stage. Similar procedures have been advocated by (Sharma &

Adhikary, 2018), based on this operating characteristic curve and accept-reject rules for two and three-stage screening procedures had been derived by (Roseberry & Gehan 1964). Mixed sampling product control for costly or destructive items by (Schilling, 1967, 1982). Based on this screening procedure and switching the rule of the variable to attribute gives an idea for creating a new concept in a double sampling plan. Generally, we are going to the second sample when the defective lies in between two acceptance numbers, but in this procedure (Soundarajan & Vijayagaghavan, 1992).

Implementation of a New Screening Procedure in the Double Sampling Plan

Fig 3 shows flow chart for DSP_{NSP}. The procedure for implementing to arrive at a decision about the lot is described in the following steps:

Step 1: We draw a random sample (first sample) of size n_1 from the lot received from the supplier or the final assembly.

Step 2: We inspect each and every unit of the sample and classify it as defective or non-defective. At the end of the inspection, we count the number of defective units found in the sample. Suppose the number of defective units found in the first sample is d_1.

Step 3: We compare the number of defective units (d_1) found in the first sample with the stated acceptance numbers c_1 and c_2.

Step 4: We take the decision on the basis of the first sample as follows:

Step 5: If $d_1 > c_2$ but nearer value, we can also draw a second random sample of size n_{22} from the lot. We inspect each and every unit of the third sample and count the number of defective units found in it. Suppose the number of defective units found in the third sample is d_{22}.

Step 6: We combine the number of defective units (d_1 and d_{22}) found in both samples and consider $d_1 + d_{22}$ for taking the decision about the lot on the basis of the third sample.

Step 7: If $d_1 + d_{22} \leq c_2$, we accept the lot otherwise reject the lot.

Figure 3. Flow chart of D SP$_{NSP}$

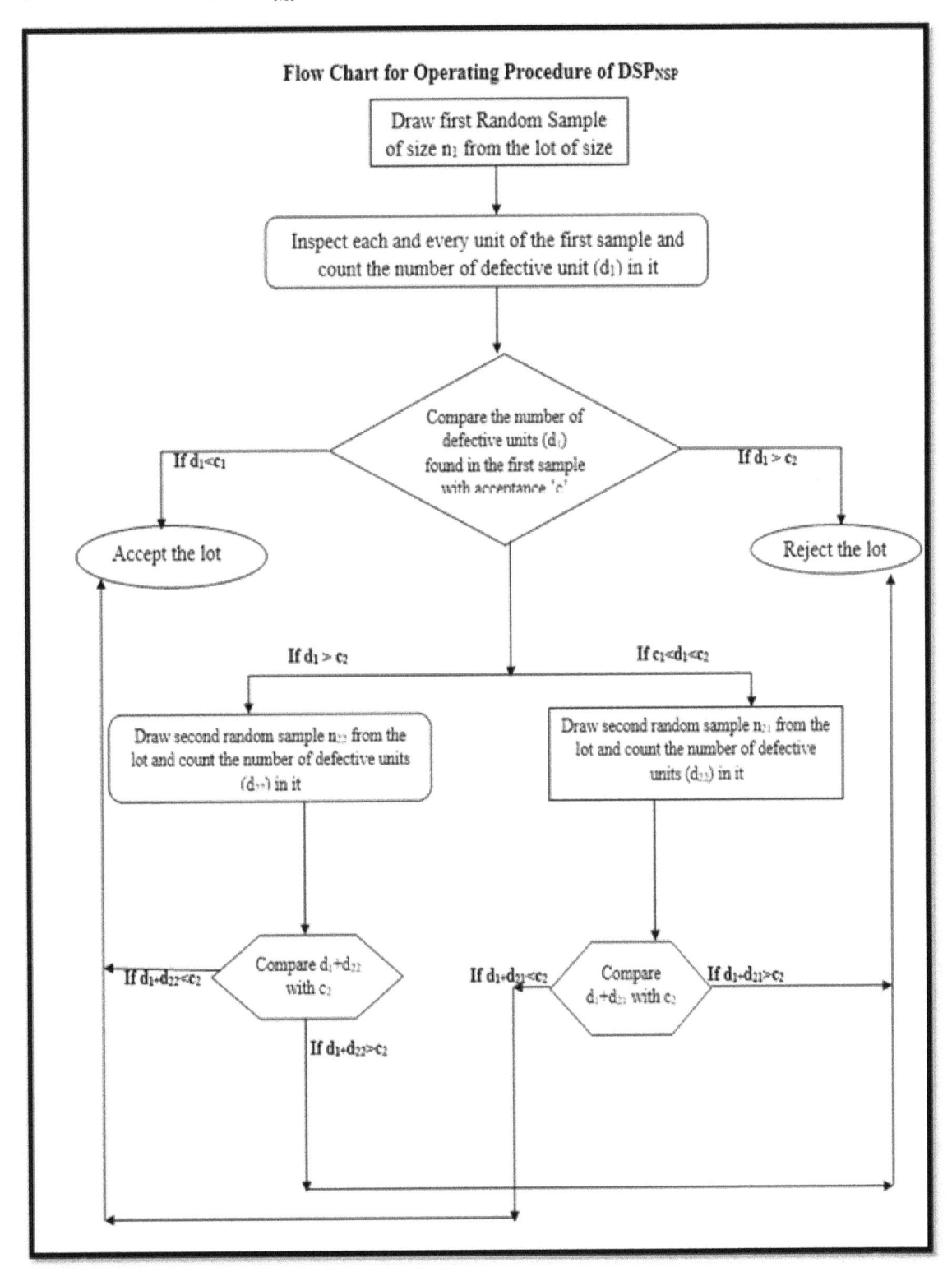

Operating Characteristic (OC) Curve

The operating characteristic (OC) curve displays the discriminatory power of the sampling plan. That is, it shows the probability that a lot submitted with a certain fraction of defective will either be accepted or rejected. in a double sampling plan, the decision of acceptance or rejection of the lot is taken on the basis of two samples. The lot is accepted on the first sample if the number of defective units (d_1) in the first sample is less than the acceptance number c1. The lot is accepted on the second sample if the number of defective units ($d_1 + d_2$) in both samples is greater than c_1 and less than or equal to the acceptance number c_2. Therefore, if $Pa_1(p)$ and $Pa_2(p)$ denote the probabilities of accepting a lot on the first sample and the second sample, respectively, the probability of accepting a lot of quality level p is given by

$$P_a(p) = P_{a1}(p) + P_{a2}(p) \tag{1}$$

Under Poisson model the OC function of the Conditional double sampling plan is

$$P_a(p) = \sum_{r=0}^{c_1} \frac{e^{-n_1 p}(n_1 p)^r}{r!} + \left[\sum_{k=c_1+1}^{c_2} \frac{e^{-n_1 p}(n_1 p)^k}{k!} \left\{ \sum_{r=0}^{c_2-k} \frac{e^{-n_2 p}(n_2 p)^r}{r!} \right\} \right] \tag{2}$$

The OC function of the STDS plan is

$$P_a(p) = (1-\theta)e^{-np} + \theta(e^{-np} + np\,e^{-np}) \tag{3}$$

The OC function of the NSDSP is

$$P_a(p) = P_{a1}(p) + (P_{a21}(p) + P_{a22}(p)) \tag{4}$$

OPTIMISTIC MACHINE LEARNING ALGORITHM IN MEDICAL FIELD

Machine learning (ML) has revolutionized various industries, and its application in healthcare is particularly transformative. The medical field, characterized by its complexity and high-stakes decision-making, presents unique challenges for ensuring accuracy, precision, and safety in processes like diagnostics, treatment planning, and quality control. One innovative approach to leveraging ML in healthcare is the development of an *optimistic machine learning algorithm*—a model designed to err on the side of caution while dynamically adapting to uncertain situations. In the context of medical applications, this approach can be critical in ensuring patient safety, optimizing resource allocation, and improving the quality of care.

Optimistic Machine Learning

Optimistic machine learning refers to an ML algorithm designed to handle uncertainty in decision-making while maintaining a focus on reducing errors that have significant negative consequences. In healthcare, errors such as misdiagnoses, incorrect treatments, or the acceptance of defective medical products can lead to severe repercussions, including harm to patients or regulatory violations. An optimistic ML algorithm aims to reduce both *false positives* (e.g., accepting a defective product or making an incorrect diagnosis) and *false negatives* (e.g., rejecting a good product or failing to detect a disease). This is particularly useful in situations where the cost of mistakes is high, such as in medical product manufacturing, clinical trials, and diagnostic testing. By integrating optimism into the model, the algorithm cautiously manages risk by prioritizing safety and quality.

Application in Medical Quality Control

In medical quality control, where acceptance sampling and inspection processes are used to evaluate products such as medical devices, pharmaceuticals, and diagnostic kits, the risk of accepting faulty products (consumer risk) or rejecting acceptable products (producer risk) is a critical concern. Traditionally, methods like the Double Sampling Plan (DSP) have been used to manage these risks. However, these methods rely on fixed statistical tables that do not adapt to real-time data, which can result in inefficient or inaccurate decision-making.

By integrating an optimistic machine learning algorithm into the DSP, medical quality controllers can improve the process of determining whether a batch of products should be accepted or rejected. The algorithm can learn from historical inspection data, optimize sample sizes, and calculate the risks more precisely, thus making the acceptance or rejection process more efficient and reliable. This results in reduced inspection time and cost, while maintaining high standards of quality and safety in medical products.

Features of the Optimistic Machine Learning Algorithm

1. **Risk Management:** The algorithm optimizes decisions by balancing producer and consumer risks. In the medical field, managing these risks is critical to avoid defective products entering the market or valuable, high-quality products being discarded unnecessarily. The algorithm learns from data patterns and adjusts its predictions in real time, ensuring the minimization of risks without sacrificing accuracy.
2. **Real-Time Adaptation:** Unlike traditional methods that rely on fixed parameters, an optimistic ML algorithm can adapt dynamically to real-time data. As new information is collected from product inspections or medical diagnostics, the model updates its predictions, making it more robust in handling unexpected variations or defects that may arise in medical products.
3. **Cautious Decision-Making:** The algorithm incorporates a cautious approach when making decisions about whether to accept or reject a product. This ensures that when uncertainty exists, the algorithm errs on the side of caution, reducing the likelihood of errors that could lead to significant negative outcomes. This cautious optimism is critical in healthcare environments where precision and safety are paramount.
4. **Flexibility Across Medical Products:** One of the strengths of an optimistic ML algorithm is its ability to adapt to different types of medical products, whether they are diagnostic tools, surgical instruments, or pharmaceuticals. Each product category has different risk profiles, and the algorithm can be fine-tuned to account for these variations, providing customized risk management solutions for each type of product.

5. **Automated Decision-Making:** By automating the decision-making process, the algorithm reduces the reliance on human inspectors, thereby minimizing human error and improving the speed of decision-making. This is especially valuable in large-scale medical manufacturing processes, where hundreds or thousands of products need to be inspected in a short time.

Advantages

1. **Improved Efficiency:** The optimistic ML algorithm reduces the time and effort required to make accurate decisions in medical product quality control. By automating the process and using real-time data to optimize sample sizes, the algorithm allows for faster inspections without sacrificing quality.
2. **Enhanced Accuracy:** With the ability to learn from data and dynamically adjust its predictions, the optimistic ML algorithm significantly reduces the likelihood of errors in accepting or rejecting products. This leads to fewer defective products reaching the market and a lower risk of rejecting acceptable products, thus optimizing resource use.
3. **Cost Reduction:** By optimizing the sampling process and reducing the need for large sample sizes, the algorithm minimizes the cost of inspections. Additionally, reducing errors can save manufacturers from costly recalls or regulatory penalties associated with defective medical products.
4. **Scalability:** The algorithm is scalable and can be implemented across a variety of medical fields, from large pharmaceutical companies to small medical device manufacturers. As it learns from new data, its accuracy and reliability improve over time, making it suitable for both small-scale and large-scale operations.

Broader Implications in Healthcare

Beyond quality control in medical product manufacturing, optimistic machine learning algorithms have broader implications in the healthcare sector. They can be applied in clinical decision-making, where similar trade-offs between risks (such as false positives and false negatives) exist. For instance, in diagnostic imaging, an optimistic ML algorithm could be used to assist radiologists in interpreting scans more accurately, ensuring that abnormalities are detected while minimizing false alarms. In drug discovery, optimistic ML algorithms could help researchers balance the risks of pursuing certain drug candidates by optimizing clinical trial designs. In this context, the algorithm could predict the likelihood of success or failure for a new drug based on historical data from past trials, helping pharmaceutical companies allocate resources more effectively. Additionally, optimistic machine learning models could be applied to patient risk assessment, where they could assist healthcare providers in identifying patients who are at higher risk of complications during treatments or surgeries. The algorithm's ability to learn from patient data would enable it to provide personalized risk assessments that can improve treatment outcomes.

The integration of an optimistic machine learning algorithm in the medical field represents a major advancement in quality control and decision-making. By combining the predictive power of machine learning with the rigorous statistical methods used in traditional quality control processes, such as the Double Sampling Plan, the algorithm offers a powerful solution for managing risks and improving the efficiency of medical product inspections. Its ability to adapt to real-time data, automate decision-making, and balance producer and consumer risks makes it an invaluable tool in a field where accuracy, safety, and quality are paramount. As healthcare continues to evolve and generate more complex data, the role of machine learning algorithms—particularly optimistic models—will become increasingly important in ensuring that the products and treatments delivered to patients meet the highest standards of quality and safety.

CONCLUSION AND OUTLOOK

In the evolving landscape of the medical field, ensuring the highest quality standards in products like pharmaceuticals, medical devices, and diagnostic tools is crucial for both patient safety and regulatory compliance. The integration of machine learning into traditional statistical quality control methods, particularly through the use of an *optimistic machine learning algorithm*, represents a significant advancement in risk management and decision-making. This chapter introduced a pioneering approach where the Double Sampling Plan (DSP) is enhanced with machine learning capabilities, allowing for dynamic, data-driven decision-making while managing producer and consumer risks efficiently. The optimistic machine learning algorithm serves to address the limitations of conventional sampling techniques. By automating the decision-making process and using real-time data, the algorithm reduces inspection time and cost, while maintaining a high standard of product quality. It minimizes errors in accepting defective products or rejecting quality ones, thus balancing the critical producer and consumer risks in medical quality control. Moreover, the flexibility of the algorithm allows it to be applied across various types of medical products, providing customized solutions for each category.

The integration of machine learning in this context also brings added benefits such as increased efficiency, cost reduction, and scalability. The MLA's ability to adapt to evolving data, learn from historical trends, and automate decisions allows medical professionals to optimize their processes without sacrificing the critical safety and quality requirements that are foundational to healthcare. Looking forward, the use of machine learning algorithms in quality control will continue to grow as healthcare industries increasingly rely on complex data systems. The optimistic machine learning algorithm introduced in this chapter could be further refined and expanded to handle even more sophisticated risk profiles, incorporating additional quality parameters and real-time feedback loops from ongoing production processes.

Future developments may also explore how these algorithms can be integrated into broader healthcare applications, such as patient risk assessment, diagnostic decision-making, and even treatment planning. With the increasing complexity of medical products and the rise of personalized medicine, the demand for intelligent, adaptable systems that can manage uncertainty will only become more critical. In addition, regulatory bodies may need to establish new standards to assess and validate the use of machine learning in quality control systems, ensuring that these algorithms meet the rigorous safety and effectiveness criteria required in healthcare. Collaboration between industry leaders, healthcare professionals, and regulatory agencies will be essential in fostering innovation while ensuring that machine learning systems remain trustworthy and reliable. Ultimately, the optimistic machine learning algorithm represents just the beginning of a new era in medical quality control, where AI and machine learning work hand in hand with traditional methodologies to ensure that healthcare products not only meet but exceed the highest standards of quality and safety. This approach paves the way for more efficient, precise, and cost-effective processes, positioning the medical field to better handle future challenges while safeguarding patient health.

REFERENCES

Acharya N. (2005). Construction of conditional double sampling plans using intervened random effect Poisson distribution. *Proceedings volume of SJYSDNS, 1*, 57-61.

Aggarwal, C. C. (2015). *Data Mining: The Textbook*. Springer. DOI: 10.1007/978-3-319-14142-8

Anderson, R. (2020). Statistical quality control using deep learning techniques. *Journal of Quality Technology*, 52(3), 220–232.

Baker, R. C., & Brost, R. W. (1978). Conditional double sampling plan. *Journal of Quality Technology*, 10(4), 1–11. DOI: 10.1080/00224065.1978.11980843

Balamurali, S., & Subramani, S. (2012). Conditional variable double sampling plan for Weibull distributed life times under sudden death testing. *Bonfring International Journal of Data Mining*, 2(3), 12–15. DOI: 10.9756/BIJDM.1343

Bertsimas, D., Dunn, J., Mundru, N., & Velmahos, G. (2020). Machine learning in medical decision-making: Algorithms, challenges, and opportunities. *Operations Research for Health Care*, 26, 100275.

Bishop, C. M. (2006). *Pattern Recognition and Machine Learning*. Springer.

Box, G. E. P., Hunter, J. S., & Hunter, W. G. (2005). *Statistics for Experimenters: Design, Innovation, and Discovery* (2nd ed.). Wiley.

Chakraborty, S., & Guha, S. (2021). Applications of machine learning in medical imaging and diagnostics. *Nature Machine Intelligence*, 3(2), 101–110.

Chatterjee, S., & Hadi, A. S. (2015). *Regression Analysis by Example* (5th ed.). Wiley.

Dodge, H. F., & Romig, H. G. (1959). *Sampling Inspection Tables—Single and Double Sampling*. John Wiley & Sons.

Dumicic, K. (2012). Decision making based on single and double acceptance sampling plans for assessing quality of lots. *Business Systems Research*, 3(2).

Duncan, A. J. (1986). *Quality Control and Industrial Statistics* (5th ed.). Homewood Publisher.

Fleuren, W. W., Alkema, W., Vervloet, M. G., & Maas, A. H. E. M. (2017). Machine learning for the prediction of cardiac risk in a clinical population. *Heart (British Cardiac Society)*, 103(11), 899–906.

Goodfellow, I., Bengio, Y., & Courville, A. (2016). *Deep Learning*. MIT Press.

Govindaraju, K. (1991). Fractional acceptance number single sampling plan. *Communications in Statistics. Simulation and Computation*, 20(1), 173–190. DOI: 10.1080/03610919108812947

Hamaker. (1950). *Double Sampling Plan*. Engineering Statistics Handbook.

Hastie, T., Tibshirani, R., & Friedman, J. (2009). *The Elements of Statistical Learning: Data Mining, Inference, and Prediction* (2nd ed.). Springer. DOI: 10.1007/978-0-387-84858-7

Jordan, M. I., & Mitchell, T. M. (2015). Machine learning: Trends, perspectives, and prospects. *Science*, 349(6245), 255–260. DOI: 10.1126/science.aaa8415 PMID: 26185243

Kelleher, J. D., Mac Namee, B., & D'Arcy, A. (2020). *Fundamentals of Machine Learning for Predictive Data Analytics* (2nd ed.). MIT Press.

Kim, K. J., Kim, S., & Kim, J. (2019). Optimizing quality control in the healthcare supply chain using statistical quality control and machine learning. *Journal of Healthcare Engineering*, 20.

Meeker, W. Q., & Escobar, L. A. (2014). *Statistical Methods for Reliability Data*. Wiley.

Mitchell, T. M. (1997). *Machine Learning*. McGraw-Hill.

Montgomery, D. C. (2012). *Introduction to Statistical Quality Control* (7th ed.). Wiley.

Pearl, J., & Mackenzie, D. (2018). *The Book of Why: The New Science of Cause and Effect*. Basic Books.

Radhakrishnan, R., & Sekkizhar, J. (2007). A New Screening Procedure on Double Sampling Plan for Costly or Destructive items. *International Journal of Statistics and Management System*, 2(1-2), 88–97.

Roseberry, T. D., & Gehan, E. A. (1964). Operating characteristic curves and accept-reject rules for two and three stage screening procedures. *Biometrics*, 20(1), 73–84. DOI: 10.2307/2527618

Schilling, E. G. (1967). A general method for determining the operating characteristics of mixed variables–attribute sampling plans single side specifications, S.D. known. Ph.D Dissertation, Rutgers – The State University, New Brunswick, NJ.

Schilling, E. G. (1982). *Acceptance Sampling in Quality Control*. Chapman and Hall/CRC.

Sharma, S. K., & Adhikary, P. K. (2018). Machine learning algorithms for medical applications: A review. *International Journal of Recent Technology and Engineering*, 7(6), 128–133.

Soundarajan, V., & Vijayagaghavan, R. (1992). Procedures and tables for the construction and selection of conditional double sampling plans. *Journal of Applied Statistics*, 19(3), 329–338. DOI: 10.1080/02664769200000030

Uma, G., & Manjula, D. (2019). A technical study on varieties of sampling plan and implementation of new screening tri-sampling plan. *International Journal of Research in Advent Technology*, 5(Special Issue), 232–237.

Vapnik, V. N. (1995). *The Nature of Statistical Learning Theory*. Springer. DOI: 10.1007/978-1-4757-2440-0

Venkatasubramanian, V., Rengaswamy, R., & Kavuri, S. N. (2003). A review of process fault detection and diagnosis: Part I. *Computers & Chemical Engineering*, 27(3), 293–311. DOI: 10.1016/S0098-1354(02)00160-6

Xu, W., Gu, Y., & Cai, W. (2018). Medical data quality control based on machine learning. *Journal of Medical Systems*, 42(7).

Zhang, J., & Zhan, M. (2017). Machine learning in rock mechanics and geomechanics. *Advances in Civil Engineering*, 20, 12–17.

Zou, J., Huss, M., Abid, A., Mohammadi, P., Torkamani, A., & Telenti, A. (2019). A primer on deep learning in genomics. *Nature Genetics*, 51(1), 12–18. DOI: 10.1038/s41588-018-0295-5 PMID: 30478442

Chapter 21
Transforming Global Healthcare:
Unleashing Generative AI and IoMT in the 21st Century

Rajrupa Ray Chaudhuri
Brainware University, India

ABSTRACT

The global healthcare environment is poised for a revolution because to the convergence of Generative Artificial Intelligence (AI) and the Internet of Medical Things (IoMT). This article investigates how these technologies can improve healthcare delivery efficiency, enable tailored treatment regimens, and improve diagnostic accuracy. A summary of the development of healthcare technology across time is provided, emphasizing the significant advancements in AI and IoMT. Through case studies, the application of generative AI to drug development, customized medicine, and predictive analytics is explored; the influence of IoMT on telemedicine, remote patient monitoring, and real-time data analytics is also covered. The amalgamation of Generative AI with IoMT holds potential to elevate clinical results, augment operational efficacy, and augment healthcare accessible, specifically in marginalized areas. However, there are drawbacks such as socioeconomic inequality, privacy and problems with data quality. Strong cybersecurity defenses, data governance are needed in future development.

1. INTRODUCTION

1.1. Overview

1.1.1. Generative AI and IoMT's Potential to Revolutionize Healthcare

The combination of the Internet of Medical Things (IoMT) and Generative Artificial Intelligence (AI) is poised to propel the healthcare industry towards a technological revolution. From drug development to individualized treatment plans, generative AI—a branch of AI focused on producing new content from existing data—has the potential to transform every aspect of human endeavor. In addition, real-time

DOI: 10.4018/979-8-3693-6180-1.ch021

Copyright ©2025, IGI Global. Copying or distributing in print or electronic forms without written permission of IGI Global is prohibited.

data collection and monitoring are made possible by IoMT, or the network of medical devices and apps linked to healthcare IT systems over the internet. This is revolutionizing patient care. When combined, these technologies have the potential to drastically alter how healthcare services are thought about and delivered, as well as to improve the effectiveness and efficiency of healthcare delivery.

Figure 1. Overview of AI and IoMT

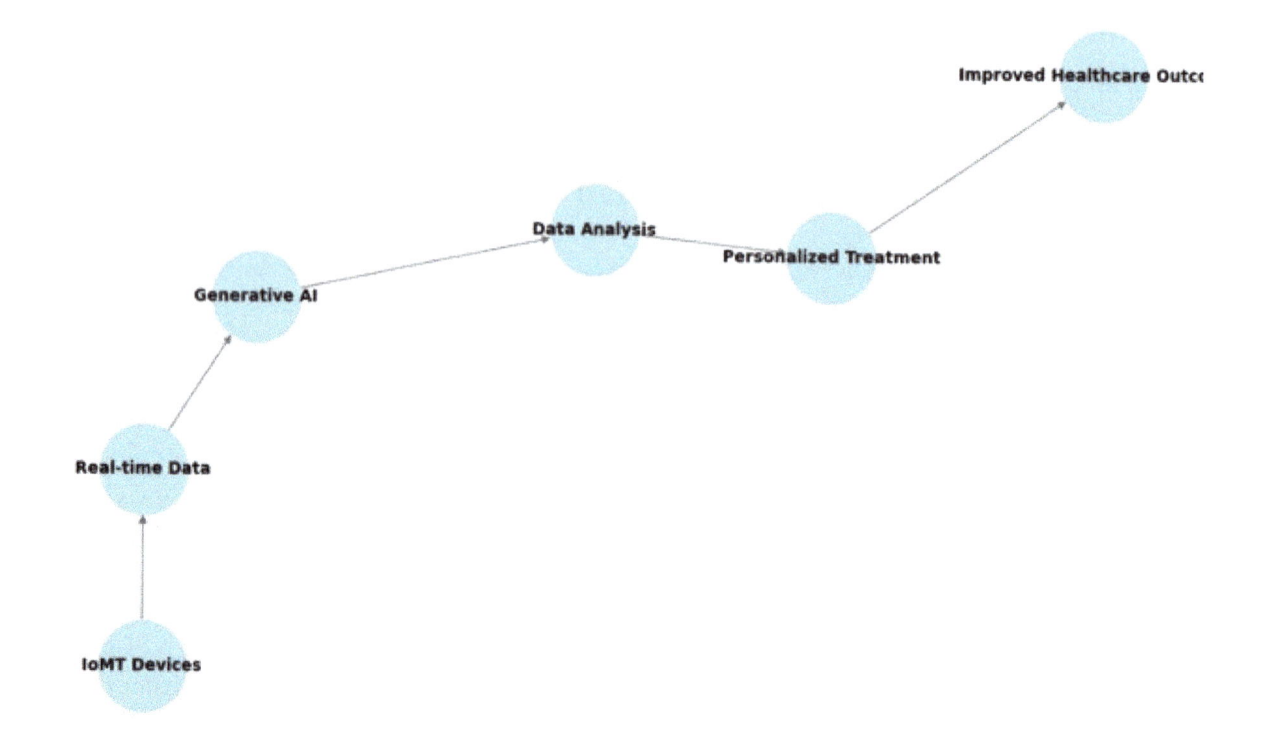

1.2. Context

1.2.1. The State of Global Healthcare Today and the Requirement for Innovation in Technology

The world's healthcare system is currently dealing with hitherto unseen issues, such as aging populations, growing expenses, and notable gaps in access to care. Global healthcare systems are under increased strain as a result of the COVID-19 pandemic, which has also revealed weaknesses and made pre-existing problems worse. There is a serious scarcity of healthcare personnel and inadequate healthcare infrastructure in many locations, especially in low- and middle-income countries. These difficulties highlight the critical need for creative solutions that can improve patient outcomes, improve healthcare delivery, and lower the cost of treatment. Technology innovation is increasingly viewed as a vital route to overcome these obstacles and guaranteeing that healthcare systems can fulfill the demands of the twenty-first century, especially through AI and IoMT, (Da Silva, 2024).

1.3. Objectives

1.3.1. Goals of the Chapter

The purpose of this chapter is to examine how IoMT and generative AI are revolutionizing healthcare around the world, (Okonji, Yunusov, & Gordon, 2024). It will specifically look at how new technologies might improve diagnostic precision, allow for more individualized treatment plans, and facilitate more effective healthcare delivery to solve today's problems. Together with their potential to lessen healthcare inequities and provide access to high-quality care globally, these technologies also raise ethical and regulatory questions that will be covered in this chapter. Readers will have a thorough understanding of the opportunities and problems presented by IoMT and Generative AI in defining the future of healthcare by the end of this chapter.

2. THE EVOLUTION OF HEALTHCARE TECHNOLOGY

2.1. Historical Background

2.1.1. A Synopsis of Technological Progress in Healthcare

Over the past few centuries, there have been enormous changes to healthcare due to technical developments that have profoundly altered the diagnosis, treatment, and management of diseases. Important inventions like the stethoscope, anesthesia, and antiseptics were developed in the 19th century, and these developments set the foundation for contemporary medical procedures. Antibiotics, MRIs, and X-rays are examples of groundbreaking discoveries made throughout the 20th century. The discovery of DNA also served as a catalyst for the rapid advancement of genetics and biotechnology. These developments paved the way for the emergence of electronic health records (EHRs), telemedicine, and the first steps toward medical robotics and artificial intelligence (AI) during the late 20th and early 21st centuries, (Khubchandani *et al.*, 2023) (Nah *et al.*, 2023).

Figure 2. Timeline of technological advancements in healthcare

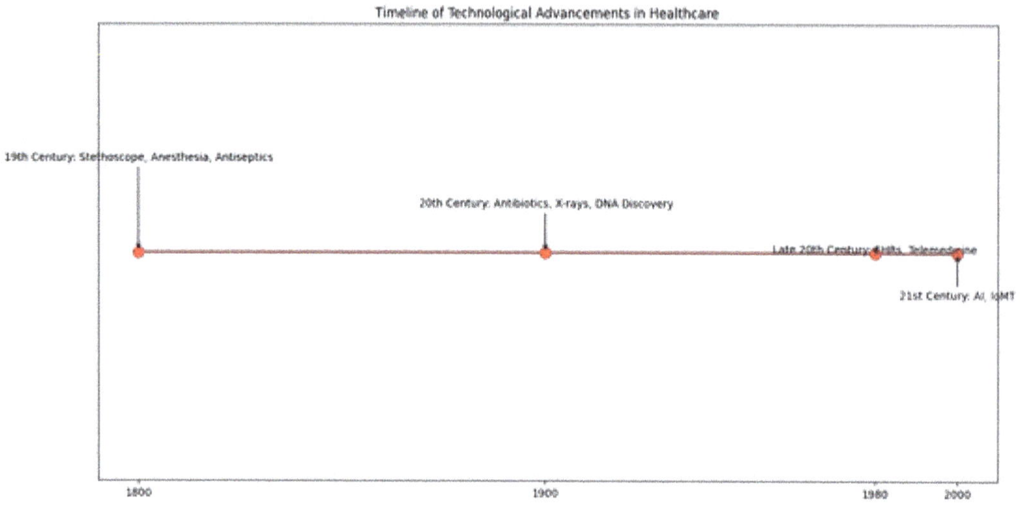

2.2. Rise of AI and IoMT

2.2.1. Overview of AI and IoMT Technologies and Their Earlier Uses in the Medical Field

Healthcare technology is entering a new age with the development of artificial intelligence (AI) and the Internet of Medical Things (IoMT), (Kumar *et al.*, 2024). In the early 2000s, artificial intelligence (AI), especially as it related to machine learning and deep learning, started to acquire popularity in the healthcare sector, (Daneshvar *et al.*, 2024) (Morley *et al.*, 2022) (Manickam *et al.*, 2022). In order to improve diagnosis accuracy and turnaround times, algorithms used in diagnostic imaging were taught to identify patterns in medical pictures like MRIs and X-rays. Concurrently, the Internet of Medical Things (IoMT) surfaced as a crucial element of healthcare innovation, utilizing medical devices' connectivity to gather, transfer, and evaluate patient data instantaneously. Early uses of IoMT included remote monitoring of long-term illnesses including diabetes and heart disease, which made it possible to provide hitherto unachievable continuous care and early intervention.

2.3. Current Landscape

2.3.1. A Summary of AI and IoMT's Current Status in Healthcare

AI and IoMT are leading the way in healthcare innovation today, with a plethora of expanding applications, (Da Silva, 2024c). AI is currently being used in many areas of healthcare, including robotic surgery, personalized medicine, predictive analytics, and drug development. Prominent firms in the artificial intelligence (AI) healthcare sector comprise IBM Watson Health, Google Health, and precision medicine-focused start-ups like Tempus. IoMT has changed as well; by 2028, it is expected that the worldwide IoMT market would have grown to over $250 billion. Technological developments in wearables, smart health devices, and telehealth platforms that facilitate easy patient monitoring and data-driven decision-making are the main drivers of this rise, (Moshawrab *et al.*, 2023). Smart implants, AI-powered diagnostics, and real-time health analytics are just a few examples of the innovations that are revolutionizing and personalizing patient care in an efficient way.

3. GENERATIVE AI IN HEALTHCARE

3.1. Concept and Mechanisms: What is Healthcare Generative AI and How Does It Operate?

The term "generative AI" describes a kind of artificial intelligence that uses patterns discovered in pre-existing datasets to produce new content—text, graphics, or other types of data. It works by using machine learning models that can produce original, new data that closely mimics the input data, like variational autoencoders (VAEs) and generative adversarial networks (GANs). Generative AI is used in healthcare to provide new medical insights, model patient situations, and even create new molecular structures for drug development, (Capobianco, 2023). In order to find patterns and produce fresh theories or solutions that would not be apparent through conventional research, these models analyze enormous volumes of healthcare data, including medical records, imaging tests, and genomic data.

3.2. Uses

3.2.1. Analyzing Generative AI's Effect on Healthcare

1. **Drug Discovery**: The development of new drugs is one of the most well-known uses of generative AI in healthcare. It can take years and billions of dollars to introduce a novel treatment to the market using traditional drug discovery methods, which are also pricey. This procedure is sped up by generative AI, which creates new molecules with the potential to be therapeutics by examining enormous chemical databases, (Trinkley *et al.*, 2024). To drastically reduce the time needed for drug development, businesses such as Insilico Medicine and Atomwise are utilizing artificial intelligence (AI) to forecast molecular structures and model potential interactions between novel medications and biological targets.
2. **Personalized Medicine**: Personalized medicine is being revolutionized by generative AI, which facilitates the development of customized treatment regimens that take into account an individual's own genetic composition, way of life, and medical backgrounds, (Chinta *et al.*, 2024). Healthcare providers can create highly individualized care plans that maximize positive results and limit negative effects by using AI-driven models to examine patient data and forecast how the patient could react to various therapies, (Moujahid, Aouad, & Zbakh, 2023).
3. **Predictive Analytics**: Forecasting disease development, patient outcomes, and future complications is made easier with the use of Generative AI in predictive analytics. AI can identify people who have a higher chance of contracting specific diseases, like diabetes or heart disease, and recommend

early detection or preventive actions by creating data-driven models. Using proactive care and early identification, this application is especially helpful in treating chronic illnesses and cutting healthcare expenses.

Figure 3. Generative AI in drug discovery process

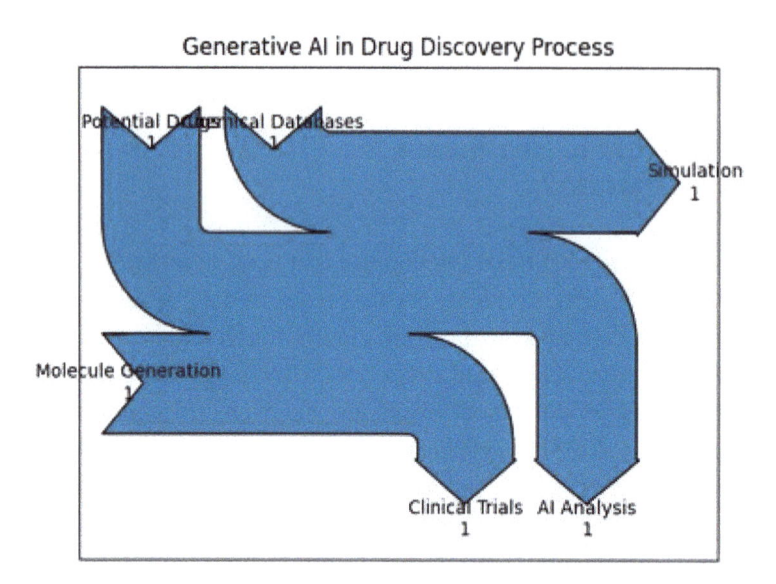

3.2.2. Case Studies: Practical Instances of Healthcare Generative AI

1. **Insilico Medicine's AI-Driven Drug Discovery**: Leading AI-powered drug discovery company Insilico Medicine has created multiple therapeutic candidates with the use of generative AI. Their efforts to create novel molecules for the treatment of fibrosis are one noteworthy example; they employed AI to create drug-like compounds that are presently undergoing clinical testing. This example demonstrates how generative artificial intelligence (AI) can expedite the drug discovery process and lower the expenses related to introducing novel medicines to the market.
2. **DeepMind's AlphaFold**: DeepMind's AlphaFold, an artificial intelligence system that predicts protein shapes with amazing accuracy, is another ground-breaking example. Comprehending protein folding is essential for developing new drugs and comprehending diseases from a molecular perspective. It has been acknowledged that AlphaFold's capacity to produce precise predictions of protein structures represents a noteworthy advancement that may result in novel therapies for a number of illnesses, (Chinta *et al.*, 2024) (Da Silva, 2024b).

3. **IBM Watson's Oncology Platform**: Oncologists may create tailored treatment plans for patients with cancer with the help of IBM Watson's Oncology platform, which uses Generative AI. Watson makes customized therapy suggestions for each patient by evaluating patient data, including genetic information and health records. Several healthcare facilities have adopted this AI-driven strategy, showcasing the potential of generative AI to improve patient outcomes and clinical decision-making.

4. THE INTERNET OF MEDICAL THINGS (IOMT)

4.1. Overview

4.1.1. Defining IoMT and Its Components

The term "Internet of Medical Things" (IoMT) describes the networked ecosystem of medical equipment and software that interacts online with healthcare IT systems. IoMT collects, analyzes, and transmits patient data in real time by integrating wearable technology, remote monitoring systems, smart medical equipment, and healthcare applications. The following are the main elements of IoMT, (Dwivedi, Mehrotra, & Chandra, 2022):

1. **Wearable Devices** These are portable devices, such as fitness trackers, smartwatches, and biosensors, that keep an eye on a range of health indicators, including blood sugar, heart rate, and physical activity, (Moshawrab *et al.*, 2023). Sensors that can gather data continually and transmit it to healthcare providers for monitoring and analysis are frequently seen in wearable technology.
2. **Remote Monitoring Systems**: These devices provide remote patient monitoring, frequently in real-time, for healthcare providers. They are especially helpful in the treatment of long-term illnesses like diabetes, high blood pressure, and cardiac issues. Devices can, for instance, send information about a patient's blood pressure or glucose levels straight to their doctor, allowing for prompt actions.
3. **Smart Medical Equipment**: This group comprises smart pill dispensers, insulin pumps, and linked inhalers, among other cutting-edge medical equipment. These devices carry out their intended tasks as well as gather and send usage data, which may be examined to enhance patient compliance and treatment optimization.

In order to improve patient outcomes and operational efficiency in healthcare settings, IoMT has the potential to completely transform the industry by enabling continuous monitoring, eliminating the need for in-person visits, and supporting data-driven decision-making.

4.2. Applications

4.2.1 Exploring the Impact of IoMT in Healthcare

1. **Remote Patient Monitoring**: With IoMT, patients can stay in their homes and have their health conditions continuously monitored. Healthcare practitioners may now follow patients' health data in real time with the use of devices like connected blood pressure cuffs, glucose sensors, and wearable ECG monitors. This enables more individualized care and early diagnosis of potential difficulties.

For instance, enabling more proactive health care and minimizing the need for frequent hospital visits, remote monitoring has proven especially helpful for older patients and those with chronic diseases.
2. **Telemedicine**: IoMT is essential to telemedicine because it provides the infrastructure required for online consultations. During telehealth visits, healthcare providers can access real-time data through IoMT, which enhances the precision of diagnosis and treatment plans. For example, in a virtual consultation, a physician can evaluate wearable device data to determine the patient's current state of health and modify the treatment plan as necessary. This particular use has gained significant importance in light of the COVID-19 epidemic, which hastened the global deployment of telemedicine.
3. **Real-Time Data Analytics**: In order to obtain insights into patient health trends and outcomes, IoMT generates enormous amounts of data that may be evaluated in real-time. By processing this data using advanced analytics systems, patterns and possible health problems can be predicted, enabling early intervention, (Zhang *et al.*, 2023). When a high-risk patient is at risk of having a heart attack or stroke, real-time analytics can notify medical professionals in advance, allowing for a quick intervention that may save lives.

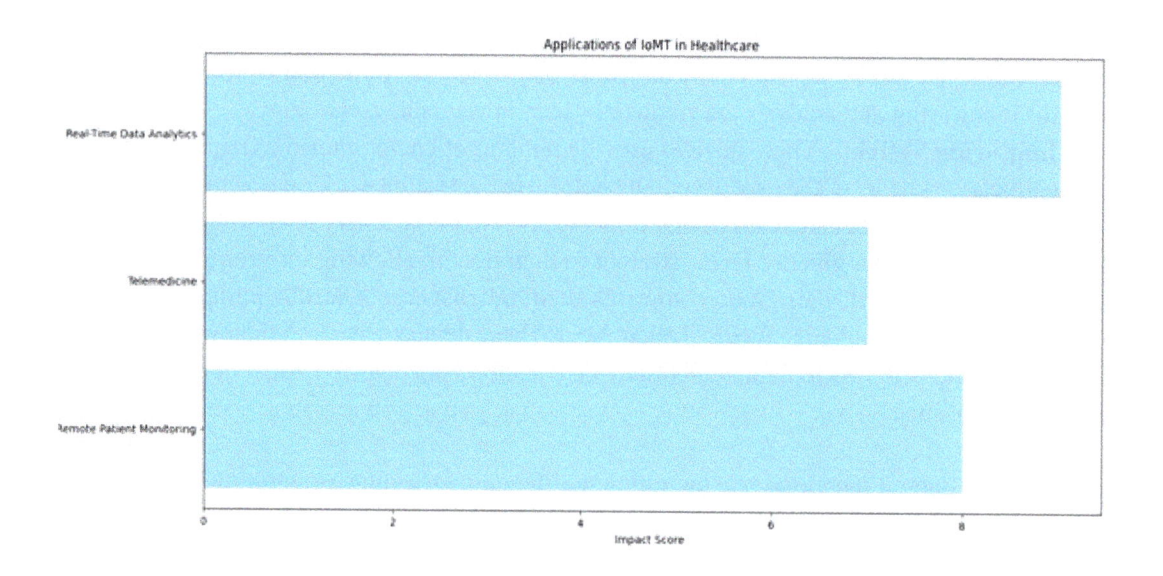

Figure 4. Application of IoMT in healthcare

4.3. Case Studies

4.3.1. Successful IoMT Implementations in Healthcare

1. **Philips HealthSuite**: HealthSuite, an IoMT platform developed by Philips, links millions of wearable sensors, medical equipment, and healthcare apps. Real-time health data analytics and remote patient monitoring are made possible by the platform, (Bak *et al.,* 2023). HealthSuite, for example, has been utilized in remote cardiac care programs, where patients with heart issues are monitored from home, resulting in improved patient outcomes and a significant decrease in hospital readmissions.
2. **Medtronic's Remote Monitoring for Diabetes**: Leading medical device manufacturer Medtronic has created a diabetes patient remote monitoring system based on IoMT. With the help of an insulin pump and a continuous glucose monitor (CGM), the system may automatically modify insulin delivery in response to current glucose readings. With this combined strategy, individuals with diabetes now have better glucose control and a lower risk of complications
3. **GE Healthcare's Smart Imaging Systems**: By integrating IoMT into its medical imaging systems, GE Healthcare has made it possible to continuously monitor and analyze the operation of imaging equipment. This intelligent system can anticipate maintenance needs, saving downtime and guaranteeing that imaging equipment is always available for vital tests. Hospital operational effectiveness and patient throughput have increased because to the real-time data from these systems.

5. INTEGRATION OF GENERATIVE AI AND IOMT

5.1. Synergy

5.1.1. The Synergistic Relationship Between Generative AI and IoMT

The Internet of Medical Things (IoMT) and Generative AI together offer a potent synergy that is revolutionizing healthcare delivery. Generative AI uses the massive volumes of real-time patient data that IoMT devices continuously gather to produce fresh insights, forecasts, and individualized treatment regimens. This combination gives healthcare practitioners the ability to make data-driven decisions with previously unheard-of accuracy and speed, leading to more effective and efficient healthcare solutions. These technologies work well together because they can enhance one another. Generative AI analyzes and interprets the vast amounts of data collected by IoMT to produce actionable insights that improve patient care and streamline healthcare operations.

Data Utilization: How IoMT Data Enhances Decision-Making Through Generative AI

IoMT devices, like smart medical equipment, wearable health monitors, and remote patient monitoring systems, capture a wealth of data that can be leveraged to improve healthcare decision-making. This data is analyzed by generative AI models, which then produce individualized treatment recommendations, forecast results, and spot patterns. For example, blood sugar levels are monitored throughout the day using continuous glucose monitors (CGMs), which are employed in the management of diabetes. By analyzing this data, generative AI can improve glycemic management by forecasting changes in glucose levels and making suggestions for insulin modifications. Furthermore, the AI can model various therapy situations, enabling medical professionals to customize interventions for specific patients, ultimately resulting in more effective and individualized care.

Figure 5. Integration of generative AI and IoMT in healthcare

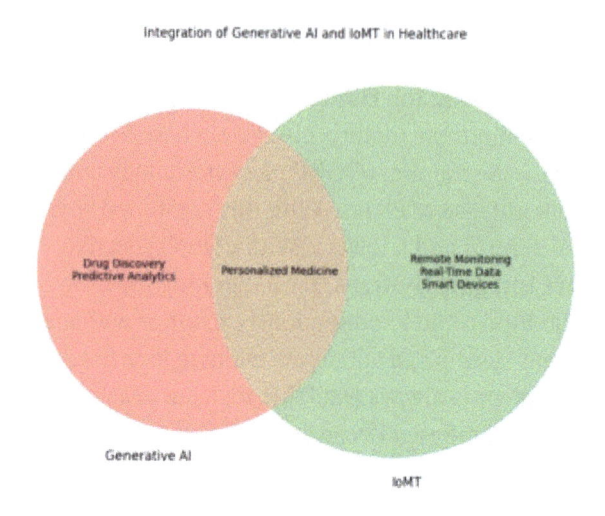

5.2. Examples

5.2.1. AI and IoMT Working Together in Clinical Settings

Remote Patient Monitoring and AI-Driven Predictive Analytics: The integration of IoMT and Generative AI is especially noticeable in remote patient monitoring systems in clinical settings. For instance, wearable technology that tracks vital signs like blood pressure and heart rate may be used by individuals with long-term cardiac issues. These gadgets send their data in real time to healthcare experts, who use Generative AI algorithms to analyze it and forecast any negative outcomes, like heart attacks, before they happen. Early interventions made possible by this predictive capacity lower hospital admission rates and enhance patient outcomes.

1. **Personalized Cancer Treatment**: In the field of cancer, for instance, real-time monitoring of a patient's response to treatment is possible thanks to IoMT devices. With this information, generative AI may simulate several treatment plans and forecast their effectiveness according to the patient's particular genetic profile and present state of health, (Moujahid, Aouad, & Zbakh, 2023) (Abbasian et al., 2024). AI-generated models have been utilized in the creation of individualized cancer treatment regimens, assisting physicians in selecting the most effective treatments with the fewest side effects that are catered to the specific needs of each patient.

2. **AI-Enhanced Medical Imaging**: In the field of medical imaging, Internet of Medical Things (IoMT) devices, such smart imaging systems, gather precise patient images, (Liao *et al.,* 2023). Generative AI then analyzes these images to find anomalies that might not be evident to the human eye. This integration increases diagnosis accuracy, especially in complex instances where early identification is crucial, such early-stage malignancies. AI is also capable of predicting how found anomalies may develop, which helps doctors decide on the best course of action.

These illustrations show how merging IoMT and Generative AI in healthcare has the potential to be revolutionary. More accurate, timely, and individualized medical care is now possible because to AI's capacity to evaluate and learn from the constant stream of data produced by IoMT devices. This will eventually improve patient outcomes and streamline healthcare systems.

6. IMPACT ON GLOBAL HEALTHCARE

6.1. Clinical Results: Enhanced Patient Safety, Treatment Precision, and Diagnostics

By raising treatment precision, improving diagnostic accuracy, and supporting patient safety, the combination of Generative AI with IoMT has greatly enhanced clinical outcomes. Compared to conventional approaches, AI-driven diagnostic technologies have proven to be more accurate in early disease detection, such as cancer. AI algorithms trained on enormous datasets can find deeply ingrained patterns in medical imaging that human radiologists would overlook, resulting in earlier and more precise diagnoses.

Generative AI makes it possible to build customized medicine, which customizes therapies to the unique characteristics of each patient, resulting in more precise therapy delivery. This tailored strategy improves treatment efficacy and lowers the risk of negative medication reactions. AI algorithms, for example, can forecast a patient's reaction to a particular medication based on their genetic profile, resulting in safer and more efficient treatment regimens.

The continuous monitoring features that IoMT devices offer have greatly improved patient safety. By notifying healthcare professionals promptly when a patient's condition deteriorates, these devices enable preventive measures to be taken before difficulties arise. Through the early detection and resolution of problems, remote monitoring of patients with chronic heart disease, for instance, has been demonstrated to lower hospital readmission rates.

6.2. Operational Efficiency: Cutting Costs and Streamlining Healthcare Processes

By optimizing workflows, cutting expenses, and enhancing resource management, AI and IoMT are completely changing the way healthcare operates. Healthcare practitioners can concentrate more on patient care by automating repetitive processes like scheduling, billing, and data entry, which boosts operational efficiency. For instance, AI-driven systems can anticipate patient admissions, discharges, and the need for particular resources, which helps enhance hospital operations and guarantee that personnel and equipment are used efficiently.

In addition to inventory management and supply chain optimization, artificial intelligence (AI) has predictive capabilities that minimize waste and guarantee the availability of critical goods at the appropriate time. big healthcare systems are especially in need of this since inefficiencies can result in big cost overruns. Reducing the necessity for frequent in-person visits is another benefit of using IoMT for remote patient monitoring. This eases the strain on healthcare facilities and lowers associated expenditures like hospital stays and transportation.

6.3. Accessibility: Increasing Access to Medical Care in Underserved Areas

IoMT and generative AI have the potential to greatly increase healthcare accessible, particularly in underserved and distant areas, (Gupta *et al.,* 2024). Thanks to this technology, people living in remote or underdeveloped areas can receive medical consultations and follow-up without having to make lengthy trips to medical facilities. IoMT devices, for instance, can be used to monitor patients with chronic diseases at remote locations. AI can then analyze the data and give patients or local healthcare providers useful insights.

Moreover, by using automated systems to provide precise diagnoses, AI-driven diagnostic technologies can make up for the dearth of specialty physicians in these areas. An AI-powered smartphone app, for instance, has the ability to evaluate photos of a skin lesion and offer an early diagnosis, which can be life-saving in places where dermatologists are hard to come by. These technologies not only expand access to healthcare services but also help reduce health inequities by offering previously underserved communities high-quality care.

Generative AI and IoMT integration has the potential to revolutionize healthcare globally by increasing access to care, optimizing operational efficiency, and improving clinical outcomes—especially in traditionally underserved locations.

7. CHALLENGES AND LIMITATIONS

7.1. Privacy and Security Concerns

Although IoMT and generative AI significantly improve healthcare, they also raise serious privacy and security issues, (Kamalov *et al.,* 2023). Data privacy becomes increasingly important as more sensitive health data is gathered and processed. Data breaches and illegal access to personal health information are two of the biggest hazards connected to the implementation of IoMT devices, according to a 2023 study by Cui *et al.* (2023). Similar to this, strong encryption and access control procedures are required when using Generative AI to create and manage medical data in order to prevent data exploitation.

7.2. Data Quality and Computational Challenges

The quality of the data utilized has a major impact on how well Generative AI and IoMT work. Biased or insufficient data can produce unreliable conclusions and ineffectual therapy suggestions. According to recent research, one major obstacle facing AI-driven healthcare solutions is guaranteeing high-quality, diversified, and representative datasets (Smith *et al.*, 2024) (Martin *et al.*, 2024). Additionally, these systems' scalability and performance may be hampered by computational constraints like processor power and algorithmic complexity.

7.3. Socio-economic, Cultural, and Ethical Implications

Socioeconomic and cultural issues are also brought up by the use of IoMT and Generative AI in healthcare. Health inequities across various socioeconomic groups can be exacerbated by unequal access to new technologies. Inequalities in digital literacy and technology access can impact healthcare equity, (Khubchandani *et al.*, 2023). To guarantee that these technologies are well-received and efficiently employed by a wide range of demographics, culturally aware methodologies are required. To emphasizes the importance of ethical considerations, such as informed permission and data ownership, it is critical to establish the boundary and frameworks that ensure the patient autonomy, protect the sensitive information by promoting the transparency in how data is used and shared within healthcare domain.

7.4. Strategies for Addressing These Challenges

To tackle these obstacles, a diverse strategy is needed. Adopting cutting-edge cybersecurity solutions and putting in place robust data governance frameworks are crucial for reducing privacy and security threats. Strict validation procedures and the utilization of a variety of datasets to increase AI model accuracy are key components of improving data quality. Inclusive policies that guarantee fair access to technology and advance digital literacy can help alleviate socioeconomic and cultural issues. In order to protect patient rights and data integrity, ethical standards and laws should be put in place to regulate the use of AI and IoMT.

8. FUTURE DIRECTIONS AND INNOVATIONS

8.1. Emerging Trends in Generative AI and IoMT

Both the Internet of Medical Things (IoMT) and Generative AI are rapidly changing fields. In order to construct more complex health monitoring systems, emerging trends involve integrating AI with cutting-edge IoMT devices, (Da Silva, 2024b). For instance, it is now possible for IoMT devices to detect health issues before they become serious thanks to recent advancements in AI-driven predictive analytics. Plus, real-time data processing and latency reduction are made possible by the rise of edge computing in IoMT, which is essential for prompt medical interventions.

8.2. Potential Advancements and Their Impact on Healthcare

Personalized medicine and diagnostics are about to undergo a revolutionary change because to advances in generative AI, including more precise image production and enhanced natural language processing. Improved AI models should improve health outcomes by offering more accurate disease forecasts and customizing treatments based on each patient's genetic profile (Smith *et al.*, 2024) (Martin *et al.*, 2024). It is projected that IoMT will greatly improve patient monitoring and health management with the development of next-generation wearable devices with better sensors and longer battery lives (Lee & Chen, 2023) (Qin et al., 2023). These developments should result in more proactive and preventive healthcare strategies, which will lessen the strain on global healthcare systems.

8.3. Opportunities for Further Research and Development

In the fields of IoMT and generative AI, there are numerous interesting avenues for further study and advancement. Investigating AI algorithms that can more efficiently manage large-scale and diversified health data sets is a significant opportunity, as it addresses the present shortcomings in computing efficiency and data quality. The creation of privacy-preserving methods, such federated learning, to guarantee data security while using shared medical data is another crucial field, (Chaddad, Wu, & Desrosiers, 2024). Furthermore, to guarantee that AI and IoMT are implemented fairly and responsibly, study on the ethical and cultural ramifications of these technologies in various healthcare settings is essential.

9. STRATEGIC ADOPTION AND IMPLEMENTATION

9.1. Recommendations for Healthcare Professionals and Institutions

Prioritizing a few crucial measures will help healthcare practitioners and institutions utilize Generative AI and IoMT technology more successfully. To make sure that employees are competent in using these cutting-edge instruments, they need first make investments in education and training. According to recent studies on healthcare data breaches, putting in place thorough cybersecurity measures to safeguard patient data is also essential, (Wasserman & Wasserman, 2022). Furthermore, encouraging multidisciplinary cooperation between IT professionals and medical professionals might improve the assimilation and application of these technologies.

9.2. Best Practices for Integrating These Technologies

For successful integration of IoMT and generative AI few best practices are essential. It is crucial to establish explicit data governance frameworks to control privacy and data quality. Maintaining and updating technology systems regularly is also essential to stay up to date with security standards and improvements. Moreover, identifying possible problems and streamlining integration procedures can be achieved by testing new technologies in controlled settings before their widespread adoption.

9.3. Considerations for Global Healthcare Systems

Adopting Generative AI and IoMT technology necessitates resolving a number of factors for global healthcare systems. Preventing the widening of health inequities requires ensuring fair access to these technologies across all areas and socio-economic groups. Furthermore, for these technologies to be used effectively, they must be modified to satisfy local regulatory needs and cultural settings (Johnson & Patel, 2023) (Patel et al., 2023). Global cooperation and information exchange can help various healthcare systems embrace best practices and standards.

10. CONCLUSION

This chapter focused on the revolutionary effects of generative artificial intelligence (AI) and the Internet of Medical Things (IoMT) on the global healthcare system, highlighting their contributions to improved real-time patient monitoring, individualized treatment plans, and medical diagnosis. While there are many advantages to these developments, like better illness prediction and operational efficiencies, their full potential cannot be achieved unless issues with data privacy, security, and socioeconomic inequality are resolved. These technologies, which have the potential to completely transform healthcare outcomes globally, must be adopted and distributed fairly. To that end, strategic measures such as strong data governance and interdisciplinary collaboration are needed

REFERENCES

Abbasian, M., Khatibi, E., Azimi, I., Oniani, D., Abad, Z. S. H., Thieme, A., Sriram, R., Yang, Z., Wang, Y., Lin, B., Gevaert, O., Li, L. J., Jain, R., & Rahmani, A. M. (2024). Foundation metrics for evaluating effectiveness of healthcare conversations powered by generative AI. *NPJ Digital Medicine*, 7(1), 82. Advance online publication. DOI: 10.1038/s41746-024-01074-z PMID: 38553625

Bak, M. R., Ploem, M. C., Tan, H. L., Blom, M. T., & Willems, D. L. (2023). Towards trust-based governance of health data research. *Medicine, Health Care, and Philosophy*, 26(2), 185–200. DOI: 10.1007/s11019-022-10134-8 PMID: 36633724

Capobianco, J. P. (2023). The New Era of Global Services: A Framework for Successful Enterprises in Business Services and IT. References. (2023). In *Emerald Publishing Limited eBooks* (pp. 203–226). DOI: 10.1108/9781837536269

Chaddad, A., Wu, Y., & Desrosiers, C. (2024). Federated Learning for Healthcare Applications. *IEEE Internet of Things Journal*, 11(5), 7339–7358. DOI: 10.1109/JIOT.2023.3325822

Chinta, S. V., Wang, Z., Zhang, X., Viet, T. D., Kashif, A., Smith, M. A., & Zhang, W. (2024). AI-Driven Healthcare: A Survey on Ensuring Fairness and Mitigating Bias. *arXiv (Cornell University)*. https://doi.org//arxiv.2407.19655DOI: 10.48550

Cui, A., Zhang, T., Xiao, P., Fan, Z., Wang, H., & Zhuang, Y. (2023). Global and regional prevalence of vitamin D deficiency in population-based studies from 2000 to 2022: A pooled analysis of 7.9 million participants. *Frontiers in Nutrition*, 10, 1070808. Advance online publication. DOI: 10.3389/fnut.2023.1070808 PMID: 37006940

Da Silva, R. G. L. (2024). The advancement of artificial intelligence in biomedical research and health innovation: Challenges and opportunities in emerging economies. *Globalization and Health*, 20(1), 44. Advance online publication. DOI: 10.1186/s12992-024-01049-5 PMID: 38773458

Da Silva, R. G. L. (2024b). The advancement of artificial intelligence in biomedical research and health innovation: Challenges and opportunities in emerging economies. *Globalization and Health*, 20(1), 44. Advance online publication. DOI: 10.1186/s12992-024-01049-5 PMID: 38773458

Da Silva, R. G. L. (2024c). The advancement of artificial intelligence in biomedical research and health innovation: Challenges and opportunities in emerging economies. *Globalization and Health*, 20(1), 44. Advance online publication. DOI: 10.1186/s12992-024-01049-5 PMID: 38773458

Daneshvar, N., Pandita, D., Erickson, S., Sulmasy, L. S., & DeCamp, M. (2024). Artificial Intelligence in the Provision of Health Care: An American College of Physicians Policy Position Paper. *Annals of Internal Medicine*, 177(7), 964–967. DOI: 10.7326/M24-0146 PMID: 38830215

Dwivedi, R., Mehrotra, D., & Chandra, S. (2022). Potential of Internet of Medical Things (IoMT) applications in building a smart healthcare system: A systematic review. *Journal of Oral Biology and Craniofacial Research*, 12(2), 302–318. DOI: 10.1016/j.jobcr.2021.11.010 PMID: 34926140

Gupta, P., Ding, B., Guan, C., & Ding, D. (2024). Generative AI: A systematic review using topic modelling techniques. *Data and Information Management*, 100066(2), 100066. Advance online publication. DOI: 10.1016/j.dim.2024.100066

Kamalov, F., Pourghebleh, B., Gheisari, M., Liu, Y., & Moussa, S. (2023). Internet of Medical Things Privacy and Security: Challenges, Solutions, and Future Trends from a New Perspective. *Sustainability (Basel)*, 15(4), 3317. DOI: 10.3390/su15043317

Khubchandani, J., Sharma, S., England-Kennedy, E., Pai, A., & Banerjee, S. (2023). Emerging technologies and futuristic digital healthcare ecosystems: Priorities for research and action in the United States. *Journal of Medicine, Surgery, and Public Health*, 1, 100030. DOI: 10.1016/j.glmedi.2023.100030

. Kim, J. Y., Boag, W., Gulamali, F., Hasan, A., Hogg, H. D. J., Lifson, M., Mulligan, D., Patel, M., Raji, I. D., Sehgal, A., Shaw, K., Tobey, D., Valladares, A., Vidal, D., Balu, S., & Sendak, M. (2023). *Organizational Governance of Emerging Technologies: AI Adoption in Healthcare.* DOI: 10.1145/3593013.3594089

Kumar, V., Saini, D., Rastogi, S., Raman, R., Verma, A., & Meenakshi, R. (2024).. . *Development of Medical IOT System for the Prediction of Heart Disease.*, 10, 951–956. DOI: 10.1109/ICACITE60783.2024.10617362

Liao, J., Li, X., Gan, Y., Han, S., Rong, P., Wang, W., Li, W., & Zhou, L. (2023). Artificial intelligence assists precision medicine in cancer treatment. *Frontiers in Oncology*, 12, 998222. Advance online publication. DOI: 10.3389/fonc.2022.998222 PMID: 36686757

Manickam, P., Mariappan, S. A., Murugesan, S. M., Hansda, S., Kaushik, A., Shinde, R., & Thipperudraswamy, S. P. (2022). Artificial Intelligence (AI) and Internet of Medical Things (IoMT) Assisted Biomedical Systems for Intelligent Healthcare. *Biosensors (Basel)*, 12(8), 562. DOI: 10.3390/bios12080562 PMID: 35892459

Martin, S. S., Aday, A. W., Almarzooq, Z. I., Anderson, C. A., Arora, P., Avery, C. L., Baker-Smith, C. M., Gibbs, B. B., Beaton, A. Z., Boehme, A. K., Commodore-Mensah, Y., Currie, M. E., Elkind, M. S., Evenson, K. R., Generoso, G., Heard, D. G., Hiremath, S., Johansen, M. C., Kalani, R., & Palaniappan, L. P. (2024). 2024 Heart Disease and Stroke Statistics: A Report of US and Global Data From the American Heart Association. *Circulation*, 149(8). Advance online publication. DOI: 10.1161/CIR.0000000000001209 PMID: 38264914

Morgan, J. (2020). Meeting the greatest challenges for leaders of the future. *Leader to Leader*, 2020(96), 19–26. DOI: 10.1002/ltl.20500

Morley, J., Murphy, L., Mishra, A., Joshi, I., & Karpathakis, K. (2022). Governing Data and Artificial Intelligence for Health Care: Developing an International Understanding. *JMIR Formative Research*, 6(1), e31623. DOI: 10.2196/31623 PMID: 35099403

Moshawrab, M., Adda, M., Bouzouane, A., Ibrahim, H., & Raad, A. (2023). Smart Wearables for the Detection of Cardiovascular Diseases: A Systematic Literature Review. *Sensors (Basel)*, 23(2), 828. DOI: 10.3390/s23020828 PMID: 36679626

Moujahid, F. E., Aouad, S., & Zbakh, M. (2023). Smart Healthcare Development Based on IoMT and Edge-Cloud Computing: A Systematic Survey. In *Lecture notes on data engineering and communications technologies* (pp. 575–593). DOI: 10.1007/978-3-031-27762-7_52

Nah, F. F. H., Zheng, R., Cai, J., Siau, K., & Chen, L. (2023). Generative AI and ChatGPT: Applications, challenges, and AI-human collaboration. *Journal of Information Technology Case and Application Research*, 25(3), 277–304. DOI: 10.1080/15228053.2023.2233814

Okonji, O. R., Yunusov, K., & Gordon, B. (2024). *Applications of Generative AI in Healthcare: algorithmic, ethical, legal and societal considerations*. DOI: 10.36227/techrxiv.171527587.75649430/v1

Patel, N. J., Wang, X., Fu, X., Kawano, Y., Cook, C., Vanni, K. M. M., Qian, G., Banasiak, E., Kowalski, E., Zhang, Y., Sparks, J. A., & Wallace, Z. S. (2023). Factors associated with COVID-19 breakthrough infection among vaccinated patients with rheumatic diseases: A cohort study. *Seminars in Arthritis and Rheumatism*, 58, 152108. DOI: 10.1016/j.semarthrit.2022.152108 PMID: 36347211

Qin, S., Chan, S. L., Gu, S., Bai, Y., Ren, Z., Lin, X., Chen, Z., Jia, W., Jin, Y., Guo, Y., Hu, X., Meng, Z., Liang, J., Cheng, Y., Xiong, J., Ren, H., Yang, F., Li, W., Chen, Y., & Verset, G. (2023). Camrelizumab plus rivoceranib versus sorafenib as first-line therapy for unresectable hepatocellular carcinoma (CARES-310): A randomised, open-label, international phase 3 study. *Lancet*, 402(10408), 1133–1146. DOI: 10.1016/S0140-6736(23)00961-3 PMID: 37499670

Trinkley, K. E., An, R., Maw, A. M., Glasgow, R. E., & Brownson, R. C. (2024). Leveraging artificial intelligence to advance implementation science: Potential opportunities and cautions. *Implementation Science : IS*, 19(1), 17. Advance online publication. DOI: 10.1186/s13012-024-01346-y PMID: 38383393

Wasserman, L., & Wasserman, Y. (2022). Hospital cybersecurity risks and gaps: Review (for the non-cyber professional). *Frontiers in Digital Health*, 4, 862221. Advance online publication. DOI: 10.3389/fdgth.2022.862221 PMID: 36033634

Zhang, A., Wu, Z., Wu, E., Wu, M., Snyder, M. P., Zou, J., & Wu, J. C. (2023). Leveraging physiology and artificial intelligence to deliver advancements in health care. *Physiological Reviews*, 103(4), 2423–2450. DOI: 10.1152/physrev.00033.2022 PMID: 37104717

Chapter 22
Navigating the Convergence of IoMT and Generative AI in Global Healthcare:
Opportunities, Challenges, and Ethical Considerations

Muhammad Usman Tariq
https://orcid.org/0000-0002-7605-3040
Abu Dhabi University, UAE & University College Cork, Ireland

ABSTRACT

This chapter examines the transformative potential of combining Generative AI with the Internet of Medical Things (IoMT) in healthcare. IoMT's capacity to empower ceaseless wellbeing observing and ongoing information assortment, joined with Generative man-made intelligence's high-level prescient and logical power, guarantees huge progressions in diagnostics, patient administration, and customized medication. The chapter focuses on case studies that demonstrate improved healthcare delivery and outcomes as it examines novel applications of these technologies. Be that as it may, it additionally addresses basic difficulties like security, security, and moral situations, including information insurance, algorithmic predisposition, and patient independence. Systems for beating these hindrances, particularly in asset compelled settings, are talked about, accentuating the requirement for hearty moral structures and administrative approaches.

INTRODUCTION

The application of IoMT, coupled with Generative AI, in global healthcare is inaugurating a new era in medical science. IoMT is defined as the interstate connection of commonly used medical instruments and software tools engaged in data collection and transmission over the Internet. Another segment of AI is called generative AI, which consists of sophisticated machine-learning tools that enable new content and draw new conclusions from gigabytes of information. Altogether, these technologies are determining new approaches in healthcare, diagnostics, and patient care and opening up solutions on the one hand and controversies/ethical issues on the other. IoMT covers virtually any type of device,

DOI: 10.4018/979-8-3693-6180-1.ch022

including wearable health monitors, smart implants, and connected medical equipment, which collect vast amounts of patient data (Affia et al., 2023). Such devices help in the constant monitoring of health status, real-time identification of abnormal conditions, and supervision of patients at a distance. For example, wrist-wearables such as smartwatches may track heart rate, steps taken, and sleep quality, which may help doctors know when a patient is developing severe conditions (Lakhan et al., 2024). Advanced generators, such as insulin pumps and pacemakers, provide adequate data and enable wholesale changes which will help to improve the quality of the care provided to patients.

At the same time, emergent generative AI is changing the way this data is leveraged. Such systems can help diagnose diseases, recommend the right treatment, including drug prescription, and even estimate the patient's prognosis. For instance, in radiology, generative AI can diagnose images, meaning the ability to diagnose diseases such as cancer or bone fractures with massive accuracy beyond that of human radiologists (Gou et al., 2024). In addition, AI-enabled chatbots and virtual health assistants have become common tools for engage/patient education, responding to health-related questions/queries and chronic disease self-management, and decreasing the workload of human health care providers (Gupta et al., 2024). There are great possibilities for improving the healthcare system owing to the overlap between IoMT and generative AI. One use is in Intelligent Predictive Analytics where the IoMT devices collect patient data that are streamed and analysed by AI algorithms for the prognosis of adverse events. For instance, AI for predicting complications arising from diabetes from the measurement of glucose levels from IoMT can help intervene and develop corrective measures tailored for the patient (Husnain et al., 2023). This integration not only enhances the patient's well-being but also increases the efficiency of healthcare delivery systems, as they decrease hospitalisation relapses and ER visits.

Furthermore, the effectiveness of these technologies is more significant in the management of patients, mainly those with chronic ailments. For instance, in dealing with cardiovascular diseases, IoMT devices constantly measure and send other data to an AI system that forecasts instances of heart failure. These predictions allow healthcare providers to manage the condition a little early, so that severe outcomes cannot be expected (Marima et al., 2023). Likewise, generative AI can help in developing effective rehabilitation schedules for strokes by integrating data collected from IoMT-based physical therapy equipment with the help of physical therapists to guarantee an individual approach and consider a patient's progress as well as their requirements (Tariq, 2024). Nevertheless, the integration of IoMT and generative AI has certain drawbacks and ethical issues. Another issue is the protection of data and privacy because the constant status of patients' health information creates high vulnerability to data theft and unauthorised access (Omidian, 2024). This process means that medical institutions employ tight security standards, and local laws require stringent protection of patients' data. Moreover, bioethical considerations lead to problems concerning the disclosure of AI decision-making procedures. Some AI algorithms are opaque, and this raises questions on how they arrive at a certain decision, which is not good for healthcare providers and patients because they cannot give full trust to such systems (İncegil et al., 2023). Furthermore, the use of sophisticated devices has intensified health inequalities in society. In LMICs, the availability of IoMT devices and AI-enabled healthcare tools can be constrained, affecting the equitable distribution between the rich and the poor (Rahman et al., 2024). Eradicating these gaps calls for collaborations to achieve fair distribution of technologies, as well as creating solutions to fit most health settings, which are also inexpensive to implement. The growing burden of chronic and acute diseases globally necessitates innovative approaches in healthcare delivery. Advancements in technology, particularly the integration of IoMT and generative AI, have emerged as crucial tools to address these challenges. These technologies are vital not only for improving patient outcomes but also for reducing costs and optimising healthcare delivery. This discussion seeks to contribute by highlighting the integration of IoMT and generative AI in the global healthcare context, with a focus on their applications, benefits, and ethical considerations.

BACKGROUND

The Internet of Medical Things (IoMT) is an essential paradigm in today's healthcare systems that provides innovative applications that augment patient care delivery and healthcare systems. IoMT is defined as a system of medical devices and applications linked through Internet technology to gather, analyse, and disseminate patient healthcare data. Healthcare technology has benefited several different healthcare environments, heading from home care to elevated diagnostic equipment, and has created real value to steward the healthcare digitalisation process (Govardanan et al., 2024). A good example of IoMT is remote patient monitoring, also known as RPM. In turn, RPM uses wearable gadgets and home-based sensors to check the patient's vital status and other factors without interruption. For instance, smartwatches and fit trackers can monitor the heart rate, blood pressure, and glucose levels and relay them to doctors and nurses in real time. This open and continuous flow of information enables early intervention, thus minimising the rate of readmission to hospitals and the management of chronic diseases. Thus, IoMT devices in diabetes care can read glucose levels and the use of insulin and note potential problems before they reach an acute stage (Rahman et al., 2024).

Another massive application is in smart hospitals, where the Internet of Medical Things is used to optimise hospital functionalities and patient satisfaction. Other smart hospital systems involve the utilisation of IoMT devices to track hospital assets, patient flow, and equipment usage. For example, connected devices can monitor the location and status of a hospital's critical medical equipment to guarantee readiness and functionality at the right time. Further, with the help of systems involving IoMT, the admission and discharge processes, as well as the transfer of patients, exhibited more organizational efficiency in healthcare facilities. One example of its success comes from a hospital that integrates an IoMT system into its work; this system led to a 20% decrease in the patient's wait time and a 15% increase in OR use (Marima et al., 2023). The IoMT is also vital for the provision of personalised medicine. They also assist in the management of big data by gathering information on patients, thereby assisting in treatment customisation according to patient needs. Smart inhalers for asthma patients can also be monitored when the inhalers are used and the conditions under which they are used, and recommendations can be made on how to avoid the conditions that trigger an asthma attack. Likewise, IoMT-integrated pacemakers can also check the patients' heart conditions and adapt the pacemaker's functioning according to real-time data, providing individualised medical treatment for specific cardiovascular issues (Azrour et al., 2024).

What intensifies IoMT is that it can be complemented with artificial intelligence (AI). Thus, the data collected and generated by IoMT devices can be analysed using AI to develop trends and health prognoses. For example, IoMT devices based on AI can identify early stages of sepsis in patients with in-hospital mortality. In another case, an IoMT system that had integrated AI was again able to predict the health status of patients within the intensive care unit and was able to instigate early intervention; thus, the results showed reduced mortality rates (Putra et al., 2024). Another area that IoMT influences is telemedicine, which enables virtual consultations and diagnostic services. IoMT devices also allow patient information to be received by healthcare providers during telemedicine sessions to ensure proper diagnosis and treatment. These are essential in regions where access to healthcare facilities may be very limited, which makes sense in such regions. The health information provided by IoMT devices guarantees that a particular patient is treated as urgently as possible and as necessary all over the location (Govardanan et al., 2024).

The realisation of IoMT in healthcare is not devoid of challenges, as is highlighted below. The risk management of data breaches and privacy protection must be prioritised because IoMT systems transfer comprehensive healthcare data easily. It is mandatory and wise to establish strong cybersecurity and adhere to the rules to safeguard the patient's information and build trust and confidence in IoMT devices (Patruni & Humayun, 2024).

Generative AI for Medical Data Synthesis and Image Analysis

Generative Artificial Intelligence (AI) has been developing into a useful asset in medicine, particularly for synthesising medical data and improving medical imaging. Generative AI relates to AI models that could generate new content, such as new images, new text, or new audio based on learned data. In healthcare, these capabilities are used to create artificial medical data for academic application and knowledgeable human resources and to optimize healthcare picture resolution for better work and improved treatment (Rahman et al., 2024; Putra et al., 2024). From this perspective, generative AI has been widely used for the synthesis of medical data. Health information, particularly patient information, is private and lacks the same permissiveness in terms of access to health training and research as other data. Consequently, generative AI can generate synthetic datasets that contain statistical characteristics like real patient data while protecting patients' rights. For instance, AI algorithms can create authentic patient datasets with specific data triggers masked for confidentiality purposes, enabling researchers to create and improve new medical paradigms and algorithms. These synthetic data are important because they are used to train AI systems to help them learn from various datasets without necessarily using actual patient data (patients' records) (Azrour et al., 2024, Patruni & Humayun, 2024).

Currently, generative AI is at the forefront of changing how images are handled in medical imaging applications. Through AI algorithms, the acquired images can be improved to calibrate the necessary and accurate diagnosis of diseases by these professionals. For example, the improved image resolution of poor-quality medical images can be achieved using generative adversarial networks (GANs). Owing to their training on high-resolution images, GANs can improve the quality of images at lower resolutions, facilitating better analyses. This capability is highly useful in radiology, because fine and crisp images are relevant for precise diagnosis (Gupta et al., 2024; Gou et al., 2024).

Another crucial area served by generative AI is enhancing diagnostic functions with the help of superior image processing. Artificial intelligence-based tools can read X-rays, MRIs, and CT scans and can detect patterns or defects that the human naked eye may not see. For instance, the identification of disease precursors, such as cancer, using AI in histopathological image analysis. Such algorithms can identify suspicious areas, which would be beneficial to radiologists when making accurate diagnoses. One of the most famous use cases concerns AI application to mammography and shows better effectiveness than radiologists in identifying cases of breast cancer, which enables earlier and more efficient diagnosis (Varnosfaderani & Forouzanfar, 2024). Another crucial area of utilisation is the use of big data in the field of predictive analysis. Thus, generative AI can help identify disease trends and predict patient outcomes based on the statistics provided. For example, it is possible to use AI models to simulate what may happen to a patient with a specific disease and to come up with the best treatment package. Such simulations are useful to clinicians to be able to prepare for possible adverse outcomes and adjust the treatment plan to those ends, thus increasing the patient's quality of life and lowering healthcare expenditures (Marima et al., 2023; Govardanan et al., 2024)

To this end, generative AI also improves surgical planning and training. Surgeons can use AI-conducted 3D models in patients' anatomy to better understand the approaching surgery, as such often requires detailed visualisation of the operational area. These models can be derived from quality medical imaging data and can provide details of the structures to be operated upon and possible difficulties that could be faced in the operation. Furthermore, synthetic data and models are very helpful in teaching and training medical students and residents because they can work on the issues on this package with many realistic scenarios without having to violate patients' rights while at the same time enduring many procedural formalities (Rahman et al., 2024). As beneficial as the generative AI mechanism might be used in medical data synthesis and image analysis, this approach is not without its setbacks. The veracity and credibility of the AI data and images should be preserved as much as possible because accurate information is needed in patient diagnosis and treatment plans. In addition, the ethical issues that entail data privacy and synthetic data must be closely monitored to ensure the patients' privacy and regulatory approvals in health terms that were given by Affia et al. (2023) and Gupta et al. (2024), respectively. Therefore, as generative AI has been clearly demonstrated, it is possible to provide new and more efficient systems for medical data synthesis and image analysis. This study examines how generative AI affects the healthcare system through the production of synthetic datasets, enhancement of image quality, increased diagnostic accuracy, and powering of surgical planning. Over time, their application has been bound to change clinical practices and improve the delivery of healthcare services (Tariq, 2024).

Privacy and Security Issues in IoMT

The Internet of Medical Things (IoMT) has caused rapid development in healthcare, as it has increased the opportunities for patient monitoring, diagnosis, and treatment using connected devices and systems. However, this technological advancement comes with a lot of merits, it has however brought about a lot of issues in the privacy and security. They also carry health data and become vulnerable to hacking and data theft, because IoMT devices create concerns regarding the confidentiality, integrity, and availability of patient data (Affia et al., 2023). The main privacy concern of IoMT devices is the large amount of personal health information that they create and transmit. These devices constantly record information on the patient's status, including vital signs, usage of prescribed medications, and other parameters, and data are often transferred through open networks. For example, modern devices, including smart watches and fitness bracelets, track heart rate, sleep, and activity, and share this information with doctors and other applications. Lack of strong data encryption and safe communication channels, this information can fall into the wrong hands of people with an inflicting intent, with a probable consequence of unlawful utilisation of confidential health-related information (Gupta et al., 2024).

Another major problem is unauthorised access to not only patient information, but also IoMT devices. Most IoMT devices have poor security elements, including appropriate authentication and timely software updates, hence becoming vulnerable to hacking. This makes them vulnerable to attacks, and once intruded, hackers get access to larger healthcare networks and more significant breaches. For instance, the hacker may control an IoMT insulin pump, as well as the patient's records and every related system present in the healthcare network (Azrour et al., 2024). There is also security issues associated with the integration of IoMT devices in hospital systems. The vast continuum of IoMT includes a wide and complex array of medical devices in hospitals, from MRIs to systems monitoring patients. The presence of this network means that if one of the devices is penetrated, it becomes a link through which attackers gain access to other networks. One such incident was the ransomware attack on a hospital where the IoMT devices were infected and the patient data encrypted, further leading to the halt of critical services and posing potential threats to the patients' lives. This shows that it is time for more elaborate security solutions to be implemented to address the threats affecting IoMT devices and the networks they use (Rahman et al., 2024).

To enhance the privacy and security of the data collected and shared by different actors in an IoMT ecosystem, it is possible to deploy the following strategies: First, encryption is essential. Because the information exchanged between IoMT devices and healthcare systems needs to be communicated to other devices or systems, this information should be encrypted so as not to be decrypted by unauthorised users. Full data protection guarantees that even if information is captured, it cannot be understood or altered in some way. In addition, using security features such as transmitted layer security or TLS can also increase the security of the data during its transfer (Govardanan et al., 2024). Second, authentication plays a significant role in enforcing the security of IoMT devices. Multifactor authentication (MFA) is a widely used security technique that enhances the security of an application or system by requesting the user to input two or more pieces of verification information. For example, a healthcare provider that needs to retrieve patient information using an applied IoMT device will need a password and code received for the mobile application. This extra measure of protection increases the level of challenges an attacker may encounter in obtaining actual data (Patruni & Humayun, 2024).

Other essential procedures are also crucial for enhancing the security of IoMT devices, including software updates and patching. Therefore, manufacturers need to check devices frequently to close the gaps and enhance security. Both the healthcare facilities' IT departments and manufacturers of different IoMT devices should implement strong patch management mechanisms to ensure that all devices are patched and updated. This approach also assists in preventing attacks on discovered vulnerabilities, making the computation of the latter relatively risk-free (Varnosfaderani and Forouzanfar, 2024). Another useful prevention technique is network segmentation to defend IoMT ecosystems. Networking separation minimises the extent to which cyberattacks can affect a given healthcare organisation because the network can be compartmentalised. A castle with walls that have different levels of strength implies that if one level is penetrated, the attacker cannot easily expand to other areas. For instance, IoMT devices may be wired upon a different network than that of the various crucial hospital systems, so that if an attack occurs, most of the systems would not be significantly affected (Putra et al., 2024).

CLINICAL DATA COLLECTION AND ANALYSIS

The combination of the Web of Clinical Things (IoMT) and man-made consciousness (computer-based intelligence) in medical services has altered the techniques for gathering and breaking down clinical information. Wearable devices, smart implants, and interconnected medical equipment are just a few examples of devices that can benefit from these technologies' real-time data collection and continuous monitoring capabilities. For instance, wearable devices such as fitness trackers and smartwatches continuously collect information about a patient's vital signs, levels of physical activity, and sleep patterns to provide a complete picture of their health (Gupta et al., 2024).

These data are sent to healthcare providers, making it possible to keep an eye on things and spot problems before they become serious. AI plays a crucial role in analysing the vast amounts of data generated by IoMT devices. AI calculations can process and decipher this information to recognise examples and relationships that may not be promptly clear to human clinicians. AI algorithms, for instance, can predict blood sugar trends based on data from continuous glucose monitors, thereby allowing personalised diabetes management recommendations. Patient outcomes are significantly improved by this predictive capability, which enables interventions to be more precise and timelier (Putra et al., 2024). Personalised medicine and clinical decision-making are profoundly affected by real-time data analysis. Healthcare providers can make data-driven decisions tailored to each patient's needs by integrating IoMT and AI. Real-time data analysis enables prompt intervention by facilitating the early detection of anomalies. For instance, continuous monitoring devices can detect irregular heart rhythms in cardiac patients and immediately notify healthcare providers, potentially preventing severe cardiac events (Azrour et al., 2024).

Furthermore, personalised medicine is enhanced by the capacity to analyse data in real time and consider each patient's individual characteristics. To create individualised treatment plans, AI algorithms can incorporate data from various sources, such as medical history, lifestyle factors, and genetic information. This method ensures that the treatments work better and meet the patient's specific needs. For instance, customised malignant growth treatment plans can be created by breaking down cancer qualities and anticipating what various therapies will mean to the patient's condition (Varnosfaderani and Forouzanfar, 2024).

GENERATIVE AI FOR PERSONALIZED MEDICINE AND DRUG DISCOVERY

Generative man-made intelligence is at the forefront of changing customised medication and medication disclosure, offering remarkable experiences and abilities to foresee illnesses and alter treatment plans. Data from various sources, including genomic sequences, electronic health records, and lifestyle information, can be analysed using AI models to identify patterns and predict the onset and progression of diseases. For instance, genetic predispositions and environmental factors can be used by AI to predict the likelihood of developing particular diseases. According to Husnain et al. (2023), this predictive capability enables healthcare providers to develop proactive and individualised treatment plans, thereby enhancing patient outcomes and lowering healthcare costs. In customised medication, artificial intelligence's capacity to coordinate and dissect assorted informational indexes empowers the customisation of treatment plans custom-made to a singular's novel hereditary cosmetics and well-being profile. For instance, in oncology, AI can predict which therapies will be most effective for a particular patient by analysing genetic mutations in cancer cells. Precision oncology reduces the trial-and-error process commonly associated with cancer therapy by ensuring that patients receive targeted treatments with a higher success rate (Rahman et al., 2024). AI can also monitor how patients respond to treatment in real time, making it possible to dynamically adjust treatment plans based on the most recent data and increasing treatment efficacy while decreasing side effects. Generative AI also accelerates drug discovery, significantly reducing the time and money required to bring new drugs to the market. AI can streamline various stages of the traditional drug discovery process, which can take over a decade and cost billions of US dollars. AI algorithms can predict how various compounds interact with potential drug targets, identify potential drug targets from biological data, and optimise the design of new drugs.

According to Govardanan et al. (2024), generative models can generate novel molecular structures with the desired properties, accelerating the initial stages of drug development. Owing to this capability, promising drug candidates can be quickly identified and subjected to additional testing and refinement. AI's involvement of AI in the creation of COVID-19 treatment options is a notable illustration of its influence on drug discovery. The rapid identification of candidates for clinical trials was made possible using AI models to screen existing drugs for their potential to be effective against the virus. In addition to expediting the discovery process, this strategy provides valuable insights into the mechanism of action of drugs (Omidian, 2024).

In addition, AI has the potential to improve the safety and efficacy of new treatments by assisting in the prediction of potential adverse effects and toxicity. AI-driven drug discovery has profound effects on global health. AI has the potential to address unmet medical needs and improve health outcomes worldwide by accelerating the development of new medications and optimising treatment plans. For instance, AI can assist in locating affordable and efficient treatments for prevalent diseases in low-resource settings, thereby enhancing healthcare accessibility and equity (Sindhwani et al., 2024) In addition, AI has the potential to make it easier to develop methods of personalized medicine that are tailored to the genetic and environmental contexts of various populations, thereby promoting healthcare that is both more inclusive and more efficient.

CHALLENGES IN SCALING IOMT AND GENERATIVE AI SOLUTIONS

The broad reception of the Web of Clinical Things (IoMT) and generative simulated intelligence in medical services is laden with difficulties that envelop infrastructural, administrative, and financial boundaries. To fully utilise these technologies and transform global healthcare delivery, these obstacles must be overcome. The integration of diverse and frequently incompatible healthcare systems is a primary infrastructure challenge associated with scaling IoMT and AI solutions. The volume and complexity of data generated by IoMT devices cannot be handled by the outdated systems of many healthcare providers. This contradiction creates huge obstructions for consistent information sharing and interoperability, which are pivotal for viable computer-based intelligence-driven investigation and navigation. For example, incorporating wearable well-being screens with emergency clinic data frameworks requires vigorous information reconciliation systems that can deal with various information configurations and correspondence conventions (Lakhan et al., 2024). Without normalised conventions, the information gathered from IoMT gadgets might remain siloed, restricting its convenience for extensive medical care investigations. Administrative obstacles also present significant difficulties in the reception of IoMT and man-made intelligence in medical care. Concerns regarding privacy, security, and ethical implications arise when patient data are used, particularly in AI applications. Patient consent and data protection are subject to stringent regulations such as the General Data Protection Regulation (GDPR) in Europe and the Health Insurance Portability and Accountability Act (HIPAA) in the United States. These regulations are necessary for the protection of patient information; however, they can also slow down the implementation of new technologies because developers must navigate complicated compliance landscapes (Rauniyar et al., 2023).

Additionally, the lack of specific regulatory frameworks for AI in healthcare hinders innovation and adoption by creating uncertainty for developers and healthcare providers. The substantial initial investment required for infrastructure and technology is another obstacle to scaling IoMT and AI solutions. Executing IoMT gadgets across medical service settings requires significant monetary assets to procure gadgets, guarantee availability, and keep up with the frameworks. Health disparities are exacerbated because many healthcare facilities, particularly those in low- and middle-income nations, lack resources to invest in these technologies (Sindhwani et al., 2024). Additionally, preparing medical care experts to utilise and decipher information from IoMT gadgets and simulated intelligence frameworks requires significant exertion and assets, which may not be achievable in asset-obliged settings. Notwithstanding these difficulties, there are various opportunities to scale IoMT and artificial intelligence advancements across different financial settings. A single open door lies in the improvement of reasonable and versatile IoMT arrangements customised for low-asset conditions. Without the need for a lot of infrastructure, innovations such as low-cost wearable sensors and mobile health apps can provide essential health-monitoring capabilities (Affia et al., 2023). For instance, versatile well-being applications that influence artificial intelligence to break down information from essential IoMT gadgets can offer significant well-being bits of knowledge and backing preventive consideration, reducing the weight of medical care offices.

Additionally, public-private partnerships are crucial in overcoming financial obstacles to the expansion of IoMT and AI. These technologies can be funded and implemented in underserved areas through collaboration among governments, nonprofit organisations, and private businesses. According to Varnosfaderani and Forouzanfar (2024), initiatives that concentrate on developing digital health infrastructure and providing healthcare workers with training have the potential to significantly boost the capacity to implement IoMT and AI solutions. Moreover, worldwide associations and improvement offices can support such drivers through awards and specialised help, guaranteeing that headways in medical service innovation benefit a more extensive population. In addition, IoMT systems that are more secure and robust are becoming possible owing to advancements in AI research. For instance, federated learning improves data privacy and security by allowing AI models to be trained across multiple decentralised devices without sharing raw data (Govardanan et al., 2024).

Decision-Making Systems for IoMT Applied to Medical Sensors

The integration of the Internet of Medical Things (IoMT) sensors and decision-making systems is a revolutionary strategy for improving healthcare delivery. These cutting-edge systems use data gathered from a variety of medical sensors to support clinical decisions, enhance patient outcomes, and provide real-time insights. By using man-made intelligence-driven examinations, these frameworks offer remarkable abilities for diagnosing, checking, and treating ailments. Dynamic frameworks in IoMT are intended to handle huge amounts of information created by clinical sensors, such as wearable gadgets, implantable sensors, and remote checking apparatuses. Vital health metrics, such as heart rate, blood pressure, glucose levels, and oxygen saturation, were continuously collected by these sensors and sent to cloud-based platforms for analysis. For instance, electrocardiogram (ECG) sensors in wearable devices such as smartwatches can detect irregular heart rhythms and alert patients and healthcare providers to potential cardiac issues before they become serious (Affia et al., 2023). Such continuous checking and investigation empower opportune intercessions, diminishing the gamble of difficulties and working on tolerant results. Computer-based intelligence-driven dynamic frameworks investigate sensor information using AI calculations to recognise examples and peculiarities that might demonstrate medical problems. Based on individual patient data, these systems can predict disease progression, suggest preventative measures, and recommend customised treatment plans. For example, artificial intelligence calculations can break down glucose levels from consistent glucose screens (CGMs) in diabetic patients, anticipating hyperglycaemic or hypoglycaemic events, and providing suggestions for insulin measurement changes (Govardanan et al., 2024). This degree of accuracy and personalisation in treatment improves patient security and enhances helpful results.

The capacity of AI-driven sensor analysis to enhance clinical decision making through predictive analytics is one of its primary advantages. Based on the historical and current data, predictive models can predict patient outcomes and assist clinicians in making informed decisions regarding patient care. For instance, predictive analytics can be utilised to identify patients who are at a high risk of being readmitted to the hospital. As a result, healthcare providers can implement specific interventions to prevent readmission (Lakhan et al., 2024). These systems help to make healthcare delivery more efficient and effective by anticipating potential health issues. Furthermore, dynamic frameworks for IoMT sensors improve the proficiency of medical care activities by robotising routine errands and providing noteworthy bits of knowledge. Automated systems can continuously monitor patient data and notify healthcare professionals of significant deviations from normal parameters. Healthcare workers are free to concentrate on more challenging and crucial tasks because of this burden reduction. For instance, remote checking frameworks can follow post-careful patient recuperation progress, naturally informing clinical staff of any indications of contamination or intricacies, consequently guaranteeing opportune clinical considerations (Rauniyar et al., 2023). This works on quiet consideration and upgrades the general productivity of medical service offices. Additionally, the development of smart hospitals, in which interconnected systems and devices collaborate to provide seamless and comprehensive patient care, is aided by the integration of AI with IoMT sensors. Shrewd clinic conditions use information from different sources, including IoMT sensors, electronic wellbeing records (EHRs), and imaging frameworks, to create an all-encompassing perspective on quiet wellbeing.

To support clinical workflows, optimise resource allocation, and improve patient outcomes, AI-driven decision-making systems analyse these integrated data. According to Sindhwani et al. (2024), smart infusion pumps can automatically adjust medication dosages based on real-time patient data, ensuring that drugs are delivered accurately and safely. Patient safety and clinical efficacy are enhanced by this level of automation and precision of treatment. The implementation of decision-making systems in IoMT also makes it easier to move toward value-based care, which focuses on lowering healthcare costs, while simultaneously improving patient outcomes. By empowering early discovery and intercession, these frameworks can forestall expensive hospitalisation and entanglement.

In addition, the consistent checking and information examination capacities of IoMT sensors support constant illness for executives, decreasing the requirement for continuous in-person visits and permitting patients to deal with their circumstances at home (Varnosfaderani & Forouzanfar, 2024). Patients' quality of life is enhanced, and healthcare systems are spared from additional strain. In conclusion, sophisticated decision-making systems that use data from IoMT sensors have a significant impact on improving healthcare delivery (Tariq, 2025).

Wearable IoMT Devices for Smart Healthcare

The application of solutions related to wearable devices makes a definite improvement in the concept of smart healthcare, providing constant health tracking and customised patient care and control within the Internet of Medical Things (IoMT). Smartwatches, fitness trackers, implantable sensors, and other similar devices receive and store data regarding the state of a person's health, which means that such a state can be controlled in advance. Being constantly connected, the wearable IoMT devices' main function is real-time health monitoring. Smart watches, for instance, still have sensors for tracking physiological factors, such as heart rate, activity, sleep, and even blood oxygen levels. For instance, the Apple watch, which has an electrocardiogram (ECG) sensor, can detect atrial fibrillation stoke, increasing the risk (Affia et al., 2023). If the device records any abnormality in the heart rate, an alert is raised to the user to warrant a visit to the doctor. Such monitoring is particularly useful for clients with chronic diseases as it will help identify other health complications in a timely manner and seek medical help.

Other components of smart healthcare include the use of smart bands, such as Fitbit and Garmin gadgets. These wearables record the amount of daily motion; thus, they essentially endorse an active lifestyle. Logging the results of the activities carried out in terms of steps, calories, and exercise intensity is crucial in managing weight, cardiovascular diseases, and exercise. Because they involve goal setting and monitoring of activity rates, these devices ensure that individuals become active, change their lifestyle, and hence assist in long-term chronic disease management. Another type of wearable IoMT gadget is implantable sensors, such as implants, which have also displayed promising performance in the supervision of chronic ailments. For instance, continuous glucose monitors (CGMs) are widely used by patients with diabetes to monitor blood glucose levels during the day. Smart CGMs such as Dexcom G6 provide constant glucose values, directionality, and alarm for hyperglycaemia or hypoglycaemia to help the patient adjust their food intake and prescribed insulin (Govardanan et al., 2024). Such an extent of monitoring not only enhances glycaemic regulation but also decreases thresholds for serious diabetic complications.

Again, it is not only in individual healthcare that wearable IoMT devices will be presented but also in other areas of healthcare. For instance, remote patient monitoring (RPM) is an application where wearables play a significant role. RPM technologies help to store information regarding patients' health by wearing a digital device and facilitate the management of patients with chronic diseases through non-face-to-face interactions. For example, patients with heart fallowing can wear devices which will show their heart rate and blood pressure. The gathered information is delivered to the latter to interpret and modify patient care if needed (Lakhan et al., 2024). This form of monitoring is continuous and completely remote; hence, it reduces the number of visits to the hospital, reduces inconvenience to the patients, and enables timely management of any complications. Wearable IoMT devices also play an important role in the prevention of diseases, because possible threats to the health of users can be easily detected before escalating to the entrepreneurial level. For instance, modern wristbands that track sleep may record sleep apnea, which, if untreated, causes hypertension and heart diseases. The identification of these symptoms through wearables allows the user to consult a doctor and make relevant changes in his or her lifestyle to avoid the worsening of such diseases (Rauniyar et al., 2023).

In addition, wearable devices act as key instruments for research and clinical trials, as they offer real and current results of the patient's physiological status. The benefit of these data is especially helpful to researchers who want to compare the impact of a new treatment or intervention. For example, clinical trial wearables applied in cardiovascular medications allow consistent tracking of the participant's heart rate and other essential data, offering an accurate impression of the drug's benefit and side effects (Sindhwani et al., 2024). This constant data collection is even more accurate and extensive than sporadic periodic examinations during clinic visits. There is increasing medical literature evidence demonstrating the effectiveness of wearable IoMT devices in healthcare. For instance, a study in which TG utilised wearable ECG monitors for patients with atrial absorption indicated a decrease in stroke rates (Affia et al., 2023). In another study, patients with diabetes using CGM showed better glycaemic control and fewer hypoglycaemic events (Govardanan et al., 2024). These examples unfathomed the impact of wearable devices in improving patients' quality of life and the efficiency of the provision of health care.

Socio-Economic Challenges of Smart Health Using Generative AI

GA's role in enhancing the functionalities of smart health solutions can be discussed as a revolutionary avenue for change with strong socio-economic implications. These challenges emerge, especially when the focal areas touch on issues such as healthcare facilities, service accessibility, and disparities in accessibility between the developed and developing regions. These concerns are important, especially given that Generative AI is set to infiltrate all sectors of the healthcare system; hence, it becomes relevant to assess the socio-economic impacts that Generative AI must provide fairness to all population groups.

The management of social and economic risks entails identifying several significant issues, one of which is the digital divide. Technological tools for delivering modern healthcare solutions include Generative AI; however, resources such as digital networks and fast internet connectivity are crucial. In many low-income and rural regions, such infrastructure is either lacking or very poor; hence, the availability of sophisticated solutions is restricted. For example, patients in rural areas may not have adequate connectivity to sustain telemedicine solutions or continuous data streaming from IoMT devices, thereby disfranchising these demographics regarding opportunities for smart health innovations (Affia et al., 2023). This digital divide widens health inequalities, and those who are already worst-off such that their health can barely tolerate any further pressure from any angle will be worse off due to their inability to embrace these modern health interventions. Economic hurdles also arise as another factor that affects the fairness of smart health interventions. The generation of web services containing the Generative AI systems and IoMT devices would entail high cost during implementation for understaffed regions. Another hindrance may be the inability of clinics and hospitals located in economically disadvantaged regions to spend time on technology and trainers who can help implement these solutions in practice. This financial limitation does not simply hinder the integration of Av-based healthcare, but also impacts the possible enhancements to patients' health in these societies. For instance, elite city hospitals may have infrastructural provisions to hire state-of-the-art AI diagnosis and individual treatment charts, but they may still be basic healthcare facilities with old-fashioned methodologies in rural areas; therefore, they are likely to deliver vastly different quality of service (Govardanan et al., 2024).

The discussion of the socioeconomic effects of smart health solutions depends on healthcare equality. Generative AI holds the possibility of changing how patient-specific treatment is applied because of a patient's unique genetics and medical background. However, the issue that has emerged due to these is essential is the distribution of these benefits fairly. Patients living in developed areas or areas that can afford more premium health insurance are privileged to receive advanced treatment, while those in underdeveloped areas receive less treatment. This has the potential to widen the gap with one side of society, benefiting from advanced technology in the management of diseases, while the other side continues to die from easily preventable and manageable diseases (Sindhwani et al., 2024).

It is apparent that another socioeconomic challenge is the job threat. This poses the threat of displacing some of the human personnel in the healthcare sector, especially those whose duties are to engage in repetitive work, such as data entry duties or initial evaluation of patients. This could be costly, especially for communities in which employment in the health sector is the main source of income. For example, if the AI systems assume the responsibility of carrying out radiological assessments, then many radiologists and other related personnel are likely to lose their jobs, resulting in more unemployment and strain on families and costs within the economy (Lakhan et al., 2024). Another determinant is the culture and society of community users, where smart health technologies are adapted to the provision of care. There may be some regions that may not embrace artificial intelligence health because of negative attitudes towards the use of technology or because of conventional medicine. This resistance manifests itself in the form of culture and can hinder the uptake of useful technologies as well as their potential economic influence. Challenges of these barriers include the failure to realise the potential of smart health solutions, especially for the mentioned communities; learning and building trust within these communities is key to overcoming such barriers to attain the intended benefits of all the relevant stakeholders (Rauniyar et al., 2023).

Nevertheless, this chapter identified the possibilities of reducing the socioeconomic effects of smart health solutions. More emphasis can be placed on closing the gap for the discordance and provision of quality healthcare technology solutions and access to the communities experiencing disparities through policy intercessions and focused funding. International organizations and governments can substantially contribute to developing the necessary infrastructure and subsidising the implementation of Generative AI in zones with low coverage. For instance, general schemes that support the availability of affordable or even free Internet connections in rural zones will improve the applicability of telemedicine and other distant health checkouts (Affia et al., 2023). In addition, engaging technology developers, healthcare service providers, and community-based organizations may help enhance implementation strategy inclusiveness. Adaptive solutions suitable for specialised population types as well as addressing the cultural components and making the solutions easily available would go a long way to mitigate socioeconomic issues. For example, communicating and solving artificial intelligence (AI) health applications in different languages and in consideration of cultural barriers increases its acceptance level and usage among various groups (Sindhwani et al., 2024).

Ethical Implications of AI-Driven Healthcare Decision-Making

Healthcare is one of the areas that benefits most from AI, as it has great potential for enhancing patients' quality of life, making clinical processes more efficient, and reducing expenses. Nevertheless, it also brings about great ethical issues that need to be discussed and solved. Issues involved in bias, patient self-determination, and consent can also be categorised among the available concerns. It is crucial to create sound ethical principles and protocols to help regulate AI and IOMT systems to ensure appropriateness in the medical setting and fairness in others. This chapter evaluates several ethical issues regarding the use of Artificial Intelligence in the health sector: whistle blower, bias, and conflicts of interest rank high. AI systems can improve their performance by learning from the data given to them; consequently, if the datasets input to such systems are tainted by bias, any AI that operates on the data will expound the bias. For instance, if an AI diagnostic tool is trained on a specific set of patient data, it will likely yield poor results for patients with different demographics. This can lead to misdiagnoses or the recommendation of an improper course of action for underrepresented patients (Sindhwani et al.,

2024). To counteract this, diverse gender-balanced datasets must be used to train AI, and these algorithms need to be updated to provide equal performance across genders for all patients.

Self-determination by the patient is another conflict of ethical principles that is evident in healthcare. The use of Artificial Intelligence in healthcare decision-making can be a way to marginalise patients in their own treatment processes. For example, the use of AI makes it possible to prescribe a course of treatment based on statistics and risk factors that do not consider the patient's desires, beliefs, or situations. Thus, it is crucial to consider that patients must remain in control of their treatment choices. This offers them understandable information about the use of AI in their care and allows them to engage the doctor in questioning or enhancing AI recommendations (Lakhan et al., 2024).

Thus, informed consent is closely connected with the concept of patient autonomy and is considered one of the primary ethical principles in medicine. Finally, another interaction between AI and human life, specifically in the healthcare domain, is the enhancement of the already problematic informed consent process. It was discussed that patients should be informed not only of the usual consequences of the decision on the choice of therapy but also about the involvement of AI systems in the process. This encompasses knowledge on how their data are utilised in the AI processes, the process that the AI adopts in arriving at a conclusion, and the limitations and uncertainties inherent in the AI's recommendations. Thus, it is vital to make this information easily available and understandable to maintain patients' trust in their physicians and to let the patients make informed decisions regarding their health (Govardanan et al., 2024). Several frameworks and guidelines have been proposed to address these ethical issues. The framework focuses on so many principles such as openness, responsibility, and equity. Transparency is achieved when the operations and decisions of AI systems are understandable and accessible to patients and caregivers. This can be achieved with the help of explainable AI (XAI) tools and methodologies that show how decisions arrive. Accountability ensures that there is a way of pointing out that something is wrong and is a way of correcting the system if it has distorted information about certain aspects or groups. This may include the execution of frequent audits and cooperation with bodies supervising the performance and application of AI in healthcare facilities (Sindhwani et al., 2024).

Another essential principle is fairness, which entails efforts to eradicate unfairness in AI systems as well as the striving for equal availability of the effects of AI solutions in the healthcare sphere. These may involve things like using other datasets apart from the traditional ones to train the AI models, engaging the stakeholder's groups, and providing extra services and facilities to the minority groups to ensure they benefit from the AI in health care (Rauniyar et al., 2023). However, some guidelines have not been provided, such as data privacy and security. Many IoMT devices and AI systems deal with elevated volumes of sensitive health data. It must be noted that these data are likely to attract several attempts at breach; therefore, any measure that can prevent breaching of this data must be adopted. Measures necessary in a program to protect patient data include implementing strong data encryption, access controls, and periodic assessment for security risks. In addition, patients should be made aware of how their data is used and have rights and control over data confidentiality and privileges (Affia et al., 2023).

IoMT-Enabled Healthcare Infrastructure in Resource-Constrained Settings

IoMT, which is the connection of medical devices through the Internet, has the potential to change healthcare delivery, especially in developing countries. Opportunely, such a conception as IoMT indicates promising opportunities for introducing improvements to important aspects of healthcare, such as availability, quality, and effectiveness. This section details possible ways of applying IoMT solutions, particularly in regions with few resources, and considers how such solutions can compensate for the absent healthcare dependencies. Another solution aimed at the efficient implementation of IoMT solutions in regions with limited access to resources is the use of affordable and simple devices. Portable and wearable IoMT devices, smartwatches, mobile health (mHealth) applications, and remote monitoring sensors can be provided to patients in remote areas for constant health checks without multiple hospital visits. For instance, in rural areas of India, mobile health units connected with IoMT devices have helped in the management of chronic illnesses such as diabetes and hypertension-sparing patient trips over long distances for healthcare facilities (Lakhan et al., 2024). Another efficient approach, in this case, is the connectivity of IoMT with telemedicine platforms. Telemedicine coupled with IoMT can provide real-time insights of the patient to healthcare providers, which assists them in making decisions remotely. This is especially important when there is a general lack of hospitals, and any form of specialised treatment is a luxury that most cannot afford. For instance, in the regions of Sub-Saharan Africa, telemedicine services involving IoMT gadgets have been applied to treat infectious diseases, such as tuberculosis and HIV/AIDS. Remote monitoring gadgets are used to ensure patient compliance with regimes and check their vitals, while teleconsultations make it easy for healthcare professionals to review patients' plans and tweak them if necessary (Govardanan et al., 2024).

The challenges associated with the use of IoMT are Power source, weak internet connection, and weak internet connectivity. Solving these issues requires the integration of new strategies for the utilisation of solar-powered IoMT devices and low-bandwidth communication methods. Solar-powered health monitoring devices for patients' health help provide continuous monitoring of health care even in places with little assurance of power supply. Furthermore, employing technologies that consume low bandwidth, such as LoRaWAN, can help in passing health information from the far reaches of the world to central health information systems (Affia et al., 2023). In addition, IoMT reduces healthcare disparities because it strengthens the capacity of CHWs. Currently, CHWs are regarded as the mainstay of PHC implementation in a myriad of resource-limited environments. Supplying them with IoMT devices will transform them into providing adequate care to their clients. For example, in Kenya, CHWs with portable phones and diagnostic devices such as malaria and anaemia diagnosis screens have been able to cover various geographical regions. The collected data are channelled to central health facilities for analysis to detect diseases at an early stage (Sindhwani et al., 2024). IoMT has the potential to enhance health outcomes by making decisions easier and allocating resources based on the data. In asset-compelled settings, medical care assets are often restricted and should be apportioned effectively. IoMT gadgets create enormous volumes of well-being information that can be examined to recognise patterns, anticipate flare-ups, and designate assets where they are generally required. For instance, IoMT-enabled surveillance systems have been utilised in several low-income nations during the COVID-19 pandemic to track infection rates and oversee the distribution of medical supplies and personnel (Rauniyar et al., 2023). IoMT deployment in resource-constrained settings requires community involvement and training. Nearby people should be associated with the preparation and execution of IoMT tasks to guarantee that they meet the requirements and social settings of the population. Preparing programs for medical care suppliers and patients using the most proficient method to utilise IoMT gadgets can upgrade the reception and effect of these innovations. In Ethiopia, people group well-being programs that remembered preparing for IoMT gadgets for maternal and younger well-being have prompted huge enhancements in pre-birth and post-pregnancy care (Sindhwani et al., 2024). Overall, IoMT offers groundbreaking potential for further development of medical care in asset-compelled settings. Systems, for example, sending savvy gadgets, coordinating IoMT with telemedicine, tending to network difficulties, enabling local area well-being labourers, working in an information-driven direction, and drawing in nearby networks can assist with crossing over medical care holes and improve well-being results in underserved regions. IoMT has the potential to play a pivotal role in achieving global health equity and ensuring that even communities with the fewest resources have access to high-quality health care.

CONCLUSION

The combination of the Web of Clinical Things (IoMT) and generative man-made intelligence holds groundbreaking potential for worldwide medical care. The delivery of healthcare, diagnostics, patient management, and personalised medicine that these technologies promise to revolutionise Generative AI uses connected devices for continuous monitoring and data collection, and IoMT uses these data to build sophisticated models that can predict diseases, tailor treatment plans, and speed up drug discovery. Together, they have the potential to make healthcare more effective, accurate, and accessible, particularly in settings with limited resources. IoMT applications are currently having huge effects in different medical care settings, from wearable gadgets that screen persistent circumstances to telemedicine stages that provide distant discussions.

In underserved communities, where traditional healthcare infrastructure may be lacking, these innovations are bridging gaps in healthcare delivery. For instance, in rustic regions, versatile wellbeing units furnished with IoMT gadgets have diminished the requirement for patients to travel significant distances for normal check-ups, while telemedicine administration has empowered the far-off administration of irresistible illnesses. Be that as it may, the arrangement of IoMT and Generative man-made intelligence in medical care presents additional difficulties, especially concerning protection, security, and moral contemplations. Data breaches and unauthorised access pose serious concerns when large amounts of sensitive health data are collected and analysed. Furthermore, the potential for predisposition to computer-based intelligence calculations, the gamble of subverting patient independence, and the intricacies of informed assent require cautious thought and powerful moral structures.

Methodologies to resolve these issues incorporate assorted datasets for preparing artificial intelligence models, guaranteeing straightforwardness and responsibility in the direction of computer-based intelligence, and executing rigid information security measures. Enhancing the security of IoMT devices, developing ethical guidelines that address the unique challenges posed by these technologies, and developing AI models that are more inclusive, and representative should be the primary focuses of future research. Policymakers should attempt to create administrative structures that guarantee protected and enhanced utilisation of IoMT and Generative simulated intelligence in medical services. This includes supporting the implementation of these technologies in environments with limited resources, and establishing standards for data privacy, security, and AI transparency. Patients should be educated about the advantages and disadvantages of IoMT and AI tools, and healthcare providers should be trained in their use. Local area commitment is fundamental for the effective execution of these advances, guaranteeing that they meet the necessities and social settings of the populace they serve.

Furthermore, progressing the checking and assessment of IoMT and computer-based intelligence applications in medical care can help distinguish and resolve any arising issues, guaranteeing that these advancements will proceed to develop and get to the next level. In conclusion, the application of IoMT and Generative AI to healthcare presents great potential for enhancing patient care, enhancing health outcomes, and reducing access disparities to healthcare. We can maximise their benefits and create a healthcare system that is more equitable and effective by addressing the difficulties and ethical considerations associated with these technologies and encouraging collaboration among researchers, policymakers, healthcare providers, and communities. Utilising these cutting-edge technologies to provide everyone with personalised, data-driven, and accessible healthcare is key to the industry's future success.

REFERENCES

Affia, A. A. O., Finch, H., Jung, W., Samori, I. A., Potter, L., & Palmer, X. L. (2023). IoT health devices: Exploring security risks in the connected landscape. *IoT*, 4(2), 150–182. DOI: 10.3390/iot4020009

Aftab, M., Nadeem, A., Zhang, C., Dong, Z., Jiang, Y., & Liu, K. (2024). Advancements and challenges in artificial intelligence applications in healthcare delivery systems.

Alalawi, S., Alalawi, M., & Alrae, R. (2024, August). Privacy preservation for the IoMT using federated learning and blockchain technologies. In *The International Conference on Innovations in Computing Research* (pp. 713-731). Cham: Springer Nature Switzerland. DOI: 10.1007/978-3-031-65522-7_62

Azrour, M., Mabrouki, J., Guezzaz, A., Ahmad, S., Khan, S., & Benkirane, S. (Eds.). (2024). *IoT, machine learning and data analytics for smart healthcare*. CRC Press.

Gou, F., Liu, J., Xiao, C., & Wu, J. (2024). Research on artificial-intelligence-assisted medicine: A survey on medical artificial intelligence. *Diagnostics (Basel)*, 14(14), 1472. DOI: 10.3390/diagnostics14141472 PMID: 39061610

Govardanan, C. S., Murugan, R., Yenduri, G., Gurrammagari, D. R., Bhulakshmi, D., Kandati, D. R., ... & Jhaveri, R. H. (2024). The amalgamation of federated learning and explainable artificial intelligence for the Internet of Medical Things: A review. *Recent Advances in Computer Science and Communications (Formerly: Recent Patents on Computer Science)*, 17(4), 1-19.

Gupta, P., Ding, B., Guan, C., & Ding, D. (2024). Generative AI: A systematic review using topic modelling techniques. *Data and Information Management*, 8(2), 100066. DOI: 10.1016/j.dim.2024.100066

Husnain, A., Rasool, S., Saeed, A., Gill, A. Y., & Hussain, H. K. (2023). AI'S healing touch: Examining machine learning's transformative effects on healthcare. *Journal of Wood Science*, 2(10), 1681–1695.

İncegil, D., Kayral, İ. H., & Şenel, F. Ç. (2023). The new era: Transforming healthcare quality with artificial intelligence. In *Algorithmic discrimination and ethical perspective of artificial intelligence* (pp. 183–202). Springer Nature Singapore.

Khang, A. (Ed.). (2024). *AI-driven innovations in digital healthcare: Emerging trends, challenges, and applications: Emerging trends, challenges, and applications*.

Lakhan, A., Hamouda, H., Abdulkareem, K. H., Alyahya, S., & Mohammed, M. A. (2024). Digital healthcare framework for patients with disabilities based on deep federated learning schemes. *Computers in Biology and Medicine*, 169, 107845. DOI: 10.1016/j.compbiomed.2023.107845 PMID: 38118307

Lilhore, U. K., Simaiya, S., Poongodi, M., & Dutt, V. (Eds.). (2024). *Federated learning and privacy-preserving in healthcare AI*. IGI Global. DOI: 10.4018/979-8-3693-1874-4

Maleki Varnosfaderani, S., & Forouzanfar, M. (2024). The role of AI in hospitals and clinics: Transforming healthcare in the 21st century. *Bioengineering (Basel, Switzerland)*, 11(4), 337. DOI: 10.3390/bioengineering11040337 PMID: 38671759

Marengo, A. (2023). The future of AI in IoT: Emerging trends in intelligent data analysis and privacy protection.

Marima, R., Mtshali, N., Phillips, P., Molefi, T., Khanyile, R., Mbita, Z., & Dlamini, Z. (2023). Health informatics applications in healthcare and society 5.0. In *Society 5.0 and next generation healthcare: Patient-focused and technology-assisted precision therapies* (pp. 31–49). Springer Nature Switzerland. DOI: 10.1007/978-3-031-36461-7_2

Mathur, S., Bhattacharjee, S., Sehgal, S., & Shekhar, R. (2024). Role of artificial intelligence and internet of things in neurodegenerative diseases. In *AI and neuro-degenerative diseases: Insights and solutions* (pp. 35–62). Springer Nature Switzerland. DOI: 10.1007/978-3-031-53148-4_2

McDonnell, K. J. (2023). Leveraging the academic artificial intelligence ecosystem to advance the community oncology enterprise. *Journal of Clinical Medicine*, 12(14), 4830. DOI: 10.3390/jcm12144830 PMID: 37510945

Omidian, H. (2024). Synergizing blockchain and artificial intelligence to enhance healthcare. *Drug Discovery Today*, 29(9), 104111. DOI: 10.1016/j.drudis.2024.104111 PMID: 39034026

Patruni, M. R., & Humayun, A. G. (2024). PPAM-mIoMT: A privacy-preserving authentication with device verification for securing healthcare systems in 5G networks. *International Journal of Information Security*, 23(1), 679–698. DOI: 10.1007/s10207-023-00762-3

Prithivraj, S., Lighittha, P. R., & Priya, L. (2024, April). Privacy preservation and confidentiality assurance in critical healthcare networks: Navigating complex data challenges within. In *Conference Proceedings: Encryptcon-An International Research Conference on CyberSecurity* (p. 10). Shashwat Publication.

Putra, K. T., Arrayyan, A. Z., Hayati, N., Damarjati, C., Bakar, A., & Chen, H. C. (2024). A review on the application of Internet of Medical Things in wearable personal health monitoring: A cloud-edge artificial intelligence approach. *IEEE Access : Practical Innovations, Open Solutions*, 12, 21437–21452. DOI: 10.1109/ACCESS.2024.3358827

Rahman, A., Debnath, T., Kundu, D., Khan, M. S. I., Aishi, A. A., Sazzad, S., Sayduzzaman, M., & Band, S. S. (2024). Machine learning and deep learning-based approach in smart healthcare: Recent advances, applications, challenges and opportunities. *AIMS Public Health*, 11(1), 58–109. DOI: 10.3934/publichealth.2024004 PMID: 38617415

Rajawat, A. S., Goyal, S. B., Bedi, P., Jan, T., Whaiduzzaman, M., & Prasad, M. (2023). Quantum machine learning for security assessment on the Internet of Medical Things (IoMT). *Future Internet*, 15(8), 271. DOI: 10.3390/fi15080271

Rauniyar, A., Hagos, D. H., Jha, D., Håkegård, J. E., Bagci, U., Rawat, D. B., & Vlassov, V. (2023). Federated learning for medical applications: A taxonomy, current trends, challenges, and future research directions. *IEEE Internet of Things Journal*.

Sachin, D. N., Annappa, B., & Ambesange, S. (2024). Federated learning for digital healthcare: Concepts, applications, frameworks, and challenges. *Computing*, 106(9), 1–38. DOI: 10.1007/s00607-024-01317-7

Saudagar, A. K. J., Kumar, A., & Khan, M. B. (2024). Mediverse beyond boundaries: A comprehensive analysis of AR and VR integration in medical education for diverse abilities. *Journal of Disability Research*, 3(1), 20230066. DOI: 10.57197/JDR-2023-0066

Sindhwani, N., Tanwar, S., Rana, A., & Kannan, R. (Eds.). (2024). *Smart technologies in healthcare management: Pioneering trends and applications*. CRC Press. DOI: 10.1201/9781003330523

Srivastava, J., Routray, S., Ahmad, S., & Waris, M. M. (2022). Internet of Medical Things (IoMT)-based smart healthcare system: Trends and progress.

Tariq, M. U. (2024). Integration of IoMT for Enhanced Healthcare: Sleep Monitoring, Body Movement Detection, and Rehabilitation Evaluation. In Liu, H., Tripathy, R., & Bhattacharya, P. (Eds.), *Clinical Practice and Unmet Challenges in AI-Enhanced Healthcare Systems* (pp. 70–95). IGI Global., DOI: 10.4018/979-8-3693-2703-6.ch004

Tariq, M. U. (2024). Social Innovations for Improving Healthcare. In Chandan, H. (Ed.), *Social Innovations in Education, Environment, and Healthcare* (pp. 302–317). IGI Global., DOI: 10.4018/979-8-3693-2569-8.ch015

Tariq, M. U. (2024). Application of blockchain and Internet of Things (IoT) in modern business. In Sinha, M., Bhandari, A., Priya, S., & Kabiraj, S. (Eds.), *Future of customer engagement through marketing intelligence* (pp. 66–94). IGI Global., DOI: 10.4018/979-8-3693-2367-0.ch004

Tariq, M. U. (2024). AI and IoT in flood forecasting and mitigation: A comprehensive approach. In Ouaissa, M., Ouaissa, M., Boulouard, Z., Iwendi, C., & Krichen, M. (Eds.), *AI and IoT for proactive disaster management* (pp. 26–60). IGI Global., DOI: 10.4018/979-8-3693-3896-4.ch003

Tariq, M. U. (2025). The Belmont Report: Guiding Ethical Principles in Human Research. In Throne, R. (Ed.), *IRB, Human Research Protections, and Data Ethics for Researchers* (pp. 245–268). IGI Global Scientific Publishing., DOI: 10.4018/979-8-3693-3848-3.ch010

Tariq, M. U., & Sergio, R. P. (2025). Nurturing Digital Citizenship in Society 5.0 Through AI and Computational Intelligence Education. In Pandey, R., Srivastava, N., Prasad, R., Prasad, J., & Garcia, M. (Eds.), *Open AI and Computational Intelligence for Society 5.0* (pp. 59–84). IGI Global Scientific Publishing., DOI: 10.4018/979-8-3693-4326-5.ch003

Ullah, I., Khan, I. U., Ouaissa, M., Ouaissa, M., & El Hajjami, S. (Eds.). (2024). *Future communication systems using artificial intelligence, internet of things and data science*. CRC Press. DOI: 10.1201/9781032648309

Vishwakarma, V. K. (2024). Navigating challenges and unlocking opportunities: The convergence of IoT and AI in India.

KEY TERMS AND DEFINITIONS

Internet of Medical Things (IoMT): A network of interconnected medical devices and software that collect, analyse, and transmit health data in real time to improve healthcare delivery.

Generative AI: Advanced machine learning systems capable of creating new content, making predictions, and deriving insights from vast datasets for applications such as diagnostics and drug discovery.

Personalized Medicine: Tailored medical treatment and care designed for individual patients based on their unique clinical data and genetic profiles.

Real-Time Data Analysis: The immediate processing and interpretation of data collected by IoMT devices to support timely clinical decision-making.

Ethical AI: The application of artificial intelligence in a manner that upholds principles of fairness, transparency, autonomy, and data privacy in healthcare settings.

Chapter 23
Transformative Insights:
Integrating IoMT With Generative AI for Personalized Medicine and Drug Discovery

Hina Bansal
https://orcid.org/0000-0003-1683-1581
Amity University, Noida, India

Banashree Bondhopadhyay
https://orcid.org/0000-0002-6679-7791
Amity Institute of Biotechnology, Amity University, Noida, India

Seneha Santoshi
https://orcid.org/0000-0001-8893-2221
Amity Institute of Biotechnology, Amity University, Noida, India

Himansu
https://orcid.org/0009-0007-9553-8020
Amity University, Noida, India

Rajbeen Mazumder
https://orcid.org/0009-0003-7791-1558
Amity University, Noida, India

ABSTRACT

The rapid increase of generative AI aligned with IoMT promotes the medical and healthcare industry with its numerous applications such as in precision medicine (PM), drug discovery, disease diagnosis, etc. In the past decade, acceptance of AI remoulded the ongoing innovations in the medical industry. As the world grapples with chronic illnesses and lifestyle disorders burdening hospitals and clinics, AI succors by lessening the load. Nevertheless, its limitations like data security and privacy are a cause for worry. IoMT consists of a sensor, or wearable connected via the internet to the data recorder. This chapter attempts to comprehend the goals, outcome, future perspective, and tribulations of alignment of Generative AI with IoMT. The integration of Generative AI and IoMT in healthcare offers transformative outcomes, including enhanced diagnostic accuracy through precise and timely analyses. These innovations promise better outcomes and greater efficiency, but it's essential to prioritize ethics, protect

DOI: 10.4018/979-8-3693-6180-1.ch023

patient data, and ensure compliance as they become part of everyday care.

INTRODUCTION

Convergence of two cutting- edge innovations in health and medicine nowadays—the AI and IoMT Manufactured Insights—promises to be revolutionary in its outcome, well-balanced to reset understanding care and healthcare deliverance frameworks. The integration of IoMT and Generative AI symbolizes an urgent crossroads in restorative advancement, exuding incomparable openings for modifying demonstrative preciseness, customize treatment modalities, and aligning healthcare operations. (Zhang & Kamel Boulos, 2023).

The utilize of innovation in healthcare, frequently alluded to as healthtech or computerized wellbeing. It includes a wide extent of apparatuses, frameworks, and advancements to outline and stride the understanding care, streamline forms, upgrade productivity, and also develop restorative investigation. IoMT envelops an organization where therapeutic gadgets, sensors, and frameworks are interconnected to gather and transmit wellbeing information. This arrange encourages farther checking, determination, and treatment. Gadgets inside IoMT run from wearable wellness trackers to implantable therapeutic gadgets and shrewd healing center hardware. Generative AI includes calculations, competent of producing modern information, pictures, or substance by learning designs from existing information. In healthcare, generative AI is utilized for errands like therapeutic picture era, sedate revelation, and personalized treatment proposals (N. Tommarello et al. 2024).

The combination of Generative AI and IoMT extends much prospective across various medical industries. By joining IoMT devices with Generative AI algorithms, healthcare professionals and clinicians will be able to take the benefit of analytics in real-time information to achieve high demonstrative precision, minimal personalized treatment methods, and optimize healthcare operations. Moreover, this integration encourages patients to engage actively in their healthcare journey, furthermore towards preventive and proactive healthcare standards (Kannan, 2023). The current chapter will loiter around the tribulations, moral considerations and related disputes adjoining the integration of generative AI and IoMT in healthcare. It tries to expand on how this convergence modified the face of precision medicine and drug discovery by assessment of the amalgation, surveying the coordinated effect, analyzing the enhancement of healthcare workflow and moral and administrative contemplations with customer engagement and empowerment. It also enlightens the future perspective and challenges.

The blending of IoMT and Generative AI in healthcare speaks to the integration of real-time wellbeing information from IoMT gadgets with progressed AI calculations. These calculations can create significant bits of knowledge, expectations, and personalized mediations. This merging engages healthcare suppliers to utilize broad quiet information to upgrade determination precision, make inventive medicines, and streamline healthcare conveyance forms.

Objective

The point of examining the merging of IoMT and Generative AI in healthcare is to pick up a comprehensive understanding of the suggestions, openings, and challenges inborn in this combination. The objective is to bring together Generative AI and the Internet of Medical Things (IoMT) to make healthcare smarter and more efficient. By combining AI's ability to analyze data and generate insights with IoMT's real-time monitoring and connectivity, we can provide more accurate diagnoses, predict health issues earlier, and support doctors in making faster decisions. This approach also helps reduce administrative work, allowing healthcare providers to focus more on patients. At its core, this integration aims to create a connected and reliable healthcare system that prioritizes patient care with various applications, addresses ethical considerations, other limitations and meets all necessary regulations. Through a deliberate examination, the goals include:

- **Assessment of Integration Achievability:** Survey the specialized practicality and potential points of interest of amalgamating IoMT gadgets with Generative AI calculations inside healthcare situations.
- **Examination of Clinical Affect:** Investigate the coordinate consequences on clinical workflows, understanding care forms, and restorative comes about emerging from the amalgamation of IoMT and Generative AI advances.
- **Investigation of Upgraded Healthcare Streamlining:** Scrutinize how the merging streamlines healthcare operations, including conclusion, treatment arranging, and asset allotment, driving to increased operational productivity and cost-effectiveness.
- **Examination of Personalized Pharmaceutical Openings:** Test the potential for leveraging IoMT-derived information and Generative AI analytics to customize treatment methodologies, refine helpful intercessions, and lift understanding results through exactness pharmaceutical techniques.

GENERATIVE AI

Generative AI is a subset of hoax insights techniques that are adhered on creating new information and substance determined from designs and existing data. Inside the healthcare space, Generative AI algorithms have high potency in ability to look through large persistent data to forecast result, observe designs, and keep up clinical decision-making processes (Sai et al., 2024). Figure 1 is Illustrating the various types of Generative AI.

Figure 1. Types of generative AI

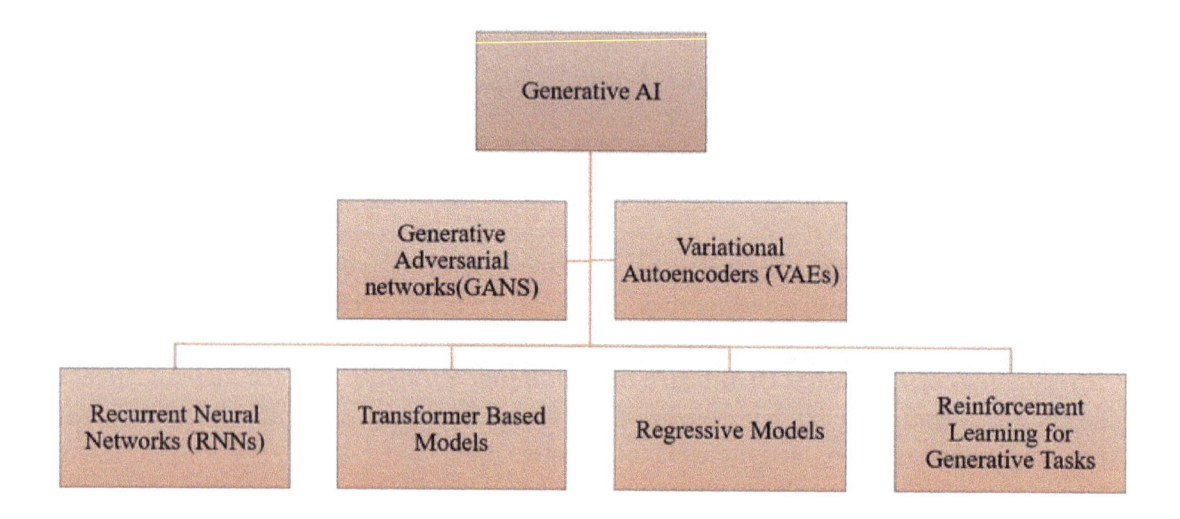

Generative Adversarial Networks (GANS)

GANs are a course of machine learning systems outlined for producing manufactured information through a one-of-a-kind competitive handle including two neural systems: the generator; and the discriminator. The generator is capable of creating engineered information, which can incorporate pictures, content, or sound. It begins with arbitrary clamour and changes this clamour into information that mirrors real-world tests. The generator's essential objective is to form information that's so reasonable that it can hoodwink the discriminator into considering it honest to goodness.

Discriminator on the other hand, acts as a classifier. Its assignment is to assess information and decide whether it is genuine (credibility check) or unreal (generated by the creator). The differentiator acquires skill in distinguishing unobtrusive contrasts between the genuine and manufactured information, making stride its precision over time.

The interaction between these two systems is associated to an amusement where both players ceaselessly upgrade their methodologies. The generator tries to deliver superior and more practical information to defeat the discriminator, whereas the discriminator gets way better at identifying the fake information produced by the generator. This continuous competition drives both systems to move forward (Wenzel M,2013).

Variational Autoencoders (VAEs)

(VAEs) are generative models that encrypts input information into a lower-dimensional idle space and translate it to reproduce the initial information. Not at all like conventional autoencoders, VAEs learn probabilistic representations, empowering them to produce modern samples from the learned dispersion. The method begins with an encoder that changes the input information into an idle space representation, regularly taking after a Gaussian conveyance.

The decoder at that point remakes the input information from the idle factors. By optimizing both the encoder and decoder, VAEs precisely replicate input information whereas keeping up an important inactive space. This permits VAEs to create unused information tests that take after the preparing information but are not indistinguishable to any particular occurrence.

VAEs are especially profitable in picture era, making modern pictures by inspecting and interpreting idle factors. They are moreover connected to content and sound era, creating coherent and important yields. In general, VAEs are effective instruments for encoding, reproducing and creating information over different areas (Singh A et al.2021).

Autoregressive Models

Autoregressive models (AM) are a lesson of generative models that make information consecutively, one component at a time, whereas considering already produced components. This step-by-step prepare guarantees each modern component adjusts relevantly with the past ones, making the arrangement coherent. The centre rule is foreseeing the likelihood of another component based on prior components utilizing conditional likelihood. In content era, models like GPT (Generative Pre-trained Transformer) anticipate the following word or character based on the starting input, overhauling the arrangement iteratively. Autoregressive models depend intensely on preparing information to memorize designs and structures, empowering them to produce arrangements that reflect the subtleties of the preparing information. They exceed expectations in characteristic dialect preparing, making coherent and relevantly fitting substance, and have applications in picture era and music composition. Their capacity to conditionally produce components based on earlier setting makes them imperative in progressing AI and machine learning (Burant CJ,2022).

Recurrent Neural Networks (RNNs)

RNNs are specialized neural networks that draw plans to grasp sequential data, and speech recognition, enabling them ideal for errands like natural language processing, and time-series analysis. RNNs keeps a concealed state that apprehends information about preceding element in an order, enabling them to use pertinent past information for errands such as time series forecasting and language modelling. In generative tasks, RNNs predict the succeeding element in an order based on preceding element. For example, in text generation, an RNN predicts the next character or word in a sentence, iteratively generating coherent text from an initial input (Das S et al.2023). However, RNNs face challenges with long sequences due to the vanishing gradient problem, where gradients become very small during training, hindering the network's ability to learn long-range dependencies. To address this, advanced RNN variants like Long Short-Term Memory (LSTM) networks and Gated Recurrent Units (GRUs) were developed.

LSTMs introduce gates—input, forget, and output gates—that regulate information flow, allowing important information to be retained over long periods while discarding irrelevant data. This structure helps LSTMs capture long-range dependencies effectively.

GRUs simplify the LSTM architecture by combining the input and forget gates into a single update gate and using a reset gate to control the influence of the previous hidden state. This reduces computational complexity while still managing long-term dependencies and mitigating the vanishing gradient problem.

Both LSTMs and GRUs have proven effective in applications like language modelling, speech recognition, machine translation, and time-series prediction, making them valuable tools for advanced generative models and sequence-based tasks (Das S et al.2023).

Transformer Based Models

Transformers, exemplified by models just like the GPT arrangement, have revolutionized NLP (Natural Language Programme) and generative errands. Their ubiquity stems from a few key developments and capabilities that set them separated from prior models like RNNs Table1is representing the application of NLP and Generative Errands.

Table 1. Applications of NLP and generative errands

S.No.	Feature	Description
1	Content Era	Models like GPT-3 produce extensive, coherent, and meaningful content, valuable for writing, narrating, and content creation.
2	Machine Interpretation	Transformers record nexus connections among words in various languages, controlling state-of-the-art interpretation frameworks.
3	Summarization	They condense long reports into brief summaries while retaining key information and context
4	Address Replying	Transformers understand and generate detailed responses to complex queries by considering the full context of the input.8
5	Assumption Examination	They analyse content to determine sentiment, useful in areas like social media monitoring and customer feedback analysis.
6	The GPT Arrangement	Developed by OpenAI, these models are pre-trained on vast amounts of text data and fine-tuned for specific tasks. GPT-3, with 175 billion parameters, generates human-like text that is relevant and coherent over long passages.

Features and Working of TBM

1. **Consideration Instruments:**

Consideration instrument presents at the centre of Transformers, especially for self-attention. It permits to weigh the significance of distinctive components in an arrangement relative to each other and enabling it to consider the complete setting while making expectations. Unlike RNNs, which prepare arrangements step-by-step and battle with long-term conditions, self-attention calculates weights (consideration scores) that measure the centrality of each word to each other word within the arrangement (Zhang S et al.2023).

2. **Parallelization:**

Transformers, moreover, have a parallelizable design. Unlike RNNs, which handle arrangements consecutively, Transformers handle all components of a grouping at the same time. The self-attention component makes this conceivable, permitting proficient computation on present-day equipment like GPUs and TPUs. This parallelization radically speeds up preparation times, making it attainable to prepare on expansive datasets.

3. **Taking Care of Long Groupings:**

Transformers exceed expectations at taking care of long groupings by capturing long-range conditions through self-attention. Whereas RNNs endure from the vanishing slope issue, making it hard to learn long-term conditions, Transformers keep up the setting of the complete arrangement all through handling. Typically, significant for errands like content era, where keeping up coherence and setting over long entries is basic.

Reinforcement Learning for Generative Tasks

Reinforcement Learning has shown its strength and flexibility in integrating human preconceptions from a variety of perspectives, including contradictory learning, main rules, and learned reward models, to create a more effective model. It has also served as a competitive option to introduce new training signals by developing new objectives that utilize new signals. As a result, reinforcement learning has emerged as a trending research area and challenged the limitations of generative AI in both model conception and deployment (Table 2). Transformers, exemplified by models just like the GPT arrangement, have revolutionized characteristic dialect preparing (NLP) and generative errands. Their ubiquity stems from a few key developments and capabilities that set them separated from prior models like RNNs (Korshunova M et al.2022).

Table 2. Depiction of reinforcement learning for generative AI

S.No.	Aspect	Description
1	Agent and Environment Interaction	In RL, an agent takes actions in an environment to achieve a goal. For generative tasks, actions involve generating data samples (e.g., text, images, music). Environment provides feedback/rewards based on the quality of generated samples.
2	Reward Mechanism	Crucial for guiding the learning process - In text generation, rewards can be based on user feedback, grammatical correctness, coherence, or relevance. Designing an appropriate reward function is essential.
3	Applications in Text Generation	Notable application of RL in generative tasks. Traditional text generation models can be fine-tuned using RL to produce contextually appropriate and user-aligned text. Example: Chatbots improving responses through user interactions.

continued on following page

Table 2. Continued

S.No.	Aspect	Description
4	Other Applications	Applied to image synthesis, music composition, game level generation. In each case, the agent learns to produce content meeting certain quality or novelty criteria. - Example: RL refining details in generated images.
5	Challenges and Advancements	RL offers powerful mechanisms for improving generative models but also presents challenges (e.g., need for high-quality feedback, computational complexity). - Ongoing research aims to develop more efficient algorithms and explore new applications.

INTERNET OF MEDICAL THINGS (IoMT)

The Internet of Medical Things (IoMT) merges widespread connectivity, communication and working out with ambient intelligence, creating a cyber-physical framework where actual-world elements stay interconnected. The IoMT has altered numerous industries, counting healthcare, transportation and agriculture. Hospitals can be stressful for both aged and children. With the world's population steadily increasing, traditional patient-doctor appointments are becoming less efficient, making smart healthcare essential. Smart healthcare can be utilized in various ways, from monitoring a baby's temperature to trailing crucial signs in the hexagenerians and older. The complications and price of these implementations depend on the essential valuables, functionality, and sophistication of the gadgets and applications involved. Additionally, smart healthcare intersects with technologies like big data, VLSI, machine learning, embedded systems, artificial intelligence and cloud computing.

With its capabilities in identification, location, sensing, and connectivity, the IoMT plays a crucial role in smart healthcare. In healthcare systems, Internet of Medical Things applications range from calibrating medical equipment to personalized monitoring. It is essential in managing chronic diseases and tracking daily physical activities to support fitness goals. Moreover, the IoMT facilitates monitoring the production process and tracing the delivery of healthcare equipment.

IoMT enables users to seamlessly integrate electronic devices, smartphones, and tablets, facilitating both physical and wireless communication. This connectivity enables the management of numerous devices and extends internet benefits such as data sharing, remote access, and in relevance to other domains including transportation, agriculture, healthcare, surveillance, and others.

Internet of Medical Things-based architectonics are utilized to gather healthcare data from users, acting as a conduit between doctors and patients through remote access. This capability enables continuous monitoring of patients and remote consultations. By integrating cloud computing, processors, microcontrollers, actuators, and sensors, the Internet of Medical Things ensures precise results and enhances medical accessibility for everyone (N. Tommarello et al.2024).

Working of Internet of Medical Things (IoMT)

The convergence and occupancy of internet into our surrounding has opened the way for Internet of Medical Things systems and applications into our existence often. The majority of Internet of Medical Things systems appeal in the subsequent major layers that merge devices, various technologies, systems interconnected and sensors via wireless or wired connection and electronics (Figure 2). The functionality and structure of each layer is depicted.

Figure 2. Architectonics of IoMT

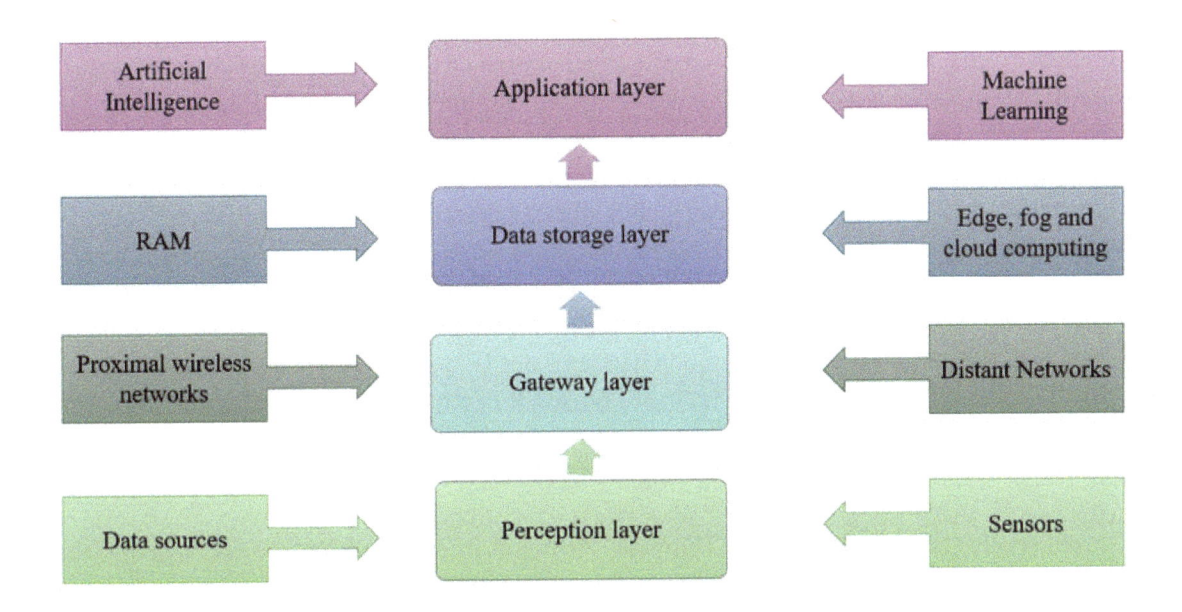

INTEGRATION OF IOMT AND GENERATIVE AI

The IoMT engineering has been well-received within the restorative space because of its capacity to bolster communication among various restorative gadgets, counting choice activities that are generative AI-enabled. Fastened by endless sums of information, capabilities of analytics and enhancements in AI, the numerous conceivable outcomes of joining in these advances are leaping up in present day medicine. Internet of Medical Things is characterized as the collective arrange of associated gadgets and the innovation that allows them to make contact with each one. Within the restorative industry, Internet of Medical Things is in some cases alluded to as the Web of Restorative things. Nevertheless, there are obvious tribulations to appropriation within the restorative field which will not continuously be clear, particularly in context of security and morals.

Artificial Intelligence Assisted Healthcare Devices

A) CGM (ceaseless glucose monitor) is an IoMT gadget, which computes an individual's sugar level via a sensor, transmits the perusing to the transmitter, and after that transmits the perusing to the patient's cell phone. During this, in the event that the perusing is out of run then it will be alarmed so a choice can be made on how to read the sugar reading. Such innovation not as it were but helps in malady and moves forward day to day administration of the condition (Reddy N et al. 2023).

B) Artificial Intelligence assisted- Computerized diagnosis are the recent trends in radiology. QuatX a computerized diagnosis device enabled by AI helps in detecting abnormalities in breast with high resolution imaging. It selects area or regions of concern aligning with user's preferences in Magnetic Resonance Imaging of Breast. Thereby, aids in early detection of myeloma tissues (Pennello G et al. 2023).

C) ContaCT is another device that assists in computed tomography of the cerebrum. It alerts the brain specialist about any possible huge vessel obstruction or stroke. Similarly, Viz ICH alerts the medical staff and doctors about possible cerebral haemorrhage (Pennello G et al.2023).

D) BPPW (Blood Pressure Predict Wristband) device is centred on less consumption of power. This Band is incorporated with a sensor that measures the blood pressure of the individual by the pulse rate at the radial artery. It then aligns the parameter with the one established with the AI framework and aids in keeping a track (Tan P et al. 2022).

E) Additionally, Internet of Medical Things & Artificial Intelligence have joined together to make AIoMT (Artificial Intelligence of Medical Things). AIoMT is progressing and quiet often observed within the therapeutic industry. In common, therapeutic Gen AI help can diminish stretch on both doctors and patients. An understanding with a chronic ailment can utilize an Artificial Intelligence-enabled Internet of Medical Things framework to manage therapy in the absence of genuine time by a doctor. Therapeutic rebellions, for instance, stethoscopes, blood weight and smart thermometers can interface to the Web and utilize Gen AI to help health-care experts in precise analysis and malady verdicts. Smartwatches and wellness trackers can collect vitals to create judgments and provide inputs approximately of a person in general wellbeing. These gadgets have the competence to progress in general quality of life for patient (Priyan Malarvizhi Kumar,2018).

ADVANTAGES OF IOMT AND GEN AI

Mechanical foundation has continuously been the bedrock of health-care progressions. The AIoMT based apparatuses are presently engaged in a lot more evolutionary part in medical industry, hoisting the contemporary restorative space a lot quicker than at any time recently. The advantages of Artificial Intelligence of Medical Things (AIoMT) are various. These incorporates moving forward decision-making, improved remedial care availability, early expectation and location, diminished stretch for patients and doctors, and brought down costs. Also, helpful information capacity is made conceivable by AIoMT gadgets and empowers doctors to store abundant information with simple access (S. Alian et al.2018). few examples are as follows:

I. Usage of Artificial Intelligence of Medical Things in diabetes control, emphasise the possibility of integrating IoMT innovation with prescient models. The AI framework could be a way to deliver insulin via a pump which communicates with a CGM. Machine Learning calculations analyse the blood sugar perusing, anticipates what the blood sugar will be cantered on the existing slant, and consequently alters delivery of insulin on that forecast. Such a closed-loop framework has been demonstrated to enormously make strides the standard of life for Diabetic patients (type 1) by lessening the stress of consistent blood glucose observing. The choices of the AI framework can be nullified by the persistent, achieving a Level 2 basic framework. Consequently, advances comparative to this are getting to be prevalent within the therapeutic industry because to their halfway autonomy.

II. GI (Gastroenterology) that is ponder of the stomach related framework, and hepatology which is the ponder of the liver and gallbladder, moreover have their claim illustrations illustrating Artificial Intelligence's ability to save lives with minimal intervention. (Machine Learning & (Artificial Intelligence) software systems as of now help within the treatment and administration of liver and stomach illnesses. In a ML & AI model of 2012, were utilized to distinguish patients with ulcerative Crohn's illness and colitis with the help of endoscopic images, with a normal exactness of ninety percent. These frameworks can be used to distinguish high-risk patients who are incapable of being identified with standard emphasizing AI abilities', screening over triumphing innovation. Another illustration is in anaesthesiology, which needs the investigation of complex information, where ML calculations studied patients' EEG signals to look at their condition beneath anaesthesia. The calculations utilized in anaesthesiology incorporate profound learning neural systems, that collaborates to move forward exactness in anticipating the individual's condition.

BENEFITS OF AIoMT IN DRUG DISCOVERY

i. **Expediting drug discovery** - A bIoMTech (*Insilco* Pharmaceutical), company centred in China, has the ability to display pan-fibrotic inhibitor, INS018_055 and the primary sedate found and planned with Gen AI. The company has moved to Stage 1 trials within two years. The conventional medicate revelation handle would take twofold this time.

ii. **Streamlining budgets** - Conventional sedate disclosure and improvement are costly. The normal R&D use for an expansive pharmaceutical company is evaluated at $6.16 billion per sedate. The previously mentioned *Insilco* medication progressed its INS018_055 to Stage 2 clinical trials, investing as it were one-tenth of the sum it would take with the conventional strategy.

iii. **Enabling customization** - Gen AI models can consider the hereditary cosmetics to decide how person patients will respond to choose drugs. They can distinguish biomarkers demonstrating illness arrange and seriousness to consider these variables amid sedate revelation.

iv. **Drug Success predictability** - Around ninety percent of drugs fall flat clinical trials. It would be cheaper and more proficient to dodge taking each sedate candidate there. *Insilico* medication, pioneers in Gen AI-driven medicate improvement, built a generative AI instrument named inClinico that can anticipate clinical trial results for distinctive new drugs. Over a 7 year consider, this apparatus illustrated 79% forecast precision comparison to clinical trial comes about.

v. **Addressing data constraints** – Top notch information is rare within the pharma and medical spaces, and it do not continuously conceivable to utilize the accessible information due to security concerns. Generative AI in sedate disclosure can prepare exquisite information and synthesize practical information focuses to prepare encourage and progress show precision.

LIMITATIONS OF IOMT AND GEN AI

Whereas AIoMT presents unused and promising openings in wellbeing care, there stay challenges to be tended to. Inquire about, advancement, and administrative endeavours to address concerns with respect to unwavering quality, generalizability, security, and maintainability are in progress. It is clear that transformative developments are promoting independent restorative innovations; in any case, current innovative impediments are a downside. These restrictions incorporate information protection, constrained information accessibility, one-sided information sets, persistent damage, and machine mistake (S. Greene et al .2016).

Understanding security -is of most extreme significance in wellbeing care. Individual's need to get that their information safe and at the risk of breachment. When original Artificial Intelligence of Medical Things frameworks are sent in wellbeing care, the chances of the information being compromised is distant more prominent than most patients get it or are willing to endure since of the challenges of these frameworks. Not as it were does unprotected persistent protection increment the plausibility of persistent segregation by expanding information inclination, but it moreover effects ever-lasting wellbeing care costs.

Reliability-The gigantic sums of information and the concluded designs by AIoMT frameworks exemplify inside them the predispositions of our community, building their utilization in wellbeing care a potential for moral suggestions. Subsequently, such arrangements may not be seen as reliable as those derived by prepared doctors. Forecasts from AIoMT frameworks are as it were as great as the information they get. When that information appeared to have inclinations, the coming about expectations are not ideal.

Measurability-Another obstacle is that present innovation can't measure or control outside variables, making it troublesome to adjust. Hence, the unwavering quality of Artificial Intelligence of Medical Things can be debased since of changes within the patient's surrounding that are troublesome for the calculations to identify. The AI framework utilized in diabetic patients is an illustration of an Artificial Intelligence of Medical Things gadget utilized in medication with impediments that can be credited to its calculation. In a recursive delivery of insulin framework is planned to alter insulin level centred on sugar levels, the calculation misconstrued what the individual is effectively doing or how it may influence their future blood sugar level. For illustration, it cannot to the extent of sum of work out of the individuals or the sort of nourishment they're devouring, so it may regulate the off-base sum of insulin. This sort of blunder can result in hypo or hyperglycaemia, which can be deadly.

Legitimate issues - AIoMT in therapeutics too has legitimate impediments. Harm and blunder which are inevitable in pharmaceutical, but when an issue does happen due to innovation, legitimate measures must be considered. When doctors are held responsible rather than the innovation, they may get to be at risk.

IoMT is creating quick and is progressively being embraced in healthcare. It is evident that caution ought to proceed to be utilized with Artificial Intelligence centred innovation. By virtue of their basic nature, medical systems should be guaranteed to be dependable and keep up such unwavering quality all through their utilization. AIoMT has the potential to create restorative care more secure, more effective, reasonable, and less unpleasant for doctors and patients alike, consequently progressing medical care conveyance. Be that as it may, in spite of their guarantee to help doctors in malady conclusion and treatment suggestion, AIoMT systems have more prominent related chance than predominant innovation. Moreover, restorative innovation still has much work to go some time recently it can be completely believed by clinicians. Meanwhile, analysts are proceeding to act on Artificial Intelligence of Medical Things more dependable by creating new vision to overcome their confinements.

APPLICATIONS OF IOMT AND GEN AI

Precision Medicine

The field of accuracy pharmaceutical is additionally encountering quick development. Accuracy medication is maybe best depicted as a wellbeing care development including what the National Investigate Committee at first called the advancement of "a Modern Scientific classification of human illness based on atomic biology," or an insurgency in wellbeing care activated by information picked up from human genome sequencing. The field, since has advanced to acknowledge how the crossing point of multi-omic information integrated with social behavioural determinants, therapeutic history and natural information absolutely attributes wellbeing states, illness states, and restorative alternatives for influenced people.

Accuracy pharmaceutical provides medical suppliers the capacity to find and display data that either approves or modifies the direction of a therapeutic choice from one that is centred on the prove for the normal understanding, to one that is based upon individual's one-of-a-kind characteristics. It encourages a clinician's conveyance of care personalized for each quiet. Exactness medication disclosure enables conceivable outcomes that would something else have been unrealized.

Propels in exactness medication show into substantial wellfare, for instance early discovery of illness and planning precision medications are getting to be more widespread in wellbeing care. The control of accuracy medication to precision care is empowered by a few information analytics innovations and collection. In specific, the meeting of high-throughput sequencing and worldwide selection of E-Health Records gives researchers a phenomenal opportunity to determine unused phenotypes from biomarker information and real-world clinical. These phenotypes, integrated with information from the E-Health Records, may approve the require for extra medications or may progress analyze of malady variations.

Maybe the foremost well-studied effect of accuracy medication on wellbeing care nowadays is genotype-guided treatment. Clinicians have utilized genotype information as a guideline to assist decide the proper dose of warfarin. The Clinical Pharmacogenetics Execution Consortium distributed genotype-based medicate rules to assist clinicians optimize medicate treatments with genetic test comes about. Genomic profiling of tumors can illuminate focused on therapy plans for patients with lung and breast cancer. Accuracy pharmaceutical, coordinates into healthcare, has the potential to surrender more exact analyze, anticipate infection hazard some time recently side effects happen, and plan customized treatment plans that maximize security and effectiveness. The slant toward empowering the utilize of accuracy medication by building up information storehouses isn't confined to the Joined together States; cases from Biobanks in numerous nations, such as the UK Biobank, BioBank Japan, and Australian Genomics Wellbeing Organization together illustrate the control of changing demeanors toward exactness medication on a worldwide scale.

In spite of the fact that there is much guarantee for precision medication and AI, more work still has to be done to test, approve, and alter treatment hones. Analysts confront challenges of receiving bound together information groups (e.g., Quick Healthcare Interoperability Assets), obtaining sufficient and high quality labelled information for preparing calculations, and tending to administrative, security, and sociocultural prerequisites (Johnson KB et al.2020).

Drug Discovery

In drug discovery Generative AI has 5 key applications (Figure 3):

1. Molecule and compound generation
2. Biomarker identification
3. Prediction of Drug-target interaction
4. Drug combination and repurposing
5. Prediction of drug side effects

Figure 3. IoMT and gen AI applications in drug discovery

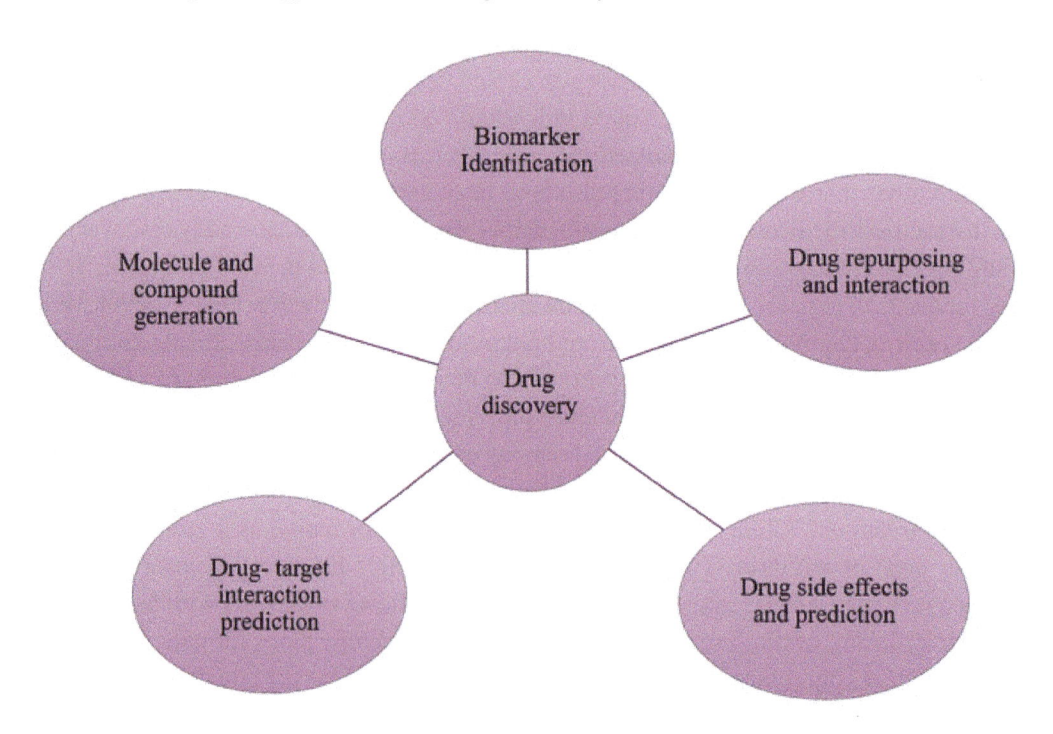

1) **Molecule and Compound Generation**

One of the prevailing applications of Gen AI in drug discovery is in compound and molecule generation. Generative AI models can:

- **Generate Novel, Valid Molecules Optimized for a Specific Purpose**

Gen AI calculations can prepare on 3-D shapes of atoms and their properties to create innovative particles with the required characteristics, for instance official to a particular receptor.

- **Perform Multi-Objective Molecule Optimization**

Frameworks that are prepared on chemical responses information can anticipate intelligent among chemical compounds and suggest modifications to particle characteristics that will adjust their profile regarding engineered possibility, power, security, and other components.

- **Screen Compounds**

Generative AI in sedate disclosure can not as it were create a expansive set of virtual compounds but too offer assistance analysts assess them hostile to organic targets and discover the ideal compatible.

- **Encouraging Genuine Instances**

Insilico Pharmaceutical utilized Gen-AI to create ISM6331—a particle that can aim progressed strong cancer cells. Amid this explore, the AI show produced > 6,000 potential atoms which were also reviewed to recognize the foremost strong contender. The winning ISM6331 appears guarantee as a pan-TEAD inhibitor in opposite to TEAD proteins that tumors got to advance and stand up to drugs. In preclinical thinks about, ISM6331 demonstrated to be exceptionally effective and secure for utilization. Adaptyv Bio, a bIoMTech venture centred in Europe, depends on Gen-AI for protein designing. But they do not halt at fair creating practical protein plans. The venture includes a protein building workcell where researchers, in conjunction with AI, compose exploratory conventions and create the proteins outlined by calculations.

2) **Biomarker Identification**

Biomarkers are atoms that unobtrusively show certain forms within the human body. A few biomarkers point to ordinary organic forms, and a few flag the nearness of a malady and reflect its seriousness.

In sedate revelation, biomarkers are for the most part utilized to recognize potential restorative targets for personalized medicines. They can moreover offer assistance select the ideal understanding populace for medical trials. Individuals with identical biomarkers have comparative properties and are at comparative stages of the illness that shows in comparative ways. To put it another way, this empowers the revelation of profoundly precision drugs.

In this angle of medicate disclosure, the part of generative AI is to ponder endless proteomics and genomics datasets to distinguish suitable biomarkers comparing to diverse infections and after that explore for these markers in patients. Calculations can recognize biomarkers in restorative pictures, such as MRIs and CAT looks, and other sorts of quiet information (Manickam P et al. 2022).

3) **Prediction of Drug-Target Interaction**

Gen AI frameworks comprehend from medicate structures, known drug-target and quality expression profiles intelligent to mimic atom intelligent and foresee the authoritative partiality of modern sedate compounds and their target proteins. Gen AI can quickly run target proteins in opposite to gigantic repositories of chemical structures to discover any archive atoms that can tie to the target. In case none is discovered, they can create new compounds and validate their ligand-receptor interaction quality. For example, analysts from Tufts College and MIT thought up an emerging approach to assessing drug-target intelligent utilizing ConPLex, a huge dialect demonstrate. One extraordinary privilege of this Gen AI calculation is that it can run contender medicate atoms in opposite to the target protein without having to compute the particle structure, assessing over 100 million compounds in a single day. Another vital highlight of ConPLex is that it can dispose of bait elements—imposter compounds that are exceptionally comparative to an real medicate but can't be associated with the target. Researchers utilized this Gen AI calculation on more than four thousand candidate particles to test their authoritative liking to a set of protein kinases. ConPLex recognizes 19 suitable drug-target sets. The investigate group tried these comes about and discovered that twelve of them have colossally solid authoritative capability. So solid that indeed a modest sum of medicate can restrain the target protein.

4) **Drug Combining and Repurposing**

Gen AI calculations can hunt for modern restorative usage of existing, affirmed drugs. Reusing existing drugs is much speedier than turning to the conventional sedate improvement approach. Moreover, these drugs were as of now tried and have a built-up security profile. In expansion to repurposing a single sedate, generative AI in medicate disclosure can anticipate which sedate combinations can be viable for treating a clutter.
Real-Life Cases:

- A group of analysts tested with utilizing Gen AI to discover sedate candidates for Alzheimer's illness via repurposing. The show recognized 20 promising drugs. The researchers tried the beat 10 candidates on patients over the age of sixty-five. Three of the medicate contendors, to be specific simvastatin, metformin and losartan were related with decreasing Alzheimer's dangers.
- Analysts assessed the possibility of Gen AI for finding drugs which can be repurposed to address the sort of dementia that tends to go with Parkinson's illness. Their framework executed on the IBM Watson Wellbeing information and mimicked distinctive cohorts of people who did and did not take the contendor sedate. They moreover regarded contrasts in sexual orientation, concurrent diseases, and other pertinent qualities.

5) **Prediction of Drug Side Effects**

Generative Artificial Intelligence models can total information and reenact atom intuitive to anticipate potential side impacts and the probability of their event, permitting researchers to pick the most secure candidates. Here is how Generative AI does that.

- **Anticipating Chemical Structures:** Generative AI in medicate revelation can analyze novel particle structures and figure their chemical reactivity and properties. A few auxiliary highlights are generally related with unfavourable responses.
- **Analyzing Organic Pathways:** These models can decide which natural forms can be influenced by the medicate particle. As atoms connected in a cell, they can make byproducts or result in cell changes.
- **Coordination Omics Information:** Generative AI can allude to proteomic, genomic and sorts of Omics information to "understand" how diverse hereditary makeups can react to the candidate sedate.
- **Anticipating Unfavorable Occasions:** These calculations can think about noteworthy drug-adverse occasion affiliations to figure potential side impacts.
- **Recognizing Poisonous Quality:** Medicate atoms can tie to non-target proteins, which can lead to poisonous quality. By assessing drug-protein intelligent, Generative AI models can anticipate such occasions and their results.

IMPLANTABLE DEVICES AND WEARABLES

Developments and innovations within the biomedical field offer assistance improve wellbeing care quality. Be that as it may, the nanotechnology's potential needs a distinct comprehension, and more significant information via AI is vital for craved affectability and microfabrication. Uniting the interface between AI-empowered and nanotechnology frameworks interfaces with IoMT innovation is basic for creating inventive care strategies, including nanorobotics and nanomedicine. The utilities of nanotechnology-empowered portable uninterrupted vigilance gadgets are prevalent within the medical segment. Progressed wearable gadgets are nano-enabled sensor implanted, empowering the gadget to screen biological metrics persistently. A broad clinical information set needs AI examination and preparing for precise conclusion and guess. The microfabricated gadgets connects a wide range of investigate zones, counting biomedical and nanotechnology designing, to outwit the tribulations in conclusion and remedies (operations and focused on medicate treatment). The presentation of progressed 2-dimensional utilitarian materials such as Mxenes, borophene, and graphene has empowered the era of emerging generation bio-portable gadgets with progressed spatIoMTemporal highlights. As of late, MXene-consolidated e-skin-centred sensors for checking person's movement centred on the weight modulation rule have moreover been detailed.

The sustainable Mxene weight portables illustrated great air permeability. The portables can be interfaced with remote shrewd detecting gadgets for down to earth applications, counting human motion observing, sustainable implanted devices, shrewdly electronic skins, and restorative observing. MXene has advanced as amazing meddle fabric in healthcare and natural gas detecting with momentous affectability and finesse. Within the case of glucose checking, the impedance properties and characteristic heterogeneous electron exchange characteristics of MXene have been explored for creating emerging generation glucose-detection gadgets. Coordinate and fast blood-sugar estimation is essential for overseeing diabetes mellitus in a precision way. The chemical and physical properties of Mxene offer assistance in upgrading the affectability of the detecting gadgets for medical biology, natural, and nourishment analytics utility. Making crossover nanocomposite materials byintegrating a 2-Dimensional Mxene with 1D nanoparticles for upgrading the attachment soundness on the transceiver surface for prolonged observing has too been endeavoured. The frontier combination of a 2-Dimensional Mxene/1D graphene nanoribbon has been explored for creating the specified weight sensor with an progressed life cycle. ML tactics were employed for preparing the portable for identifying different sitting stances with >95curacy. Sharma et al. as of late highlighted the significance of 2D borophene frameworks upheld by IoMT smartphone-supported high-performance applications (Z. A. Khan et al.2011).

Telemedicine

Artificial Intelligence's application in telemedicine has provided a remarkable tool in making diagnoses and recommended health interventions with unwavering accuracy (Figure 4). Coupled with advanced data analytics, these technologies have dwindled the margin for human error, subsequently creating a safer, more efficient health infrastructure AI-powered telemedicine has been proving advantageous in many ways – from its potential to assess patient symptoms remotely, triage and follow-up on their condition, to even offering therapeutic recommendations. Leading tech like IBM Watson, for example, employs AI in deciphering patient symptoms, accessing extensive research data to provide a predictive diagnosis, thus mitigating the challenges of geographical barriers (Manickam P et al. 2022).

Figure 4. Illustration of AI enabled wearables deciphering of patient's symptoms and predictive diagnosis

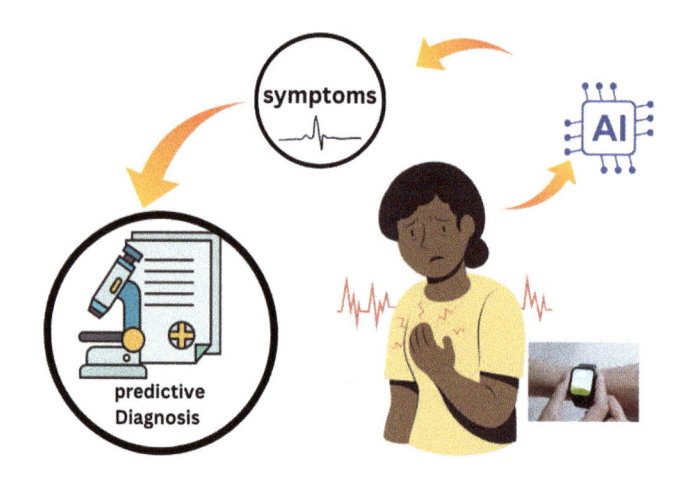

Smart Operating Rooms

IoMT empowered working room known as "Keen Cyber Working Theater" that had open resource interface for the network innovation for interfacing therapeutic devices. Another working theatre that has been created incorporates later generations organizing office known as OPeLiNK communication interface showing intraoperative MRI (Magnetic Resonance Imaging). Keen Working rooms with Automated framework that can replicate hand movements of a specialist by expanded degrees of opportunity through haptic upheld upgraded sensing capacity, tissue acknowledgment and real-time conclusion. The accuracy of operation is additionally upgraded owing to decrease in hand tremor and improved visualization given by high-resolution 3-D video pictures.

One of the concepts prevalently so-called tele-surgery is picking up ubiquity where operating methods are done indeed when specialist and the persistent are at extraordinary separations, by utilizing automated arm intervened imitation of the doctor's real hand movements to the surgical disobedient over the patient's organ.

Crossover Working rooms permit specialists to do combined open, negligibly obtrusive, catheter-centred and/or image-guided strategies within the similar agent setting. Utilization of Radio Frequency Identification for operation to progress for envison of the operation strategy and progress the security by ideal utilization of surgical devices.

Augmented Reality framework can too be utilized to imagine volumetric data anticipated upon the patient's organ amid surgery. Essentially, inner pathology of strong organs can moreover be visualized without entry point utilizing inlay unreal pictures. To expel tumors more effectively, the surgical group can utilize high-definition, 3-dimensional, real-time picture direction (Z. A. Khan et al.2011).

Tele-Dentistry

The utilization of broadcast communications in dentistry through organizing and sharing computerized data (utilizing phone, photographs, or recordings), further separations investigation of clinical data and pictures for workup and removed interviews encouraging conveyance of verbal well-being care and verbal well-being instruction administrations is the unused rising concept named 'Tele-dentistry'. It requires ownership of a smartphone by the persistent having satisfactory Web get to and a cloud-centred tele dentistry stage by the dental specialist that can bolster the spilling of recordings in real-time with the office to store and forward the photographs and gathered clinical information from the E-Health Record. This stage can total all the information for farther assessment and suggestion for the treatment by the dental practitioner.

The American Dental Affiliation too issued an approach on tele-dentistry that provides direction on the modalities to be taken after. It will improve the common hone of tele-dentistry.

Despite the progress, more research is required to decide the innovation needs and sorts of oral medical issues that can be securely tended to utilizing tele-dentistry. (Tommarello et al. 2024)

Ambient Assisted Living

AAL is Artificial intelligence-backed living where maturing individuals are helped to survive autonomously, with comfort & security inside their domestic. The most important reason of Ambient Assisted Living is a real-time observation so that when a therapeutic crisis happens, arrangements for human service-like help can be created.

It uses progressed incorporation of different frameworks like Artificial Intelligence, huge information examination, machine learning for activity, and surrounding acknowledgment together with observing the vitals like heart rate, blood weight, respiratory rate, etc.

A mechanized secluded design for security and communication has been created utilizing IPv6-based low-power remote individual region systems (6LoWPAN). For communication, dialogical communication benefits utilizing RFID and NFC have been utilized for setting up an association among understanding and medical attendants. Checking of persistent health & conditions crises in aged individuals can moreover be done by a crisis locator created to help and caution the attendants.

Internet of Medical Things-centred medical frameworks utilizing aided robots can too be engaged to track standard of indoor discuss and prompt cautions to the medical attendants whenever there is a diminishment within the discuss quality underneath a quality value. So also, to identify liquid admissions distinctive wearable, savvy holders, surface and inserted sensors can be utilized especially in aged patients (N. Tommarello et al. 2024).

I-Robotics

An IoMT-aided mechanical framework could be a keen environment comprising numerous interconnected progressed coordinates frameworks comprising people, robots and the Internet of Medical Things system. The framework generally employs a cloud-robotic framework which could get to a huge sum of information and prepare the data utilizing detecting, computing, and memory to perform particular assignments.

The improvement of mechanical innovation points to realize humanoid mechanization in order to decrease human intercession. The framework utilizes ML (Machine Learning) calculations to program and prepare robots/machines to execute on the premise of patient's well-being data information gotten through the network among well-being experts or by utilizing the brilliant calculations to execute within the therapeutic environment.

'Lio', is a medical robot that employs a concoction of visual, sound mechanical sensors, laser, and ultrasound to maintain a strategic distance from collision independently. This empowers secure routes for patients and staff in a health center. Essentially, "Guido", an E-walker was created for outwardly disabled individuals and employs the map-centered route framework to form an outline of the encompassing to retrieve the location and utilize a crash shirking calculation to make a way to achieve the goal excluding barriers.

Additionally, a robot a.k.a "Nao Robot" is competent in connecting to the patients after dissecting the restorative information and instructing them about the crucial status of their body, anticipate the chance of heart maladies within the future and suggest the essential changes within the way of life to dodge related complications.

Alternatively, Internet of Medical Things-assisted automated framework empowers recording of particular movements by the practitioners to be reproduced in patients with imperfect appendage movements. 'ROBIN', a rehabilitative robot gives steadiness to the trunk amid locomotory changes and encourage basic hands & arm developments for coming to and getting a handle on things.

Separated from those specified, a few benefit robots for aged like JoHOBBIT, PT2, CAESAR, Care-o-Bot, and Aibo, with offer assistance of Internet of medical things innovations (sensors, RFID, GPS, infrared, and portable sensors) interfaces the aged with wellbeing experts and family individuals in this manner supporting in keeping up a quality of life by giving updates, drop location, and meddle with other domestic appliances.

In clinics moreover, independent robots (I- robots) are being utilized for biomedical waste management and sanitization. In expansion I- robots can convey pharmaceutical, nourishment, or restorative supplies to patients. A wheeled telepresence robot has been evolved that can execute face-to-face (virtually) quiet appraisal conjointly perform symptomatic tests after collecting the swab tests from the patients (Dwivedi R et al.2022).

Advantages of Existing Works (Performance Metrics)

- **Enhanced Diagnostic Accuracy:** Integration of IoMT and Generative AI allows for real-time analysis of health data, leading to more precise and timely diagnoses.
- **Personalized Treatments:** IoMT devices paired with Generative AI enable tailored treatment plans based on a patient's unique profile, improving outcomes and reducing adverse effects.
- **Operational Efficiency:** Automating data analysis and healthcare workflows minimizes costs and improves resource allocation.
- **Drug Discovery Optimization:** Generative AI significantly reduces the time and cost for drug discovery, enhancing molecule generation and predicting drug-target interactions effectively.
- **Remote and Continuous Monitoring:** IoMT devices facilitate patient tracking, especially for chronic illnesses and remote populations, ensuring better access to healthcare.
- **Proactive Health Management:** Data insights from IoMT enhance patient engagement and preventive healthcare practices.

Disadvantages of Existing Works (Performance Metrics)

- **Data Privacy Concerns:** Handling large volumes of sensitive health data increases the risk of breaches, undermining patient trust.
- **Reliability Issues:** AI systems may misinterpret data due to biases or contextual limitations, leading to errors in diagnosis or treatment.
- **Limited Generalizability:** Current AI models often rely on specific datasets, which may not account for diverse populations or conditions.
- **Legal and Ethical Challenges:** Ambiguities in accountability for AI-driven errors and compliance with privacy regulations pose significant obstacles.
- **High Dependency on Technology:** IoMT systems require robust infrastructure and constant connectivity, which might not be accessible in underdeveloped regions.
- **Computational Complexity:** Advanced AI models demand significant computational resources, making them costly to implement at scale.

ETHICAL CONSIDERATIONS

As rising advances hold on in reshaping the healthcare scene, it gets to be basic to scrutinize the moral and lawful measurements going with these headways. Tending to significant viewpoints such as protection, information security, administrative compliance, and impartial get to gets to be foremost in exploring the advancing crossing point of innovation and healthcare.

Privacy and Data Security

The raising digitization of healthcare information and the integration of technology-driven arrangements emphasize the basic significance of prioritizing understanding security and guaranteeing vigorous information security measures. Healthcare organizations confront the basic of executing rigid shields to shield delicate quiet data from the dangers of information breaches and unauthorized get to. Fundamental measures envelop encryption conventions, secure arrange foundation, and immovable adherence to security directions, exemplified by the Wellbeing Protections Compactness and Responsibility Act (HIPAA), all of which are significant in maintaining understanding believe and keeping up the most extreme privacy.

Regulatory Compliance and Patient Consent

Guaranteeing moral hones in healthcare innovation requires strict compliance with legitimate and administrative systems. Adherence to rules, such as the Common Information Security Control (GDPR), is foundational. Getting educated quiet assent for the collection, capacity, and utilization of information could be a pivotal angle of moral healthcare hones. Straightforward communication with respect to the utilization of information and unequivocal assent for sharing or investigate purposes are indispensably moral contemplations that request cautious consideration and usage.

AI and Automation's Ethical Implications in Healthcare

The developing integration of AI and robotization in healthcare sparkles basic moral request. Concerns encompassing calculation inclination, responsibility for AI choices, and the potential for work relocation require fastidious investigation. Maintaining moral guidelines in AI-driven healthcare requests measures such as guaranteeing straightforwardness in AI calculations, tending to predisposition in preparing information, and building up express rules for human oversight. These contemplations are crucial in exploring the moral complexities that emerge with the expanding dependence on fake insights inside the healthcare space.

Ensuring Equitable Access to Healthcare Technology

. As innovation unquestionably coordinating into healthcare, guaranteeing impartial get to for all people, independent of geographic area or financial status, rises as an basic. Moral contemplations command tending to the advanced separate by giving preparing and back for underserved communities. Moreover, creating arrangements to bridge the crevice between mechanical progressions and get to care gets to be vital, underscoring the commitment to inclusivity in healthcare. These moral objectives are principal to cultivating a healthcare scene that's not as it were innovatively progressed but too generally open.

CONTRIBUTIONS

- The platform for researching the integration of IoMT and Generative AI in Healthcare needs to have some basic measures for a comprehensive appraisal:
- Specialized Integration: Assess the amalgamation of devices using IoMT with the calculations of Generative AI in the delivery of healthcare and measure the features that give credence to this integration, such as compatibility, interoperability, and versatility
- Healthcare Workflow Improvement: Analyze how the combination of IoMT and Generative AI enhances healthcare workflows, progressing proficiency in information examination, decision-making bolster, and asset allotment.

- Moral and Administrative Contemplations: Examine moral angles like information protection, security, and quiet assent, nearby adherence to administrative benchmarks .
- Value and Openness: Degree to which the meeting of IoMT and Generative AI advances reasonable get to healthcare administrations, tending to incongruities affected by topography, financial status, and mechanical get to.
- Understanding Engagement and Empowerment: Look at how this merging engages patients to lock in in their care through custom fitted intercessions, instruction, and decision-making apparatuses.
- Future Viewpoint and Challenges: Survey up-and-coming patterns, potential applications, and tireless obstacles, counting specialized restrictions and roads for assist investigate and progress.

- The future of healthcare is unfolding before us. The merging of the Internet of Medical Things (IoMT) and Generative Artificial Intelligence (Gen AI) is transforming how we think about and deliver care. This isn't just about new technology—it's a revolutionary shift toward personalized, proactive healthcare.

- Imagine a device that constantly monitors your vital signs, offering real-time insights to help you stay on top of your health. Or envision a world where AI-driven analytics and smart devices work together to provide tailored treatments and enable remote care. These innovations are no longer a distant dream; they're quickly becoming part of our reality.

- But with these advancements comes a need for caution. As we integrate these technologies, we must carefully consider ethical issues like data security, ensuring fair access, and protecting patient consent. By addressing these concerns, we can ensure a more patient-centered and sustainable healthcare system.

- The impact of IoMT and Gen AI will be broad and transformative. We can expect improvements in operational efficiency, cost reductions, more accurate diagnoses, and stronger patient engagement. At the same time, we must face challenges like privacy risks, potential biases in AI models, and technical limitations that need to be addressed.

- Looking ahead, there are even more exciting possibilities. From using optical sensors for activity recognition to creating IoMT-driven solutions for elderly care, the potential applications are vast.

- Ultimately, the integration of IoMT and Gen AI has the power to reshape healthcare as we know it. By embracing these technologies and tackling their challenges head-on, we can create a healthcare system that is more efficient, effective and focused on the needs of patients.

IMPACT AND SIGNIFICANCE

The merging of IoMT and Generative AI in healthcare stands to apply a significant and far-reaching impact over different spaces:

- *Increased Healthcare Productivity*

Coordination IoMT gadgets with Generative AI calculations optimizes forms like determination, treatment arranging, and quiet observing, reinforcing operational proficiency and asset assignment in healthcare situations.

- *Raised Quiet Results*

Through encouraging exact analyze and personalized treatment plans, the amalgamation of IoMT and Generative AI holds the guarantee of progressing persistent results, relieving treatment complications, and cultivating by and large way better wellbeing comes about for people.

- ***Strengthening of Healthcare Specialists***

Healthcare experts pick up get to to advanced choice bolster apparatuses and information analytics capabilities advertised by Generative AI, engaging them to form educated clinical choices and convey predominant care to their patients.

- ***Upgraded Persistent Engagement and Independence***

Prepared with IoMT gadgets coordinates with Generative AI-driven apparatuses, patients accomplish more profound bits of knowledge into their wellbeing status, empowering them to effectively take part in overseeing their well-being and making well-informed choices with respect to their treatment.

- ***Movement in Populace Wellbeing Administration***

Leveraging the combined potential of IoMT and Generative AI, healthcare frameworks can gather more profound experiences into populace wellbeing patterns, recognize helpless populaces, and actualize focused on intercessions to upgrade open wellbeing results.

Generally, the meeting of IoMT and Generative AI holds the potential to convert healthcare conveyance by refining proficiency, opening up understanding results, enabling both patients and healthcare suppliers, and progressing techniques for populace wellbeing administration.

FINDINGS

The merging of Generative AI and IoMT in medical industry presents numerous transformative conceivable results:

1. Improved Symptomatic Accuracy

Aligning AI with IoMT information empowered the medical and health space suppliers to comprehend more precisely and conveniently analyse, ensuing upgrading continuous outcomes and boosting early medication for multiple conditions.

2. Custom-fitted Treatment Procedures:

By examining wider information gathered by Generative AI, IoMT devices can define precise treatment fits to each patient's therapeutic history, inclinations, and well-defined properties This customization optimizes regenerative approaches and minimizes hostile impacts.

3. Optimized Healthcare Forms:

The merging of IoMT and Generative AI aligns decision-making, multiple healthcare approaches, and computing information examination. This robotization boosts operational effectiveness and yields fetched investment funds for healthcare teachers.

Research Gaps

1. Data Privacy and Security
   - **Challenge**: Data protection of patients remains a concern including use of Generative AI, which needs a large data set for training. The threat of leaks and unauthorized access erodes trust in these systems.
   - **Research Gap**: Advancements in encryption, federated learning frameworks, and differential privacy techniques for IoMT-Generative AI systems.
2. Bias and Reliability in AI Models
   - **Challenge:** An IoMT systems may collect data that might include an underlying social or systemic bias that can influence the accuracy and unbiased nature of AI predictions on stereotyping groups of people.
   - **Research Gap:** Developing unbiased training datasets and models resistant to biased data.
3. Integration and Interoperability
   - **Challenge**: The lack of standardization is proving to be a roadblock as current IoMT and Generative AI systems do not integrate seamlessly across devices and platforms.
   - **Research Gap**: Explore universal protocols and frameworks for greater interoperability while ensuring the authenticity of data.
4. Ethical Considerations
   - **Challenge**: Concerns over accountability, the transparency of AI decision-making, and fair access to these powerful systems.
   - **Research Gap**: Establishing ethical policies, interpretable methods, and cost-effective solutions for disadvantaged communities.
5. Regulatory and Compliance Challenges
   - **Challenge**: Dealing with different regulatory environments like GDPR or HIPAA for data use in healthcare apps.
   - **Research Gap**: Develop internationally acceptable regulatory structures which keep pace with the ever-changing landscape of AI technology.
6. Scalability and Real-World Implementation
   - **Challenge**: IoMT-Generative AI integration scaling in the context of diverse and resource-constrained settings such as rural healthcare systems.
   - **Research Gap**: Studying cost-effective and adaptable implementations of IoMT-Generative AI in low-resource environments.
7. Limited Dataset Availability
   - **Challenge**: There is a scarcity of high-quality labeled datasets in healthcare due to privacy issues and the complicated nature of obtaining informed consent.
   - **Research Gap**: Applying Generative AI for synthetic data generation and augmentation an its advantage over limited datasets.
8. Lack of Real-Time Feedback

- **Challenge**: In critical situations like emergencies, many IoMT systems have not yet been optimized to provide real-time feedback.
- **Research Gap**: Exploring real-time analytics and decision-making algorithms that can be applied to IoMT architecture.

Consequences of Limitations on Findings

1. Impact on Diagnostic Accuracy
   - **Limitation**: Incomplete or non-representative data from IoMT devices leads to biases in AI models.
   - **Consequence**: Diagnostic tools can exhibit low accuracy, especially in relation to underrepresented groups, making them less effective in the real world.
2. Data Privacy Concerns
   - **Limitation**: Struggles for data security and abiding by regulations: HIPAA and GDPR
   - **Consequence**: Patient trust in healthcare systems can be diminished through data breaches, as can present legal and ethical dilemmas and deter adoption by healthcare providers and patients.
3. Integration and Interoperability Issues
   - **Limitation**: IoMT devices often lack standardized protocols for seamless communication with AI systems.
   - **Consequence**: Inefficient integration may result in fragmented healthcare workflows, reducing the operational benefits of the system.
4. Reliability and Scalability Challenges
   - **Limitation**: Current IoMT systems may not handle variable environmental or patient conditions effectively.
   - **Consequence**: Findings might not generalize across diverse healthcare settings, limiting scalability to resource-constrained or rural areas.
5. Ethical and Legal Ambiguities
   - **Limitation**: Ambiguities around accountability in AI-driven decisions and insufficient regulatory clarity.
   - **Consequence**: Legal disputes and ethical pushback can delay or inhibit the deployment of these technologies in critical healthcare environments.
6. Lack of High-Quality Datasets
   - **Limitation**: Insufficient availability of annotated, high-quality datasets for training AI models.
   - **Consequence**: The effectiveness of generative AI in personalized treatments and predictive analytics may remain theoretical without robust data validation.
7. Cost and Accessibility Barriers
   - **Limitation**: High development and operational costs for AI-IoMT systems.
   - **Consequence**: Limited accessibility in low-income regions or among marginalized populations, contradicting the goal of equitable healthcare delivery.
8. Technological Dependence Risks
   - **Limitation**: Over-reliance on AI-IoMT systems without adequate human oversight.

- **Consequence**: Potential errors or malfunctions could lead to adverse patient outcomes, undermining confidence in the technology.

FUTURE DEVELOPMENT

1. Optical sensor centred human activity detection models have possible applications in healthcare ranges and medical. There is a model for care of senior citizens by acknowledging 6 irregular exercises; forward drop, in reverse drop, chest torment, swoon, upchuck, and migraine, chosen from the standard of living exercises of elderly individuals. Protection of elderly individuals is guaranteed by consequently extricating the twofold outlines from video exercises. Two issues are tended to in be inquired about, which diminish detection precision amid the method of anomalous human activity detection models advancement. To begin with, the issue of ceaseless changing remove of a moving individual from 2 perspectives is settled by utilizing the R-transform. R-transform extricates intermittent, scale and interpretation of constant highlights from the arrangements of exercises. Moment, the tall similitudes in stances of distinctive exercises is essentially moved forward by utilizing the part discriminant examination. KDA increments separation between diverse classes of exercises by utilizing non-linear procedure. Covered up Markov show (Gee) is utilized for preparing and acknowledgment of tasks. The framework is assessed opposed direct discriminant investigation on the first outline highlights and LDA on the R-transform highlights. Normal acknowledgment rate of 95.8% demonstrates the achievability of the framework for care aged people at domestic. (Z. A. Khan et al.2011)
2. There is an open-air checking framework for aged individuals, that transmits data on biological signals and falling occasions to a medical centre at whenever needed and from any input. while differentiating at the same time the event of any falling occasion, along with the relative ECG (electrocardiogram) flag of the client, a concurrent strategy is proposed with the aim of improving the precision of discovery and reaction time. A healthcare box is utilized to decide the relative position of the understanding through a worldwide situating framework for drop location; additionally, an ECG flag procurement string is received to extend the accuracy of the drop discovery framework. Joining a exact outline into the checking framework encourages contemplating of a patient of the right area and encompassing surrounding utilizing the versatile show. Agreeing to exploratory comes about centred on four thousand tests, effective discovery time with the concurrent strategy was diminished by 38 percent, subsequently expanding protect openings for elderly patients who are at chance
3. savvy domestic situations that not as it were to transmit alarms, but moreover dispatches communication models, including audio help and visuals. Such network may permit more seasoned grown-ups to connected with the system without an issue of a learning bend. The recommended Internet of Medical Things-centred drop location framework will empower medical staff and families to be quickly informed of the occasion and distantly screen the person. Coordinates inside a keen domestic surrounding, the recommended Internet of Medical Things-centred drop location framework can make strides the life's standard of living within more seasoned grown-ups.
4. An upgraded drop location model is put forward for elderly people observing that is centred on smart probes fastened to the body and coping with buyer domestic model. With triple-pronged, unforeseen stumbles could be detected within the domestic healthcare surroundings. By utilizing data gathered from an accelerometer, card IoMT achometer, and smart probes, the impacts of descents

can be registered and identified from usual day-by-day exercises. Implications of a test bunch of thirty reliable individuals, it was concluded that the suggested drop location model can achieve an accurate elevation positioning of 97.5%, whereas the precision and vulnerability are 96.8% and 98.1% singularly. Hence, this framework can reliably be formed and sent into a buyer item for utilization as a veteran person noticing device with tall exactness

5. An adaptable tier-3 engineering to reserve and prepare such a colossal magnitude of wearable sensor information. One-Tier centers on the collection of information from IoMT portable sensor gadgets. Two-tier employs Apache HBase for putting away the huge magnitude of portable IoMT sensor information in cloud computing. In expansion, three-tier employs Apache Mahout for creating the calculated relapse expectation show for heart illnesses. At long last, ROC investigation is executed to recognize the foremost essential health factors to induce cardiac illness.

6. A decisive diabetes management suggestion framework particularly for AI individuals. It prescribes sound life fashion to clients to battle for their diabetes. Much appreciated to the extremely common utilization of cell phones in most AI tribes, we select cell phones as the stage to supply savvy precision support for virtual patients. With coordination, the virtual users' cognitive profile with common clinical diabetes suggestion and rules, the framework can make personalized suggestions (e.g., nourishment admissions and endurance activity) centred on the uncommon financial, social, and topographical status especially to AI Individuals. The proposed framework was actualized as versatile utilizations. Assessments performed by utilizing case ponders and human master confirmation illustrate the viability of the framework (J. Wang et al. 2014).

CONCLUSION

The rise of the Web of Restorative Things (IoMT) and Generative AI in healthcare means a significant change inside the industry. By leveraging interconnected gadgets and modern AI calculations, healthcare suppliers can provide care that's more custom-made, proficient, and impactful for patients. IoMT gadgets encourage persistent checking and information gathering, empowering healthcare experts to form educated choices in real-time. In the interim, Generative AI contributes to made strides symptomatic exactness, treatment strategizing, and pharmaceutical advancement, on a very basic level reshaping different features of healthcare arrangement. Together, IoMT and Generative AI hold a guarantee for considerably upgrading persistent results, streamlining workflows, and on a very basic level reshaping the conveyance and encounter of healthcare. As these innovations advance, it gets to be basic for partners to prioritize moral contemplations, information security, and administrative adherence to guarantee their moral and impartial joining into healthcare frameworks around the world.

REFERENCES

Alian, S., Li, J., & Pandey, V. (2018). (n.d) "A Personalized Recommendation System to Support Diabetes Self-Management for American Indians. *IEEE Access : Practical Innovations, Open Solutions*, 6, 73041–73051. DOI: 10.1109/ACCESS.2018.2882138

Burant, C. J. (2022, December). A Methodological Note: An Introduction to Autoregressive Models. *International Journal of Aging & Human Development*, 95(4), 516–522. DOI: 10.1177/00914150211066554 PMID: 34866432

Das, S., Tariq, A., & Santos, T.. (2023 Jul 23). Recurrent Neural Networks (RNNs): Architectures, Training Tricks, and Introduction to Influential Research. In Colliot, O. (Ed.), *Machine Learning for Brain Disorders* [Internet]. Humana., Available from https://www.ncbi.nlm.nih.gov/books/NBK597502/ , DOI: 10.1007/978-1-0716-3195-9_4

Dwivedi, R., Mehrotra, D., & Chandra, S. (2022, March-April). Potential of Internet of Medical Things (IoMT) applications in building a smart healthcare system: A systematic review. *Journal of Oral Biology and Craniofacial Research*, 12(2), 302–318. DOI: 10.1016/j.jobcr.2021.11.010 PMID: 34926140

Greene, S., Thapliyal, H., & Carpenter, D. (2016) "IoMT-Based Fall Detection for Smart Home Environments," IEEE International Symposium on Nanoelectronic and Information Systems (iNIS), Gwalior, India, pp. 23-28, DOI: 10.1109/iNIS.2016.017

Johnson, K. B., Wei, W. Q., Weeraratne, D., Frisse, M. E., Misulis, K., Rhee, K., Zhao, J., & Snowdon, J. L. (2021, January). Precision Medicine, AI, and the Future of Personalized Health Care. *Clinical and Translational Science*, 14(1), 86–93. DOI: 10.1111/cts.12884 PMID: 32961010

Khan, Z. A., & Sohn, W. (2011). Abnormal human activity recognition system based on R-transform and kernel discriminant technique for elderly home care. *IEEE Transactions on Consumer Electronics*, 57(4), 1843–1850.

Korshunova, M., Huang, N., Capuzzi, S., Radchenko, D. S., Savych, O., Moroz, Y. S., Wells, C. I., Willson, T. M., Tropsha, A., & Isayev, O. (2022, October 18). Generative and reinforcement learning approaches for the automated de novo design of bioactive compounds. *Communications Chemistry*, 5(1), 129. DOI: 10.1038/s42004-022-00733-0 PMID: 36697952

Kumar, P. M., & Gandhi, U. D. (2018). A novel three-tier Internet of Medical Things architecture with machine learning algorithm for early detection of heart diseases (Vol. 65). Computers & Electrical Engineering., https://www.sciencedirect.com/science/article/pii/S0045790617328410, , ISSN 0045-7906. DOI: 10.1016/j.compeleceng.2017.09.001

Manickam, P., Mariappan, S. A., Murugesan, S. M., Hansda, S., Kaushik, A., Shinde, R., & Thipperudraswamy, S. P. (2022, July 25). Artificial Intelligence (AI) and Internet of Medical Things (IoMT) Assisted Biomedical Systems for Intelligent Healthcare. *Biosensors (Basel)*, 12(8), 562. DOI: 10.3390/bios12080562 PMID: 35892459

. Pennello G, Samuelson F(2023).AI–Enabled Medical Devices and Diagnostics: Statistical Challenges and Opportunities from a Regulatory Perspective; AMSTATNEWS; American statistical association.

Reddy, N., Verma, N., & Dungan, K. (2023). *Monitoring technologies-continuous glucose monitoring, mobile technology, biomarkers of glycemic control.* Endotext. [Internet]

Singh, A., & Ogunfunmi, T. (2021, December 28). An Overview of Variational Autoencoders for Source Separation, Finance, and Bio-Signal Applications. *Entropy (Basel, Switzerland)*, 24(1), 55. DOI: 10.3390/e24010055 PMID: 35052081

Tan, P., Xi, Y., Chao, S., Jiang, D., Liu, Z., Fan, Y., & Li, Z. (2022, April 11). An Artificial Intelligence-Enhanced Blood Pressure Monitor Wristband Based on Piezoelectric Nanogenerator. *Biosensors (Basel)*, 12(4), 234. DOI: 10.3390/bios12040234 PMID: 35448294

. N. Tommarello and R. Deek. (2024) "The Convergence of the Internet of Medical Things and Artificial Intelligence in Medicine: Assessing the Benefits, Challenges, and Risks" in Computer, vol. 57, no. 02, pp. 95-99, DOI: 10.1109/MC.2023.3321188

Wang, J., Zhang, Z., Li, B., Lee, S., & Sherratt, R. S. (2014, February). An enhanced fall detection system for elderly person monitoring using consumer home networks. *IEEE Transactions on Consumer Electronics*, 60(1), 23–29. DOI: 10.1109/TCE.2014.6780921

Wang, L.-H., Hsiao, Y.-M., Xie, X.-Q., & Lee, S.-Y. (2016, May). An outdoor intelligent healthcare monitoring device for the elderly. *IEEE Transactions on Consumer Electronics*, 62(2), 128–135. DOI: 10.1109/TCE.2016.7514671

Wenzel, M. (2023). (2023 Jul 23). Generative Adversarial Networks and Other Generative Models. In Colliot, O. (Ed.), *Machine Learning for Brain Disorders* [Internet]. Humana., Available from https://www.ncbi.nlm.nih.gov/books/NBK597493/, DOI: 10.1007/978-1-0716-3195-9_5

Zhang, S., Fan, R., Liu, Y., Chen, S., Liu, Q., & Zeng, W. (2023, January 11). Applications of transformer-based language models in bioinformatics: A survey. *Bioinformatics Advances*, 3(1), vbad001. Advance online publication. DOI: 10.1093/bioadv/vbad001 PMID: 36845200

Compilation of References

Aavula, R.. (2022). Design and Implementation of sensor and IoT based Remembrance system for closed one. *Telematique*, 21(1), 2769–2778.

Abbasian, M., Khatibi, E., Azimi, I., Oniani, D., Abad, Z. S. H., Thieme, A., Sriram, R., Yang, Z., Wang, Y., Lin, B., Gevaert, O., Li, L. J., Jain, R., & Rahmani, A. M. (2024). Foundation metrics for evaluating effectiveness of healthcare conversations powered by generative AI. *NPJ Digital Medicine*, 7(1), 82. Advance online publication. DOI: 10.1038/s41746-024-01074-z PMID: 38553625

Abhangrao, C. M. (2024). Internet of Things in Mechatronics for Design and Manufacturing: A Review. *Journals of Mechatronics Machine Design and Manufacturing*, 6(1).

Abidi, S. S. R., & Abidi, S. R. (2019, July). Intelligent health data analytics: A convergence of artificial intelligence and big data. *Healthcare Management Forum*, 32(4), 178–182. DOI: 10.1177/0840470419846134 PMID: 31117831

Abu-salih, B., AL-Qurishi, M., Alweshah, M., AL-Smadi, M., Alfayez, R., & Saadeh, H. (2023). Healthcare knowledge graph construction: A systematic review of the state-of-the-art, open issues, and opportunities. *Journal of Big Data*, 10(1), 81. DOI: 10.1186/s40537-023-00774-9 PMID: 37274445

Acharya N. (2005). Construction of conditional double sampling plans using intervened random effect Poisson distribution. *Proceedings volume of SJYSDNS, 1*, 57-61.

Adams, J., & Smith, G. (2022). Challenges in AI integration. *Healthcare Analytics Journal*, 6(3), 144–158. DOI: 10.1080/20479700.2022.1836799

Adams, N. R., & Taylor, O. B. (2024) "AI in Surgery: The Role of IoMT for Precision and Safety," in *2024 International Conference on Surgical Robotics and AI (ICSRAI)*, Boston, USA, pp. 36-41.

Adeniyi, E. A., Ogundokun, R. O., & Awotunde, J. B. (2021). IoMT-based wearable body sensors network healthcare monitoring system. *IoT in healthcare and ambient assisted living*, 103-121.

Affia, A. A. O., Finch, H., Jung, W., Samori, I. A., Potter, L., & Palmer, X. L. (2023). IoT health devices: Exploring security risks in the connected landscape. *IoT*, 4(2), 150–182.

Aftab, M., Nadeem, A., Zhang, C., Dong, Z., Jiang, Y., & Liu, K. (2024). Advancements and challenges in artificial intelligence applications in healthcare delivery systems.

Aggarwal, C. C. (2015). *Data Mining: The Textbook*. Springer. DOI: 10.1007/978-3-319-14142-8

Aghabiglou, A., Chu, C. S., Dabbech, A., & Wiaux, Y. (2024). The R2D2 deep neural network series paradigm for fast precision imaging in radio astronomy. *arXiv preprint arXiv:2403.05452*.

Ahmed, A., Khan, M. M., Singh, P., Batth, R. S., & Masud, M. (2022). IoT-Based Real-Time Patients Vital Physiological Parameters Monitoring System Using Smart Wearable Sensors. *Neural Computing & Applications*, 35(7), 5595. DOI: 10.1007/s00521-022-07090-y PMID: 35440847

Ahmed, F. R., & Hassan, G. S. (2024) "Data Security Challenges in IoMT Systems," in *2024 International Conference on Information Security and Privacy (ICISP)*, Cairo, Egypt, pp. 11-16.

Ahmed, J., Nguyen, T. N., Ali, B., Javed, M. A., & Mirza, J. (2023). On the Physical Layer Security of Federated Learning Based IoMT Networks. *IEEE Journal of Biomedical and Health Informatics*, 27(2), 691–697. Advance online publication. DOI: 10.1109/JBHI.2022.3173947 PMID: 35536821

Ahmed, S. F., Alam, M. S. B., Afrin, S., Rafa, S. J., Rafa, N., & Gandomi, A. H. (2024). Insights into Internet of Medical Things (IoMT): Data fusion, security issues and potential solutions. *Information Fusion*, 102, 102060. DOI: 10.1016/j.inffus.2023.102060

Ahmed, S. T., Kumar, V. V., Singh, K. K., Singh, A., Muthukumaran, V., & Gupta, D. (2022). 6G enabled federated learning for secure IoMT resource recommendation and propagation analysis. *Computers & Electrical Engineering*, 102, 108210. DOI: 10.1016/j.compeleceng.2022.108210

Ahmed, Y. A. E., Yue, B., Gu, Z., & Yang, J. (2023). An overview: Big data analysis by deep learning and image processing. *International Journal of Quantum Information*, 21(7), 2340009. DOI: 10.1142/S0219749923400099

Ajagbe, S. A., Awotunde, J. B., Adesina, A. O., Achimugu, P., & Kumar, T. A. (2022). Internet of medical things (IoMT): applications, challenges, and prospects in a data-driven technology. *Intelligent Healthcare: Infrastructure, Algorithms and Management*, 299-319.

Akinrinola, O., Okoye, C. C., Ofodile, O. C., & Ugochukwu, C. E. (2024). Navigating and reviewing ethical dilemmas in AI development: Strategies for transparency, fairness, and accountability. *GSC Advanced Research and Reviews, 18*(3), 050-058.

Akram, M., & Sharma, P. (2024, January). Diabetic Retinopathy Detection Using Voting Classification Method. In *2024 IEEE 1st Karachi Section Humanitarian Technology Conference (KHI-HTC)* (pp. 1-11). IEEE. DOI: 10.1109/KHI-HTC60760.2024.10482074

Alalawi, S., Alalawi, M., & Alrae, R. (2024, August). Privacy preservation for the IoMT using federated learning and blockchain technologies. In *The International Conference on Innovations in Computing Research* (pp. 713-731). Cham: Springer Nature Switzerland. DOI: 10.1007/978-3-031-65522-7_62

Alamgir, A., Mousa, O., & Shah, Z. (2021). Artificial intelligence in predicting cardiac arrest: Scoping review. *JMIR Medical Informatics*, 9(12), e30798. DOI: 10.2196/30798 PMID: 34927595

Al-Garadi, M. A., Mohamed, A., Al-Ali, A. K., Du, X., Ali, I., & Guizani, M. (2020). A Survey of Machine and Deep Learning Methods for Internet of Things (IoT) Security. *IEEE Communications Surveys and Tutorials*, 22(3), 1646–1685. Advance online publication. DOI: 10.1109/COMST.2020.2988293

Alhaidari, F., Rahman, A., & Zagrouba, R. (2023). Cloud of Things: Architecture, applications and challenges. *Journal of Ambient Intelligence and Humanized Computing*, 14(5), 5957–5975. DOI: 10.1007/s12652-020-02448-3

Alhaj, T. A., Abdulla, S. M., Iderss, M. A. E., Ali, A. A. A., Elhaj, F. A., Remli, M. A., & Gabralla, L. A. (2022). A survey: To govern, protect, and detect security principles on internet of medical things (IoMT). *IEEE Access : Practical Innovations, Open Solutions*, 10, 124777–124791. DOI: 10.1109/ACCESS.2022.3225038

Ali, A., Al-rimy, B. A. S., Tin, T. T., Altamimi, S. N., Qasem, S. N., & Saeed, F. (2023). Empowering Precision Medicine: Unlocking Revolutionary Insights through Blockchain-Enabled Federated Learning and Electronic Medical Records. *Sensors (Basel)*, 23(17), 7476. DOI: 10.3390/s23177476 PMID: 37687931

Ali, A., Hashim, A., Saeed, A., Aftab, A. K., Ting, T. T., Assam, M., Yazeed, Y. G., & Mohamed, H. G. (2023). Blockchain-Powered Healthcare Systems: Enhancing Scalability and Security with Hybrid Deep Learning. *Sensors (Basel)*, 23(18), 7740. DOI: 10.3390/s23187740 PMID: 37765797

Alian, S., Li, J., & Pandey, V. (2018). (n.d) "A Personalized Recommendation System to Support Diabetes Self-Management for American Indians. *IEEE Access : Practical Innovations, Open Solutions*, 6, 73041–73051. DOI: 10.1109/ACCESS.2018.2882138

Ali, M., Naeem, F., Tariq, M., & Kaddoum, G. (2023). Federated Learning for Privacy Preservation in Smart Healthcare Systems: A Comprehensive Survey. *IEEE Journal of Biomedical and Health Informatics*, 27(2), 778–789. Advance online publication. DOI: 10.1109/JBHI.2022.3181823 PMID: 35696470

Al-Jarrah, O. Y., Yoo, P. D., Muhaidat, S., Karagiannidis, G. K., & Taha, K. (2015). Efficient machine learning for big data: A review. *Big Data Research*, 2(3), 87–93. DOI: 10.1016/j.bdr.2015.04.001

Al-Maani, M., Frisbie, G., Shippy, F., Tiseo, M., Darwish, O., & Abualkibash, M. 2022. "A Classifier to Detect Number of Machines Performing DoS Attack Against Arduino Oplà Device in IoT Environment." In *Proceedings - 2022 5th International Conference on Advanced Communication Technologies and Networking, CommNet 2022*, DOI: 10.1109/CommNet56067.2022.9993816

Almalki, J., Al Shehri, W., Mehmood, R., Alsaif, K., Alshahrani, S. M., Jannah, N., & Khan, N. A. (2022). Enabling blockchain with IoMT devices for healthcare. *Information (Basel)*, 13(10), 448. DOI: 10.3390/info13100448

Almansour, N. A., Syed, H. F., Khayat, N. R., Altheeb, R. K., Juri, R. E., Alhiyafi, J., Alrashed, S., & Olatunji, S. O. (2019). Neural network and support vector machine for the prediction of chronic kidney disease: A comparative study. *Computers in Biology and Medicine*, 109, 101–111. DOI: 10.1016/j.compbiomed.2019.04.017 PMID: 31054385

Alowais, S. A., Alghamdi, S. S., Alsuhebany, N., Alqahtani, T., Alshaya, A. I., Almohareb, S. N., Aldairem, A., Alrashed, M., Bin Saleh, K., Badreldin, H. A., Al Yami, M. S., Al Harbi, S., & Albekairy, A. M. (2023). Revolutionizing healthcare: The role of artificial intelligence in clinical practice. *BMC Medical Education*, 23(1), 689. DOI: 10.1186/s12909-023-04698-z PMID: 37740191

Alrubayyi, H., Alshareef, M. S., Nadeem, Z., Abdelmoniem, A. M., & Jaber, M. (2024). Security Threats and Promising Solutions Arising from the Intersection of AI and IoT: A Study of IoMT and IoET Applications. *Future Internet*, 16(3), 85. Advance online publication. DOI: 10.3390/fi16030085

Alsaffar, A. A., Pham, H. P., Hong, C. S., Huh, E. N., & Aazam, M. (2016). An architecture of IoT service delegation and resource allocation based on collaboration between fog and cloud computing. *Mobile Information Systems*, 2016(1), 6123234. DOI: 10.1155/2016/6123234

Alshammari, T. S. (2024). Applying machine learning algorithms for the classification of sleep disorders. *IEEE Access : Practical Innovations, Open Solutions*, 12, 36110–36121. DOI: 10.1109/ACCESS.2024.3374408

Al-Turjman, F., Nawaz, M. H., & Ulusar, U. D. (2020). Intelligence in the Internet of Medical Things era: A systematic review of current and future trends. *Computer Communications*, 150, 644–660.

Alturki, R., Alyamani, H. J., Ikram, M. A., Rahman, M. A., Alshehri, M. D., Khan, F., & Haleem, M. (2021). Sensor-Cloud Architecture: A Taxonomy of Security Issues in Cloud-Assisted Sensor Networks. *IEEE Access : Practical Innovations, Open Solutions*, 9, 89344–89359. Advance online publication. DOI: 10.1109/ACCESS.2021.3088225

Alwahedi, F., Aldhaheri, A., Ferrag, M. A., Battah, A., & Tihanyi, N. (2024). Machine learning techniques for IoT security: Current research and future vision with generative AI and large language models. *Internet of Things and Cyber-Physical Systems*, 4, 167–185. DOI: 10.1016/j.iotcps.2023.12.003

Alzoubi, A. A., AlSuwaidi, A., & Alzoubi, H. M. (2024). Analyzing the Approaches for Discovering Privacy and Security Breaches in IoMT. In *Technology Innovation for Business Intelligence and Analytics (TIBIA) Techniques and Practices for Business Intelligence Innovation* (pp. 345–355). Springer Nature Switzerland. DOI: 10.1007/978-3-031-55221-2_23

Alzubi, O. A., Alzubi, J. A., Shankar, K., & Gupta, D. (2021). Blockchain and artificial intelligence enabled privacy-preserving medical data transmission in Internet of Things. *Transactions on Emerging Telecommunications Technologies*, 32(12), e4360. Advance online publication. DOI: 10.1002/ett.4360

Aman, A. H. M., Hassan, W. H., Sameen, S., Attarbashi, Z. S., Alizadeh, M., & Latiff, L. A. (2021). IoMT amid COVID-19 pandemic: Application, architecture, technology, and security. *Journal of Network and Computer Applications*, 174, 102886. DOI: 10.1016/j.jnca.2020.102886 PMID: 34173428

Amann, J., Blasimme, A., Vayena, E., Frey, D., & Madai, V. I. (2020). Explainability for artificial intelligence in healthcare: A multidisciplinary perspective. *BMC Medical Informatics and Decision Making*, 20(1), 1–9. DOI: 10.1186/s12911-020-01332-6 PMID: 33256715

Amiri, Z., Heidari, A., Darbandi, M., Yazdani, Y., Jafari Navimipour, N., Esmaeilpour, M., Sheykhi, F., & Unal, M. (2023). The Personal Health Applications of Machine Learning Techniques in the Internet of Behaviors. *Sustainability (Basel)*, 15(16), 12406. DOI: 10.3390/su151612406

Anderson, J., & Smith, R. (2022). Radiological AI in cancer detection. *Journal of Clinical Imaging*, 15(3), 120–134. DOI: 10.1000/jci.2022.120

Anderson, R. (2020). Statistical quality control using deep learning techniques. *Journal of Quality Technology*, 52(3), 220–232.

Anjana, G., Nisha, K. L., & Sankar, A. (2024). Improving sepsis classification performance with artificial intelligence algorithms: A comprehensive overview of healthcare applications. *Journal of Critical Care*, 83, 154815. DOI: 10.1016/j.jcrc.2024.154815 PMID: 38723336

Archana Shreee, S., Maheshwari, B., & Jeevitha Sai, G. (2023) "A Novel Method of Identification of Delirium in Patients from Electronic Health Records Using Machine Learning," 2023 World Conference on Communication & Computing (WCONF), RAIPUR, India, 2023, pp. 1-6.

Ardila, D., Kiraly, A. P., Bharadwaj, S., Choi, B., Reicher, J. J., Peng, L., Tse, D., Etemadi, M., Ye, W., Corrado, G., Naidich, D. P., & Shetty, S. (2019). End-to-End Lung Cancer Screening with Three-Dimensional Deep Learning on Low-Dose Chest Computed Tomography. *Nature Medicine*, 25(6), 954–961. DOI: 10.1038/s41591-019-0447-x PMID: 31110349

Ariffin, N. A., Yunus, A. M., & Kadir, I. K. (2021). The role of big data in the healthcare industry. *Journal of Islamic*, 6(36), 235–245.

Arrieta, A. B., Díaz-Rodríguez, N., Del Ser, J., Bennetot, A., Tabik, S., Barbado, A., & Herrera, F. (2020). Explainable Artificial Intelligence (XAI): Concepts, taxonomies, opportunities and challenges toward responsible AI. *Information Fusion*, 58, 82–115. DOI: 10.1016/j.inffus.2019.12.012

Asan, O., Bayrak, A. E., & Choudhury, A. (2020). Artificial intelligence and human trust in healthcare: Focus on clinicians. *Journal of Medical Internet Research*, 22(6), e15154. DOI: 10.2196/15154 PMID: 32558657

Ashfaq, A., Sant'Anna, A., Lingman, M., & Nowaczyk, S. (2019). Readmission prediction using deep learning on electronic health records. *Journal of Biomedical Informatics*, 97, 103256. Advance online publication. DOI: 10.1016/j.jbi.2019.103256 PMID: 31351136

Ashfaq, Z., Rafay, A., Mumtaz, R., Hassan Zaidi, S. M., Saleem, H., Raza Zaidi, S. A., Mumtaz, S., & Haque, A. (2022). A review of enabling technologies for the Internet of Medical Things (IoMT) ecosystem. *Ain Shams Engineering Journal*, 13(4), 101660. DOI: 10.1016/j.asej.2021.101660

Ashok, M., Madan, R., Joha, A., & Sivarajah, U. (2022). Ethical framework for Artificial Intelligence and Digital technologies. *International Journal of Information Management*, 62, 102433. DOI: 10.1016/j.ijinfomgt.2021.102433

Ashreetha, B., Gowda, D., Anandaram, H., Nithya, B. A., Gupta, N., & Verma, B. K. (2023, February). IoT Wearable Breast Temperature Assessment System. In 2023 7th International Conference on Computing Methodologies and Communication (ICCMC) (pp. 1236-1241). IEEE.

Askar, N. A., Habbal, A., Mohammed, A. H., Sajat, M. S., Yusupov, Z., & Kodirov, D. (2022). Architecture, Protocols, and Applications of the Internet of Medical Things (IoMT). *Journal of Communication*, 17(11), 900–918. Advance online publication. DOI: 10.12720/jcm.17.11.900-918

Awad, A., Trenfield, S. J., Pollard, T. D., Ong, J. J., Elbadawi, M., McCoubrey, L. E., Goyanes, A., Gaisford, S., & Basit, A. W. (2021). Connected healthcare: Improving patient care using digital health technologies. *Advanced Drug Delivery Reviews*, 178, 113958. DOI: 10.1016/j.addr.2021.113958 PMID: 34478781

Ayaz, M., & Muhammad, F. P. (2023). Transforming Healthcare Analytics with FHIR: A Framework for Standardizing and Analyzing Clinical Data. *Health Care*, 11(12), 1729. PMID: 37372847

Azrour, M., Mabrouki, J., Guezzaz, A., Ahmad, S., Khan, S., & Benkirane, S. (Eds.). (2024). *IoT, machine learning and data analytics for smart healthcare*. CRC Press.

Baby, P. S., & Vital, T. P. (2015). Statistical analysis and predicting kidney diseases using machine learning algorithms. *International Journal of Engineering Research & Technology (Ahmedabad)*, 4(7), 206–210.

Bahri, S., Zoghlami, N., Abed, M., & Tavares, J. M. R. (2018). Big data for healthcare: A survey. *IEEE Access : Practical Innovations, Open Solutions*, 7, 7397–7408. DOI: 10.1109/ACCESS.2018.2889180

Baker, R. C., & Brost, R. W. (1978). Conditional double sampling plan. *Journal of Quality Technology*, 10(4), 1–11. DOI: 10.1080/00224065.1978.11980843

Bak, M. R., Ploem, M. C., Tan, H. L., Blom, M. T., & Willems, D. L. (2023). Towards trust-based governance of health data research. *Medicine, Health Care, and Philosophy*, 26(2), 185–200. DOI: 10.1007/s11019-022-10134-8 PMID: 36633724

Balamurali, S., & Subramani, S. (2012). Conditional variable double sampling plan for Weibull distributed life times under sudden death testing. *Bonfring International Journal of Data Mining*, 2(3), 12–15. DOI: 10.9756/BIJDM.1343

Bao, Y., Tang, Z., Li, H., & Zhang, Y. (2019). Computer vision and deep learning–based data anomaly detection method for structural health monitoring. *Structural Health Monitoring*, 18(2), 401–421. DOI: 10.1177/1475921718757405

Baptist, M. A., Aisyah, F. A. H., Abdillah, S. F., Othman, I. W., & Abdullah, N. J. (2023). Unravelling the Web of Issues and Challenges in Healthcare Cybersecurity for a Secure Tomorrow. *Business and Economic Review*, 13(4), 59. Advance online publication. DOI: 10.5296/ber.v13i4.21341

Baronzio, G., Parmar, G., & Baronzio, M. (2015, July 23). Overview of methods for overcoming hindrance to drug delivery to tumors, with special attention to tumor interstitial fluid. *Frontiers in Oncology*, 5, 165. DOI: 10.3389/fonc.2015.00165 PMID: 26258072

Batko, K. (2023). Digital social innovation based on Big Data Analytics for health and well-being of society. *Journal of Big Data*, 10(1), 171. DOI: 10.1186/s40537-023-00846-w

Beam, A. L., & Kohane, I. S. (2018). Big data and machine learning in health care. *Journal of the American Medical Association*, 319(13), 1317–1318. DOI: 10.1001/jama.2017.18391 PMID: 29532063

Behura, A., Sahu, S., & Kabat, M. R. (2021). Advancement of Machine Learning and Cloud Computing in the Field of Smart Health Care. *Machine Learning Approach for Cloud Data Analytics in IoT*, 273-306.

Berros, N., Mendili, F. E., Filaly, Y., & Idrissi, Y. E. B. E. (2023). Enhancing Digital Health Services with Big Data Analytics. *Big Data and Cognitive Computing*, 7(2), 64. DOI: 10.3390/bdcc7020064

Bertsimas, D., Dunn, J., Mundru, N., & Velmahos, G. (2020). Machine learning in medical decision-making: Algorithms, challenges, and opportunities. *Operations Research for Health Care*, 26, 100275.

Bhalla, N., Jolly, P., Formisano, N., & Estrela, P. (2016). Introduction to biosensors. *Essays in Biochemistry*, 60(1), 1–8. DOI: 10.1042/EBC20150001 PMID: 27365030

Bharati, S., Podder, P., Mondal, M. R. H., & Paul, P. K. (2021). Applications and challenges of cloud integrated IoMT. Cognitive Internet of Medical Things for Smart Healthcare: Services and Applications, 67-85.

Bhardwaj, A., Mangat, V., Vig, R., Halder, S., & Conti, M. (2021). Distributed Denial of Service Attacks in Cloud: State-of-the-Art of Scientific and Commercial Solutions. *Computer Science Review*, 39, 100332. Advance online publication. DOI: 10.1016/j.cosrev.2020.100332

Bhatkar, A. P., & Kharat, G. (2015). Detection of Diabetic Retinopathy in Retinal Images Using MLP Classifier. In *Proceedings of the IEEE International Symposium on Nanoelectronic and Information Systems*, Indore, India, pp. 331–335. DOI: 10.1109/iNIS.2015.30

Bhattacharyya, D., Stephen Neal Joshua, E., & Thirupathi Rao, N. (2023). Medical Image Analysis of Lung Cancer CT Scans Using Deep Learning with Swarm Optimization Techniques. *Machine Intelligence, Big Data Analytics, and IoT in Image Processing: Practical Applications*, 23-50.

Bhatti, D. S., & Saleem, S. (2020). Ephemeral secrets: Multi-party secret key acquisition for secure ieee 802.11 mobile ad hoc communication. *IEEE Access : Practical Innovations, Open Solutions*, 8, 24242–24257. DOI: 10.1109/ACCESS.2020.2970147

Bhone, A. (2024). Medconnect (Android App): Linking Doctors, Patients, and Prescriptions Digitally. *International Journal for Research in Applied Science and Engineering Technology*, 12(2), 697–702. Advance online publication. DOI: 10.22214/ijraset.2024.58409

Bhushan, B., Kumar, A., Agarwal, A. K., Kumar, A., Bhattacharya, P., & Kumar, A. (2023). Towards a secure and sustainable Internet of Medical Things (IoMT): Requirements, design challenges, security techniques, and future trends. *Sustainability (Basel)*, 15(7), 6177. DOI: 10.3390/su15076177

Bidgoli, H. (2023). Integrating Information Technology to Healthcare and Healthcare Management: Improving Quality, Access, Efficiency, Equity, and Healthy Lives. *American Journal of Management*, 23(3), 111–131. DOI: 10.33423/ajm.v23i3.6362

Bilal, A., Zhu, L., Deng, A., Lu, H., & Wu, N. (2022). AI-Based Automatic Detection and Classification of Diabetic Retinopathy Using U-Net and Deep Learning. *Symmetry*, 14(7), 1427. DOI: 10.3390/sym14071427

BioNomadix. (2024). BioNomadix: Physiology Ware. Retrieved from https://www.biopac.com/product-category/research/bionomadix-wireless-physiology/

Bishop, C. M. (2006). *Pattern Recognition and Machine Learning*. Springer.

Blasiak, A., Khong, J., & Kee, T. (2020, April 1). CURATE. AI: Optimizing personalized medicine with artificial intelligence. *SLAS Technology*, 25(2), 95–105. DOI: 10.1177/2472630319890316 PMID: 31771394

Bloom, D. E., Cafiero, E. T., Jané-Llopis, E., Abrahams-Gessel, S., Bloom, L. R., Fathima, S., ... (2011)., The global economic burden of non-communicable diseases, Geneva: Harvard School of Public Health and World Economic Forum.

Box, G. E. P., Hunter, J. S., & Hunter, W. G. (2005). *Statistics for Experimenters: Design, Innovation, and Discovery* (2nd ed.). Wiley.

Brown, A., & Patel, R. (2021). AI for scheduling in hospitals. *Medical Informatics Journal*, 24(2), 125–138. DOI: 10.1080/17538157.2021.1892448

Brown, D., Davis, M., & Lee, C. (2023) "Enhancing Medical Equipment Reliability through Predictive Maintenance and IoT," *2023 IEEE International Conference on Emerging Technologies and Factory Automation (ETFA)*, Berlin, Germany, pp. 453-459.

Brown, G., & Davis, K. (2024) "Integrating AI and IoMT for Smart Hospital Management," in *2024 IEEE Conference on Smart Healthcare Systems (ICSHS)*, San Francisco, USA, pp. 27-32.

Brown, N. (2015). *In silico medicinal chemistry: computational methods to support drug design*. Royal Society of Chemistry.

Brown, P., & Zhang, L. (2021). AI for pathology diagnostics. *Nature Medicine*, 27(5), 451–462. DOI: 10.1038/s41591-021-01345-6

BrowserStack. (2024). BrowserStack Cloud Web. Retrieved from https://www.browserstack.com

Bumgarner, J. M., Lambert, C. T., Cantillon, D. J., Cantillon, D., Rooney, L., Tarakji, K. G., & Wazni, O. M. (2018). Assessing the accuracy of an artificial intelligence–based ECG algorithm for detecting atrial fibrillation. *American Heart Journal*, 207, 94–100.

Burant, C. J. (2022, December). A Methodological Note: An Introduction to Autoregressive Models. *International Journal of Aging & Human Development*, 95(4), 516–522. DOI: 10.1177/00914150211066554 PMID: 34866432

Cabello, J. C., Karimipour, H., Jahromi, A. N., Dehghantanha, A., & Parizi, R. M. (2020). Big-data and cyber-physical systems in healthcare: Challenges and opportunities. *Handbook of Big Data Privacy*, 255-283.

Califf, R. M. (2018). Biomarker definitions and their applications. *Experimental Biology and Medicine*, 243(3), 213–221. DOI: 10.1177/1535370217750088 PMID: 29405771

Campbell, J., & Brown, P. (2021). Bias in AI algorithms. *Journal of AI Ethics*, 4(1), 78–91. DOI: 10.1007/s43681-021-00027-1

Campbell, T., & Johnson, M. (2020). Deep learning in medical imaging. *IEEE Transactions on Medical Imaging*, 39(8), 2350–2364. DOI: 10.1109/TMI.2020.2978562

Cano, M. D., & Cañavate-Sanchez, A. (2020). Preserving data privacy in the internet of medical things using dual signature ECDSA. *Security and Communication Networks*, 2020(1), 4960964. DOI: 10.1155/2020/4960964

Capobianco, J. P. (2023). The New Era of Global Services: A Framework for Successful Enterprises in Business Services and IT. References. (2023). In *Emerald Publishing Limited eBooks* (pp. 203–226). DOI: 10.1108/9781837536269

Cellina, M., Cè, M., Alì, M., Fazzini, D., Oliva, G., & Papa, S. (2023). Digital Twins: The New Frontier for Personalized Medicine? *Applied Sciences (Basel, Switzerland)*, 13(13), 7940. DOI: 10.3390/app13137940

Chaddad, A., Wu, Y., & Desrosiers, C. (2024). Federated Learning for Healthcare Applications. *IEEE Internet of Things Journal*, 11(5), 7339–7358. DOI: 10.1109/JIOT.2023.3325822

Chakraborty, S., & Guha, S. (2021). Applications of machine learning in medical imaging and diagnostics. *Nature Machine Intelligence*, 3(2), 101–110.

Chakrasali, S. V., Kumar, C., Chaturvedi, A., & Jaisudhan Pazhani, A. A. (2023). Computer vision based healthcare system for identification of diabetes & its types using AI, Measurement. *Sensors (Basel)*, 27, 10075.

Chan, H. S., Shan, H., Dahoun, T., Vogel, H., & Yuan, S. (2019). Advancing drug discovery via artificial intelligence. *Trends in Pharmacological Sciences*, 40(8), 592–604.

Char, D. S., Shah, N. H., & Magnus, D. (2018). Implementing machine learning in health care—Addressing ethical challenges. *The New England Journal of Medicine*, 378(11), 981–983. DOI: 10.1056/NEJMp1714229 PMID: 29539284

Chatrati, S. P., Hossain, G., Goyal, A., Bhan, A., Bhattacharya, S., Gaurav, D., & Tiwari, S. M. (2022). Smart home health monitoring system for predicting type 2 diabetes and hypertension. *Journal of King Saud University. Computer and Information Sciences*, 34(3), 862–870. DOI: 10.1016/j.jksuci.2020.01.010

Chatterjee, S., & Hadi, A. S. (2015). *Regression Analysis by Example* (5th ed.). Wiley.

Cheatham, B., Javanmardian, K., & Samandari, H. (2019). Confronting the risks of artificial intelligence. *The McKinsey Quarterly*, 2(38), 1–9.

Chen, C. P., & Zhang, C. Y. (2014). Data-intensive applications, challenges, techniques and technologies: A survey on Big Data. *Information sciences, 275*, 314-347. Mayer-Schönberger, V., & Cukier, K. (2013). *Big data: A revolution that will transform how we live, work, and think*. Houghton Mifflin Harcourt.

Chen, L., Wang, H., & Liu, S. (2023) "AI-Powered Decision Support Systems for IoMT Applications," *2023 IEEE International Conference on Systems, Man, and Cybernetics (SMC)*, Istanbul, Turkey, pp. 789-794.

Chen, M., Mao, S., Zhang, Y., & Leung, V. C. (2014). *Big data: related technologies, challenges and future prospects* (Vol. 100). Springer. DOI: 10.1007/978-3-319-06245-7

Chen, T., Gupta, R., & Zhang, Y. (2023) "AI-Based Framework for Real-Time Patient Monitoring Using IoMT," *2023 IEEE International Conference on Consumer Electronics (ICCE)*, Las Vegas, USA, pp. 411-416.

Chen, W., Gu, Z., Liu, Z., Fu, Y., Ye, Z., Zhang, X., & Xiao, L. (2021). A new classification method in ultrasound images of benign and malignant thyroid nodules based on transfer learning and deep convolutional neural network. *Complexity*, 2021(1), 6296811. DOI: 10.1155/2021/6296811

Chinta, S. V., Wang, Z., Zhang, X., Viet, T. D., Kashif, A., Smith, M. A., & Zhang, W. (2024). AI-Driven Healthcare: A Survey on Ensuring Fairness and Mitigating Bias. *arXiv (Cornell University)*. https://doi.org//arxiv.2407.19655DOI: 10.48550

Chintala, S. (2024). The Application of Deep Learning in Analysing Electronic Health Records for Improved Patient Outcomes. *International Journal of Intelligent Systems and Applications in Engineering*, 12(15s).

Ciallella, H. L., & Zhu, H. (2019, March 14). Advancing computational toxicology in the big data era by artificial intelligence: Data-driven and mechanism-driven modeling for chemical toxicity. *Chemical Research in Toxicology*, 32(4), 536–547. DOI: 10.1021/acs.chemrestox.8b00393 PMID: 30907586

Clark, M., & Patel, A. (2021). AI-driven drug development. *Nature Biotechnology*, 39(9), 1235–1244. DOI: 10.1038/s41587-021-00998-0

Coglianese, C., & Lehr, D. (2019). Transparency and algorithmic governance. *Administrative Law Review*, 71(1), 1–56.

Collins, F. S., & Varmus, H. (2015). A new initiative on precision medicine. *The New England Journal of Medicine*, 372(9), 793–795. DOI: 10.1056/NEJMp1500523 PMID: 25635347

CometChat. (2024). CometChat API. Retrieved from https://www.cometchat.com/

Corbin, C. K., Maclay, R., Acharya, A., Mony, S., Punnathanam, S., Thapa, R., Kotecha, N., Shah, N. H., & Chen, J. H. (2023). DEPLOYR: A technical framework for deploying custom real-time machine learning models into the electronic medical record. *Journal of the American Medical Informatics Association : JAMIA*, 30(9), 1532–1542. DOI: 10.1093/jamia/ocad114 PMID: 37369008

Cozzio, C., Viglia, G., Lemarie, L., & Cerutti, S. (2023). Toward an integration of blockchain technology in the food supply chain. *Journal of Business Research*, 162, 113909. DOI: 10.1016/j.jbusres.2023.113909

Cozzoli, N., Salvatore, F. P., Faccilongo, N., & Milone, M. (2022). How can big data analytics be used for healthcare organization management? Literary framework and future research from a systematic review. *BMC Health Services Research*, 22(1), 1–14. DOI: 10.1186/s12913-022-08167-z PMID: 35733192

Cui, A., Zhang, T., Xiao, P., Fan, Z., Wang, H., & Zhuang, Y. (2023). Global and regional prevalence of vitamin D deficiency in population-based studies from 2000 to 2022: A pooled analysis of 7.9 million participants. *Frontiers in Nutrition*, 10, 1070808. Advance online publication. DOI: 10.3389/fnut.2023.1070808 PMID: 37006940

Da Silva, R. G. L. (2024). The advancement of artificial intelligence in biomedical research and health innovation: Challenges and opportunities in emerging economies. *Globalization and Health*, 20(1), 44. Advance online publication. DOI: 10.1186/s12992-024-01049-5 PMID: 38773458

Dahm, M. R., Raine, S. E., Slade, D., Chien, L. J., Kennard, A., Walters, G., Spinks, T., & Talaulikar, G. (2024). Older patients and dialysis shared decision-making. Insights from an ethnographic discourse analysis of interviews and clinical interactions. *Patient Education and Counseling*, 122, 108124. Advance online publication. DOI: 10.1016/j.pec.2023.108124 PMID: 38232671

Daneshvar, N., Pandita, D., Erickson, S., Sulmasy, L. S., & DeCamp, M. (2024). Artificial Intelligence in the Provision of Health Care: An American College of Physicians Policy Position Paper. *Annals of Internal Medicine*, 177(7), 964–967. DOI: 10.7326/M24-0146 PMID: 38830215

Dankan Gowda, V., Swetha, K. R., Namitha, A. R., Manu, Y. M., Rashmi, G. R., & Veera Sivakumar, C. (2018). IOT Based Smart Health Care System to Monitor Covid-19 Patients.

Dash, S., Shakyawar, S. K., Sharma, M., & Kaushik, S. (2019). Big data in healthcare: Management, analysis and future prospects. *Journal of Big Data*, 6(1), 1–25. DOI: 10.1186/s40537-019-0217-0

Das, P. K., A, D. V., Meher, S., Panda, R., & Abraham, A. (2022). A systematic review of recent advancements in deep and machine learning-based detection and classification of acute lymphoblastic leukemia. *IEEE Access : Practical Innovations, Open Solutions*, 10, 81741–81763. DOI: 10.1109/ACCESS.2022.3196037

Das, S., Samal, T. K., Mohanta, B. K., & Nayak, A. 2023. "Emerging Cyber Threats in Healthcare: A Study of Attacks in IoMT Ecosystems." In *7th International Conference on I-SMAC (IoT in Social, Mobile, Analytics and Cloud), I-SMAC 2023 - Proceedings*, DOI: 10.1109/I-SMAC58438.2023.10290147

Das, S., Tariq, A., & Santos, T.. (2023 Jul 23). Recurrent Neural Networks (RNNs): Architectures, Training Tricks, and Introduction to Influential Research. In Colliot, O. (Ed.), *Machine Learning for Brain Disorders* [Internet]. Humana., Available from https://www.ncbi.nlm.nih.gov/books/NBK597502/ , DOI: 10.1007/978-1-0716-3195-9_4

Dasta, J. F. (1992). Application of artificial intelligence to pharmacy and medicine. *Hospital Pharmacy*, 27(4), 312–315.

Davenport, T., & Kalakota, R. (2019). The potential for artificial intelligence in Healthcare. *Future Healthcare Journal*, 6(2), 94–98. DOI: 10.7861/futurehosp.6-2-94 PMID: 31363513

de Almeida, P. G. R., dos Santos, C. D., & Farias, J. S. (2021). Artificial intelligence regulation: A framework for governance. *Ethics and Information Technology*, 23(3), 505–525.

de Behrends, M. R. (2021). Treating Cognitive Symptoms of Generalized Anxiety Disorder Using EMDR Therapy With Bilateral Alternating Tactile Stimulation. *Journal of EMDR Practice and Research*, 15(1), 44–59. DOI: 10.1891/EMDR-D-20-00026

De Fauw, J., Ledsam, J. R., Romera-Paredes, B., Nikolov, S., Tomasev, N., Blackwell, S., & Suleyman, M. (2018). Clinically applicable deep learning for diagnosis and referral in retinal disease. *Nature Medicine*, 24(9), 1342–1350. DOI: 10.1038/s41591-018-0107-6 PMID: 30104768

De, A., & Mishra, S. (2022). Augmented intelligence in mental health care: sentiment analysis and emotion detection with health care perspective. *Augmented Intelligence in Healthcare: A Pragmatic and Integrated Analysis*, 205–235.

Deb, D., Chakraborty, S. R., Lagineni, M., & Singh, K. 2020. "Security Analysis of MITM Attack on SCADA Network." In *Communications in Computer and Information Science*, DOI: 10.1007/978-981-15-6318-8_41

DeFronzo, R. A., Ferrannini, E., Zimmet, P., ... (2015). International Textbook of Diabetes Mellitus, Wiley-Blackwell, 2 (4).

Devi, J. S., Sreedhar, M. B., Arulprakash, P., Kazi, K., & Radhakrishnan, R. (2022). A path towards child-centric Artificial Intelligence based Education. *International Journal of Early Childhood*, 14(3), 9915–9922.

Devika, G., & Karegowda, A. G. (2021). Deep Learning in IoT: Introduction, Applications, and Perspective in the Big Data Era. In *Deep Learning Applications and Intelligent Decision Making in Engineering* (pp. 1-54). IGI Global.

Dhagarra, D., Goswami, M., & Kumar, G. (2020). Impact of trust and privacy concerns on technology acceptance in healthcare: An Indian perspective. *International Journal of Medical Informatics*, 141, 104164. DOI: 10.1016/j.ijmedinf.2020.104164 PMID: 32593847

Dhanwe, S. S.. (2024). AI-driven IoT in Robotics: A Review. *Journal of Mechanisms and Robotics*, 9(1), 41–48.

Dhinakaran, D., Srinivasan, L., Udhaya Sankar, S. M., & Selvaraj, D. (2024). QUANTUM-BASED PRIVACY-PRESERVING TECHNIQUES FOR SECURE AND TRUSTWORTHY INTERNET OF MEDICAL THINGS: AN EXTENSIVE ANALYSIS. *Quantum Information & Computation*, 24(3–4), 227–266. Advance online publication. DOI: 10.26421/QIC24.3-4-3

Dhivya, S., & Prabha, D. (2022, March). A Novel Approach on Chronic Kidney Disease Prediction Using Machine Learning. In *2022 International Conference on Advanced Computing Technologies and Applications (ICACTA)* (pp. 1-6). IEEE.

Dhiyya, A. J. A. (2022). Architecture of IoMT in healthcare. *The Internet of Medical Things (IoMT) Healthcare Transformation*, 161-172.

Dicuonzo, G., Galeone, G., Shini, M., & Massari, A. (2022). Towards the Use of Big Data in Healthcare: A Literature Review. *Health Care*, 10(7), 1232. PMID: 35885759

Dincer, C., Bruch, R., Kling, A., Dittrich, P. S., & Urban, G. A. (2017). Multiplexed point-of-care testing – xPOCT. *Trends in Biotechnology*, 35(8), 728–742. DOI: 10.1016/j.tibtech.2017.03.013 PMID: 28456344

Ding, B. (2018). Pharma Industry 4.0: Literature review and research opportunities in sustainable pharmaceutical supply chains. *Process Safety and Environmental Protection*, 119, 115–130. DOI: 10.1016/j.psep.2018.06.031

Dinges, S. S., Hohm, A., Vandergrift, L. A., Nowak, J., Habbel, P., Kaltashov, I. A., & Cheng, L. L. (2019). Cancer Metabolomic Markers in Urine: Evidence, Techniques and Recommendations. *Nature Reviews. Urology*, 16(6), 339–362. DOI: 10.1038/s41585-019-0185-3 PMID: 31092915

Dinov, I. D. (2016). Volume and value of big healthcare data. *Journal of Medical Statistics and Informatics*, 4(1), 3. Advance online publication. DOI: 10.7243/2053-7662-4-3 PMID: 26998309

Dixit, A. J., & Kazi, M. K. (2015). Iris recognition by daugman's algorithm–an efficient approach. Journal of applied Research and Social Sciences, 2(14), 1-4.

Dixit, A. J. (2014). A review paper on iris recognition. Journal GSD International society for green. *Sustainable Engineering and Management*, 1(14), 71–81.

Docker. (2024). Docker: Containerize an application. Retrieved from https://www.docker.com

Dodge, H. F., & Romig, H. G. (1959). *Sampling Inspection Tables—Single and Double Sampling*. John Wiley & Sons.

Duch, W., Swaminathan, K., & Meller, J. (2007, May 1). Artificial intelligence approaches for rational drug design and discovery. *Current Pharmaceutical Design*, 13(14), 1497–1508. DOI: 10.2174/138161207780765954 PMID: 17504169

Dulhare, U. N., & Ayesha, M. (2016, December). Extraction of action rules for chronic kidney disease using Naïve bayes classifier. In *2016 IEEE International Conference on Computational Intelligence and Computing Research (ICCIC)* (pp. 1-5). IEEE. DOI: 10.1109/ICCIC.2016.7919649

Dumicic, K. (2012). Decision making based on single and double acceptance sampling plans for assessing quality of lots. *Business Systems Research*, 3(2).

Duncan, A. J. (1986). *Quality Control and Industrial Statistics* (5th ed.). Homewood Publisher.

Dwivedi, R., Mehrotra, D., & Chandra, S. (2022). Potential of Internet of Medical Things (IoMT) applications in building a smart healthcare system: A systematic review. *Journal of Oral Biology and Craniofacial Research*, 12(2), 302–318. DOI: 10.1016/j.jobcr.2021.11.010 PMID: 34926140

Dyte. (2024). Dyte API. Retrieved from https://dyte.io/

Elbadawi, M., Gaisford, S., & Basit, A. W. (2021). Advanced machine-learning techniques in drug discovery. *Drug Discovery Today*, 26(3), 769–777. DOI: 10.1016/j.drudis.2020.12.003 PMID: 33290820

Elhoseny, M., Shankar, K., & Uthayakumar, J. (2019). Intelligent diagnostic prediction and classification system for chronic kidney disease. *Scientific Reports*, 9(1), 9583. DOI: 10.1038/s41598-019-46074-2 PMID: 31270387

Elhoseny, M., Thilakarathne, N. N., Alghamdi, M. I., Mahendran, R. K., Gardezi, A. A., Weerasinghe, H., & Welhenge, A. (2021). Security and privacy issues in medical internet of things: Overview, countermeasures, challenges and future directions. *Sustainability (Basel)*, 13(21), 11645. DOI: 10.3390/su132111645

Elswah, D. K., Elnakib, A. A., & Moustafa, H. E. d (2020). Automated diabetic retinopathy grading using resnet; *Proceedings of the 2020 37th National Radio Science Conference (NRSC)*; Cairo, Egypt. 8–10; pp. 248–254. DOI: 10.1109/NRSC49500.2020.9235098

Erdem, A., Morales-Narváez, E., & Dincer, C. (2020). Paper-based plasmonic biosensors for point-of-care applications. *Chemical Reviews*, 120(17), 8832–8853.

Eschenbrenner, B., & Brenden, R. (2022). Deriving Value from Big Data Analytics in Healthcare: A Value-focused Thinking Approach. *AIS Transactions on Human-Computer Interaction*, 14(3), 289–313. DOI: 10.17705/1thci.00170

Escorcia-Gutierrez, J., Mansour, R. F., Leal, E., Villanueva, J., Jimenez-Cabas, J., Soto, C., & Soto-Díaz, R. (2023). Privacy Preserving Blockchain with Energy Aware Clustering Scheme for IoT Healthcare Systems. *Mobile Networks and Applications*. Advance online publication. DOI: 10.1007/s11036-023-02115-9

Esteva, A., Kuprel, B., Novoa, R. A., Ko, J., Swetter, S. M., Blau, H. M., & Thrun, S. (2017). Dermatologist-level classification of skin cancer with deep neural networks. *Nature*, 542(7639), 115–118. DOI: 10.1038/nature21056 PMID: 28117445

Estrela, V. V., Monteiro, A. C. B., França, R. P., Iano, Y., Khelassi, A., & Razmjooy, N. (2018). Health 4.0: applications, management, technologies and review: array. *Medical Technologies Journal*, 2(4), 262–276.

Evans, J. M., Newton, R. W., Ruta, D. A., MacDonald, T. M., & Morris, A. D. (2000). Socio-economic status, obesity and prevalence of type 1 and type 2 diabetes mellitus. *Diabetic Medicine*, 17(6), 478–480. DOI: 10.1046/j.1464-5491.2000.00309.x PMID: 10975218

Evans, L., & Martin, G. (2020). AI for diabetes risk prediction. *Journal of Medical Systems*, 44(4), 32–41. DOI: 10.1007/s10916-020-1532-8

Eyeleko, A. H., & Feng, T. (2023). A Critical Overview of Industrial Internet of Things Security and Privacy Issues Using a Layer-Based Hacking Scenario. *IEEE Internet of Things Journal*, 10(24), 21917–21941. Advance online publication. DOI: 10.1109/JIOT.2023.3308195

Ezhilarasi, K., Hussain, D. M., Sowmiya, M., & Krishnamoorthy, N. (2023). Crop information retrieval framework based on LDW-ontology and SNM-BERT techniques. *Information Technology and Control*, 52(3), 731–743. DOI: 10.5755/j01.itc.52.3.31945

Faaique, M. (2024). Overview of Big Data Analytics in Modern Astronomy. *International Journal of Mathematics, Statistics, and Computer Science*, 2, 96–113. DOI: 10.59543/ijmscs.v2i.8561

Feng, W., Wu, H., Ma, H., Tao, Z., Xu, M., Zhang, X., Lu, S., Wan, C., & Liu, Y. (2024). Applying contrastive pre-training for depression and anxiety risk prediction in type 2 diabetes patients based on heterogeneous electronic health records: A primary healthcare case study. *Journal of the American Medical Informatics Association : JAMIA*, 31(2), 445–455. Advance online publication. DOI: 10.1093/jamia/ocad228 PMID: 38062850

Ferrucci, D. A., Levas, A., Bagchi, S., Gondek, D., & Mueller, E. T. (2013). Watson: Beyond jeopardy! *Artificial Intelligence*, 199, 93–105. DOI: 10.1016/j.artint.2012.06.009

Fiani, F., Russo, S., & Napoli, C. (2023). An advanced solution based on machine learning for remote emdr therapy. *Technologies*, 11(6), 172. DOI: 10.3390/technologies11060172

Firth, N. C., Atrash, B., Brown, N., & Blagg, J. (2015, June 22). MOARF, an integrated workflow for multiobjective optimization: Implementation, synthesis, and biological evaluation. *Journal of Chemical Information and Modeling*, 55(6), 1169–1180. DOI: 10.1021/acs.jcim.5b00073 PMID: 26054755

Fleuren, W. W., Alkema, W., Vervloet, M. G., & Maas, A. H. E. M. (2017). Machine learning for the prediction of cardiac risk in a clinical population. *Heart (British Cardiac Society)*, 103(11), 899–906.

Floridi, L., Cowls, J., Beltrametti, M., Chatila, R., Chazerand, P., Dignum, V., Luetge, C., Madelin, R., Pagallo, U., Rossi, F., Schafer, B., Valcke, P., & Vayena, E. (2018). AI4People—an ethical framework for a good AI society: Opportunities, risks, principles, and recommendations. *Minds and Machines*, 28(4), 689–707. DOI: 10.1007/s11023-018-9482-5 PMID: 30930541

Frank, K. J., & Dieckert, J. P. (1996). Clinical review of diabetic eye disease: A primary care perspective. *Southern Medical Journal*, 89(2), 463–470. DOI: 10.1097/00007611-199605000-00002 PMID: 8638169

Gang, L., Chutatape, O., & Krishnan, S. M. (2002). Detection and measurement of retinal vessels in fundus images using amplitude modified second-order Gaussian filter. *IEEE Transactions on Biomedical Engineering*, 49(2), 4–37. DOI: 10.1109/10.979356 PMID: 12066884

Garg, N., Wazid, M., Singh, J., Singh, D. P., & Das, A. K. (2022). Security in IoMT-driven Smart Healthcare: A Comprehensive Review and Open Challenges. *Security and Privacy*, 5(5), e235. Advance online publication. DOI: 10.1002/spy2.235

Gawanmeh, A., Mohammadi-Koushki, N., Mansoor, W., Al-Ahmad, H., & Alomari, A. (2020). Evaluation of MAC protocols for vital sign monitoring within smart home environment. *Arabian Journal for Science and Engineering*, 45(12), 11007–11017. DOI: 10.1007/s13369-020-04915-7

Gaytan, J. C. T. (2022). A literature survey of security and privacy issues in internet of medical things. International Journal of Computations, Information and Manufacturing (IJCIM), 2(2).

GBD 2015 Risk Factors Collaborators (2016). Global, regional, and national comparative risk assessment of 79 behavioural, environmental and occupational, and metabolic risks or clusters of risks, 1990-2015: a systematic analysis for the Global Burden of Disease Study 2015. Lancet; 388: 1659-1724; DOI: http://dx.doi.org/ (16)31679-8.DOI: 10.1016/S0140-6736

Gelkopf, M., Mazor, Y., & Roe, D. (2022). A systematic review of patient-reported outcome measurement (PROM) and provider assessment in mental health: Goals, implementation, setting, measurement characteristics and barriers. *International Journal for Quality in Health Care : Journal of the International Society for Quality in Health Care*, 34(Supplement_1), ii13–ii27. DOI: 10.1093/intqhc/mzz133 PMID: 32159763

Geneiatakis, D., Kounelis, I., Neisse, R., Nai-Fovino, I., Steri, G., & Baldini, G. 2017. "Security and Privacy Issues for an IoT Based Smart Home." In *2017 40th International Convention on Information and Communication Technology, Electronics and Microelectronics, MIPRO 2017 - Proceedings*, DOI: 10.23919/MIPRO.2017.7973622

Ghafar, M. H. B. A., Abdullah, N. A. B., Razak, A. H. A., Ali, M. S. A. B. M., & Al-Junid, S. A. M. (2022, December). Chronic Kidney Disease Prediction based on Data Mining Method and Support Vector Machine. In *2022 IEEE 10th Conference on Systems, Process & Control (ICSPC)* (pp. 262-267). IEEE.

Gheorghe, A. V., Pyne, J. C., Sisti, J., Keating, C. B., Katina, P. F., & Edmonson, W. (2023). Critical Space Infrastructure: A Complex System Governance Perspective. *International Journal of Cyber Diplomacy*, 4, 15–28. DOI: 10.54852/ijcd.v4y202302

Ghubaish, A., Salman, T., Zolanvari, M., Unal, D., Al-Ali, A., & Jain, R. (2020). Recent advances in the internet-of-medical-things (IoMT) systems security. *IEEE Internet of Things Journal*, 8(11), 8707–8718. DOI: 10.1109/JIOT.2020.3045653

Ginter, P. M., Duncan, W. J., & Swayne, L. E. (2018). *The strategic management of health care organizations*. john wiley & sons.

Git. (2024). Git. Retrieved from https://git-scm.com

Goga, N., Boiangiu, C.-A., Vasilateanu, A., Popovici, A.-F., Dragoi, M.-V., Popovici, R., ... Hadar, A. (2022). An Efficient System for Eye Movement Desensitization and Reprocessing (EMDR) Therapy: A Pilot Study.

Golberg, D. E. (1989). Genetic algorithms in search, optimization, and machine learning. Addion wesley, 1989(102), 36.

Goldstein, B. A., Navar, A. M., Pencina, M. J., & Ioannidis, J. P. A. (2017). Opportunities and challenges in developing risk prediction models with electronic health records data: A systematic review. *Journal of the American Medical Informatics Association : JAMIA*, 24(1), 198–208. DOI: 10.1093/jamia/ocw042 PMID: 27189013

Goldstein, E. V., Bailey, E. V., & Wilson, F. A. (2024). Poverty and Suicidal Ideation Among Hispanic Mental Health Care Patients Leading up to the COVID-19 Pandemic. *Hispanic Health Care International; the Official Journal of the National Association of Hispanic Nurses*, 22(1), 6–10. Advance online publication. DOI: 10.1177/15404153231181110 PMID: 37312509

Golombek, S. K., May, J. N., Theek, B., Appold, L., Drude, N., Kiessling, F., & Lammers, T. (2018). Tumor targeting via EPR: Strategies to enhance patient responses. *Advanced Drug Delivery Reviews*, 130, 17–38.

Goodfellow, I., Bengio, Y., & Courville, A. (2016). *Deep Learning*. MIT Press.

Gou, F., Liu, J., Xiao, C., & Wu, J. (2024). Research on artificial-intelligence-assisted medicine: A survey on medical artificial intelligence. *Diagnostics (Basel)*, 14(14), 1472. DOI: 10.3390/diagnostics14141472 PMID: 39061610

Govardanan, C. S., Murugan, R., Yenduri, G., Gurrammagari, D. R., Bhulakshmi, D., Kandati, D. R., ... & Jhaveri, R. H. (2024). The amalgamation of federated learning and explainable artificial intelligence for the Internet of Medical Things: A review. *Recent Advances in Computer Science and Communications (Formerly: Recent Patents on Computer Science)*, 17(4), 1-19.

Govindaraju, K. (1991). Fractional acceptance number single sampling plan. *Communications in Statistics. Simulation and Computation*, 20(1), 173–190. DOI: 10.1080/03610919108812947

Gowda, D., Bakshi, F., Gahana, A., Naik, A. B., & Navya, H. G. (2021, December). Covid-19 Prevention Kit Based on an Infrared Touchless Thermometer and Distance Detector. In 2021 5th International Conference on Electronics, Communication and Aerospace Technology (ICECA) (pp. 358-362). IEEE.

Gowda, D., Lokesh, M., Viraj, H. P., Mailapur, R. V., & Mahendra, K. (2023, June). Implementation of GUI based Vital Track Ambulance for Patient Health Monitoring. In *2023 8th International Conference on Communication and Electronics Systems (ICCES)* (pp. 1417-1424). IEEE.

Gowda, D., Shekhar, R., Prasad, K., Kumar, P. S., Gangadharan, S., & Srividya, C. N. (2023, October). Scalable and Reliable Cloud-Based UV Monitoring for Public Health Applications. In *2023 4th IEEE Global Conference for Advancement in Technology (GCAT)* (pp. 1-8). IEEE.

Greene, S., Thapliyal, H., & Carpenter, D. (2016) "IoMT-Based Fall Detection for Smart Home Environments," IEEE International Symposium on Nanoelectronic and Information Systems (iNIS), Gwalior, India, pp. 23-28, DOI: 10.1109/iNIS.2016.017

Green, J. O., & Black, L. M. (2024) "Optimizing Healthcare Delivery with IoMT and AI," in *2024 International Conference on Health Care Systems Engineering (ICHSE)*, Paris, France, pp. 30-35.

Green, M., Lopez, F., & Brown, T. (2023) "AI and IoMT: A Synergistic Approach to Personalized Medicine," *2023 IEEE International Conference on Computational Intelligence and Virtual Environments for Measurement Systems and Applications (CIVEMSA)*, Milan, Italy, pp. 110-115.

Green, R., & Evans, J. (2021). Regulation of AI in healthcare. *Healthcare Policy Journal*, 16(1), 45–56. DOI: 10.12927/hcpol.2021.26420

Green, S., & Lopez, J. (2020). Operational efficiency via AI. *Health Care Management Review*, 45(3), 189–202. DOI: 10.1097/HMR.0000000000000260

Greenwood-Lee, J., Jewett, L., Woodhouse, L., & Marshall, D. A. (2018). A categorisation of problems and solutions to improve patient referrals from primary to specialty care. *BMC Health Services Research*, 18(1), 1–16. DOI: 10.1186/s12913-018-3745-y PMID: 30572898

Gtmetrix. (2024). Gtmetrix: Web Peformance and Monitoring. Retrieved from https://gtmetrix.com

Gunarathne, W. H. S. D., Perera, K. D. M., & Kahandawaarachchi, K. A. D. C. P. (2017, October). Performance evaluation on machine learning classification techniques for disease classification and forecasting through data analytics for chronic kidney disease (CKD). In *2017 IEEE 17th international conference on bioinformatics and bioengineering (BIBE)* (pp. 291-296). IEEE.

Gund, V. D.. (2023). PIR Sensor-Based Arduino Home Security System. *Journal of Instrumentation and Innovation Sciences*, 8(3), 33–37.

Gupta, V., & Yang, H. (2024). Study protocol for factors influencing the adoption of ChatGPT technology by startups: Perceptions and attitudes of entrepreneurs. *PLoS ONE, 19*(2 February). DOI: 10.1371/journal.pone.0298427

Gupta, B. B., Chaudhary, P., Chang, X., & Nedjah, N. (2022). Smart defense against distributed Denial of service attack in IoT networks using supervised learning classifiers. *Computers & Electrical Engineering*, 98, 107726. DOI: 10.1016/j.compeleceng.2022.107726

Gupta, N. S., & Kumar, P. (2023). Perspective of artificial intelligence in healthcare data management: A journey towards precision medicine. *Computers in Biology and Medicine*, 162, 107051. DOI: 10.1016/j.compbiomed.2023.107051 PMID: 37271113

Gupta, P., Ding, B., Guan, C., & Ding, D. (2024). Generative AI: A systematic review using topic modelling techniques. *Data and Information Management*, 100066(2), 100066. Advance online publication. DOI: 10.1016/j.dim.2024.100066

Gupta, R., Koli, N., Mahor, N., & Tejashri, N. (2020, June). Performance analysis of machine learning classifier for predicting chronic kidney disease. In *2020 International Conference for Emerging Technology (INCET)* (pp. 1-4). IEEE. DOI: 10.1109/INCET49848.2020.9154147

Gupta, S., Johnson, K., & Wang, Y. (2023) "Hybrid Cloud and Edge Computing for Scalable IoT Healthcare Solutions," *2023 IEEE International Conference on Cloud Computing Technology and Science (CloudCom)*, London, UK, pp. 210-215.

Gupta, S., Sapre, N., & Sapre, N. S. (2015). In silico de novo design of novel NNRTIs: A bio-molecular modelling approach. *RSC Advances*, 5(19), 14814–14827. DOI: 10.1039/C4RA15478A

Gururaj, B. (2022) "An Integrated IoT Technology for Health and Traffic Monitoring System with Smart Ambulance," *2022 IEEE North Karnataka Subsection Flagship International Conference (NKCon)*, Vijaypur, India, 2022, pp. 1-6.

Habchi, Y., ... "Machine learning and vision transformers for thyroid carcinoma diagnosis: A review." arXiv preprint arXiv:2403.13843 (2024).

Habib, M., Wang, Z., Qiu, S., Zhao, H., & Murthy, A. S. (2022). Machine learning-based healthcare system for investigating the association between depression and quality of life. *IEEE Journal of Biomedical and Health Informatics*, 26(5), 2008–2019. DOI: 10.1109/JBHI.2022.3140433 PMID: 34986108

Haleem, A., Javaid, M., Singh, R. P., & Suman, R. (2022). Medical 4.0 technologies for healthcare: Features, capabilities, and applications. *Internet of Things and Cyber-Physical Systems*, 2, 12–30. DOI: 10.1016/j.iotcps.2022.04.001

Halli, U. M. (2022). Voltage Sag Mitigation Using DVR and Ultra Capacitor. *Journal of Semiconductor Devices and Circuits.*, 9(3), 21–31p.

Halli, U. M. (2022a). Nanotechnology in IoT Security, *Journal of Nanoscience. Nanoengineering & Applications*, 12(3), 11–16.

Halli, U. M. (2022b). Nanotechnology in E-Vehicle Batteries. *International Journal of Nanomaterials and Nanostructures.*, 8(2), 22–27.

Hamaker. (1950). *Double Sampling Plan*. Engineering Statistics Handbook.

Hameed, S. S., Hassan, W. H., Latiff, L. A., & Ghabban, F. (2021). A systematic review of security and privacy issues in the internet of medical things; the role of machine learning approaches. *PeerJ. Computer Science*, 7, e414. DOI: 10.7717/peerj-cs.414 PMID: 33834100

Han, T., Jiang, D., Zhao, Q., Wang, L., & Yin, K. (2018). Comparison of random forest, artificial neural networks and support vector machine for intelligent diagnosis of rotating machinery. *Transactions of the Institute of Measurement and Control*, 40(8), 2681–2693. DOI: 10.1177/0142331217708242

Haque, R. U., & Hasan, A. T. (2021). Privacy-preserving multivariant regression analysis over blockchain-based encrypted IoMT data. In *Artificial Intelligence and Blockchain for Future Cybersecurity Applications* (pp. 45–59). Springer International Publishing. DOI: 10.1007/978-3-030-74575-2_3

Harish, K. P., Dhivyanchali, M. N., Devi, K. N., Krishnamoorthy, N., Sree, R. D., & Dharanidharan, R. (2023, January). Smart Diagnostic System For Early Detection And Prediction Of Polycystic Ovary Syndrome. In *2023 International Conference on Computer Communication and Informatics (ICCCI)* (pp. 1-6). IEEE. doi:DOI: 10.1109/CSNT57126.2023.10134748

Harris, A., & Green, B. (2021). Natural language processing in EHRs. *Journal of Health Informatics*, 12(4), 85–98. DOI: 10.1016/j.jhi.2021.02.001

Harris, S., & Clark, T. (2021). Ethics in AI decision-making. *Health Ethics Journal*, 12(3), 98–112. DOI: 10.1111/hej.2034

Harvey, P., Toutsop, O., Kornegay, K., Alale, E., & Reaves, D. (2020, December). Security and privacy of medical internet of things devices for smart homes. In 2020 7th International Conference on Internet of Things: Systems, Management and Security (IOTSMS) (pp. 1-6). IEEE.

Hassan, M., Awan, F. M., Naz, A., deAndrés-Galiana, E. J., Alvarez, O., Cernea, A., Fernández-Brillet, L., Fernández-Martínez, J. L., & Kloczkowski, A. (2022). Innovations in Genomics and Big Data Analytics for Personalized Medicine and Health Care: A Review. *International Journal of Molecular Sciences*, 23(9), 4645. DOI: 10.3390/ijms23094645 PMID: 35563034

Hastie, T., Tibshirani, R., & Friedman, J. (2009). *The Elements of Statistical Learning: Data Mining, Inference, and Prediction* (2nd ed.). Springer. DOI: 10.1007/978-0-387-84858-7

Hebbar, S., & Vandana, B. (2023). Artificial Intelligence in Future Telepsychiatry and Psychotherapy for E-Mental Health Revolution. In *Computational Intelligence in Medical Decision Making and Diagnosis* (pp. 39–60). CRC Press. DOI: 10.1201/9781003309451-3

Hegde, S. K., Hegde, R., Hombalimath, V., Palanikkumar, D., Patwari, N., & Gowda, V. D. (2023, January). Symmetrized Feature Selection with Stacked Generalization based Machine Learning Algorithm for the Early Diagnosis of Chronic Diseases. In 2023 5th International Conference on Smart Systems and Inventive Technology (ICSSIT) (pp. 838-844). IEEE.

He, K., Zhang, X., Ren, S., & Sun, J. (2016). Deep residual learning for image recognition. In *Proceedings of the IEEE conference on computer vision and pattern recognition* (pp. 770-778).

Hernandez-Jaimes, M. L., Martinez-Cruz, A., Ramírez-Gutiérrez, K. A., & Feregrino-Uribe, C. (2023). Artificial Intelligence for IoMT Security: A Review of Intrusion Detection Systems, Attacks, Datasets and Cloud–Fog–Edge Architectures. *Internet of Things : Engineering Cyber Physical Human Systems*, 23, 100887. Advance online publication. DOI: 10.1016/j.iot.2023.100887

Hernandez, O. W., & Ruiz, P. D. (2024) "Leveraging IoMT for Predictive Health Analytics," in *2024 IEEE International Conference on Computational Intelligence in Healthcare (ICCIH)*, São Paulo, Brazil, pp. 25-30.

Higgins, O., Short, B. L., Chalup, S. K., & Wilson, R. L. (2023). Artificial intelligence (AI) and machine learning (ML) based decision support systems in mental health: An integrative review. *International Journal of Mental Health Nursing*, 32(4), 966–978. DOI: 10.1111/inm.13114 PMID: 36744684

Hilbert, M. (2016). Big data for development: A review of promises and challenges. *Development Policy Review*, 34(1), 135–174. DOI: 10.1111/dpr.12142

Hireche, R., Mansouri, H., & Pathan, A. S. K. (2022). Security and privacy management in Internet of Medical Things (IoMT): A synthesis. *Journal of cybersecurity and privacy*, 2(3), 640-661.

Hireche, R., Mansouri, H., & Pathan, A. S. K. (2022). Security and privacy management in Internet of Medical Things (IoMT): A synthesis. *Journal of Cybersecurity and Privacy*, 2(3), 640–661. DOI: 10.3390/jcp2030033

Holmes, J. H., & Durbin, D. R. (2020). Emergency medical services: Using data to advance pediatric emergency care. *Pediatrics*, 145(Supplement_2), S111–S117.

Holmes, J., Sacchi, L., & Bellazzi, R. (2004). Artificial intelligence in medicine. *Annals of the Royal College of Surgeons of England*, 86(5), 334–338. DOI: 10.1308/147870804290 PMID: 15333167

Hosny, A., Parmar, C., Quackenbush, J., Schwartz, L. H., & Aerts, H. J. (2018). Artificial intelligence in radiology. *Nature Reviews. Cancer*, 18(8), 500–510. DOI: 10.1038/s41568-018-0016-5 PMID: 29777175

Hossain, E., Rana, R., Higgins, N., Soar, J., Barua, P. D., Pisani, A. R., & Turner, K. (2023). Natural Language Processing in Electronic Health Records in relation to healthcare decision-making: A systematic review. In *Computers in Biology and Medicine* (Vol. 155). DOI: 10.1016/j.compbiomed.2023.106649

Hotkar, P. R., Kulkarni, V., Kamble, P., & Kazi, K. S. (2019). Implementation of Low Power and area efficient carry select Adder. International Journal of Research in Engineering. *Science and Management*, 2(4), 183–184.

Houssein, E. H., Gad, A. G., Hussain, K., & Suganthan, P. N. (2021). Major advances in particle swarm optimization: Theory, analysis, and application. *Swarm and Evolutionary Computation*, 63, 100868. DOI: 10.1016/j.swevo.2021.100868

Huang, X., & Nazir, S. (2020). Evaluating Security of Internet of Medical Things Using the Analytic Network Process Method. *Security and Communication Networks*, 2020, 1–14. Advance online publication. DOI: 10.1155/2020/8829595

Husnain, A., Rasool, S., Saeed, A., Gill, A. Y., & Hussain, H. K. (2023). AI'S healing touch: Examining machine learning's transformative effects on healthcare. *Journal of Wood Science*, 2(10), 1681–1695.

Huynh, T. P., & Haick, H. (2016). Self-Healing, Fully Functional, and Multiparametric Flexible Sensing Platform. *Advanced Materials*, 28(1), 138–143. DOI: 10.1002/adma.201504104 PMID: 26551539

İncegil, D., Kayral, İ. H., & Şenel, F. Ç. (2023). The new era: Transforming healthcare quality with artificial intelligence. In *Algorithmic discrimination and ethical perspective of artificial intelligence* (pp. 183–202). Springer Nature Singapore.

International Diabetes Federation. IDF Diabetes Atlas (2021), 10th Ed Brussels, Belgium. Available at: https://www.diabetesatlas.org; Last accessed on 03.02.2024

Iqbal, N., Mumtaz, R., Shafi, U., & Zaidi, S. M. H. (2021). Gray level co-occurrence matrix (GLCM) texture based crop classification using low altitude remote sensing platforms. *PeerJ. Computer Science*, 7, e536.

Iqbal, W., Abbas, H., Daneshmand, M., Rauf, B., & Bangash, Y. A. (2020). An In-Depth Analysis of IoT Security Requirements, Challenges, and Their Countermeasures via Software-Defined Security. *IEEE Internet of Things Journal*, 7(10), 10250–10276. Advance online publication. DOI: 10.1109/JIOT.2020.2997651

Iyer, V., Desai, G., & Patil, N. (2023) "Role of Wearable IoT Devices in Remote Health Monitoring," 2023 IEEE International Conference on Internet of Things (iThings), Beijing, China, pp. 334-339.

Iyortsuun, N. K., Kim, S.-H., Jhon, M., Yang, H.-J., & Pant, S. (2023). A Review of Machine Learning and Deep Learning Approaches on Mental Health Diagnosis. []. MDPI.]. *Health Care*, 11, 285. PMID: 36766860

Jadhav, M. R., & Kaur, M. (2023) "Predictive Modeling of Dental Health Outcomes Based on Fluoride Concentrations using AI," *2023 3rd International Conference on Smart Generation Computing, Communication and Networking (SMART GENCON)*, Bangalore, India, 2023, pp. 1-7.

Jadhav, V. L. (2024). Detection of Fire in the Environment via a Robot Based Fire Fighting System Using Sensors, *International Journal of Advanced Research in Science* [IJARSCT]. *Tongxin Jishu*, 4(4), 410–418.

Jain, L. (2023). Artificial Intelligence and Machine Learning for Healthcare.

Jalal, A. H., Alam, F., Roychoudhury, S., Umasankar, Y., Pala, N., & Bhansali, S. (2018). Prospects and Challenges of Volatile Organic Compound Sensors in Human Healthcare. *ACS Sensors*, 3(7), 1246–1263. DOI: 10.1021/acssensors.8b00400 PMID: 29879839

Javaid, M. A., Ahmed, A. S., Durand, R., & Tran, S. D. (2016). Saliva as a Diagnostic Tool for Oral and Systemic Diseases. *Journal of Oral Biology and Craniofacial Research*, 6(1), 67–76. DOI: 10.1016/j.jobcr.2015.08.006 PMID: 26937373

Jeevan, K., & Sathisha, B. M. (2020) "Implementation of IoT Based Wireless Electronic Stethoscope," *2020 Third International Conference on Multimedia Processing, Communication & Information Technology (MPCIT)*, pp. 103-106.

Jeevitha Sai, G. (2023) "A Novel Method of Identification of Delirium in Patients from Electronic Health Records Using Machine Learning," *2023 World Conference on Communication & Computing (WCONF)*, Raipur, India, 2023, pp. 1-6.

Jeyavel, J., Parameswaran, T., Mannan, J. M., & Hariharan, U. (2021). Security vulnerabilities and intelligent solutions for IoMT systems. Internet of Medical Things: Remote Healthcare Systems and Applications, 175-194.

Jha, R., Bhattacharjee, V., & Mustafi, A. (2022). Increasing the prediction accuracy for thyroid disease: A step towards better health for society. *Wireless Personal Communications*, 122(2), 1921–1938. DOI: 10.1007/s11277-021-08974-3

Jha, S., & Topol, E. J. (2021). Adapting to Artificial Intelligence: Radiologists and Pathologists as Information Specialists. *Journal of the American Medical Association*, 316(22), 2353–2354. DOI: 10.1001/jama.2016.17438 PMID: 27898975

Johari, A. A., Abd Wahab, M. H., & Mustapha, A. (2019, November). Two-class classification: Comparative experiments for chronic kidney disease. In *2019 4th International Conference on Information Systems and Computer Networks (ISCON)* (pp. 789-792). IEEE.

Johnson, B. K., & Lee, T. (2024) "Real-Time Analytics for IoMT in Chronic Disease Management," in *2024 International Conference on Biomedical Engineering and Informatics (ICBEI)*, London, UK, pp. 45-50.

Johnson, K. B., Wei, W. Q., Weeraratne, D., Frisse, M. E., Misulis, K., Rhee, K., Zhao, J., & Snowdon, J. L. (2021, January). Precision Medicine, AI, and the Future of Personalized Health Care. *Clinical and Translational Science*, 14(1), 86–93. DOI: 10.1111/cts.12884 PMID: 32961010

Johnson, K., & White, F. (2021). AI in global health. *Global Health Journal (Amsterdam, Netherlands)*, 7(4), 132–143. DOI: 10.1016/j.ghj.2021.06.004

Jones, D., & Roberts, K. (2022). AI for EHR data structuring. *Health Data Science Journal*, 9(2), 210–223. DOI: 10.1093/hdsj/hdac021

Jones, R. T., & Clark, S. U. (2024) "Data Privacy and Security in IoMT-Based Healthcare," in *2024 International Conference on Cybersecurity in Healthcare Systems (ICCHS)*, Berlin, Germany, pp. 18-23.

Jordan, M. I., & Mitchell, T. M. (2015). Machine learning: Trends, perspectives, and prospects. *Science*, 349(6245), 255–260. DOI: 10.1126/science.aaa8415 PMID: 26185243

Juhn, Y., & Liu, H. (2020). Artificial intelligence approaches using natural language processing to advance EHR-based clinical research. *The Journal of Allergy and Clinical Immunology*, 145(2), 463–469. DOI: 10.1016/j.jaci.2019.12.897 PMID: 31883846

Junejo, A. K., Komninos, N., & McCann, J. A. (2021). A Secure Integrated Framework for Fog-Assisted Internet-of-Things Systems. *IEEE Internet of Things Journal*, 8(8), 6840–6852. Advance online publication. DOI: 10.1109/JIOT.2020.3035474

Jurcik, T., Jarvis, G. E., Doric, J. Z., Krasavtseva, Y., Yaltonskaya, A., Ogiwara, K., & Grigoryan, K. (2023). Adapting mental health services to the COVID-19 pandemic: reflections from professionals in four countries. In *How the COVID-19 Pandemic Transformed the Mental Health Landscape* (pp. 3–28). Routledge. DOI: 10.4324/9781003352235-2

JWT. (2024). JSON Web Tokens Standard. Retrieved from https://jwt.io

Kakhi, K., Alizadehsani, R., Kabir, H. D., Khosravi, A., Nahavandi, S., & Acharya, U. R. (2022). The internet of medical things and artificial intelligence: Trends, challenges, and opportunities. *Biocybernetics and Biomedical Engineering*, 42(3), 749–771. DOI: 10.1016/j.bbe.2022.05.008

Kamalov, F., Pourghebleh, B., Gheisari, M., Liu, Y., & Moussa, S. (2023). Internet of Medical Things Privacy and Security: Challenges, Solutions, and Future Trends from a New Perspective. *Sustainability (Basel)*, 15(4), 3317. DOI: 10.3390/su15043317

Kaptan, S. K., Kaya, Z. M., & Akan, A. (2024). Addressing mental health need after COVID-19: A systematic review of remote EMDR therapy studies as an emerging option. *Frontiers in Psychiatry*, 14, 1336569. DOI: 10.3389/fpsyt.2023.1336569 PMID: 38250261

Karale Aishwarya, A.. (2023). Smart Billing Cart Using RFID, YOLO and Deep Learning for Mall Administration. *International Journal of Instrumentation and Innovation Sciences*, 8(2).

Kar, S. S., & Maity, S. P. (2018). Automatic Detection of Retinal Lesions for Screening of Diabetic Retinopathy. *IEEE Transactions on Biomedical Engineering*, 65(3), 1–9. DOI: 10.1109/TBME.2017.2707578 PMID: 28541892

Kasat, K., Shaikh, N., Rayabharapu, V. K., & Nayak, M. (2023). Implementation and Recognition of Waste Management System with Mobility Solution in Smart Cities using Internet of Things, *2023 Second International Conference on Augmented Intelligence and Sustainable Systems (ICAISS)*, Trichy, India, 2023, pp. 1661-1665, DOI: 10.1109/ICAISS58487.2023.10250690

Kashyap, H., Ahmed, H. A., Hoque, N., Roy, S., & Bhattacharyya, D. K. (2015). Big data analytics in bioinformatics: A machine learning perspective. *arXiv preprint arXiv:1506.05101*.

Kashyap, H., Ahmed, H. A., Hoque, N., Roy, S., & Bhattacharyya, D. K. (2016). Big data analytics in bioinformatics: Architectures, techniques, tools and issues. *Network Modeling and Analysis in Health Informatics and Bioinformatics*, 5(1), 1–28. DOI: 10.1007/s13721-016-0135-4

Kaur, R., & Ahmed, S. (2022). AI in personalized cancer treatment. *Journal of Precision Oncology*, 5(3), 256–270. DOI: 10.1007/s41669-021-00162-3

Kaur, S., Singla, J., Nkenyereye, L., Jha, S., Prashar, D., Joshi, G. P., El-Sappagh, S., Islam, M. S., & Islam, S. R. (2020). Medical diagnostic systems using artificial intelligence (ai) algorithms: Principles and perspectives. *IEEE Access : Practical Innovations, Open Solutions*, 8, 228049–228069. DOI: 10.1109/ACCESS.2020.3042273

Kauser, S. H., Gowda, D., Tanguturi, R. C., & CH, V. (2023, June). Implementation of Machine Learning Approach for Detecting Cardiovascular Diseases. In 2023 3rd International Conference on Intelligent Technologies (CONIT) (pp. 1-6). IEEE.

Kaushal, R., Bates, D. W., & Poon, E. G. (2003). Health information technology: A national imperative. *Health Affairs*, 22(4), 117–126.

Kavitha, R., Gowda, D., Vishal, B. R., Shankar, M. U., & Kabilan, A. M. (2023, May). Cardiovascular Disease Prediction Using LSTM Algorithm based On Cytokines. In 2023 4th International Conference for Emerging Technology (INCET) (pp. 1-5). IEEE.

Kavitha, R., Gowda, V. D., Kumar, R. K., & Pandidurai, M. (2023, July). Design of IoT based Rural Health Helper using Natural Language Processing. In 2023 4th International Conference on Electronics and Sustainable Communication Systems (ICESC) (pp. 328-333). IEEE.

Kavitha, R., Kumar, A., Kalpana, V., & Hariram, V. (2023) "Artificial Intelligence based Health Monitoring System on IoTH platform," *2023 Second International Conference on Augmented Intelligence and Sustainable Systems (ICAISS)*, Trichy, India, pp. 1458-1463.

Kawale, S. R., & Diwan, S. P. (2022) "Intelligent Breast Abnormality Framework for Detection and Evaluation of Breast Abnormal Parameters," *2022 International Conference on Edge Computing and Applications (ICECAA)*, pp. 1503-1508.

Kazi K S, (2023). IoT based Healthcare system for Home Quarantine People, *Journal of Instrumentation and Innovation sciences*, 18(1), pp. 1- 8

Kazi K., (2022b). Model for Agricultural Information system to improve crop yield using IoT, *Journal of open Source development*, 9(2), pp. 16 – 24.

Kazi Kutubuddin S. L., (2022c). Business Mode and Product Life Cycle to Improve Marketing in Healthcare Units, *E-Commerce for future & Trends*, 9(3), pp. 1-9.

Kazi Kutubuddin, S. L. (2022a). Predict the Severity of Diabetes cases, using K-Means and Decision Tree Approach. *Journal of Advances in Shell Programming*, 9(2), 24–31.

Kazi Kutubuddin, S. L. (2022b). A novel Design of IoT based 'Love Representation and Remembrance' System to Loved One's. *Gradiva Review Journal*, 8(12), 377–383.

Kazi, K. (2024b). Modelling and Simulation of Electric Vehicle for Performance Analysis: BEV and HEV Electrical Vehicle Implementation Using Simulink for E-Mobility Ecosystems. *In L. D., N. Nagpal, N. Kassarwani, V. Varthanan G., & P. Siano (Eds.), E-Mobility in Electrical Energy Systems for Sustainability (pp. 295-320). IGI Global.* Available at: https://www.igi-global.com/gateway/chapter/full-text-pdf/341172DOI: 10.4018/979-8-3693-2611-4.ch014

Kazi, K. (2022). Hybrid optimum model development to determine the Break. *Journal of Multimedia Technology & Recent Advancements*, 9(2), 24–32.

Kazi, K. (2022). Smart Grid energy saving technique using Machine Learning. *Journal of Instrumentation Technology and Innovations*, 12(3), 1–10.

Kazi, K. (2022a). Reverse Engineering's Neural Network Approach to human brain. *Journal of Communication Engineering & Systems*, 12(2), 17–24.

Kazi, K. (2024). Complications with Malware Identification in IoT and an Overview of Artificial Immune Approaches. *Research & Reviews. The Journal of Immunology : Official Journal of the American Association of Immunologists*, 14(01), 54–62.

Kazi, K. (2024). Nanotechnology in Medical Applications: A Study. *Nano Trends-A Journal of Nano Technology & Its Applications.*, 26(02), 1–11.

Kazi, K. (2024a). AI-Driven IoT (AIIoT) in Healthcare Monitoring. In Nguyen, T., & Vo, N. (Eds.), *Using Traditional Design Methods to Enhance AI-Driven Decision Making* (pp. 77–101). IGI Global., available at https://www.igi-global.com/chapter/ai-driven-iot-aiiot-in-healthcare-monitoring/336693, DOI: 10.4018/979-8-3693-0639-0.ch003

Kazi, K. (2024a). Machine Learning (ML)-Based Braille Lippi Characters and Numbers Detection and Announcement System for Blind Children in Learning. In Sart, G. (Ed.), *Social Reflections of Human-Computer Interaction in Education, Management, and Economics*. IGI Global., DOI: 10.4018/979-8-3693-3033-3.ch002

Kazi, K. (2025b). Machine Learning-Driven-Internet of Things(MLIoT) Based Healthcare Monitoring System. In Wickramasinghe, N. (Ed.), *Impact of Digital Solutions for Improved Healthcare Delivery*. IGI Global.

Kazi, K. (2025c). *AI-Driven-IoT (AIIoT) based Decision-Making in Drones for Climate Change: KSK Approach. Recent Theories and Applications for Multi-Criteria Decision-Making*. IGI Global.

Kazi, K. (2025c). AI-Powered-IoT (AIIoT) based Decision Making System for BP Patient's Healthcare Monitoring: KSK Approach for BP Patient Healthcare Monitoring. In Aouadni, S., & Aouadni, I. (Eds.), *Recent Theories and Applications for Multi-Criteria Decision-Making*. IGI Global.

Kazi, K. (2025c). Moonlighting in Carrier. In Tunio, M. N. (Ed.), *Applications of Career Transitions and Entrepreneurship*. IGI Global.

Kazi, K. S. (2017). Significance and Usage of Face Recognition System. *Scholarly Journal for Humanity Science and English Language*, 4(20), 4764–4772.

Kazi, K. S. (2022a). IoT-Based Healthcare Monitoring for COVID-19 Home Quarantined Patients. *Recent Trends in Sensor Research & Technology*, 9(3), 26–32.

Kazi, K. S. (2023a). Detection of Malicious Nodes in IoT Networks based on Throughput and ML. *Journal of Electrical and Power System Engineering*, 9(1), 22–29.

Kazi, K. S. (2024). Artificial Intelligence (AI)-Driven IoT (AIIoT)-Based Agriculture Automation. In Satapathy, S., & Muduli, K. (Eds.), *Advanced Computational Methods for Agri-Business Sustainability* (pp. 72–94). IGI Global., DOI: 10.4018/979-8-3693-3583-3.ch005

Kazi, K. S. (2024). Machine Learning-Based Pomegranate Disease Detection and Treatment. In Zia Ul Haq, M., & Ali, I. (Eds.), *Revolutionizing Pest Management for Sustainable Agriculture* (pp. 469–498). IGI Global., DOI: 10.4018/979-8-3693-3061-6.ch019

Kazi, K. S. (2024a). Computer-Aided Diagnosis in Ophthalmology: A Technical Review of Deep Learning Applications. In Garcia, M., & de Almeida, R. (Eds.), *Transformative Approaches to Patient Literacy and Healthcare Innovation* (pp. 112–135). IGI Global., Available at https://www.igi-global.com/chapter/computer-aided-diagnosis-in-ophthalmology/342823, DOI: 10.4018/979-8-3693-3661-8.ch006

Kazi, K. S. (2024b). IoT Driven by Machine Learning (MLIoT) for the Retail Apparel Sector. In Tarnanidis, T., Papachristou, E., Karypidis, M., & Ismyrlis, V. (Eds.), *Driving Green Marketing in Fashion and Retail* (pp. 63–81). IGI Global., DOI: 10.4018/979-8-3693-3049-4.ch004

Kazi, K. S. (2025). IoT Technologies for the Intelligent Dairy Industry: A New Challenge. In Thandekkattu, S., & Vajjhala, N. (Eds.), *Designing Sustainable Internet of Things Solutions for Smart Industries* (pp. 321–350). IGI Global., DOI: 10.4018/979-8-3693-5498-8.ch012

Kazi, K. S. L. (2018). Significance of Projection and Rotation of Image in Color Matching for High-Quality Panoramic Images used for Aquatic study. *International Journal of Aquatic Science*, 9(2), 130–145.

Kazi, K. S. L. (2023a). IoT-based weather Prototype using WeMos. *Journal of Control and Instrumentation Engineering*, 9(1), 10–22.

Kazi, K. S. L. (2023c). Analysis for Field distribution in Optical Waveguide using Linear Fem method, *Journal of Optical communication. Electronics (Basel)*, 9(1), 23–28.

Kazi, K. S. L. (2023h). IoT based Healthcare Monitoring for COVID- Subvariant JN-1. *Journal of Electronic Design Technology*, 4(3).

Kazi, K. S. L. (2023i). Smart Motion Detection System using IoT: A NodeMCU and Blynk Framework. *Journal of Microelectronics and Solid State Devices*, 10(3).

Kazi, K. S. L. (2023j). Nanotechnology in Precision Farming: The Role of Research. *International Journal of Nanomaterials and Nanostructures*, 9(2). Advance online publication. DOI: 10.37628/ijnn.v9i2.1051

Kazi, K. S. L. (2023k). Home Automation System Based on GSM. *Journal of VLSI Design Tools & Technology*, 13(3), 7–12p. DOI: 10.37591/jovdtt.v13i3.7877

Kazi, K. S. L. (2024). Nanotechnology in BattleField: A Study. Journal of Nanoscience. *Nanoengineering & Applications*, 14(2), 18–30p.

Kazi, K. S. L. (2024). Nanotechnology in BattleField: A Study. Journal of Nanoscience. *Nanoengineering & Applications.*, 14(2), 18–30p.

Kazi, K. S. L. (2024). Review of Biopolymers in Agriculture Application: An Eco-Friendly Alternative. *International Journal of Composite and Constituent Materials.*, 10(1), 50–62p.

Kazi, K. S. L. (2024f). Blynk IoT-Powered Water Pump-Based Smart Farming. *Recent Trends in Semiconductor and Sensor Technology*, 1(1), 8–14.

Kazi, K. S. L. (2024g). Impact of Solar Penetrations in Conventional Power Systems and Generation of Harmonic and Power Quality Issues. *Advance Research in Power Electronics and Devices*, 1(1), 10–16.

Kazi, K. S. L. (2024r). Intelligent Watering System(IWS) for Agricultural Land Utilising Raspberry Pi. *Recent Trends in Fluid Mechanics*, 10(2), 26–31.

Kazi, K. S. L. (2024s). IoT and Sensor-based Smart Agriculturing Driven by NodeMCU. *Research & Review: Electronics and Communication Engineering*, 1(2), 25–33.

Kazi, K. S. L. (2024v). Smart Agriculture based on AI-Driven-IoT(AIIoT): A KSK Approach, *Advance Research in Communication Engineering and its. Innovations*, 1(2), 23–32.

Kazi, K. S. S. L. (2024). Polymer Applications in Energy Generation and Storage: A Forward Path. Journal of Nanoscience. *Nanoengineering & Applications.*, 14(2), 31–39p.

Kazi, S. S. L. (2023b). Integrating IoT and Mechanical Systems in Mechanical Engineering Applications. *Journal of Mechanisms and Robotics*, 8(3), 1–6.

Kazi, S. S. L. (2023c). IoT Changing the Electronics Manufacturing Industry. *Journal of Analog and Digital Communications*, 8(3), 13–17.

Kazi, S. S. L. (2023d). IoT in the Electric Power Industry. *Journal of Controller and Converters*, 8(3), 1–7.

Kazi, S. S. L. (2023e). Review of Integrated Battery Charger (IBC) for Electric Vehicles (EV). *Journal of Advances in Electrical Devices*, 8(3), 1–11.

Kazi, S. S. L. (2023f). ML in the Electronics Manufacturing Industry. *Journal of Switching Hub*, 8(3), 9–13.

Kazi, S. S. L. (2023g). IoT in Electrical Vehicle: A Study. *Journal of Control and Instrumentation Engineering*, 9(3), 15–21.

Kazi, S. S. L. (2023h). PV Power Control for DC Microgrid Energy Storage Utilisation. *Journal of Digital Integrated Circuits in Electrical Devices*, 8(3), 1–8.

Kazi, S. S. L. (2023i). Electronics with Artificial Intelligence Creating a Smarter Future: A Review. *Journal of Communication Engineering and Its Innovations*, 9(3), 38–42.

Kazi, S. S. L. (2023j). Dispersion Compensation in Optical Fiber: A Review. *Journal of Telecommunication Study*, 8(3), 14–19.

Kazi, S. S. L. (2023k). IoT Based Arduino-Powered Weather Monitoring System. *Journal of Telecommunication Study*, 8(3), 25–31.

Kazi, S. S. L. (2023l). Arduino Based Weather Monitoring System. *Journal of Switching Hub*, 8(3), 24–29.

Kazi, S. S. L. (2023m). Accepting Internet of Nano-Things: Synopsis, Developments, and Challenges. *Journal of Nanoscience. Nanoengineering & Applications.*, 13(2), 17–26p. DOI: 10.37591/jonsnea.v13i2.1464

Kazi, S. S. L. (2023n). Nanomedicine as a Potential Therapeutic Approach to COVID-19. *International Journal of Applied Nanotechnology.*, 9(2), 27–35p.

Kazi, S.. (2023a). Fruit Grading, Disease Detection, and an Image Processing Strategy. *Journal of Image Processing and Artificial Intelligence*, 9(2), 17–34.

Keating, C. B., & Katina, P. F. (2019). Complex system governance: Concept, utility, and challenges. *Systems Research and Behavioral Science*, 36(5), 687–705. DOI: 10.1002/sres.2621

Keating, C. B., Katina, P. F., Bradley, J. M., Hodge, R., & Pyne, J. C. (2023). Sustainability: A Complex System Governance Perspective. *INCOSE International Symposium*, 33(1), 1117–1131. DOI: 10.1002/iis2.13073

Keating, C. B., Katina, P. F., Chesterman, C. W., & Pyne, J. C. (Eds.). (2022). *Complex system governance: Theory and practice*. Springer International Publishing., Retrieved from https://link.springer.com/book/10.1007/978-3-030-93852-9 DOI: 10.1007/978-3-030-93852-9

Keikhosrokiani, P. (Ed.). (2022). *Big data analytics for healthcare: datasets, techniques, life cycles, management, and applications*. Academic Press.

Kelleher, J. D., Mac Namee, B., & D'Arcy, A. (2020). *Fundamentals of Machine Learning for Predictive Data Analytics* (2nd ed.). MIT Press.

Khang, A. (Ed.). (2024). *AI-driven innovations in digital healthcare: Emerging trends, challenges, and applications: Emerging trends, challenges, and applications.*

Khan, I. A., Razzak, I., Pi, D., Khan, N., Hussain, Y., Li, B., & Kousar, T. (2024). Fed-inforce-fusion: A federated reinforcement-based fusion model for security and privacy protection of IoMT networks against cyber-attacks. *Information Fusion*, 101, 102002. DOI: 10.1016/j.inffus.2023.102002

Khanna, S., & Srivastava, S. (2020). Patient-centric ethical frameworks for privacy, transparency, and bias awareness in deep learning-based medical systems. *Applied Research in Artificial Intelligence and Cloud Computing*, 3(1), 16–35.

Khan, Z. A., & Sohn, W. (2011). Abnormal human activity recognition system based on R-transform and kernel discriminant technique for elderly home care. *IEEE Transactions on Consumer Electronics*, 57(4), 1843–1850.

khan, Z. F., & Alotaibi, S. R. (2020, September). Z. F. khan and S. R. Alotaibi, "Applications of artificial intelligence and big data analytics in m-health: A healthcare system perspective,". *Journal of Healthcare Engineering*, 2020, 1–15. DOI: 10.1155/2020/8894694

Kharghani, E., Aliakbari, S., Bidad, J., & Amir, M. A. M. 2023. "A Lightweight Authentication Protocol for M2M Communication in IIoT Using Physical Unclonable Functions." In *2023 31st International Conference on Electrical Engineering, ICEE 2023,* DOI: 10.1109/ICEE59167.2023.10334808

Khatiwada, P., Yang, B., Jia, C. L., & Blobel, B. (2024). Patient-Generated Health Data (PGHD): Understanding, Requirements, Challenges, and Existing Techniques for Data Security and Privacy. *Journal of Personalized Medicine*, 14(3), 282. Advance online publication. DOI: 10.3390/jpm14030282 PMID: 38541024

Khatkar, M., Kumar, K., & Kumar, B. 2020. "An Overview of Distributed Denial of Service and Internet of Things in Healthcare Devices." In *Proceedings of International Conference on Research, Innovation, Knowledge Management and Technology Application for Business Sustainability, INBUSH 2020,* DOI: 10.1109/INBUSH46973.2020.9392171

Khezri, S., Tanha, J., & Samadi, N. (2024). An experimental review of the ensemble-based data stream classification algorithms in non-stationary environments. *Computers & Electrical Engineering*, 118, 109420. DOI: 10.1016/j.compeleceng.2024.109420

Khubchandani, J., Sharma, S., England-Kennedy, E., Pai, A., & Banerjee, S. (2023). Emerging technologies and futuristic digital healthcare ecosystems: Priorities for research and action in the United States. *Journal of Medicine, Surgery, and Public Health*, 1, 100030. DOI: 10.1016/j.glmedi.2023.100030

Khullar, D., Casalino, L. P., Qian, Y., Lu, Y., Krumholz, H. M., & Aneja, S. (2022). Perspectives of patients about Artificial Intelligence in Health Care. *JAMA Network Open*, 5(5), e2210309. DOI: 10.1001/jamanetworkopen.2022.10309 PMID: 35507346

Khurana, V. (2024). Accelerating Pace of Scientific Discovery and Innovation through Big Data Enabled Artificial Intelligence and Deep Learning. *Emerging Trends in Machine Intelligence and Big Data*, 16(1), 38–53.

Kim, B., Park, J., & Suh, J. (2020). Transparency and accountability in AI decision support: Explaining and visualizing convolutional neural networks for text information. *Decision Support Systems*, 134, 113302. DOI: 10.1016/j.dss.2020.113302

Kim, D. H., & Park, E. S. (2024) "AI-Assisted Surgery: Improving Outcomes with IoMT," in *2024 International Conference on Robotics and Automation in Medicine (ICRAM)*, Seoul, South Korea, pp. 33-38.

Kim, K. J., Kim, S., & Kim, J. (2019). Optimizing quality control in the healthcare supply chain using statistical quality control and machine learning. *Journal of Healthcare Engineering*, •••, 20.

King, R. D., Hirst, J. D., & Sternberg, M. J. (1995, March 1). Comparison of artificial intelligence methods for modeling pharmaceutical QSARS. *Applied Artificial Intelligence*, 9(2), 213–233. DOI: 10.1080/08839519508945474

Kiruthika, V., Shoba, S., Sendil, M., Nagarajan, K., & Punetha, D. (2024). Hybrid ensemble-deep transfer model for early cassava leaf disease classification. *Heliyon*, 10(16).

Kishore Kumar, R., Pandidurai, M., & Senthil Kamalesh, M. S. C. (2023) "Design of IoT based Rural Health Helper using Natural Language Processing," *2023 4th International Conference on Electronics and Sustainable Communication Systems (ICESC)*, Coimbatore, India, pp. 328-333.

Kitchin, R. (2013). Big data and human geography: Opportunities, challenges and risks. *Dialogues in Human Geography*, 3(3), 262–267. DOI: 10.1177/2043820613513388

Koene, A., Clifton, C., Hatada, Y., Webb, H., & Richardson, R. (2019). A governance framework for algorithmic accountability and transparency.

Konda, S. R. (2022). Ethical Considerations in the Development and Deployment of AI-Driven Software Systems. *INTERNATIONAL JOURNAL OF COMPUTER SCIENCE AND TECHNOLOGY*, 6(3), 86–101.

Kong, W., You, Z., Lyu, S., & Lv, X. (2024). Multi-dimensional stereo face reconstruction for psychological assistant diagnosis in medical meta-universe. *Information Sciences*, 654, 119831. DOI: 10.1016/j.ins.2023.119831

Kordzadeh, N., & Ghasemaghaei, M. (2022). Algorithmic bias: Review, synthesis, and future research directions. *European Journal of Information Systems*, 31(3), 388–409. DOI: 10.1080/0960085X.2021.1927212

Korshunova, M., Huang, N., Capuzzi, S., Radchenko, D. S., Savych, O., Moroz, Y. S., Wells, C. I., Willson, T. M., Tropsha, A., & Isayev, O. (2022, October 18). Generative and reinforcement learning approaches for the automated de novo design of bioactive compounds. *Communications Chemistry*, 5(1), 129. DOI: 10.1038/s42004-022-00733-0 PMID: 36697952

Koshiyama, A., Kazim, E., Treleaven, P., Rai, P., Szpruch, L., Pavey, G., Ahamat, G., Leutner, F., Goebel, R., Knight, A., Adams, J., Hitrova, C., Barnett, J., Nachev, P., Barber, D., Chamorro-Premuzic, T., Klemmer, K., Gregorovic, M., Khan, S., & Chatterjee, S. (2024). Towards algorithm auditing: Managing legal, ethical and technological risks of AI, ML and associated algorithms. *Royal Society Open Science*, 11(5), 230859. DOI: 10.1098/rsos.230859 PMID: 39076787

Košmerl, I., Rabuzin, K., & Šestak, M. (2020). Multi-model databases-Introducing polyglot persistence in the big data world. In *2020 43rd International Convention on Information, Communication and Electronic Technology (MIPRO)* (pp. 1724–1729). IEEE. DOI: 10.23919/MIPRO48935.2020.9245178

Kranthi, M., & Tanguturi, R. C. (2023) "Design of Intelligent Medical Integrity Authentication and Secure Information for Public Cloud in Hospital Administration," 2023 2nd International Conference on Edge Computing and Applications (ICECAA), Namakkal, India, pp. 256-261.

Krishnamoorthy, N., Kumar, V. V., Nair, C., Maheswari, A., Mishra, S., & Sinha, A. (2024). HR Analytics and Employee Attrition Prediction Using Machine Learning. In Emerging Advancements in AI and Big Data Technologies in Business and Society (pp. 79-96). IGI Global. DOI: 10.4018/979-8-3693-0683-3.ch004

Krishnamoorthy, N., Venkatesan, V. K., Swapna, B., Rawal, D., Dutta, D., & Sushil, S. (2024). Personality Prediction Based on Myers-Briggs Type Indicator Using Machine Learning. In Emerging Advancements in AI and Big Data Technologies in Business and Society (pp. 353-368). IGI Global.

Krishnamoorthy, N., Prasad, L. N., Kumar, C. P., Subedi, B., Abraha, H. B., & Sathishkumar, V. E. (2021). Rice leaf diseases prediction using deep neural networks with transfer learning. *Environmental Research*, 198, 111275. DOI: 10.1016/j.envres.2021.111275 PMID: 33989629

Kroenke, K., Alford, D. P., Argoff, C., Canlas, B., Covington, E., Frank, J. W., Haake, K. J., Hanling, S., Hooten, W. M., Kertesz, S. G., Kravitz, R. L., Krebs, E. E., Stanos, S. P.Jr, & Sullivan, M. (2019). Challenges with implementing the centers for disease control and prevention opioid guideline: A consensus panel report. *Pain Medicine*, 20(4), 724–735. DOI: 10.1093/pm/pny307 PMID: 30690556

Kumar, P. M., & Gandhi, U. D. (2018). A novel three-tier Internet of Medical Things architecture with machine learning algorithm for early detection of heart diseases (Vol. 65). Computers & Electrical Engineering., https://www.sciencedirect.com/science/article/pii/S0045790617328410, , ISSN 0045-7906. DOI: 10.1016/j.compeleceng.2017.09.001

Kumar, S. R. (2023, December). Intrusion Detection System for Defending against DoS Attacks in the IoMT Ecosystem. In 2023 4th International Conference on Communication, Computing and Industry 6.0 (C216) (pp. 1-5). IEEE.

Kumar, S. S., & Koti, M. S. (2021, December). Efficient Authentication for Securing Electronic Health Records using Algebraic Structure. In *2021 5th International Conference on Electrical, Electronics, Communication, Computer Technologies and Optimization Techniques (ICEECCOT)* (pp. 366-370). IEEE. DOI: 10.1109/ICEECCOT52851.2021.9708050

Kumar, S., Arora, A. K., Gupta, P., & Saini, B. S. 2021. "A Review of Applications, Security and Challenges of Internet of Medical Things." In *Studies in Systems, Decision and Control*, DOI: 10.1007/978-3-030-55833-8_1

Kumar, V., Kushwaha, S., Singh, I., Barik, R. K., Singh, G., & Sabraj, M. (2024). Internet of Multimedia Things (IoMT): Communication Techniques Perspective. *5G and Beyond Wireless Networks*, 147-162.

Kumar, A., Sharma, S., & Verma, P. (2023) "Data Privacy and Security in IoMT: Challenges and Solutions," *2023 IEEE International Conference on Information Privacy, Security, Risk, and Trust (PASSAT)*, San Francisco, USA, pp. 321-326.

Kumar, M., Verma, S., Kumar, A., Ijaz, M. F., & Rawat, D. B. (2022). ANAF-IoMT: A novel architectural framework for IoMT-enabled smart healthcare system by enhancing security based on RECC-VC. *IEEE Transactions on Industrial Informatics*, 18(12), 8936–8943. DOI: 10.1109/TII.2022.3181614

Kumar, R., & Tripathi, R. (2021). Towards design and implementation of security and privacy framework for Internet of Medical Things (IoMT) by leveraging blockchain and IPFS technology. *The Journal of Supercomputing*, 77(8), 7916–7955. DOI: 10.1007/s11227-020-03570-x

Kumar, S. (2019, August). Diabetic retinopathy diagnosis with ensemble deep-learning. In *Proceedings of the 3rd International Conference on Vision, Image and Signal Processing* (pp. 1-5).

Kumar, S. S., Muthukumaran, V., Devi, A., Geetha, V., & Yadav, P. N. (2023). A Quantitative Approach of Purposive Sampling Techniques for Security and Privacy Issues in IoT Healthcare Applications. In *Handbook of Research on Advancements in AI and IoT Convergence Technologies* (pp. 281–299). IGI Global. DOI: 10.4018/978-1-6684-6971-2.ch016

Kumar, S. S., & Sanjay, M. (2018). Improved Quality of Patient Care and Data Security Using Cloud Crypto System in EHR. *International Journal of Advanced Studies of Scientific Research*, 3(10).

Kumar, V., Saini, D., Rastogi, S., Raman, R., Verma, A., & Meenakshi, R. (2024).. . *Development of Medical IOT System for the Prediction of Heart Disease.*, 10, 951–956. DOI: 10.1109/ICACITE60783.2024.10617362

Kumar, Y., Ilin, A., Salo, H., Kulathinal, S., Leinonen, M. K., & Marttinen, P. (2024). Self-Supervised Forecasting in Electronic Health Records With Attention-Free Models. *IEEE Transactions on Artificial Intelligence*, 5(8), 3926–3938. Advance online publication. DOI: 10.1109/TAI.2024.3353164

Kurle, S. S., Maralbhavi, N. P., Salunke, S. U., & Chandanshive, A. A. (2017, June). Diabetic retinopathy analysis using CDR technique. In *2017 International Conference on Intelligent Computing and Control Systems (ICICCS)* (pp. 708-711). IEEE.

Kutubuddin, K. (2024c). Vehicle Health Monitoring System (VHMS) by Employing IoT and Sensors, *Grenze International Journal of Engineering and Technology,* Vol 10, Issue 2, pp- 5367-5374. Available at: https://thegrenze.com/index.php?display=page&view=journalabstract&absid=3371&id=8

Kutubuddin, K. (2024d). A Novel Approach on ML based Palmistry, *Grenze International Journal of Engineering and Technology,* Vol 10, Issue 2, pp- 5186-5193. Available at: https://thegrenze.com/index.php?display=page&view=journalabstract&absid=3344&id=8

Kutubuddin, K. (2022d). Detection of Malicious Nodes in IoT Networks based on packet loss using ML, *Journal of Mobile Computing, Communication & mobile. Networks*, 9(3), 9–16.

Kutubuddin, K. (2022e). Big data and HR Analytics in Talent Management: A Study. *Recent Trends in Parallel Computing*, 9(3), 16–26.

Kutubuddin, K. (2023a). Blockchain-Enabled IoT Environment to Embedded System a Self-Secure Firmware Model. *Journal of Telecommunication Study*, 8(1), 13–19.

Kutubuddin, K. (2023b). A Study HR Analytics Big Data in Talent Management. *Research and Review: Human Resource and Labour Management*, 4(1), 16–28.

Kutubuddin, K. (2024e). IoT based Boiler Health Monitoring for Sugar Industries, *Grenze. IACSIT International Journal of Engineering and Technology*, 10(2), 5178–5185. https://thegrenze.com/index.php?display=page&view=journalabstract&absid=3343&id=8

Kwarteng, E., & Cebe, M. (2022). A Survey on Security Issues in Modern Implantable Devices: Solutions and Future Issues. *Smart Health (Amsterdam, Netherlands)*, 25, 100295. Advance online publication. DOI: 10.1016/j.smhl.2022.100295

Kwasigroch, A., Jarzembinski, B., & Grochowski, M. (2018, May). Deep CNN based decision support system for detection and assessing the stage of diabetic retinopathy. In *2018 International Interdisciplinary PhD Workshop (IIPhDW)* (pp. 111-116). IEEE. DOI: 10.1109/IIPHDW.2018.8388337

Lakhan, A., Hamouda, H., Abdulkareem, K. H., Alyahya, S., & Mohammed, M. A. (2024). Digital healthcare framework for patients with disabilities based on deep federated learning schemes. *Computers in Biology and Medicine*, 169, 107845. DOI: 10.1016/j.compbiomed.2023.107845 PMID: 38118307

Lakhan, A., Mohammed, M. A., Nedoma, J., Martinek, R., Tiwari, P., Vidyarthi, A., Alkhayyat, A., & Wang, W. (2022). Federated-learning based privacy preservation and fraud-enabled blockchain IoMT system for healthcare. *IEEE Journal of Biomedical and Health Informatics*, 27(2), 664–672. DOI: 10.1109/JBHI.2022.3165945 PMID: 35394919

Lamberti, M. J., Wilkinson, M., Donzanti, B. A., Wohlhieter, G. E., Parikh, S., Wilkins, R. G., & Getz, K. (2019, August 1). A study on the application and use of artificial intelligence to support drug development. *Clinical Therapeutics*, 41(8), 1414–1426. DOI: 10.1016/j.clinthera.2019.05.018 PMID: 31248680

Landi, I., Glicksberg, B. S., Lee, H. C., Cherng, S., Landi, G., Danieletto, M., Dudley, J. T., Furlanello, C., & Miotto, R. (2020). Deep representation learning of electronic health records to unlock patient stratification at scale. *NPJ Digital Medicine*, 3(1), 96. Advance online publication. DOI: 10.1038/s41746-020-0301-z PMID: 32699826

Lazrek, G., Chetioui, K., Balboul, Y., Mazer, S., & El bekkali, M. (2024). An rfe/ridge-ml/dl based anomaly intrusion detection approach for securing iomt system. *Results in Engineering*, 23, 102659. DOI: 10.1016/j.rineng.2024.102659

Lee, B. G., & Chung, W. Y. (2017). Wearable Glove-Type Driver Stress Detection Using a Motion Sensor. *IEEE Transactions on Intelligent Transportation Systems*, 18(7), 1835-1844. DOI: 10.1109/TITS.2016.2617881

Lee, C. H., & Ke, Y. H. (2021). Fundus images classification for Diabetic Retinopathy using Deep Learning; *Proceedings of the 2021 The 13th International Conference on Computer Modeling and Simulation*; Melbourne, Australia. 25–27; pp. 264–270. DOI: 10.1145/3474963.3475849

Lee, D., & Yoon, S. N. (2021). Application of artificial intelligence-based technologies in the healthcare industry: Opportunities and challenges. *International Journal of Environmental Research and Public Health*, 18(1), 271. DOI: 10.3390/ijerph18010271 PMID: 33401373

Lee, D., & Zhang, Y. (2023). AI-based treatment pathways. *Future Healthcare Journal*, 10(1), 89–97. DOI: 10.7861/fhj.2022.0075

Lee, E., Ha, H., Kim, H. J., Moon, H. J., Byon, J. H., Huh, S., Son, J., Yoon, J., Han, K., & Kwak, J. Y. (2019). Differentiation of thyroid nodules on US using features learned and extracted from various convolutional neural networks. *Scientific Reports*, 9(1), 19854. DOI: 10.1038/s41598-019-56395-x PMID: 31882683

Lee, J., Little, T. D., & Helal, S. (2018). Adopting a remote patient monitoring system: Application to congestive heart failure monitoring. *Computers in Biology and Medicine*, 98, 89–96.

Lee, K. S., & Park, H. (2022). Machine learning on thyroid disease: A review. *Frontiers in Bioscience (Landmark Edition)*, 27(3), 101. DOI: 10.31083/j.fbl2703101 PMID: 35345333

Lee, S., Choi, M., & Park, D. (2023) "Challenges and Solutions in Integrating AI with IoMT for Healthcare," *2023 IEEE International Conference on Networking, Sensing, and Control (ICNSC)*, Vienna, Austria, pp. 121-126.

Leung, P. H., Chui, K. T., Lo, K., & de Pablos, P. O. (2021). A support vector machine–based voice disorders detection using human voice signal. In *Artificial Intelligence and Big Data Analytics for Smart Healthcare* (pp. 197–208). Academic Press. DOI: 10.1016/B978-0-12-822060-3.00014-0

Liao, J., Li, X., Gan, Y., Han, S., Rong, P., Wang, W., Li, W., & Zhou, L. (2023). Artificial intelligence assists precision medicine in cancer treatment. *Frontiers in Oncology*, 12, 998222. Advance online publication. DOI: 10.3389/fonc.2022.998222 PMID: 36686757

Li, H. X., & Zhang, J. Y. (2024) "Machine Learning Techniques for Real-Time Health Monitoring," in *2024 IEEE International Conference on Machine Learning and Applications (ICMLA)*, Beijing, China, pp. 39-44.

Lilhore, U. K., Simaiya, S., Poongodi, M., & Dutt, V. (Eds.). (2024). *Federated learning and privacy-preserving in healthcare AI*. IGI Global. DOI: 10.4018/979-8-3693-1874-4

Lin, H., Garg, S., Hu, J., Wang, X., Piran, M. J., & Shamim Hossain, M. (2021). Privacy-Enhanced Data Fusion for COVID-19 Applications in Intelligent Internet of Medical Things. *IEEE Internet of Things Journal*, 8(21), 15683–15693. Advance online publication. DOI: 10.1109/JIOT.2020.3033129 PMID: 35782177

Litjens, G., Kooi, T., Bejnordi, B. E., Setio, A. A. A., Ciompi, F., Ghaforian, M., van der Laak, J. A. W. M., van Ginneken, B., & Sánchez, C. I. (2017). A survey on deep learning in medical image analysis. *Medical Image Analysis*, 42, 60–88. DOI: 10.1016/j.media.2017.07.005 PMID: 28778026

Liu, J. Y. H., & Rudd, J. A. (2023). Predicting drug adverse effects using a new Gastro-Intestinal Pacemaker Activity Drug Database (GIPADD). *Scientific Reports*, 13(1), 6935. DOI: 10.1038/s41598-023-33655-5 PMID: 37117211

Liu, Q., & Chen, A. (2020). Data privacy in AI systems. *Journal of Cybersecurity in Healthcare*, 14(2), 200–212. DOI: 10.1093/csh/caq033

Liu, Y., Zhang, L., Yang, Y., Zhou, L., Ren, L., Wang, F., Liu, R., Pang, Z., & Deen, M. J. (2019). A novel cloud-based framework for the elderly healthcare services using digital twin. *IEEE Access : Practical Innovations, Open Solutions*, 7, 49088–49101. DOI: 10.1109/ACCESS.2019.2909828

Liu, Z., Zhong, S., Liu, Q., Xie, C., Dai, Y., Peng, C., Chen, X., & Zou, R. (2021). Thyroid nodule recognition using a joint convolutional neural network with information fusion of ultrasound images and radiofrequency data. *European Radiology*, 31(7), 5001–5011. DOI: 10.1007/s00330-020-07585-z PMID: 33409774

Li, W., Chai, Y., Khan, F., Jan, S. R. U., Verma, S., Menon, V. G., & Li, X. (2021). A comprehensive survey on machine learning-based big data analytics for IoT-enabled smart healthcare system. *Mobile Networks and Applications*, 26(1), 234–252. DOI: 10.1007/s11036-020-01700-6

Li, X., & Wang, Y. (2021). Patient outcomes improved via AI. *Journal of Clinical Medicine*, 10(12), 2389–2399. DOI: 10.3390/jcm10122389

Li, Y., & Chen, W. (2020). AI in drug discovery. *Drug Development Research*, 81(6), 720–732. DOI: 10.1002/ddr.21600

Li, Y., Wu, F. X., & Ngom, A. (2018). A review on machine learning principles for multi-view biological data integration. *Briefings in Bioinformatics*, 19(2), 325–340. DOI: 10.1093/bib/bbw113 PMID: 28011753

Liyakat Kazi, K. S. (2024). ChatGPT: An Automated Teacher's Guide to Learning. In Bansal, R., Chakir, A., Hafaz Ngah, A., Rabby, F., & Jain, A. (Eds.), *AI Algorithms and ChatGPT for Student Engagement in Online Learning* (pp. 1–20). IGI Global., DOI: 10.4018/979-8-3693-4268-8.ch001

Liyakat, K. S. (2022). Nanotechnology Application in Neural Growth Support System. Nano Trends: A Journal of Nanotechnology and Its Applications, 24(2), 47-55.

Liyakat, K. K. (2025). Heart Health Monitoring Using IoT and Machine Learning Methods. In Shaik, A. (Ed.), *AI-Powered Advances in Pharmacology* (pp. 257–282). IGI Global., DOI: 10.4018/979-8-3693-3212-2.ch010

Liyakat, K. K. S. (2017). Lessar methodology for network intrusion detection. *Scholarly Research Journal for Humanity Science & English Language*, 4(24), 6853–6861.

Liyakat, K. K. S. (2022). Implementation of e-mail security with three layers of authentication. *Journal of Operating Systems Development and Trends*, 9(2), 29–35.

Liyakat, K. K. S. (2023). Machine Learning Approach Using Artificial Neural Networks to Detect Malicious Nodes in IoT Networks. In Shukla, P. K., Mittal, H., & Engelbrecht, A. (Eds.), *Computer Vision and Robotics. CVR 2023. Algorithms for Intelligent Systems*. Springer., DOI: 10.1007/978-981-99-4577-1_3

Liyakat, K. K. S. (2023).Detecting Malicious Nodes in IoT Networks Using Machine Learning and Artificial Neural Networks, *2023 International Conference on Emerging Smart Computing and Informatics (ESCI)*, Pune, India, 2023, pp. 1-5, DOI: 10.1109/ESCI56872.2023.10099544

Liyakat, K. K. S. (2024). Explainable AI in healthcare. *Explainable Artificial Intelligence in Healthcare Systems*, 2024, 271–284.

Liyakat, K. K. S. (2024). Machine Learning Approach Using Artificial Neural Networks to Detect Malicious Nodes in IoT Networks. In Udgata, S. K., Sethi, S., & Gao, X. Z. (Eds.), *Intelligent Systems. ICMIB 2023. Lecture Notes in Networks and Systems* (Vol. 728). Springer., available at https://link.springer.com/chapter/10.1007/978-981-99-3932-9_12, DOI: 10.1007/978-981-99-3932-9_12

Liyakat, K. K. S., Paradeshi, K. P., Shaikh, J. A., Pandyaji, K. K., & Kadam, D. B. (2022). Development of Machine Learning based Epileptic Seizureprediction using Web of Things (WoT). *NeuroQuantology : An Interdisciplinary Journal of Neuroscience and Quantum Physics*, 20(8), 9394.

Liyakat, S. (2023). Intelligent Watering System (IWS) for Agricultural Land Utilising Raspberry Pi. *Recent Trends in Fluid Mechanics.*, 10(2), 26–31p.

Liyakat, S. S. (2024). IoT-based Alcohol Detector using Blynk. *Journal of Electronics Design and Technology*, 1(1), 10–15.

López, O. A. M., López, A. M., & Crossa, J. (2022). *Multivariate Statistical Machine Learning Methods for Genomic Prediction*. Springer International Publishing. DOI: 10.1007/978-3-030-89010-0

Lundervold, A. S., & Lundervold, A. (2019). An overview of deep learning in medical imaging focusing on MRI. *Zeitschrift für Medizinische Physik*, 29(2), 102–127. DOI: 10.1016/j.zemedi.2018.11.002 PMID: 30553609

Luo, J., Wu, M., Gopukumar, D., & Zhao, Y. (2016). Big data application in biomedical research and health care: a literature review. *Biomedical informatics insights, 8*, BII-S31559.

Lv, Z., Qiao, L., Wang, Q., & Piccialli, F. (2021). Advanced machine-learning methods for brain-computer interfacing. *IEEE/ACM Transactions on Computational Biology and Bioinformatics*, 18(5), 1688–1698. DOI: 10.1109/TCBB.2020.3010014 PMID: 32750892

M. R. G. and H. Anandaram. (2022) "Extraction of Fetal ECG Using ANFIS and the Undecimated-Wavelet Transform," 2022 IEEE 3rd Global Conference for Advancement in Technology (GCAT), pp. 1-5.

Machha Babitha, Ms.. (2022). Trends of Artificial Intelligence for online exams in education, International journal of Early Childhood special. *Education*, 14(1), 2457–2463.

Magrabi, F., Ammenwerth, E., McNair, J. B., De Keizer, N. F., Hyppönen, H., Nykänen, P., & Georgiou, A. (2019). Artificial intelligence in clinical decision support: Challenges for evaluating AI and practical implications. *Yearbook of Medical Informatics*, 28(01), 128–134.

Mahadevaiah, G., Rv, P., Bermejo, I., Jaffray, D., Dekker, A., & Wee, L. (2020). Artificial Intelligence-Based Clinical Decision Support in Modern Medical Physics: Selection, Acceptance, Commissioning, and Quality Assurance. *Medical Physics*, 47(5), 228–235. DOI: 10.1002/mp.13562 PMID: 32418341

Mahadevkar, S. V., Khemani, B., Patil, S., Kotecha, K., Vora, D. R., Abraham, A., & Gabralla, L. A. (2022). A review on machine learning styles in computer vision—Techniques and future directions. *IEEE Access : Practical Innovations, Open Solutions*, 10, 107293–107329. DOI: 10.1109/ACCESS.2022.3209825

Maistry, A., Pillay, A., & Jembere, E. (2020, September). Improving the accuracy of diabetes retinopathy image classification using augmentation. In *Conference of the South African Institute of Computer Scientists and Information Technologists 2020* (pp. 134-140). DOI: 10.1145/3410886.3410914

Majumder, S., & Deen, M. J. (2019). Smartphone Sensors for Health Monitoring and Diagnosis. *Sensors (Basel)*, 19(9), 2164. DOI: 10.3390/s19092164 PMID: 31075985

Mak, K. K., & Pichika, M. R. (2019, March 1). Artificial intelligence in drug development: Present status and future prospects. *Drug Discovery Today*, 24(3), 773–780. DOI: 10.1016/j.drudis.2018.11.014 PMID: 30472429

Maleki Varnosfaderani, S., & Forouzanfar, M. (2024). The role of AI in hospitals and clinics: Transforming healthcare in the 21st century. *Bioengineering (Basel, Switzerland)*, 11(4), 337. DOI: 10.3390/bioengineering11040337 PMID: 38671759

Malgaroli, M., Hull, T. D., Zech, J. M., & Althoff, T. (2023). Natural language processing for mental health interventions: A systematic review and research framework. *Translational Psychiatry*, 13(1), 309. DOI: 10.1038/s41398-023-02592-2 PMID: 37798296

Malik, S., & Tyagi, A. K. (Eds.). (2022). *Intelligent Interactive Multimedia Systems for E-Healthcare Applications*. CRC Press. DOI: 10.1201/9781003282112

Mallikarjun, S. D., & Kawale, S. R. (2023) "Cloud-Based Multi-Layer Security Framework for Protecting E-Health Records," *2023 International Conference on Artificial Intelligence for Innovations in Healthcare Industries (ICAIIHI)*, Raipur, India, 2023, pp. 1-7.

Mamoshina, P., Vieira, A., Putin, E., & Zhavoronkov, A. (2016). Applications of deep learning in biomedicine. *Molecular Pharmaceutics*, 13(5), 1445–1454. DOI: 10.1021/acs.molpharmaceut.5b00982 PMID: 27007977

Manickam, P., Mariappan, S. A., Murugesan, S. M., Hansda, S., Kaushik, A., Shinde, R., & Thipperudraswamy, S. P. (2022). Artificial Intelligence (AI) and Internet of Medical Things (IoMT) Assisted Biomedical Systems for Intelligent Healthcare. In *Biosensors* (Vol. 12, Issue 8). DOI: 10.3390/bios12080562

Manikandan, A., & Gayathri Narayanan, K. S. (2024). Investigations in Security Challenges and Solutions for M2M Communications—A Review. *International Journal of Electrical and Electronic Engineering and Telecommunications*, 13(1), 17–32. Advance online publication. DOI: 10.18178/ijeetc.13.1.17-32

Manivannan, D. (2024). Recent endeavors in machine learning-powered intrusion detection systems for the internet of things. *Journal of Network and Computer Applications*, 229, 103925. DOI: 10.1016/j.jnca.2024.103925

Manyika, J., Chui, M., Brown, B., Bughin, J., Dobbs, R., Roxburgh, C., & Hung Byers, A. (2011). Big data: The next frontier for innovation, competition, and productivity.

Marengo, A. (2023). The future of AI in IoT: Emerging trends in intelligent data analysis and privacy protection.

Marima, R., Mtshali, N., Phillips, P., Molefi, T., Khanyile, R., Mbita, Z., & Dlamini, Z. (2023). Health informatics applications in healthcare and society 5.0. In *Society 5.0 and next generation healthcare: Patient-focused and technology-assisted precision therapies* (pp. 31–49). Springer Nature Switzerland. DOI: 10.1007/978-3-031-36461-7_2

Marjani, M., Nasaruddin, F., Gani, A., Karim, A., Hashem, I. A. T., Siddiqa, A., & Yaqoob, I. (2017). Big IoT data analytics: architecture, opportunities, and open research challenges. *ieee access, 5*, 5247-5261.

Marques, G., Bhoi, A. K., de Albuquerque, V. H. C., & Hareesha, K. S. (2021). *IoT in healthcare and ambient assisted living* (Vol. 933). Springer. DOI: 10.1007/978-981-15-9897-5

Martinez, C. J., & Galmes, S. 2022. "Analysis of the Primary Attacks on IoMT Internet of Medical Things Communications Protocols." In *2022 IEEE World AI IoT Congress, AIIoT 2022*, DOI: 10.1109/AIIoT54504.2022.9817252

Martinez, E. L., & Santos, P. N. (2024) "Predictive Analytics for Disease Prevention Using IoMT," in *2024 International Symposium on Health Informatics (ISHI)*, Madrid, Spain, pp. 18-23.

Martin, G. L., Jouganous, J., Savidan, R., Bellec, A., Goehrs, C., Benkebil, M., Miremont, G., Micallef, J., Salvo, F., Pariente, A., & Létinier, L. (2022). Validation of Artificial Intelligence to support the automatic coding of patient adverse drug reaction reports, using Nationwide Pharmacovigilance Data. *Drug Safety*, 45(5), 535–548. DOI: 10.1007/s40264-022-01153-8 PMID: 35579816

Martín-Noguerol, T., Paulano-Godino, F., López-Ortega, R., Górriz, J. M., Riascos, R. F., & Luna, A. (2021). Artificial intelligence in radiology: Relevance of collaborative work between radiologists and engineers for building a multidisciplinary team. *Clinical Radiology*, 76(5), 317–324. DOI: 10.1016/j.crad.2020.11.113 PMID: 33358195

Martin, S. S., Aday, A. W., Almarzooq, Z. I., Anderson, C. A., Arora, P., Avery, C. L., Baker-Smith, C. M., Gibbs, B. B., Beaton, A. Z., Boehme, A. K., Commodore-Mensah, Y., Currie, M. E., Elkind, M. S., Evenson, K. R., Generoso, G., Heard, D. G., Hiremath, S., Johansen, M. C., Kalani, R., & Palaniappan, L. P. (2024). 2024 Heart Disease and Stroke Statistics: A Report of US and Global Data From the American Heart Association. *Circulation*, 149(8). Advance online publication. DOI: 10.1161/CIR.0000000000001209 PMID: 38264914

Massari, H. E., Sabouri, Z., Mhammedi, S., & Gherabi, N. (2022). Diabetes prediction using machine learning algorithms and ontology. *Journal of ICT Standardization*, 10(2), 319–337. DOI: 10.13052/jicts2245-800X.10212

Masud, M., Gaba, G. S., Alqahtani, S., Muhammad, G., Gupta, B. B., Kumar, P., & Ghoneim, A. (2021). A Lightweight and Robust Secure Key Establishment Protocol for Internet of Medical Things in COVID-19 Patients Care. *IEEE Internet of Things Journal*, 8(21), 15694–15703. Advance online publication. DOI: 10.1109/JIOT.2020.3047662 PMID: 35782176

Mathkor, D. M., Mathkor, N., Bassfar, Z., Bantun, F., Slama, P., Ahmad, F., & Haque, S. (2024). Multirole of the internet of medical things (iomt) in biomedical systems for managing smart healthcare systems: An overview of current and future innovative trends. *Journal of Infection and Public Health*, 17(4), 559–572. DOI: 10.1016/j.jiph.2024.01.013 PMID: 38367570

Mathur, S., Bhattacharjee, S., Sehgal, S., & Shekhar, R. (2024). Role of artificial intelligence and internet of things in neurodegenerative diseases. In *AI and neuro-degenerative diseases: Insights and solutions* (pp. 35–62). Springer Nature Switzerland. DOI: 10.1007/978-3-031-53148-4_2

Mbunge, E., Muchemwa, B., Jiyane, S., & Batani, J. (2021). Sensors and healthcare 5.0: Transformative shift in virtual care through emerging digital health technologies. [Special issue on Intelligent Medicine Leads the New Development of Human Health.]. *Global Health Journal (Amsterdam, Netherlands)*, 5(4), 169–177. DOI: 10.1016/j.glohj.2021.11.008

McDonnell, K. J. (2023). Leveraging the academic artificial intelligence ecosystem to advance the community oncology enterprise. *Journal of Clinical Medicine*, 12(14), 4830. DOI: 10.3390/jcm12144830 PMID: 37510945

MDN-Popstate. (2024). Window: popstate event. Retrieved from https://developer.mozilla.org/en-US/docs/Web/API/Window/popstate_event

Medhi, N., & Dandapat, S. (2016). An effective fovea detection and automatic assessment of diabetic maculopathy in color fundus images. *Computers in Biology and Medicine*, 74, 30–44. DOI: 10.1016/j.compbiomed.2016.04.007 PMID: 27174686

Meeker, W. Q., & Escobar, L. A. (2014). *Statistical Methods for Reliability Data*. Wiley.

Mehta, N., Rossi, F., & Johnson, D. (2023) "Generative AI in Healthcare: Enhancing Diagnostic Accuracy and Efficiency," *2023 IEEE International Conference on Artificial Intelligence and Machine Learning (AIML)*, Dubai, UAE, pp. 215-220.

Messinis, S., Temenos, N., Protonotarios, N. E., Rallis, I., Kalogeras, D., & Doulamis, N. (2024). Enhancing internet of medical things security with artificial intelligence: A comprehensive review. *Computers in Biology and Medicine*, 170, 108036. DOI: 10.1016/j.compbiomed.2024.108036 PMID: 38295478

Miles, J. C., & Walker, A. J. (2006, September). The potential application of artificial intelligence in transport. In IEE proceedings-intelligent transport systems (Vol. 153, No. 3, pp. 183-198). IET Digital Library.

Miller, D. D., & Brown, E. W. (2018). Artificial intelligence in medical practice: The question to the answer? *The American Journal of Medicine*, 131(2), 129–133. DOI: 10.1016/j.amjmed.2017.10.035 PMID: 29126825

Mirbabaie, M., Stieglitz, S., & Frick, N. R. (2021). Artificial intelligence in disease diagnostics: A critical review and classification on the current state of research guiding future direction. *Health and Technology*, 11(4), 693–731.

Mishna, F., Milne, E., Bogo, M., & Pereira, L. F. (2021). Responding to COVID-19: New trends in social workers' use of information and communication technology. *Clinical Social Work Journal*, 49(4), 484–494. DOI: 10.1007/s10615-020-00780-x PMID: 33250542

Mishra Sunil, B.. (2024). AI-Driven IoT (AI IoT) in Thermodynamic Engineering. *Journal of Modern Thermodynamics in Mechanical System*, 6(1), 1–8.

Mishra Sunil, B.. (2024). Nanotechnology's Importance in Mechanical Engineering. *Journal of Fluid Mechanics and Mechanical Design*, 6(1), 1–9.

Mishra Sunil, B.. (2024). Review of the Literature and Methodological Structure for IoT and PLM Integration in the Manufacturing Sector. *Journal of Advancement in Machines*, 9(1), 1–5.

Mishra, V. (2018, May 30). Artificial intelligence: The beginning of a new era in pharmacy profession. [AJP]. *Asian Journal of Pharmaceutics*, 12(02).

Miss Argonda, U. A. (2018). Review paper for design and simulation of a Patch antenna by using HFSS. *International Journal of Trends in Scientific Research and Development*, 2(2), 158–160.

Mitchell, T. M. (1997). *Machine Learning*. McGraw-Hill.

Mitesh, S. (2020). *Agile, DevOps and Cloud Computing with Microsoft Azure*. BPB Publications.

Mitra, A., Roy, U., & Tripathy, B. K. 2022. "IoMT in Healthcare Industry—Concepts and Applications." In *Studies in Computational Intelligence*, DOI: 10.1007/978-981-19-2416-3_8

MND-API. (2024). HTML5 History Application Programming Interface. Retrieved from https://developer.mozilla.org/en-US/docs/Web/API/History_API

Mohammadi-Koushki, N., & Gawanmeh, A. (2018, October). Analysis of mac protocols for real-time monitoring of heart and respiratory signals. In 2018 IEEE 43rd Conference on Local Computer Networks Workshops (LCN Workshops) (pp. 117-123). IEEE.

Mohammadi, M., Al-Fuqaha, A., Sorour, S., & Guizani, M. (2018). Deep learning for IoT big data and streaming analytics: A survey. *IEEE Communications Surveys and Tutorials*, 20(4), 2923–2960. DOI: 10.1109/COMST.2018.2844341

Mongo, D. B. (2024). MongoDB: The Developer Data Platform. Retrieved from https://www.mongodb.com

Monteiro, A. C. B., França, R. P., Arthur, R., & Iano, Y. (2021). An overview of medical Internet of Things, artificial intelligence, and cloud computing employed in health care from a modern panorama. *The Fusion of Internet of Things, Artificial Intelligence, and Cloud Computing in Health Care*, 3-23.

Montgomery, D. C. (2012). *Introduction to Statistical Quality Control* (7th ed.). Wiley.

Morgan, J. (2020). Meeting the greatest challenges for leaders of the future. *Leader to Leader*, 2020(96), 19–26. DOI: 10.1002/ltl.20500

Morley, J., Murphy, L., Mishra, A., Joshi, I., & Karpathakis, K. (2022). Governing Data and Artificial Intelligence for Health Care: Developing an International Understanding. *JMIR Formative Research*, 6(1), e31623. DOI: 10.2196/31623 PMID: 35099403

Moshawrab, M., Adda, M., Bouzouane, A., Ibrahim, H., & Raad, A. (2023). Smart Wearables for the Detection of Cardiovascular Diseases: A Systematic Literature Review. *Sensors (Basel)*, 23(2), 828. DOI: 10.3390/s23020828 PMID: 36679626

Motwani, A., Shukla, P. K., & Pawar, M. (2022). Ubiquitous and smart healthcare monitoring frameworks based on machine learning: A comprehensive review. *Artificial Intelligence in Medicine*, 134, 102431. DOI: 10.1016/j.artmed.2022.102431 PMID: 36462891

Moujahid, F. E., Aouad, S., & Zbakh, M. (2023). Smart Healthcare Development Based on IoMT and Edge-Cloud Computing: A Systematic Survey. In *Lecture notes on data engineering and communications technologies* (pp. 575–593). DOI: 10.1007/978-3-031-27762-7_52

Müller, A. C., & Guido, S. (2018). *Introduction to Machine Learning with Python: A Guide for Data Scientists*. O'Reilly Media.

Murdoch, B. (2021). Privacy and artificial intelligence: Challenges for protecting health information in a new era. *BMC Medical Ethics*, 22(1), 1–5. DOI: 10.1186/s12910-021-00687-3 PMID: 34525993

Muthu, B., Sivaparthipan, C. B., Manogaran, G., Sundarasekar, R., Kadry, S., Shanthini, A., & Dasel, A. (2020). IOT based wearable sensor for diseases prediction and symptom analysis in healthcare sector. *Peer-to-Peer Networking and Applications*, 13(6), 2123–2134. DOI: 10.1007/s12083-019-00823-2

MySQL. (2024). MySQL: Database Management System. Retrieved from https://www.mysql.com

Nagarajan, S. M., Anandhan, P., Muthukumaran, V., Uma, K., & Kumaran, U. (2022). Security framework for IoT and deep belief network-based healthcare system using blockchain technology. *International Journal of Electronic Business*, 17(3), 226–243. DOI: 10.1504/IJEB.2022.124324

Nagare, M. S., & KS, M. K. (2015). An Efficient Algorithm brain tumor detection based on Segmentation and Thresholding. Journal of Management in Manufacturing and services, 2(17), 19-27.

Nagrale, M., Pol, R. S., Birajadar, G. B., & Mulani, A. O. (2024). Internet of Robotic Things in Cardiac Surgery: An Innovative Approach. *African Journal of Biological Sciences*, 6(6), 709–725. DOI: 10.33472/AFJBS.6.6.2024.709-725

Nah, F. F. H., Zheng, R., Cai, J., Siau, K., & Chen, L. (2023). Generative AI and ChatGPT: Applications, challenges, and AI-human collaboration. *Journal of Information Technology Case and Application Research*, 25(3), 277–304. DOI: 10.1080/15228053.2023.2233814

Nair, A. K., Sahoo, J., & Raj, E. D. (2023). Privacy-preserving Federated Learning framework for IoMT based big data analysis using edge computing. *Computer Standards & Interfaces*, 86, 103720. DOI: 10.1016/j.csi.2023.103720

Narang, M., Jatain, A., & Punetha, N. (2023, November). A Survey on Detection of Man-In-The-Middle Attack in IoMT Using Machine Learning Techniques. In *International Conference on Computational Intelligence* (pp. 117-132). Singapore: Springer Nature Singapore.

Naria, I. P., & Sulistyo, S. (2022, July). Security and Privacy Issue in Internet of Things, Smart Building System: A Review. In *2022 International Symposium on Information Technology and Digital Innovation (ISITDI)* (pp. 177-180). IEEE.

Natarajan, K., Muthusamy, S., Sha, M. S., Sadasivuni, K. K., Sekaran, S., Charles Gnanakkan, C. A. R., & Elngar, A., A. (. (2024). A novel method for the detection and classification of multiple diseases using transfer learning-based deep learning techniques with improved performance. *Neural Computing & Applications*, •••, 1–19. DOI: 10.1007/s00521-024-09900-x

Natarajan, K., Vinoth Kumar, V., Mahesh, T. R., Abbas, M., Kathamuthu, N., Mohan, E., & Annand, J. R. (2024). Efficient Heart Disease Classification Through Stacked Ensemble with Optimized Firefly Feature Selection. *International Journal of Computational Intelligence Systems*, 17(1), 1–14. DOI: 10.1007/s44196-024-00538-0

Naveen, K. B., Ramesha, M., & Pai, G. N. (2020). Internet of things: Internet revolution, impact, technology road map and features. *Adv. Math. Sci. J.*, 9(7), 4405–4414. DOI: 10.37418/amsj.9.7.11

NavyaSree. V., Surarchitha, Y., Reddy, A. M., Sree, B. D., Anuhya, A., & Jabeen, H. (2022, October). Predicting the Risk Factor of Kidney Disease using Meta Classifiers. In 2022 IEEE 2nd Mysore Sub Section International Conference (MysuruCon) (pp. 1-6). IEEE.

Nazer, L. H., Zatarah, R., Waldrip, S., Ke, J. X. C., Moukheiber, M., Khanna, A. K., Hicklen, R. S., Moukheiber, L., Moukheiber, D., Ma, H., & Mathur, P. (2023). Bias in artificial intelligence algorithms and recommendations for mitigation. *PLOS Digital Health*, 2(6), e0000278. DOI: 10.1371/journal.pdig.0000278 PMID: 37347721

Neeraja, P., Kumar, R. G., Kumar, M. S., Liyakat, K. K. S., & Vani, M. S. (2024). *DL-Based Somnolence Detection for Improved Driver Safety and Alertness Monitoring. 2024 IEEE International Conference on Computing, Power and Communication Technologies (IC2PCT)*. Greater Noida., Available at https://ieeexplore.ieee.org/document/10486714, DOI: 10.1109/IC2PCT60090.2024.10486714

Nelson, K. M., Chang, E. T., Zulman, D. M., Rubenstein, L. V., Kirkland, F. D., & Fihn, S. D. (2019). Using Predictive Analytics to Guide Patient Care and Research in a National Health System. *Journal of General Internal Medicine*, 34(8), 1379–1380. DOI: 10.1007/s11606-019-04961-4 PMID: 31011959

Nerkar, P. M., Shinde, S. S., Liyakat, K. K. S., Desai, S., & Kazi, S. S. L. (2023). Monitoring fresh fruit and food using Iot and machine learning to improve food safety and quality. Tuijin Jishu/Journal of Propulsion Technology, 44(3), 2927-2931.

Neto, E. C. P., Dadkhah, S., Sadeghi, S., Molyneaux, H., & Ghorbani, A. A. (2024). A review of machine learning (ml)-based iot security in healthcare: A dataset perspective. *Computer Communications*, 213, 61–77. DOI: 10.1016/j.comcom.2023.11.002

Nguyen, M. P., & Tran, N. V. (2024) "IoMT and AI: Synergy for Personalized Healthcare," in *2024 International Conference on Advanced Healthcare Informatics (ICAHI)*, Hanoi, Vietnam, pp. 29-34.

Nida, N. (2023). Shaikh, Milind. (2023). PV Penetrations in Conventional Power System and Generation of Harmonic and Power Quality Issues: A Review. *International Journal of Power Electronics Controllers and Converters*, 9(2), 12–19p.

Nie, X., Zhang, A., Chen, J., Qu, Y., & Yu, S. (2022). Blockchain-empowered secure and privacy-preserving health data sharing in edge-based IoMT. *Security and Communication Networks*, 2022(1), 8293716. DOI: 10.1155/2022/8293716

Nikita, K.. (2020). Design of Vehicle system using CAN Protocol. *International Journal for Research in Applied Science and Engineering Technology*, 8(V), 1978–1983. DOI: 10.22214/ijraset.2020.5321

Nimmesgern, E., Norstedt, I., & Draghia-Akli, R. (2017, July). Enabling personalized medicine in Europe by the European commission's funding activities. *Personalized Medicine*, 14(4), 355–365. DOI: 10.2217/pme-2017-0003 PMID: 29749834

Ni, W., Ao, H., Tian, H., Eldar, Y. C., & Niyato, D. (2024). Fedsl: Federated split learning for collaborative healthcare analytics on resource-constrained wearable iomt devices. *IEEE Internet of Things Journal*, 11(10), 18934–18935. DOI: 10.1109/JIOT.2024.3370985

Node.js. (2024). Node.js: Cross Platform. Retrieved from https://nodejs.org/en

Nti, I. K., Adekoya, A. F., Weyori, B. A., & Keyeremeh, F. (2023). A bibliometric analysis of technology in sustainable healthcare: Emerging trends and future directions. *Decision Analytics Journal*, 8, 100292. DOI: 10.1016/j.dajour.2023.100292

O'Sullivan, S., Nevejans, N., Allen, C., Blyth, A., Leonard, S., Pagallo, U., Holzinger, K., Holzinger, A., Sajid, M. I., & Ashrafian, H. (2019). Legal, regulatory, and ethical frameworks for development of standards in artificial intelligence (AI) and autonomous robotic surgery. *International Journal of Medical Robotics and Computer Assisted Surgery*, 15(1), e1968. DOI: 10.1002/rcs.1968 PMID: 30397993

Obermeyer, Z., & Emanuel, E. J. (2016). Predicting the future—Big data, machine learning, and clinical medicine. *The New England Journal of Medicine*, 375(13), 1216–1219. DOI: 10.1056/NEJMp1606181 PMID: 27682033

Obermeyer, Z., Powers, B., Vogeli, C., & Mullainathan, S. (2019). Dissecting racial bias in an algorithm used to manage the health of populations. *Science*, 366(6464), 447–453. DOI: 10.1126/science.aax2342 PMID: 31649194

Ogunsakin, O. L., & Anwansedo, S. (2024). Leveraging Ai For Healthcare Administration: Streamlining Operations And Reducing Costs.

Okonji, O. R., Yunusov, K., & Gordon, B. (2024). *Applications of Generative AI in Healthcare: algorithmic, ethical, legal and societal considerations*. DOI: 10.36227/techrxiv.171527587.75649430/v1

Olan, F., Arakpogun, E. O., Suklan, J., Nakpodia, F., Damij, N., & Jayawickrama, U. (2022). Artificial intelligence and knowledge sharing: Contributing factors to organizational performance. *Journal of Business Research*, 145, 605–615. DOI: 10.1016/j.jbusres.2022.03.008

Oleka-Onyewuchi, C. N. C. (2023). *The New Workforce Reality: Embracing Intergenerational Collaboration That Thrives in the Age of Automation and Layoffs*. Gatekeeper Press.

Olshannikova, E., Ometov, A., Koucheryavy, Y., & Olsson, T. (2015). Visualizing Big Data with augmented and virtual reality: Challenges and research agenda. *Journal of Big Data*, 2(1), 1–27. DOI: 10.1186/s40537-015-0031-2

Omidian, H. (2024). Synergizing blockchain and artificial intelligence to enhance healthcare. *Drug Discovery Today*, 29(9), 104111. DOI: 10.1016/j.drudis.2024.104111 PMID: 39034026

Ongole, D., & Saravanan, S. (2023). Colour-based segmentation using FCM and K-means clustering for 3D thyroid gland state image classification using deep convolutional neural network structure. *International Journal of Imaging Systems and Technology*, 33(5), 1814–1826. DOI: 10.1002/ima.22900

Osman, R. A. (2024). Internet of medical things (iomt) optimization for healthcare: A deep learning-based interference avoidance model. *Computer Networks*, 248, 110491. DOI: 10.1016/j.comnet.2024.110491

Padmaja, M., Shitharth, S., Prasuna, K., Chaturvedi, A., Kshirsagar, P. R., & Vani, A. (2022). Grow of artificial intelligence to challenge security in IoT application. *Wireless Personal Communications*, 127(3), 1829–1845. DOI: 10.1007/s11277-021-08725-4

Padmasini, N., Krithika, G. K., Lithiga, P., & Akshaya, S. J. (2023). Automatic Detection and Segmentation Of Retinal Manifestations Due To Diabetic Retinopathy. *International Conference on Signal Processing, Computation, Electronics, Power and Telecommunication (IConSCEPT)*, Karaikal, India, pp. 1-6. DOI: 10.1109/IConSCEPT57958.2023.10170621

Pagespeed. (2024). Google PageSpeed Insights. Retrieved from https://pagespeed.web.dev

Pai, G. N., Pai, M. S., Gowd, V. D., & Shruthi, M. (2020, November). Internet of Things: a survey on devices, ecosystem, components and communication protocols. In 2020 4th International Conference on Electronics, Communication and Aerospace Technology (ICECA) (pp. 611-616). IEEE.

Palanikkumar, D., Mary, P. A., & Begum, A. Y. (2023) "A Novel IoT Framework and Device Architecture for Efficient Smart city Implementation," 2023 7th International Conference on Trends in Electronics and Informatics (ICOEI), Tirunelveli, India, pp. 420-426.

Palanivinayagam, A., & Damaševičius, R. (2023). Effective handling of missing values in datasets for classification using machine learning methods. *Information (Basel)*, 14(2), 92. DOI: 10.3390/info14020092

Pamadi, A. M., Ravishankar, A., Nithya, P. A., Jahnavi, G., & Kathavate, S. (2022). Diabetic Retinopathy Detection using MobileNetV2 Architecture; *Proceedings of the 2022 International Conference on Smart Technologies and Systems for Next Generation Computing (ICSTSN)*; Villupuram, India. 25–26 March 2022; pp. 1–5.

Pamadi, A. M., Ravishankar, A., Nithya, P. A., Jahnavi, G., & Kathavate, S. (2022, March). Diabetic retinopathy detection using MobileNetV2 architecture. In *2022 International Conference on Smart Technologies and Systems for Next Generation Computing (ICSTSN)* (pp. 1-5). IEEE.

Panesar, A. (2019). *Machine learning and AI for healthcare*. Apress. DOI: 10.1007/978-1-4842-3799-1

Paolone, G., Iachetti, D., Paesani, R., Pilotti, F., Marinelli, M., & Di Felice, P. (2022). A Holistic Overview of the Internet of Things Ecosystem. *IoT*, 3(4), 398–434. Advance online publication. DOI: 10.3390/iot3040022

Pardeshi, D. K. (2022). Implementation of fault detection framework for healthcare monitoring system using IoT, sensors in wireless environment. *Telematique*, 21(1), 5451–5460.

Park, J., & Wu, H. (2022). Healthcare data security in AI. *Journal of Medical Internet Research*, 24(7), e29834. DOI: 10.2196/29834 PMID: 35857347

Park, K., Lee, M., & Kim, S. (2023) "Real-Time Data Analysis in IoMT: Improving Patient Outcomes with AI," *2023 IEEE International Conference on Biomedical and Health Informatics (BHI)*, Seoul, South Korea, pp. 429-434.

Park, S., Cho, B., Kim, D., & You, I. (2022). Machine Learning Based Signaling DDoS Detection System for 5G Stand Alone Core Network. *Applied Sciences (Basel, Switzerland)*, 12(23), 12456. Advance online publication. DOI: 10.3390/app122312456

Partin, A., Brettin, T. S., Zhu, Y., Narykov, O., Clyde, A., Overbeek, J., & Stevens, R. L. (2023). Deep learning methods for drug response prediction in cancer: Predominant and emerging trends. *Frontiers in Medicine*, 10, 1086097. DOI: 10.3389/fmed.2023.1086097 PMID: 36873878

Patel, C., & Gupta, M. R. (2024) "Generative AI in Personalized Medicine: A Review," in *2024 International Conference on Medical and Health Informatics (ICMHI)*, Sydney, Australia, pp. 21-26.

Patel, H., Shah, H., Patel, G., & Patel, A. (2024). Hematologic cancer diagnosis and classification using machine and deep learning: State-of-the-art techniques and emerging research directives. *Artificial Intelligence in Medicine*, 152, 102883. DOI: 10.1016/j.artmed.2024.102883 PMID: 38657439

Patel, K., Moore, L., & Singh, H. (2023) "Next-Generation IoMT Devices and AI for Enhanced Patient Care," *2023 IEEE International Conference on Robotics and Automation (ICRA)*, Barcelona, Spain, pp. 567-572.

Patel, N. J., Wang, X., Fu, X., Kawano, Y., Cook, C., Vanni, K. M. M., Qian, G., Banasiak, E., Kowalski, E., Zhang, Y., Sparks, J. A., & Wallace, Z. S. (2023). Factors associated with COVID-19 breakthrough infection among vaccinated patients with rheumatic diseases: A cohort study. *Seminars in Arthritis and Rheumatism*, 58, 152108. DOI: 10.1016/j.semarthrit.2022.152108 PMID: 36347211

Patel, S., & Gupta, R. (2021). Machine learning models for drug repurposing. *Journal of Biomedical Informatics*, 111, 103591. DOI: 10.1016/j.jbi.2020.103591

Patel, T., & Singh, S. (2022). AI innovations in surgery. *Surgical Technology International*, 41(5), 89–102. DOI: 10.1177/1553350621104969

Patil, S., & Choudhary, S. (2023, April). Prediction of Ultrasound Kidney Imaging Using Convolution Neural Networks. In 2023 IEEE 12th International Conference on Communication Systems and Network Technologies (CSNT) (pp. 451-455). IEEE.

Patruni, M. R., & Humayun, A. G. (2024). PPAM-mIoMT: A privacy-preserving authentication with device verification for securing healthcare systems in 5G networks. *International Journal of Information Security*, 23(1), 679–698. DOI: 10.1007/s10207-023-00762-3

Pavan Kumar, I., Mahaveerakannan, R., Praveen Kumar, K., Basu, I., Anil Kumar, T. C., & Choche, M. (2022). A Design of Disease Diagnosis based Smart Healthcare Model using Deep Learning Technique. *Proceedings of the International Conference on Electronics and Renewable Systems, ICEARS 2022*. DOI: 10.1109/ICEARS53579.2022.9752063

Pavya, K., & Srinivasan, B. (2017). Feature selection algorithms to improve thyroid disease diagnosis. In 2017 International conference on innovations in green energy and healthcare technologies (IGEHT) (pp. 1-5). IEEE. DOI: 10.1109/IGEHT.2017.8094070

Pearl, J., & Mackenzie, D. (2018). *The Book of Why: The New Science of Cause and Effect*. Basic Books.

Pedro, F., Subosa, M., Rivas, A., & Valverde, P. (2019). Artificial intelligence in education: Challenges and opportunities for sustainable development.

Pelekoudas-Oikonomou, F., Ribeiro, J. C., Mantas, G., Sakellari, G., & Gonzalez, J. (2023). Prototyping a hyperledger fabric-based security architecture for iomt-based health monitoring systems. *Future Internet*, 15(9), 308. DOI: 10.3390/fi15090308

Pereira, J. C., Caffarena, E. R., & Dos Santos, C. N. (2016, December 27). Boosting docking-based virtual screening with deep learning. *Journal of Chemical Information and Modeling*, 56(12), 2495–2506. DOI: 10.1021/acs.jcim.6b00355 PMID: 28024405

Perez-Pozuelo, I., Zhai, B., Palotti, J., Mall, R., Aupetit, M., Garcia-Gomez, J. M., Taheri, S., Guan, Y., & Fernandez-Luque, L. (2020, March). "The future of sleep health: A data-driven revolution in sleep science and medicine," npj. *Digital Medicine*, 3(1), 42. Advance online publication. DOI: 10.1038/s41746-020-0244-4 PMID: 32219183

Perwej, Y., Akhtar, N., Kulshrestha, N., & Mishra, P. (2022). A Methodical Analysis of Medical Internet of Things (MIoT) Security and Privacy in Current and Future Trends. *Journal of Emerging Technologies and Innovative Research*, 9(1).

Pickering, B. (2021). Trust, but verify: Informed consent, AI technologies, and public health emergencies. *Future Internet*, 13(5), 132.

Pierce, R. L., Van Biesen, W., Van Cauwenberge, D., Decruyenaere, J., & Sterckx, S. (2022). Explainability in medicine in an era of AI-based clinical decision support systems. *Frontiers in Genetics*, 13, 903600. DOI: 10.3389/fgene.2022.903600 PMID: 36199569

Pike, E. R. (2019). Defending data: Toward ethical protections and comprehensive data governance. *Emory Law Journal*, 69, 687.

Poplin, R., Chang, P. C., Alexander, D., Schwartz, S., Colthurst, T., Ku, A., Newburger, D., Dijamco, J., Nguyen, N., Afshar, P. T., Gross, S. S., Dorfman, L., McLean, C. Y., & DePristo, M. A. (2018). A universal SNP and small-indel variant caller using deep neural networks. *Nature Biotechnology*, 36(10), 983–987. DOI: 10.1038/nbt.4235 PMID: 30247488

Pradeepa, M., ... (2022). Student Health Detection using a Machine Learning Approach and IoT, *2022 IEEE 2nd Mysore sub section International Conference (MysuruCon)*, 2022.

Pradhan, T., Nimkar, P., & Jhajharia, K. (2024). Machine Learning and Deep Learning for Big Data Analysis. In *Big Data Analytics Techniques for Market Intelligence* (pp. 209–240). IGI Global. DOI: 10.4018/979-8-3693-0413-6.ch008

Pramanik, P. K. D., Pal, S., & Mukhopadhyay, M. (2022). Healthcare big data: A comprehensive overview. *Research anthology on big data analytics, architectures, and applications*, 119-147.

Pramanik, S., Pandey, D., Joardar, S., Niranjanamurthy, M., Pandey, B. K., & Kaur, J. (2023, October). An overview of IoT privacy and security in smart cities. In *AIP Conference Proceedings* (Vol. 2495, No. 1). AIP Publishing. DOI: 10.1063/5.0123511

Prasad, K., Dekka, S., Tanguturi, R. c., & Poornima, G. (2022) "An Intelligent System for Remote Monitoring of Patients Health and the Early Detection of Coronary Artery Disease," 2022 International Conference on Smart Generation Computing, Communication and Networking (SMART GENCON), Bangalore, India, pp. 1-6.

Prasad, K. R., Karanam, S. R., Ganesh, D., Liyakat, K. K. S., Talasila, V., & Purushotham, P. (2024, May). AI in public-private partnership for IT infrastructure development. *The Journal of High Technology Management Research*, 35(1), 100496. DOI: 10.1016/j.hitech.2024.100496

Prasad, K. S. R., and N, A. K., (2024) "Design and Implementation of an AI and IoT-Enabled Smart Safety Helmet for Real-Time Environmental and Health Monitoring," *2024 IEEE International Conference on Information Technology, Electronics and Intelligent Communication Systems (ICITEICS)*, Bangalore, India, 2024, pp. 1-7.

Prasad, K., Anil Kumar, N., Reddy, N. S., & Ashreetha, B. (2023) "Technologies for Comprehensive Information Security in the IoT," *2023 International Conference for Advancement in Technology (ICONAT)*, Goa, India, pp. 1-5.

Prashant, K. Magadum (2024). Machine Learning for Predicting Wind Turbine Output Power in Wind Energy Conversion Systems, *Grenze International Journal of Engineering and Technology,* Jan Issue, Vol 10, Issue 1, pp. 2074-2080. Grenze ID: 01.GIJET.10.1.4_1 Available at: https://thegrenze.com/index.php?display=page&view=journalabstract&absid=2514&id=8

Prithivraj, S., Lighittha, P. R., & Priya, L. (2024, April). Privacy preservation and confidentiality assurance in critical healthcare networks: Navigating complex data challenges within. In *Conference Proceedings: Encryptcon-An International Research Conference on CyberSecurity* (p. 10). Shashwat Publication.

Prochazka, A., Gulati, S., Holinka, S., & Smutek, D. (2019). Patch-based classification of thyroid nodules in ultrasound images using direction independent features extracted by two-threshold binary decomposition. *Computerized Medical Imaging and Graphics*, 71, 9–18. DOI: 10.1016/j.compmedimag.2018.10.001 PMID: 30453231

Prof. Kazi Kutubuddin, S. L. (2016a). Situation Invariant face recognition using PCA and Feed Forward Neural network, *Proceeding of International Conference on Advances in Engineering, Science and Technology,* 2016, pp. 260- 263.

Prof. Kazi Kutubuddin, S. L. (2016b). An Approach on Yarn Quality Detection for Textile Industries using Image Processing, *Proceeding of International Conference on Advances in Engineering, Science and Technology,* 2016, pp. 325-330.

Puspitasari, I., Nuzulita, N., & Hsiao, C.-S. (2024). Agile User-Centered Design Framework to Support the Development of E-Health for Patient Education. In *Computer and Information Science and Engineering* (Vol. 16, pp. 131–144). Springer. DOI: 10.1007/978-3-031-57037-7_10

Putra, K. T., Arrayyan, A. Z., Hayati, N., Damarjati, C., Bakar, A., & Chen, H. C. (2024). A review on the application of Internet of Medical Things in wearable personal health monitoring: A cloud-edge artificial intelligence approach. *IEEE Access : Practical Innovations, Open Solutions*, 12, 21437–21452. DOI: 10.1109/ACCESS.2024.3358827

Qin, S., Chan, S. L., Gu, S., Bai, Y., Ren, Z., Lin, X., Chen, Z., Jia, W., Jin, Y., Guo, Y., Hu, X., Meng, Z., Liang, J., Cheng, Y., Xiong, J., Ren, H., Yang, F., Li, W., Chen, Y., & Verset, G. (2023). Camrelizumab plus rivoceranib versus sorafenib as first-line therapy for unresectable hepatocellular carcinoma (CARES-310): A randomised, open-label, international phase 3 study. *Lancet*, 402(10408), 1133–1146. DOI: 10.1016/S0140-6736(23)00961-3 PMID: 37499670

Qureshi, R., Irfan, M., Ali, H., Khan, A., Nittala, A. S., Ali, S., & Alam, T. (2023). Artificial Intelligence and Biosensors in Healthcare and its Clinical Relevance: A Review. *IEEE Access : Practical Innovations, Open Solutions*, 11, 61600–61620. DOI: 10.1109/ACCESS.2023.3285596

Radhakrishnan, R., & Sekkizhar, J. (2007). A New Screening Procedure on Double Sampling Plan for Costly or Destructive items. *International Journal of Statistics and Management System*, 2(1-2), 88–97.

Rafique, W., Qi, L., Yaqoob, I., Imran, M., Rasool, R. U., & Dou, W. (2020). Complementing IoT Services through Software Defined Networking and Edge Computing: A Comprehensive Survey. *IEEE Communications Surveys and Tutorials*, 22(3), 1761–1804. Advance online publication. DOI: 10.1109/COMST.2020.2997475

Raghunath, S., Pfeifer, J. M., Ulloa-Cerna, A. E., Nemani, A., Carbonati, T., Jing, L., vanMaanen, D. P., Hartzel, D. N., Ruhl, J. A., Lagerman, B. F., Rocha, D. B., Stoudt, N. J., Schneider, G., Johnson, K. W., Zimmerman, N., Leader, J. B., Kirchner, H. L., Griessenauer, C. J., Hafez, A., & Haggerty, C. M. (2021). Deep neural networks can predict new-onset atrial fibrillation from the 12-lead ECG and help identify those at risk of atrial fibrillation–related stroke. *Circulation*, 143(13), 1287–1298. DOI: 10.1161/CIRCULATIONAHA.120.047829 PMID: 33588584

Rahmadika, S., Astillo, P. V., Choudhary, G., Duguma, D. G., Sharma, V., & You, I. (2022). Blockchain-based privacy preservation scheme for misbehavior detection in lightweight IoMT devices. *IEEE Journal of Biomedical and Health Informatics*, 27(2), 710–721. DOI: 10.1109/JBHI.2022.3187037 PMID: 35763469

Rahman, A., Debnath, T., Kundu, D., Khan, M. S. I., Aishi, A. A., Sazzad, S., Sayduzzaman, M., & Band, S. S. (2024). Machine learning and deep learning-based approach in smart healthcare: Recent advances, applications, challenges and opportunities. *AIMS Public Health*, 11(1), 58–109. DOI: 10.3934/publichealth.2024004 PMID: 38617415

Rai, B. K., Ojha, H., & Srivastava, I. (2024, March). Diabetic Retinopathy Detection using Deep Learning Model ResNet15. In *2024 2nd International Conference on Disruptive Technologies (ICDT)* (pp. 1361-1366). IEEE. DOI: 10.1109/ICDT61202.2024.10489478

Rajadevi, R., Venkatachalam, K., Masud, M., AlZain, M. A., & Abouhawwash, M. (2023). Proof of Activity Protocol for IoMT Data Security. *Computer Systems Science and Engineering*, 44(1). Advance online publication. DOI: 10.32604/csse.2023.024537

Rajawat, A. S., Goyal, S. B., Bedi, P., Jan, T., Whaiduzzaman, M., & Prasad, M. (2023). Quantum machine learning for security assessment on the Internet of Medical Things (IoMT). *Future Internet*, 15(8), 271. DOI: 10.3390/fi15080271

Rajpurkar, P., Irvin, J., Ball, R. L., Zhu, K., Yang, B., Mehta, H., & Ng, A. Y. (2018). Deep learning for chest radiograph diagnosis: A retrospective comparison of the CheXNeXt algorithm to practicing radiologists. *PLoS Medicine*, 15(11), e1002686. DOI: 10.1371/journal.pmed.1002686 PMID: 30457988

Rakova, B., Yang, J., Cramer, H., & Chowdhury, R. (2021). Where responsible AI meets reality: Practitioner perspectives on enablers for shifting organizational practices. *Proceedings of the ACM on Human-Computer Interaction, 5*(CSCW1), 1-23. DOI: 10.1145/3449081

Ramadan, N. (2023). Healthcare predictive analytics using machine learning and deep learning techniques: A survey. *Journal of Electrical Systems and Information Technology*, 10(1), 40. DOI: 10.1186/s43067-023-00108-y

Ramesh Naidu, P., Guruprasad, N., & Dankan Gowda, V. (2020). Design and implementation of cryptcloud system for securing files in cloud. *Adv. Math. Sci. J.*, 9(7), 4485–4493. DOI: 10.37418/amsj.9.7.17

Ramesh Naidu, P., Guruprasad, N., & Dankan Gowda, V. (2021). A High-Availability and Integrity Layer for Cloud Storage, Cloud Computing Security: From Single to Multi-Clouds. *Journal of Physics: Conference Series*, 1921(1), 012072. DOI: 10.1088/1742-6596/1921/1/012072

Ranjith, C. P., Natarajan, K., Madhuri, S., Ramakrishna, M. T., Bhat, C. R., & Venkatesan, V. K. (2023). Image Processing Using Feature-Based Segmentation Techniques for the Analysis of Medical Images. *Engineering Proceedings*, 59(1), 100.

Rao, B. K., Chaturvedi, A., & Hussain, N. (2022). Industrial quality healthcare services using Internet of Things and fog computing approach, Measurement. *Sensors (Basel)*, 24, 100517.

Rath, K. C., Khang, A., Rath, S. K., Satapathy, N., Satapathy, S. K., & Kar, S. (2024). Artificial intelligence (AI)-enabled technology in medicine-advancing holistic healthcare monitoring and control systems. In *Computer Vision and AI-Integrated IoT Technologies in the Medical Ecosystem* (pp. 87–108). CRC Press. DOI: 10.1201/9781003429609-6

Rauniyar, A., Hagos, D. H., Jha, D., Håkegård, J. E., Bagci, U., Rawat, D. B., & Vlassov, V. (2023). Federated learning for medical applications: A taxonomy, current trends, challenges, and future research directions. *IEEE Internet of Things Journal*.

Ravi, A.. (2022). *Pattern Recognition- An Approach towards Machine Learning, Lambert Publications, 2022.* ISBN.

Ravindraiah, R., & Chandra Mohan Reddy, S. (2018). Exudates detection in diabetic retinopathy images using possibilistic C-means clustering algorithm with induced spatial constraint. In *Artificial Intelligence and Evolutionary Computations in Engineering Systems* [Springer Singapore.]. *Proceedings of ICAIECES*, 2017, 455–463.

Ravindraiah, R., & Reddy, S. C. M. (2020). An Instinctive Application of Spatially Weighted Possibilistic Clustering Methods for the Detection of Lesions in Diabetic Retinopathy Images in Multi-dimensional Kernel Space. *Wireless Personal Communications*, 113(1), 223–240. DOI: 10.1007/s11277-020-07186-5

Ray, P. P., Dash, D., & Kumar, N. (2020). Sensors for internet of medical things: State-of-the-art, security and privacy issues, challenges and future directions. *Computer Communications*, 160, 111–131. DOI: 10.1016/j.comcom.2020.05.029

Razdan, S., & Sharma, S. (2022). Internet of medical things (IoMT): Overview, emerging technologies, and case studies. *IETE Technical Review*, 39(4), 775–788. DOI: 10.1080/02564602.2021.1927863

React, J. S. (2024). ReactJS: Computer Program. Retrieved from https://react.dev

Reddy, B. M. (2023). Amalgamation of Internet of Things and Machine Learning for Smart Healthcare Applications–A Review. *Int. J Comp. Eng. Sci. Res, 5*, 08-36.

Reddy, N. S. (2024) "Scalable AI Solutions for IoT-based Healthcare Systems using Cloud Platforms," *2024 8th International Conference on I-SMAC (IoT in Social, Mobile, Analytics and Cloud) (I-SMAC)*, Kirtipur, Nepal, 2024, pp. 156-162.

Reddy, N., Verma, N., & Dungan, K. (2023). *Monitoring technologies-continuous glucose monitoring, mobile technology, biomarkers of glycemic control*. Endotext. [Internet]

Reddy, S., & Patwal, P. P. S. (2022) "Data Analytics and Cloud-Based Platform for Internet of Things Applications in Smart Cities," *2022 International Conference on Industry 4.0 Technology (I4Tech)*, pp. 1-6.

Reguant, R., Brunak, S., & Saha, S. (2021). Understanding inherent image features in CNN-based assessment of diabetic retinopathy. *Scientific Reports*, 11(1), 9704. DOI: 10.1038/s41598-021-89225-0 PMID: 33958686

Rehman, A., Saba, T., Haseeb, K., Larabi Marie-Sainte, S., & Lloret, J. (2021). Energy-efficient IoT e-health using artificial intelligence model with homomorphic secret sharing. *Energies*, 14(19), 6414. DOI: 10.3390/en14196414

Rehm, H. L. (2017, April). Evolving health care through personal genomics. *Nature Reviews. Genetics*, 18(4), 259–267. DOI: 10.1038/nrg.2016.162 PMID: 28138143

Revanna C R, B. Kameswara Rao and Parismita Sarma (2022), Enhanced Diagnostic Methods for Identifying Anomalies in Imaging of Skin Lesions. IJEER 10(4), pp.1077-1085.

Reza, M., Hafsha, U., Amin, R., Yasmin, R., & Ruhi, S. (2023). Improving svm performance for type ii diabetes prediction with an improved non-linear kernel: Insights from the pima dataset. *Computer Methods and Programs in Biomedicine Update*, 4, 100118. DOI: 10.1016/j.cmpbup.2023.100118

Roberts, D., & Lee, M. (2020). Ethical AI in healthcare. *Bioethics Review*, 34(6), 712–725. DOI: 10.1111/bioe.12721

Rockwern, B., Johnson, D., & Sulmasy, L. S. (2021). Health Information Privacy, Protection, and Use in the Expanding Digital Health Ecosystem: A Position Paper of the American College of Physicians. *Annals of Internal Medicine*, 174(7), 994–998. Advance online publication. DOI: 10.7326/M20-7639 PMID: 33900797

Rodrigues, J. F.Jr, Florea, L., de Oliveira, M. C., Diamond, D., & Oliveira, O. N.Jr. (2021). Big data and machine learning for materials science. *Discover Materials*, 1(1), 1–27. DOI: 10.1007/s43939-021-00012-0 PMID: 33899049

Rodriguez, L. M., & Garcia, S. T. (2024) "Challenges in IoMT Integration: A Focus on Healthcare Systems," in *2024 International Symposium on Medical Device Technologies (ISMDT)*, Mexico City, Mexico, pp. 12-17.

Roseberry, T. D., & Gehan, E. A. (1964). Operating characteristic curves and accept-reject rules for two and three stage screening procedures. *Biometrics*, 20(1), 73–84. DOI: 10.2307/2527618

Rotbei, S., Tseng, W. H., Merino-Barbancho, B., Haleem, M. S., Montesinos, L., Pecchia, L., Fico, G., & Botta, A. (2024). Evaluating impact of movement on diabetes via artificial intelligence and smart devices systematic literature review. *Expert Systems with Applications*, 257, 125058. DOI: 10.1016/j.eswa.2024.125058

Rubí, J. N. S., & Gondim, P. R. L. (2019). IoMT Platform for Pervasive Healthcare Data Aggregation, Processing, and Sharing Based on OneM2M and OpenEHR. *Sensors (Switzerland)*, 19(19). Advance online publication. DOI: 10.3390/s19194283

Rudin, C. (2019). Stop explaining black box machine learning models for high stakes decisions and use interpretable models instead. *Nature Machine Intelligence*, 1(5), 206–215. DOI: 10.1038/s42256-019-0048-x PMID: 35603010

Saadat, M. N., & Shuaib, M. (2020). Advancements in deep learning theory and applications: Perspective in 2020 and beyond. *Advances and Applications in Deep Learning, 3*.

Sachin, D. N., Annappa, B., & Ambesange, S. (2024). Federated learning for digital healthcare: Concepts, applications, frameworks, and challenges. *Computing*, 106(9), 1–38. DOI: 10.1007/s00607-024-01317-7

Sadiq, K. A., Thompson, A. F., & Ayeni, O. A. (2022). Toward healthcare data availability and security using fog-to-cloud networks. Intelligent Interactive Multimedia Systems for e-Healthcare Applications, 81-103.

Saleem, M. A., Javeed, A., Akarathanawat, W., Chutinet, A., Suwanwela, N. C., Asdornwised, W., & Kaewplung, P. (2024). Innovations in stroke identification: A machine learning-based diagnostic model using neuroimages. *IEEE Access : Practical Innovations, Open Solutions*.

Salem, O., Alsubhi, K., Shaafi, A., Gheryani, M., Mehaoua, A., & Boutaba, R. (2022). Man-in-the-Middle Attack Mitigation in Internet of Medical Things. *IEEE Transactions on Industrial Informatics*, 18(3), 2053–2062. Advance online publication. DOI: 10.1109/TII.2021.3089462

Sandra. M, Kjersti. E, Valery. N and Adrian. C (2017). Retinal Diabetes Screening through Local binary patterns. IEEE Journal of Biomedical and Health Informatics (Volume: 21, Issue: 1), pp 184 – 192, .DOI: 10.1109/JBHI.2015.2490798

Sankepally, S. R., Kosaraju, N., Reddy, V., & Venkanna, U. (2022, December). Edge intelligence based mitigation of false data injection attack in iomt framework. In *2022 OITS International Conference on Information Technology (OCIT)* (pp. 422-427). IEEE.

Saranya, P., Devi, S. K., & Bharanidharan, B. (2022). Detection of Diabetic Retinopathy in Retinal Fundus Images using DenseNet based Deep Learning Model; *Proceedings of the 2022 International Mobile and Embedded Technology Conference (MECON)*; Noida, India. 10–11 March 2022; pp. 268–272. DOI: 10.1109/MECON53876.2022.9752065

Sardar, T. H., Khatun, A., Sengupta, S., Alam, Y., & Ara, T. (2024). Machine Learning in the Healthcare Sector and the Biomedical Big Data: Techniques, Applications, and Challenges. *Big Data Computing*, 336-352.

Saudagar, A. K. J., Kumar, A., & Khan, M. B. (2024). Mediverse beyond boundaries: A comprehensive analysis of AR and VR integration in medical education for diverse abilities. *Journal of Disability Research*, 3(1), 20230066. DOI: 10.57197/JDR-2023-0066

Sayyad, L. (2023). System for Love Healthcare for Loved Ones based on IoT. Research Exploration: Transcendence of Research Methods and Methodology, 2.

Scarpato, N., Pieroni, A., Di Nunzio, L., & Fallucchi, F. (2017). E-health-IoT universe: A review. *management, 21*(44), 46.

Schilling, E. G. (1967). A general method for determining the operating characteristics of mixed variables–attribute sampling plans single side specifications, S.D. known. Ph.D Dissertation, Rutgers – The State University, New Brunswick, NJ.

Schilling, E. G. (1982). *Acceptance Sampling in Quality Control*. Chapman and Hall/CRC.

Sebastian, A., Elharrouss, O., Al-Maadeed, S., & Almaadeed, N. (2023). A survey on deep-learning-based diabetic retinopathy classification. *Diagnostics (Basel)*, 13(3), 345. DOI: 10.3390/diagnostics13030345 PMID: 36766451

Sejdic, E., & Falk, T. H. (Eds.). (2018). *Signal processing and machine learning for biomedical big data*. CRC press. DOI: 10.1201/9781351061223

Sellwood, M. A., Ahmed, M., Segler, M. H., & Brown, N. (2018, September). Artificial intelligence in drug discovery. *Future Medicinal Chemistry*, 10(17), 2025–2028. DOI: 10.4155/fmc-2018-0212 PMID: 30101607

Sengan, S., Kamalam, G. K., Vellingiri, J., Gopal, J., Velayutham, P., & Subramaniyaswamy, V. (2020). Medical information retrieval systems for e-Health care records using fuzzy based machine learning model. *Microprocessors and Microsystems*, •••, 103344.

Sgallari, F. (2013). Computer Methods in Biomechanics and Biomedical Engineering: Imaging & Visualization. *Computer Methods in Biomechanics and Biomedical Engineering. Imaging & Visualization*.

Shafik, W. (2024b). Artificial Intelligence-Enabled Internet of Medical Things (AIoMT) in Modern Healthcare Practices. In *Clinical Practice and Unmet Challenges in AI-Enhanced Healthcare Systems* (pp. 42–69). IGI Global. DOI: 10.4018/979-8-3693-2703-6.ch003

Shafik, W. (2024g). Incorporating Artificial Intelligence for Urban and Smart Cities' Sustainability. In *Maintaining a Sustainable World in the Nexus of Environmental Science and AI* (pp. 23–58). IGI Global. DOI: 10.4018/979-8-3693-6336-2.ch002

Shafik, W. (2024j). Smart Health Revolution: Exploring Artificial Intelligence of Internet of Medical Things. In *Healthcare Industry Assessment: Analyzing Risks, Security, and Reliability* (pp. 201–229). Springer. DOI: 10.1007/978-3-031-65434-3_9

Shafik, W. (2024m). Wearable medical electronics in artificial intelligence of medical things. *Handbook of Security and Privacy of Ai-Enabled Healthcare Systems and Internet of Medical Things*, 21–40. https://doi.org/DOI: 10.1201/9781003370321-2

Shafik, W. (2024a). Artificial Intelligence and Machine Learning with Cyber Ethics for the Future World. In *Future Communication Systems Using Artificial Intelligence, Internet of Things and Data Science* (pp. 110–130). CRC Press., DOI: 10.1201/9781032648309-9

Shafik, W. (2024c). Artificial Intelligence-Enabled Internet of Medical Things for Enhanced Healthcare Systems. In *Smart Healthcare Systems* (pp. 119–134). CRC Press., DOI: 10.1201/9781032698519-9

Shafik, W. (2024d). The Role of Artificial Intelligence in the Emerging Digital Economy Era. In *Artificial Intelligence Enabled Management* (pp. 33–50). De Gruyter., DOI: 10.1515/9783111172408-003

Shafik, W. (2024e). Connected healthcare—the impact of Internet of Things on medical services. In *Artificial Intelligence and Internet of Things based Augmented Trends for Data Driven Systems* (pp. 181–217). CRC Press., DOI: 10.1201/9781003497318-10

Shafik, W. (2024f). Digital healthcare systems in a federated learning perspective. In *Federated Learning for Digital Healthcare Systems* (pp. 1–35). Elsevier., DOI: 10.1016/B978-0-443-13897-3.00001-1

Shafik, W. (2024h). IoT-Enabled Secure and Intelligent Smart Healthcare. In *Secure and Intelligent IoT-Enabled Smart Cities* (pp. 308–333). IGI Global., DOI: 10.4018/979-8-3693-2373-1.ch015

Shafik, W. (2024i). Navigating Emerging Challenges in Robotics and Artificial Intelligence in Africa. In *Examining the rapid advance of digital technology in Africa* (pp. 126–146). IGI Global., DOI: 10.4018/978-1-6684-9962-7.ch007

Shafik, W. (2024k). The Future of Healthcare: AIoMT—Redefining Healthcare with Advanced Artificial Intelligence and Machine Learning Techniques. In *Artificial Intelligence and Machine Learning in Drug Design and Development* (pp. 605–634). Wiley., DOI: 10.1002/9781394234196.ch19

Shafik, W. (2024l). Toward a More Ethical Future of Artificial Intelligence and Data Science. In *The Ethical Frontier of AI and Data Analysis* (pp. 362–388). IGI Global., DOI: 10.4018/979-8-3693-2964-1.ch022

Shah, F., Li, J., Shah, Y., & Shah, F. (2017, November). Broad big data domain via medical big data. In *2017 4th International Conference on Systems and Informatics (ICSAI)* (pp. 732-737). IEEE.

Shahid, Z. (2021). Distributed Machine Learning for Anomalous Human Activity Recognition using IoT Systems.

Shah, S. U., & Mehta, T. V. (2024) "Real-Time Monitoring with IoMT and AI: A Comprehensive Review," in *2024 IEEE International Conference on Biomedical Engineering and Sciences (ICBES)*, Kuala Lumpur, Malaysia, pp. 28-33.

Shaikh, M. (2023). Machine Learning in the Production Process Control of Metal Melting. *Journal of Advancement in Machines*, 8(2).

Shaik, N. S., & Cherukuri, T. K. (2022). Hinge attention network: A joint model for diabetic retinopathy severity grading. *Applied Intelligence*, 52(13), 15105–15121. DOI: 10.1007/s10489-021-03043-5

Shakeel, T., Habib, S., Boulila, W., Koubaa, A., Javed, A. R., Rizwan, M., Gadekallu, T. R., & Sufiyan, M. (2023). A survey on COVID-19 impact in the healthcare domain: Worldwide market implementation, applications, security and privacy issues, challenges and future prospects. *Complex & Intelligent Systems*, 9(1), 1027–1058. DOI: 10.1007/s40747-022-00767-w PMID: 35668731

Shanthi, K. G., Sesha Vidhya, S., Keerthi, B., Manimegalai, S., Nisha, A., & Niviya, B. R. (2021). IOT BASED PORTABLE ARTIFICIAL ELECTRONIC OLFACTORY SYSTEM FOR THE SAFETY OF MANUAL SCAVENGERS. *Journal of Engineering and Applied Sciences (Asian Research Publishing Network)*, 16(3).

Shapiro, S. C. (1992). Artificial intelligence. Encyclopedia of Artificial intelligence: Vol. 1. *2ndedn*. Wiley.

Sharma, M., Kochhar, A., Gupta, D., & Al Zubi, J. (2021). Hybrid Intelligent System for Medical Diagnosis in Health Care. In *Intelligent Systems Reference Library* (Vol. 209). DOI: 10.1007/978-981-16-2972-3_2

Sharma, S. K., & Adhikary, P. K. (2018). Machine learning algorithms for medical applications: A review. *International Journal of Recent Technology and Engineering*, 7(6), 128–133.

Shaw, J., Rudzicz, F., Jamieson, T., & Goldfarb, A. (2019). Artificial intelligence and the implementation challenge. *Journal of Medical Internet Research*, 21(7), e13659. DOI: 10.2196/13659 PMID: 31293245

Shickel, B., Tighe, P. J., Bihorac, A., & Rashidi, P. (2018). Deep EHR: A Survey of Recent Advances in Deep Learning Techniques for Electronic Health Record (EHR) Analysis. *IEEE Journal of Biomedical and Health Informatics*, 22(5), 1589–1604. Advance online publication. DOI: 10.1109/JBHI.2017.2767063 PMID: 29989977

Shimonski, R., & Solomon, M. G. (2023). *Security Strategies in Windows Platforms and Applications*. Jones & Bartlett Learning.

Shneiderman, B. (2020). Bridging the gap between ethics and practice: Guidelines for reliable, safe, and trustworthy human-centered AI systems. [TiiS]. *ACM Transactions on Interactive Intelligent Systems*, 10(4), 1–31. DOI: 10.1145/3419764

Shortliffe, E. H., & Buchanan, B. G. (1975). A model of inexact reasoning in medicine. *Mathematical Biosciences*, 23(3-4), 351–379. DOI: 10.1016/0025-5564(75)90047-4

Shweta Nagare, Ms.. (2014). Different Segmentation Techniques for brain tumor detection: A Survey, *MM- International society for green. Sustainable Engineering and Management*, 1(14), 29–35.

Siala, H., & Wang, Y. (2022). SHIFTing artificial intelligence to be responsible in healthcare: A systematic review. *Social Science & Medicine*, 296, 114782. DOI: 10.1016/j.socscimed.2022.114782 PMID: 35152047

Sikarwar, T. S., Mehta, S., Yadav, S., & Arora, D. (2022). Factors of adoption of Artificial Intelligence (AI) and Internet of Medical Things (IOMT) amongst Healthcare Workers: A Descriptive Analysis. *International Journal of Systematic Innovation*, 7(3). Advance online publication. DOI: 10.6977/IJoSI.202209_7(3).0002

Silva, I., & Soto, M. (2022). Privacy-preserving data sharing in healthcare: An in-depth analysis of big data solutions and regulatory compliance. *International Journal of Applied Health Care Analytics*, 7(1), 14–23.

Silveira, A. C. D., Sobrinho, Á., Silva, L. D. D., Costa, E. D. B., Pinheiro, M. E., & Perkusich, A. (2022). Exploring early prediction of chronic kidney disease using machine learning algorithms for small and imbalanced datasets. *Applied Sciences (Basel, Switzerland)*, 12(7), 3673. DOI: 10.3390/app12073673

Simha, S. K., and Y, T., (2023) "Healthcare Energized by Motion: Harnessing Piezoelectric Energy in Conjunction with IoT for Medical Innovations," *2023 International Conference on Artificial Intelligence for Innovations in Healthcare Industries (ICAIIHI)*, Raipur, India, 2023, pp. 1-7.

Sindhwani, N., Tanwar, S., Rana, A., & Kannan, R. (Eds.). (2024). *Smart technologies in healthcare management: Pioneering trends and applications*. CRC Press. DOI: 10.1201/9781003330523

Singh, B. (2023). Blockchain Technology in Renovating Healthcare: Legal and Future Perspectives. In *Revolutionizing Healthcare Through Artificial Intelligence and Internet of Things Applications* (pp. 177-186). IGI Global.

Singh, B. (2024). Evolutionary Global Neuroscience for Cognition and Brain Health: Strengthening Innovation in Brain Science. In *Biomedical Research Developments for Improved Healthcare* (pp. 246-272). IGI Global.

Singh, B., & Kaunert, C. (2024). Future of Digital Marketing: Hyper-Personalized Customer Dynamic Experience with AI-Based Predictive Models. *Revolutionizing the AI-Digital Landscape: A Guide to Sustainable Emerging Technologies for Marketing Professionals*, 189.

Singh, B., & Kaunert, C. (2024). Harnessing Sustainable Agriculture Through Climate-Smart Technologies: Artificial Intelligence for Climate Preservation and Futuristic Trends. In *Exploring Ethical Dimensions of Environmental Sustainability and Use of AI* (pp. 214-239). IGI Global.

Singh, B., & Kaunert, C. (2024). Salvaging Responsible Consumption and Production of Food in the Hospitality Industry: Harnessing Machine Learning and Deep Learning for Zero Food Waste. In *Sustainable Disposal Methods of Food Wastes in Hospitality Operations* (pp. 176-192). IGI Global.

Singh, B., & Kaunert, C. (2025). Cloud Computing and IoMT in Disease Screening and Diagnosis: AI Approaches in Transmuting Healthier Homes. In B. S & S. Kadry (Eds.), *Revolutionizing Healthcare Systems Through Cloud Computing and IoT* (pp. 99-120). IGI Global. DOI: 10.4018/979-8-3693-7225-8.ch005

Singh, B., & Kaunert, C. (2025). Leveraging IoT for Patient Monitoring and Smart Healthcare: Connected Healthcare System. In B. S & S. Kadry (Eds.), *Revolutionizing Healthcare Systems Through Cloud Computing and IoT* (pp. 27-46). IGI Global. https://doi.org/DOI: 10.4018/979-8-3693-7225-8.ch002

Singh, B., Vig, K., & Kaunert, C. (2024). Modernizing Healthcare: Application of Augmented Reality and Virtual Reality in Clinical Practice and Medical Education. In Modern Technology in Healthcare and Medical Education: Blockchain, IoT, AR, and VR (pp. 1-21). IGI Global.

Singh, A., & Ogunfunmi, T. (2021, December 28). An Overview of Variational Autoencoders for Source Separation, Finance, and Bio-Signal Applications. *Entropy (Basel, Switzerland)*, 24(1), 55. DOI: 10.3390/e24010055 PMID: 35052081

Singh, B. (2023). Unleashing Alternative Dispute Resolution (ADR) in Resolving Complex Legal-Technical Issues Arising in Cyberspace Lensing E-Commerce and Intellectual Property: Proliferation of E-Commerce Digital Economy. *Revista Brasileira de Alternative Dispute Resolution-Brazilian Journal of Alternative Dispute Resolution-RBADR*, 5(10), 81–105. DOI: 10.52028/rbadr.v5i10.ART04.Ind

Singh, B. (2024). Lensing Legal Dynamics for Examining Responsibility and Deliberation of Generative AI-Tethered Technological Privacy Concerns: Infringements and Use of Personal Data by Nefarious Actors. In Ara, A., & Ara, A. (Eds.), *Exploring the Ethical Implications of Generative AI* (pp. 146–167). IGI Global., DOI: 10.4018/979-8-3693-1565-1.ch009

Singh, B. (2024). Social Cognition of Incarcerated Women and Children: Addressing Exposure to Infectious Diseases and Legal Outcomes. In Reddy, K. (Ed.), *Principles and Clinical Interventions in Social Cognition* (pp. 236–251). IGI Global., DOI: 10.4018/979-8-3693-1265-0.ch014

Singh, B., & Kaunert, C. (2024). Adventure in High Altitude of Mountainous Topographies and Health Impacts: Lensing Tourism Sustainability via Reducing Ecological and Sociocultural Footprint and Health Emergency and Medical Assistance Management. In Meraj, G., Hashimoto, S., & Kumar, P. (Eds.), *Navigating Natural Hazards in Mountainous Topographies. Disaster Risk Reduction*. Springer., DOI: 10.1007/978-3-031-65862-4_15

Singh, B., & Kaunert, C. (2024). Salvaging Responsible Consumption and Production of Food in the Hospitality Industry: Harnessing Machine Learning and Deep Learning for Zero Food Waste. In Singh, A., Tyagi, P., & Garg, A. (Eds.), *Sustainable Disposal Methods of Food Wastes in Hospitality Operations* (pp. 176–192). IGI Global., DOI: 10.4018/979-8-3693-2181-2.ch012

Singh, B., & Kaunert, C. (2025). Featuring Healthcare, Environment, and Human Rights: Applications of Artificial Intelligence in the Health Domain. In Chakraborty, S., & Satapathy, S. (Eds.), *Gender, Environment, and Human Rights: An Intersectional Exploration* (pp. 45–74). IGI Global., DOI: 10.4018/979-8-3693-6069-9.ch004

Singh, B., & Kaunert, C. (2025). Intelligent Machine Learning Solutions for Cybersecurity: Legal and Ethical Considerations in a Global Context. In Thangam, D. (Ed.), *Advancements in Intelligent Process Automation* (pp. 359–386). IGI Global., DOI: 10.4018/979-8-3693-5380-6.ch014

Singh, B., Kaunert, C., & Singh, G. (2025). Scaling Legal Framework for Plastic Pollution and Advancing Cutting Edge Water Governance: Reducing and Eliminating Marine Pollution in Alignment With SDG 14 (Life Below Water). In Gaur, N., Sharma, E., Nguyen, T., Bilal, M., & Melkania, N. (Eds.), *Societal and Environmental Ramifications of Plastic Pollution* (pp. 197–222). IGI Global., DOI: 10.4018/979-8-3693-9163-1.ch010

Singh, B., Kaunert, C., & Vig, K. (2024). Reinventing Influence of Artificial Intelligence (AI) on Digital Consumer Lensing Transforming Consumer Recommendation Model: Exploring Stimulus Artificial Intelligence on Consumer Shopping Decisions. In Musiolik, T., Rodriguez, R., & Kannan, H. (Eds.), *AI Impacts in Digital Consumer Behavior* (pp. 141–169). IGI Global., DOI: 10.4018/979-8-3693-1918-5.ch006

Singh, B., Singh, A., Kaunert, C., Arora, M. K., Lal, S., & Ravesangar, K. (2025). Unleashing the Ethical and Legal Implications of E-Business Revolution: Consumer Privacy and Security Concerns in Phase of Digital Disruption. In Taherdoost, H., Drazenovic, G., Madanchian, M., Khan, I., & Arshi, O. (Eds.), *Business Transformation in the Era of Digital Disruption* (pp. 157–180). IGI Global., DOI: 10.4018/979-8-3693-7056-8.ch006

Singh, B., Yang, T., & Fernandez, R. (2023) "Temporal Analysis in Healthcare Using LSTM Networks," *2023 IEEE International Conference on Machine Learning and Applications (ICMLA)*, Toronto, Canada, pp. 612-617.

Singh, I. J., & Verma, K. K. (2024) "AI-Driven Patient Engagement Solutions Using IoMT," in *2024 International Conference on Healthcare Innovations and Technology (ICHIT)*, Mumbai, India, pp. 51-56.

Singh, M., Sukhija, N., Sharma, A., Gupta, M., & Aggarwal, P. K. (2021). Security and privacy requirements for IoMT-based smart healthcare system: Challenges, solutions, and future scope. In *Big Data Analysis for Green Computing* (pp. 17–37). CRC Press.

Singh, N., & Kaur, L. (2015, January). A survey on blood vessel segmentation methods in retinal images. In *2015 International Conference on Electronic Design, Computer Networks & Automated Verification (EDCAV)* (pp. 23-28). IEEE. DOI: 10.1109/EDCAV.2015.7060532

Singh, P., & Kumar, H. (2021). Predictive analytics for cardiovascular disease. *The Lancet. Digital Health*, 3(7), e393–e402. DOI: 10.1016/S2589-7500(21)00028-0

Singh, R. P., Javaid, M., Haleem, A., Vaishya, R., & Ali, S. (2020). Internet of Medical Things (IoMT) for orthopaedic in COVID-19 pandemic: Roles, challenges, and applications. *Journal of Clinical Orthopaedics and Trauma*, 11(4), 713–717. DOI: 10.1016/j.jcot.2020.05.011 PMID: 32425428

Smith, A., & Doe, J. (2024) "Enhancing Patient Monitoring through IoMT and Generative AI," in *2024 IEEE International Conference on Healthcare Technologies (ICHT)*, New York, USA, pp. 10-15.

Smith, A., Nugent, C., & McClean, S. (2002). Implementation of Intelligent Decision Support Systems in Health Care. *Journal of Management in Medicine*, 16(2/3), 206–218. DOI: 10.1108/02689230210434943 PMID: 12211346

Smith, D.. (2021). Deep learning in medical imaging: A comprehensive review. *NeuroImage*, 222, 117254. DOI: 10.1016/j.neuroimage.2020.117254

Smith, J., Patel, A., & Roberts, L. (2023) "Real-Time Monitoring of Chronic Diseases Using IoMT and AI Integration," *2023 IEEE International Conference on Healthcare Informatics (ICHI)*, New York, USA, pp. 101-106.

Smith, R. G., & Farquhar, A. (2000). The road ahead for knowledge management: An AI perspective. *AI Magazine*, 21(4), 17–17.

Soundarajan, V., & Vijayagaghavan, R. (1992). Procedures and tables for the construction and selection of conditional double sampling plans. *Journal of Applied Statistics*, 19(3), 329–338. DOI: 10.1080/02664769200000030

Sowmiya, R., & Kalpana, R. (2023, April). Detection of Diabetic Retinopathy by Segmentation using U-Net with Hyper-Parameter Tuning. In *2023 2nd International Conference on Smart Technologies and Systems for Next Generation Computing (ICSTSN)* (pp. 1-5). IEEE. DOI: 10.1109/ICSTSN57873.2023.10151473

Sreenivasulu, M. D., Devi, J. S., Arulprakash, P., Venkataramana, S., & Kazi, K. S. (2022). Implementation of latest machine learning approaches for students grade prediction. *International Journal of Early Childhood*, 14(3).

Sripriyanka, G., & Mahendran, A. (2021). A study on security privacy issues and solutions in internet of medical things—A review. Intelligent IoT Systems in Personalized Health Care, 147-175.

Sripriyanka, G., & Mahendran, A. (2024). Securing IoMT: A Hybrid Model for DDoS Attack Detection and COVID-19 Classification. *IEEE Access : Practical Innovations, Open Solutions*, 12, 17328–17348. Advance online publication. DOI: 10.1109/ACCESS.2024.3354034

Srivastava, J., Routray, S., Ahmad, S., & Waris, M. M. (2022). Internet of Medical Things (IoMT)-based smart healthcare system: Trends and progress.

Srivastava, J., Routray, S., Ahmad, S., & Waris, M. M. (2022). [Retracted] Internet of Medical Things (IoMT)-Based Smart Healthcare System: Trends and Progress. *Computational Intelligence and Neuroscience*, 2022(1), 7218113. PMID: 35880061

Stephens, Z. D., Lee, S. Y., Faghri, F., Campbell, R. H., Zhai, C., Efron, M. J., & Robinson, G. E. (2015). Big data: Astronomical or genomical? *PLoS Biology*, 13(7), e1002195. DOI: 10.1371/journal.pbio.1002195 PMID: 26151137

Stitt, A. W., Curtis, T. M., Chen, M., Medina, R. J., McKay, G. J., Jenkins, A., & Lois, N. (2016). The progress in understanding and treatment of diabetic retinopathy. *Progress in Retinal and Eye Research*, 51, 156–186. DOI: 10.1016/j.preteyeres.2015.08.001 PMID: 26297071

Subramaniam, E. V. D., Srinivasan, K., Qaisar, S. M., & Pławiak, P. (2023). Interoperable IoMT approach for remote diagnosis with privacy-preservation perspective in edge systems. *Sensors (Basel)*, 23(17), 7474. DOI: 10.3390/s23177474 PMID: 37687933

Sujith, A., Sajja, G. S., Mahalakshmi, V., Nuhmani, S., & Prasanalakshmi, B. (2022). Systematic review of smart health monitoring using deep learning and artificial intelligence. [Multimedia-based Emerging Technologies and Data Analytics for Neuroscience as a Service] [NaaS]. *Neuroscience Informatics (Online)*, 2(3), 100028. DOI: 10.1016/j.neuri.2021.100028

Sukeshini, S., P., Ved, M., Chintalapti, J., & Pal, S. N. (2021). Big data analytics and machine learning technologies for HPC applications. In Evolving Technologies for Computing, Communication and Smart World: Proceedings of ETCCS 2020 (pp. 411-424). Springer Singapore.

Suleimenov, I. E., Vitulyova, Y. S., Bakirov, A. S., & Gabrielyan, O. A. (2020). Artificial Intelligence:what is it? *Proc 2020 6th Int Conf Comput Technol Appl.;*22–5. DOI: 10.1145/3397125.3397141

Suleski, T., & Ahmed, M. (2023). A Data Taxonomy for Adaptive Multifactor Authentication in the Internet of Health Care Things. *Journal of Medical Internet Research*, 25, e44114. Advance online publication. DOI: 10.2196/44114 PMID: 37490633

Swain, S., Muduli, K., Kommula, V. P., & Sahoo, K. K. (2022). Innovations in Internet of Medical Things, Artificial Intelligence, and Readiness of the Healthcare Sector Towards Health 4.0 Adoption. *International Journal of Social Ecology and Sustainable Development*, 13(1), 1–14. Advance online publication. DOI: 10.4018/IJSESD.292078

Tahir, B., Jolfaei, A., & Tariq, M. (2023). A Novel Experience-Driven and Federated Intelligent Threat-Defense Framework in IoMT. *IEEE Journal of Biomedical and Health Informatics*. Advance online publication. DOI: 10.1109/JBHI.2023.3236072 PMID: 37018715

Tan, P., Xi, Y., Chao, S., Jiang, D., Liu, Z., Fan, Y., & Li, Z. (2022, April 11). An Artificial Intelligence-Enhanced Blood Pressure Monitor Wristband Based on Piezoelectric Nanogenerator. *Biosensors (Basel)*, 12(4), 234. DOI: 10.3390/bios12040234 PMID: 35448294

Tariq, M. U. (2024). AI and IoT in flood forecasting and mitigation: A comprehensive approach. In Ouaissa, M., Ouaissa, M., Boulouard, Z., Iwendi, C., & Krichen, M. (Eds.), *AI and IoT for proactive disaster management* (pp. 26–60). IGI Global., DOI: 10.4018/979-8-3693-3896-4.ch003

Tariq, M. U. (2024). Application of blockchain and Internet of Things (IoT) in modern business. In Sinha, M., Bhandari, A., Priya, S., & Kabiraj, S. (Eds.), *Future of customer engagement through marketing intelligence* (pp. 66–94). IGI Global., DOI: 10.4018/979-8-3693-2367-0.ch004

Tariq, M. U. (2024). Integration of IoMT for Enhanced Healthcare: Sleep Monitoring, Body Movement Detection, and Rehabilitation Evaluation. In Liu, H., Tripathy, R., & Bhattacharya, P. (Eds.), *Clinical Practice and Unmet Challenges in AI-Enhanced Healthcare Systems* (pp. 70–95). IGI Global., DOI: 10.4018/979-8-3693-2703-6.ch004

Tariq, M. U. (2024). Social Innovations for Improving Healthcare. In Chandan, H. (Ed.), *Social Innovations in Education, Environment, and Healthcare* (pp. 302–317). IGI Global., DOI: 10.4018/979-8-3693-2569-8.ch015

Tariq, M. U. (2025). The Belmont Report: Guiding Ethical Principles in Human Research. In Throne, R. (Ed.), *IRB, Human Research Protections, and Data Ethics for Researchers* (pp. 245–268). IGI Global Scientific Publishing., DOI: 10.4018/979-8-3693-3848-3.ch010

Tariq, M. U., Poulin, M., & Abonamah, A. A. (2021). Achieving operational excellence through artificial intelligence: Driving forces and barriers. *Frontiers in Psychology*, 12, 686624. DOI: 10.3389/fpsyg.2021.686624 PMID: 34305744

Tariq, M. U., & Sergio, R. P. (2025). Nurturing Digital Citizenship in Society 5.0 Through AI and Computational Intelligence Education. In Pandey, R., Srivastava, N., Prasad, R., Prasad, J., & Garcia, M. (Eds.), *Open AI and Computational Intelligence for Society 5.0* (pp. 59–84). IGI Global Scientific Publishing., DOI: 10.4018/979-8-3693-4326-5.ch003

Tekale, S., Shingavi, P., Wandhekar, S., & Chatorikar, A. (2018). Prediction of chronic kidney disease using machine learning algorithm. *International Journal of Advanced Research in Computer and Communication Engineering*, 7(10), 92–96. DOI: 10.17148/IJARCCE.2018.71021

Thammarat, C., & Techapanupreeda, C. (2021, March). A secure authentication and key exchange protocol for M2M communication. In 2021 9th International Electrical Engineering Congress (iEECON) (pp. 456-459). IEEE.

Thapa, C., & Camtepe, S. (2021). Precision health data: Requirements, challenges and existing techniques for data security and privacy. *Computers in Biology and Medicine*, 129, 104130. DOI: 10.1016/j.compbiomed.2020.104130 PMID: 33271399

Thaseen, A., Unnisa, R., Sultana, N., & Madhavi, K. R., NagaJyothi, G., & Kirubakaran, S. (2023, March). Breast Cancer Detection Using Deep Learning Model. In *Proceedings of Third International Conference on Advances in Computer Engineering and Communication Systems: ICACECS 2022* (pp. 669-677). Singapore: Springer Nature Singapore. DOI: 10.1007/978-981-19-9228-5_57

TherapTapper. (2024). TheraTapper. Retrieved from https://theratapperinc.com/about-theratapper/

Thomas, E. R., Brackenridge, A., Kidd, J., Kariyawasam, D., Carroll, P., Colclough, K., & Ellard, S. (2016). Diagnosis of monogenic diabetes: 10-Year experience in a large multi-ethnic diabetes center. *Journal of Diabetes Investigation*, 7(3), 332–337. DOI: 10.1111/jdi.12432 PMID: 27330718

Thomasian, N. M., & Adashi, E. Y. (2021). Cybersecurity in the Internet of Medical Things. *Health Policy and Technology*, 10(3), 100549. Advance online publication. DOI: 10.1016/j.hlpt.2021.100549

Thompson, M., Allen, R., & Garcia, J. (2023) "Interoperability in IoMT and AI: Bridging the Gap with Standardized Protocols," *2023 IEEE International Conference on Communications (ICC)*, Paris, France, pp. 879-884.

Thompson, R. F., Valdes, G., Fuller, C. D., Carpenter, C. M., Morin, O., Aneja, S., & Deasy, J. O. (2018). Artificial intelligence in radiation oncology: A specialty-wide disruptive transformation? *Radiotherapy and Oncology : Journal of the European Society for Therapeutic Radiology and Oncology*, 129(3), 421–426. DOI: 10.1016/j.radonc.2018.05.030 PMID: 29907338

Tiwari, S. K., Kaur, J., Singla, P., & Hrisheekesha, P. N. (2022, September). A Comprehensive Review of Big Data Analysis Techniques in Health-Care. In *International Conference on Emergent Converging Technologies and Biomedical Systems* (pp. 401-420). Singapore: Springer Nature Singapore.

Topol, E. J. (2019). High-performance medicine: The convergence of human and artificial intelligence. *Nature Medicine*, 25(1), 44–56. DOI: 10.1038/s41591-018-0300-7 PMID: 30617339

Trinkley, K. E., An, R., Maw, A. M., Glasgow, R. E., & Brownson, R. C. (2024). Leveraging artificial intelligence to advance implementation science: Potential opportunities and cautions. *Implementation Science : IS*, 19(1), 17. Advance online publication. DOI: 10.1186/s13012-024-01346-y PMID: 38383393

Tsui, F., & Karam, O. (2022). *Essentials of Software Engineering* (5th ed.). Jones & Bartlett Publishers.

Tutun, S., Johnson, M. E., Ahmed, A., Albizri, A., Irgil, S., Yesilkaya, I., Ucar, E. N., Sengun, T., & Harfouche, A. (2023). An AI-based decision support system for predicting mental health disorders. *Information Systems Frontiers*, 25(3), 1261–1276. DOI: 10.1007/s10796-022-10282-5 PMID: 35669335

Tyagi, A. K., George, T. T., & Soni, G. (2023). Blockchain-Based Cybersecurity in Internet of Medical Things (IoMT)-Based Assistive Systems. In AI-Based Digital Health Communication for Securing Assistive Systems (pp. 22-53). IGI Global.

U. K N and R. V M. (2022) "Arduino based COVID-19 Suspect Detection Device," 2022 6th International Conference on Electronics, Communication and Aerospace Technology, Coimbatore, India, pp. 158-163.

Uddin, S., Khan, A., Hossain, M. E., & Moni, M. A. (2019, December). Comparing different supervised machine learning algorithms for disease prediction. *BMC Medical Informatics and Decision Making*, 19(1), 281. Advance online publication. DOI: 10.1186/s12911-019-1004-8 PMID: 31864346

Ullah, I., Khan, I. U., Ouaissa, M., Ouaissa, M., & El Hajjami, S. (Eds.). (2024). *Future communication systems using artificial intelligence, internet of things and data science*. CRC Press. DOI: 10.1201/9781032648309

Uma, G., & Manjula, D. (2019). A technical study on varieties of sampling plan and implementation of new screening tri-sampling plan. *International Journal of Research in Advent Technology*, 5(Special Issue), 232–237.

Upreti, D., Yang, E., Kim, H., & Seo, C. (2024). A comprehensive survey on federated learning in the healthcare area: Concept and applications. CMES -. *Computer Modeling in Engineering & Sciences*, 140(3), 2239–2274. DOI: 10.32604/cmes.2024.048932

Vaccari, I., Carlevaro, A., Narteni, S., Cambiaso, E., & Mongelli, M. (2022). explainable and reliable against adversarial machine learning in data analytics. *IEEE Access : Practical Innovations, Open Solutions*, 10, 83949–83970. DOI: 10.1109/ACCESS.2022.3197299

Vahida, . (2023). Deep Learning, YOLO and RFID based smart Billing Handcart. *Journal of Communication Engineering & Systems*, 13(1), 1–8.

Vaishnavi, J., Ravi, S., & Anbarasi, A. (2020). An efficient adaptive histogram based segmentation and extraction model for the classification of severities on diabetic retinopathy. *Multimedia Tools and Applications*, 79(41), 30439–30452. DOI: 10.1007/s11042-020-09288-5

Vajar, P., Emmanuel, A. L., Ghasemieh, A., Bahrami, P., & Kashef, R. (2021, October). The Internet of Medical Things (IoMT): a vision on learning, privacy, and computing. In *2021 International Conference on Electrical, Computer, Communications and Mechatronics Engineering (ICECCME)* (pp. 1-7). IEEE. DOI: 10.1109/ICECCME52200.2021.9590881

Vapnik, V. N. (1995). *The Nature of Statistical Learning Theory*. Springer. DOI: 10.1007/978-1-4757-2440-0

Veena, C., Sridevi, M., Liyakat, K. K. S., Saha, B., Reddy, S. R., & Shirisha, N. (2023). *HEECCNB: An Efficient IoT-Cloud Architecture for Secure Patient Data Transmission and Accurate Disease Prediction in Healthcare Systems, 2023 Seventh International Conference on Image Information Processing*. ICIIP., Available at https://ieeexplore.ieee.org/document/10537627, DOI: 10.1109/ICIIP61524.2023.10537627

Veiseh, O., Tang, B. C., Whitehead, K. A., Anderson, D. G., & Langer, R. (2015). Managing diabetes with nanomedicine: Challenges and opportunities. *Nature Reviews. Drug Discovery*, 14(1), 45–57. DOI: 10.1038/nrd4477 PMID: 25430866

Vemuri, P. K., Kunta, A., Challagulla, R., Bodiga, S., Veeravilli, S., Bodiga, V. L., & Rao, K. R. S. S. (2020). Artificial intelligence and internet of medical things based health-care system for real-time maternal stress - Strategies to reduce maternal mortality rate. *Drug Invention Today*, 13(7), •••.

Venkatakiran, S., Ashreetha, B., & Reddy, N. S. (2023) "Implementation of a Machine Learning-based Model for Cardiovascular Disease Post Exposure prophylaxis," *2023 International Conference for Advancement in Technology (ICONAT)*, Goa, India, pp. 1-5.

Venkatasubramanian, V., Rengaswamy, R., & Kavuri, S. N. (2003). A review of process fault detection and diagnosis: Part I. *Computers & Chemical Engineering*, 27(3), 293–311. DOI: 10.1016/S0098-1354(02)00160-6

Verbakel, J. Y.. (2020, January). Clinical Reliability of point-of-care tests to support community based acute ambulatory care. *Acute Medicine*, 19(1), 4–14. DOI: 10.52964/AMJA.0791 PMID: 32226951

Viceconti, M., Hunter, P., & Hose, R. (2015). Big data, big knowledge: Big data for personalized healthcare. *IEEE Journal of Biomedical and Health Informatics*, 19(4), 1209–1215. DOI: 10.1109/JBHI.2015.2406883 PMID: 26218867

Viderman, D., Seri, E., Aubakirova, M., Abdildin, Y., Badenes, R., & Bilotta, F. (2022). Remote Monitoring of Chronic Critically Ill Patients after Hospital Discharge: A Systematic Review. *Journal of Clinical Medicine*, 11(4), 1010. Advance online publication. DOI: 10.3390/jcm11041010 PMID: 35207287

Vishwakarma, V. K. (2024). Navigating challenges and unlocking opportunities: The convergence of IoT and AI in India.

Vlasceanu, V., Neu, W., Oram, A., Alapati, S., & Safari, an O. M. C. (2019). *An Introduction to Cloud Databases*. O'Reilly Media, Incorporated.

Wale, A. D., & Dipali, R.. (2019). Smart Agriculture System using IoT. *International Journal of Innovative Research in Technology*, 5(10), 493–497.

Wal, P., Wal, A., Verma, N., Karunakakaran, R., & Kapoor, A. (2022). Internet of medical things – the future of healthcare. *The Open Public Health Journal*, 15(1), 15. DOI: 10.2174/18749445-v15-e221215-2022-142

Wang, J., & Liu, L. (2022, December). RLWE-based Privacy-Preserving Data Sharing Scheme for Internet of Medical Things System. In 2022 3rd International Conference on Electronics, Communications and Information Technology (CECIT) (pp. 441-445). IEEE.

Wang, R., Zhang, Y., & Yang, J. (2022, October). TransPND: A Transformer Based Pulmonary Nodule Diagnosis Method on CT Image. In Chinese Conference on Pattern Recognition and Computer Vision (PRCV) (pp. 348-360). Cham: Springer Nature Switzerland DOI: 10.1007/978-3-031-18910-4_29

Wang, B., Cancilla, J. C., Torrecilla, J. S., & Haick, H. (2014). Artificial Sensing Sntelligence with Silicon Nanowires for Ultraselective Detection in the Gas Phase. *Nano Letters*, 14(2), 933–938. DOI: 10.1021/nl404335p PMID: 24437965

Wang, J., Zhang, Z., Li, B., Lee, S., & Sherratt, R. S. (2014, February). An enhanced fall detection system for elderly person monitoring using consumer home networks. *IEEE Transactions on Consumer Electronics*, 60(1), 23–29. DOI: 10.1109/TCE.2014.6780921

Wang, L.-H., Hsiao, Y.-M., Xie, X.-Q., & Lee, S.-Y. (2016, May). An outdoor intelligent healthcare monitoring device for the elderly. *IEEE Transactions on Consumer Electronics*, 62(2), 128–135. DOI: 10.1109/TCE.2016.7514671

Wang, P. Q., & Liu, Q. S. (2024) "Smart Devices and AI for Remote Patient Monitoring," in *2024 International Conference on Remote Health Monitoring Systems (ICRHMS)*, Shanghai, China, pp. 32-37.

Wang, Y., Guo, Y., Kuang, Q., Pu, X., Ji, Y., Zhang, Z., & Li, M. (2015, April). A comparative study of family-specific protein–ligand complex affinity prediction based on random forest approach. *Journal of Computer-Aided Molecular Design*, 29(4), 349–360. DOI: 10.1007/s10822-014-9827-y PMID: 25527073

Wang, Y., & Zhang, L. (2023). AI-driven biosensors for healthcare: Current trends and future perspectives. *Trends in Biotechnology*, 41(3), 230–242. DOI: 10.1016/j.tibtech.2022.11.008

Wani, R. U. Z., Thabit, F., & Can, O. (2024). Security and Privacy Challenges, Issues, and Enhancing Techniques for Internet of Medical Things: A Systematic Review. *Security and Privacy*, 7(5), e409. Advance online publication. DOI: 10.1002/spy2.409

Wasserman, L., & Wasserman, Y. (2022). Hospital cybersecurity risks and gaps: Review (for the non-cyber professional). *Frontiers in Digital Health*, 4, 862221. Advance online publication. DOI: 10.3389/fdgth.2022.862221 PMID: 36033634

WebSockets. (2024). WebSockets Protcol. Retrieved from https://websockets.spec.whatwg.org

Wei, T., Liu, S., & Du, X. (2022). Learning-based efficient sparse sensing and recovery for privacy-aware IoMT. *IEEE Internet of Things Journal*, 9(12), 9948–9959. DOI: 10.1109/JIOT.2022.3163593

White, J., & Thompson, F. (2022). AI-enhanced diagnostics. *The New England Journal of Medicine*, 386(11), 1029–1035. DOI: 10.1056/NEJMc2200211

White, R., & Davis, L. (2020). AI-driven predictive analytics in healthcare: Applications and challenges. *Journal of Predictive Analytics*, 14(3), 129–137. DOI: 10.1080/15228053.2020.1776158

Wilson, K. N., & Roberts, M. T. (2024) "Generative AI for Enhancing Diagnostic Accuracy in IoMT," in *2024 International Conference on Digital Health and Medical Analytics (ICDHMA)*, Toronto, Canada, pp. 40-45.

Wirtz, B. W., Weyerer, J. C., & Geyer, C. (2019, May 19). Artificial intelligence and the public sector—Applications and challenges. *International Journal of Public Administration*, 42(7), 596–615. DOI: 10.1080/01900692.2018.1498103

Wong, E., Backholer, K., Gearon, E., Harding, J., Freak-Poli, R., Stevenson, C., & Peeters, A. (2013). Diabetes and risk of physical disability in adults: A systematic review and meta-analysis. *The Lancet. Diabetes & Endocrinology*, 1(2), 106–114. DOI: 10.1016/S2213-8587(13)70046-9 PMID: 24622316

Wong, T. Y., Cheung, C. M. G., Larsen, M., Sharma, S., & Simó, R. (2016). Diabetic retinopathy. *Nature Reviews. Disease Primers*, 2, 1–16. PMID: 27159554

World Health Organization. (2018). Continuity and coordination of care: a practice brief to support implementation of the WHO Framework on integrated people-centred health services.

Wu, H., Patel, S., & Lin, X. (2023) "Enhancing Patient Safety through AI-Integrated IoMT Systems," *2023 IEEE International Conference on Engineering in Medicine and Biology Society (EMBC)*, Boston, USA, pp. 310-315.

Wu, X., Zhu, X., Wu, G. Q., & Ding, W. (2013). Data mining with big data. *IEEE Transactions on Knowledge and Data Engineering*, 26(1), 97–107.

Xie, J., Guo, L., Zhao, C., Li, X., Luo, Y., & Jianwei, L. (2020, December). A hybrid deep learning and handcrafted features based approach for thyroid nodule classification in ultrasound images. []. IOP Publishing.]. *Journal of Physics: Conference Series*, 1693(1), 012160.

Xu, J., Xu, H. L., Cao, Y. N., Huang, Y., Gao, S., Wu, Q. J., & Gong, T. T. (2023). The performance of deep learning on thyroid nodule imaging predicts thyroid cancer: A systematic review and meta-analysis of epidemiological studies with independent external test sets. *Diabetes & Metabolic Syndrome*, 17(11), 102891. DOI: 10.1016/j.dsx.2023.102891 PMID: 37907027

Xu, L., Gao, J., Wang, Q., Yin, J., Yu, P., Bai, B., Pei, R., Chen, D., Yang, G., Wang, S., & Wan, M. (2020). Computer-aided diagnosis systems in diagnosing malignant thyroid nodules on ultrasonography: A systematic review and meta-analysis. *European Thyroid Journal*, 9(4), 186–193. DOI: 10.1159/000504390 PMID: 32903956

Xu, W., Gu, Y., & Cai, W. (2018). Medical data quality control based on machine learning. *Journal of Medical Systems*, 42(7).

Xu, Y., Zhou, Z., Li, X., Zhang, N., Zhang, M., & Wei, P. (2021). FFU-Net: Feature Fusion U-Net for Lesion Segmentation of Diabetic Retinopathy. *BioMed Research International*, 2021(1), 6644071. DOI: 10.1155/2021/6644071 PMID: 33490274

Y. P. Liu, Z. Li, C. Xu, J. Li, and R. Liang (2019). Referable diabetic retinopathy identification from eye fundus images with weighted path for convolutional neural network. Artif. Intell. Med. 99 101694, doi: . artmed. 2019. 07. 002DOI: 10. 1016/j

Yaacoub, J. P. A., Noura, M., Noura, H. N., Salman, O., Yaacoub, E., Couturier, R., & Chehab, A. (2020). Securing internet of medical things systems: Limitations, issues and recommendations. *Future Generation Computer Systems*, 105, 581–606.

Yang, G., Wu, D., Mao, J., & Du, Y. (2024). Comprehensive resilience assessment of bridge networks using ensemble learning method. *Advances in Engineering Software*, 198, 103774. DOI: 10.1016/j.advengsoft.2024.103774

Yao, Z. J., Bi, J., & Chen, Y. X. (2018). Applying Deep Learning to Individual and Community Health Monitoring Data: A Survey. *International Journal of Automation and Computing*, 15(6), 643–655. Advance online publication. DOI: 10.1007/s11633-018-1136-9

Yazid, A. (2023). Cybersecurity and privacy issues in the internet of medical things (IoMT). *Eigenpub Review of Science and Technology*, 7(1), 1–21.

Yigitcanlar, T., Corchado, J. M., Mehmood, R., Li, R. Y. M., Mossberger, K., & Desouza, K. (2021). Responsible urban innovation with local government artificial intelligence (AI): A conceptual framework and research agenda. *Journal of Open Innovation*, 7(1), 71.

Yogita Shirdale, Ms.. (2014). Analysis and design of Capacitive coupled wideband Microstrip antenna in C and X band: A Survey, *Journal GSD-International society for green. Sustainable Engineering and Management*, 1(15), 1–7.

Yogita Shirdale, Ms.. (2016). Coplanar capacitive coupled probe fed micro strip antenna for C and X band. *International Journal of Advanced Research in Computer and Communication Engineering*, 5(4), 661–663.

Young, Q. R., & Thomas, R. S. (2024) "IoMT and AI for Emergency Response Systems," in *2024 International Conference on Emergency Medicine and Healthcare Informatics (ICEMHI)*, Houston, USA, pp. 41-46.

Zafar, S., Khan, S., Iftekhar, N., & Biswas, S. (2020). Consociate Healthcare System through Biometric Based Internet of Medical Things (BBIOMT) Approach. *EAI Endorsed Transactions on Smart Cities*, 4(10), 165499. Advance online publication. DOI: 10.4108/eai.23-6-2020.165499

Zhai, K., Yousef, M. S., Mohammed, S., Aldewik, N., & Qoronfleh, M. W. (2023). Optimizing Clinical Workflow Using Precision Medicine and Advanced Data Analytics. *Processes (Basel, Switzerland)*, 11(3), 939. DOI: 10.3390/pr11030939

Zhang, A., Wu, Z., Wu, E., Wu, M., Snyder, M. P., Zou, J., & Wu, J. C. (2023). Leveraging physiology and artificial intelligence to deliver advancements in health care. *Physiological Reviews*, 103(4), 2423–2450. DOI: 10.1152/physrev.00033.2022 PMID: 37104717

Zhang, G., & Navimipour, N. J. (2022). A comprehensive and systematic review of the IoT-based medical management systems: Applications, techniques, trends and open issues. *Sustainable Cities and Society*, 82, 103914. DOI: 10.1016/j.scs.2022.103914

Zhang, H., Hung, C. L., Chu, W. C. C., Chiu, P. F., & Tang, C. Y. (2018, December). Chronic kidney disease survival prediction with artificial neural networks. In *2018 IEEE International Conference on Bioinformatics and Biomedicine (BIBM)* (pp. 1351-1356). IEEE. DOI: 10.1109/BIBM.2018.8621294

Zhang, J., & Zhan, M. (2017). Machine learning in rock mechanics and geomechanics. *Advances in Civil Engineering*, 20, 12–17.

Zhang, L., Chen, H., & Liu, X. (2023) "Integrating IoMT with AI for Advanced Healthcare: A Future Framework," *2023 IEEE International Conference on Smart Health (ICSH)*, Tokyo, Japan, pp. 102-107.

Zhang, L., Tan, J., Han, D., & Zhu, H. (2017, November 1). From machine learning to deep learning: Progress in machine intelligence for rational drug discovery. *Drug Discovery Today*, 22(11), 1680–1685. DOI: 10.1016/j.drudis.2017.08.010 PMID: 28881183

Zhang, S., Fan, R., Liu, Y., Chen, S., Liu, Q., & Zeng, W. (2023, January 11). Applications of transformer-based language models in bioinformatics: A survey. *Bioinformatics Advances*, 3(1), vbad001. Advance online publication. DOI: 10.1093/bioadv/vbad001 PMID: 36845200

Zhang, X., Lee, V. C., Rong, J., Liu, F., & Kong, H. (2022). Multi-channel convolutional neural network architectures for thyroid cancer detection. *PLoS One*, 17(1), e0262128. DOI: 10.1371/journal.pone.0262128 PMID: 35061759

Zhavoronkov, A., Aliper, A., Kazennov, A., Zhebrak, A., Zagribelnyy, B., Lee, L. H., & Aspuru-Guzik, A. (2019). Potential COVID-19 therapeutics identified by deep learning model. *Computers & Chemical Engineering*, 140, 106973.

Zhavoronkov, A., Ivanenkov, Y. A., Aliper, A., Veselov, M. S., Aladinskiy, V. A., Aladinskaya, A. V., Terentiev, V. A., Polykovskiy, D. A., Kuznetsov, M. D., Asadulaev, A., Volkov, Y., Zholus, A., Shayakhmetov, R. R., Zhebrak, A., Minaeva, L. I., Zagribelnyy, B. A., Lee, L. H., Soll, R., Madge, D., & Aspuru-Guzik, A. (2019). Deep learning enables rapid identification of potent DDR1 kinase inhibitors. *Nature Biotechnology*, 37(9), 1038–1040. DOI: 10.1038/s41587-019-0224-x PMID: 31477924

Zhou, L., Pan, S., Wang, J., & Vasilakos, A. V. (2017). Machine learning on big data: Opportunities and challenges. *Neurocomputing*, 237, 350–361. DOI: 10.1016/j.neucom.2017.01.026

Zhou, S. K., Greenspan, H., Davatzikos, C., Duncan, J. S., Van Ginneken, B., Madabhushi, A., Prince, J. L., Rueckert, D., & Summers, R. M. (2021). A review of deep learning in medical imaging: Imaging traits, technology trends, case studies with progress highlights, and future promises. *Proceedings of the IEEE*, 109(5), 820–838. DOI: 10.1109/JPROC.2021.3054390 PMID: 37786449

Zhou, S., Zhang, R., Chen, D., & Zhu, X. (2021). A novel framework for bringing smart big data to proactive decision making in healthcare. *Health Informatics Journal*, 27(2), 14604582211024698. DOI: 10.1177/14604582211024698 PMID: 34159834

Zhou, X., Li, X., Zhang, Z., Han, Q., Deng, H., Jiang, Y., Tang, C., & Yang, L. (2022). Support vector machine deep mining of electronic medical records to predict the prognosis of severe acute myocardial infarction. *Frontiers in Physiology*, 13, 991990. DOI: 10.3389/fphys.2022.991990 PMID: 36246101

Zhu, H. (2020, January 1). Big data and artificial intelligence modeling for drug discovery. *Annual Review of Pharmacology and Toxicology*, 60(1), 573–589. DOI: 10.1146/annurev-pharmtox-010919-023324 PMID: 31518513

Zikria, Y. B., Afzal, M. K., & Kim, S. W. (2020). Internet of multimedia things (IoMT): Opportunities, challenges and solutions. *Sensors (Basel)*, 20(8), 2334. DOI: 10.3390/s20082334 PMID: 32325944

Ziwei, H., Dongni, Z., Man, Z., Yixin, D., Shuanghui, Z., Chao, Y., & Chunfeng, C. (2024). The applications of internet of things in smart healthcare sectors: A bibliometric and deep study. *Heliyon*, 10(3), e25392. DOI: 10.1016/j.heliyon.2024.e25392 PMID: 38356528

Zou, J., Huss, M., Abid, A., Mohammadi, P., Torkamani, A., & Telenti, A. (2019). A primer on deep learning in genomics. *Nature Genetics*, 51(1), 12–18. DOI: 10.1038/s41588-018-0295-5 PMID: 30478442

About the Contributors

Vinoth Kumar Venkatesan, is working as Associate Professor of School of Computer Science Engineering & Information Systems, Vellore Institute of Technology (VIT), Vellore, India. He is serving as Adjunct Professor Associated with School of Computer Science, Taylor's University, Malaysia. He has published 5 books and 105 technical articles in refereed journals. He has filled 17 domestic patents the field of IoT and Autonomous vehicles. He is serving as Associate Editor of the IEEE Access, PLOS ONE, PLOS Complex Systems, BMC medical informatics and decision making, International Journal of Pervasive Computing and Communications, International Journal of e-Collaboration (IJeC) and International Journal of Intelligent Information Systems. He served as the General Chair, a Program Committee Chair, and PC Member for major international conferences. He is the BoS and Department Advisory Committee member for more than 10 institutions in India. His current research interests include Internet of Things, Artificial Intelligence, and medical image processing. He is a fellow of IEEE (senior member) and life member of ISTE. Recently, he has been honoured as one of the 'World's Top 2% Scientists' by Stanford University, USA. This esteemed recognition reflects Dr Vinoth's exceptional contributions to the field of Artificial Intelligence and Biomedical applications, particularly their potential as new learning models designed for Medical Image based solutions.

Polinpapilinho F. Katina is an Associate Professor in the Department of Informatics and Engineering Systems at the University of South Carolina Upstate (Spartanburg, South Carolina, USA). He has served in various capacities at the National Centers for System of Systems Engineering (Norfolk, Virginia, USA), Old Dominion University (Norfolk, Virginia, USA), Politecnico di Milano (Milan, Italy), Embry-Riddle Aeronautical University (Daytona Beach, Florida, USA), The University of Alabama in Huntsville (Huntsville, Alabama, USA), and Syracuse University (Syracuse, New York, USA). He holds a B.S. in Engineering Technology (Old Dominion University, Norfolk, Virginia, USA), M.Eng. in Systems Engineering (Old Dominion University, Norfolk, Virginia, USA), and Ph.D. in Engineering Management and Systems Engineering (Old Dominion University, Norfolk, Virginia, USA). He received additional training at the Politecnico di Milano (Milan, Italy) in the Energy Department in the Nuclear Division - Laboratory of Signal Analysis and Risk Analysis. His research is focused in the areas of Complex System Governance, Critical Infrastructure Systems, Decision Making and Analysis, Emerging Technologies (e.g., IoT), Energy Systems (Smart Grids), Engineering Management, Infranomics, Manufacturing Systems, System of Systems, Systems Engineering, Systems Pathology, Systems Theory, and Systems Thinking. His profile includes nearly 200 peer-reviewed journal articles, conference proceedings, and book chapters. He has also co-authored eleven (11) books [5 monographs & 6 edited]. He is a Senior Member of IEEE and Epsilon Mu Eta (Engineering Management Honor Society), ABET Program Evaluator, and journal editor for several journals: Advanced Manufacturing (ELSP), Control and Engineering of Complex Systems Frontiers in Complex Systems (Frontiers Media SA), Cureus Journal of Engineering

(Springer/Nature), Discrete Dynamics in Nature and Society (John Wiley), International Journal of Critical Infrastructures (Inderscience), and International Journal of System of Systems Engineering (Inderscience).

Jingyuan Zhao obtained her PhD in Management Science and Engineering from University of Science and Technology of China. Dr. Zhao's research expertise includes management of technology innovation, technology strategy, behavior and information technology, regional innovation systems and global innovation networks, high-tech industries, multinational governance, and science and technology policy. She has teaching experience of 15 years at the graduate and undergraduate level. Research portfolio includes more than fifty peer-reviewed articles in highly regarded journals, authored books, multiple book chapters, and conference presentations. Dr. Zhao also has extensive industry experience and provides consulting services to major corporations such as China Mobile. She serves as editor-in-chief of International Journal of e-Collaboration(IJeC).

***

Krishna, a seasoned professional, contributing to research at VTU. His expertise shines through his prolific publications in esteemed journals such as IEEE, Scopus and UGC cared journals focusing on machine learning, data science, data mining, and computer networks. Over the span of 18 years, he has facilitated collaborations among academia, industry, and research, inspiring over 5000 students to partake in software projects. Moreover, Krishna has conducted numerous workshops and been a distinguished guest speaker at prestigious organizations in Bangalore, leaving an indelible mark on the educational landscape. His impact extends to mentoring and training over 7,000 students across various technologies, equipping them for success in the competitive corporate world.

Arunachalam Manikandan completed his B.E. in Electronics and Communication Engineering from Madurai Kamaraj University in 2004, and his Master of Engineering in Communication Systems from Anna University in 2006. He received his Ph.D. from Anna University in 2018. He has 18 years of teaching experience and has guided many UG & PG projects. He is a life member of IETE & ISTE. He has published papers in 13 international journals, 13 international conferences, and 6 national conferences. Currently he is working in M2M communication and IoT. He is currently associated with Amrita School of Engineering, Amrita Vishwa Vidhyapeetham, Coimbatore,Tamilnadu India.

Hina Bansal is an inspirational teacher and researcher with 16+ years of experience specializing in Bioinformatics/Computational Biology, working as an Assistant Professor in the centre for Bioinformatics and Computational Biology, Amity Institute of Biotechnology, Amity University, Noida since January 2008. Her research interest includes Network pharmacology, functional Genomics and Genome informatics, NGS, functional Proteomics, Molecular docking and simulation, Python, Artificial intelligence, and Machine learning. She has more than forty research publications in reputable peer reviewed journals, book, and book chapters. She has presented numerous papers in various national and international conferences. She has been an active member in organising several workshops and conferences. She is a dynamic reviewer for various peer reviewed journals including BMC Computational Biology and Scientific Reports. She is very proficient in programming languages like C, C++, Java and

Python. With her perseverance, academic excellence, research capabilities, and leadership abilities, Dr. Hina a very potential candidate.

Dankan Gowda V is currently working as an Assistant Professor in the Department of Electronics and Communication Engineering at BMS Institute of Technology and Management in Bangalore. Previously, he worked as a Research Fellow at ADA DRDO and as a Software Engineer at Robert Bosch. With a total experience of 14 years, including teaching and industry, Dr. Gowda has made significant contributions to both academia and research. He has published over 120 research papers in renowned international journals and conferences. In recognition of his innovative work, Dr. Gowda has been granted six patents, including four from Indian authorities and two international patents. His research interests primarily lie in the fields of IoT and Signal Processing, where he has conducted workshops and handled industry projects. Dr. Gowda is passionate about teaching and strives to create an engaging and effective learning environment for his students. He consistently seeks opportunities to enhance his knowledge and stay updated with the latest advancements in his field.

Herat Joshi is a leading professional in Healthcare Technology and Data Intelligence at Great River Health Systems, Iowa, USA. He excels in driving technological advancements and innovation in Healthcare Information Management, Healthcare Informatics, and Medical/Bioinformatics. Recently, he has focused on scholarly research on the integration of AI with healthcare. With a deep expertise in Project Management, he leverages AI to revolutionize project execution and outcomes. He holds a PhD in Computer Science & Engineering with expertise in Data Science and AI, an MBA, and a bachelor's degree in Computer Engineering. Herat has published multiple scholarly papers and has judged numerous national and international technical events. He is an active member of several editorial boards, contributing to the advancement of academic and industry journals.

Christian Kaunert is a Professor of International Security at Dublin City University, Ireland. He is also Professor of Policing and Security and Director of the International Centre for Policing and Security at the University of South Wales. Previously, he served as an Academic Director and Professor at the Institute for European Studies, Vrije Universiteit Brussel, a Professor of International Politics, Head of Discipline in Politics, and the Director of the European Institute for Security and Justice, a Jean Monnet Centre for Excellence, at the University of Dundee. He was awarded a large Horizon 2020 research grant on Terrorist Radicalisation processes – Mindb4Act, a large Horizon Europe Marie Curie Doctoral Network EUGLOCTER, and a Jean Monnet Network EUCTER, alongside several Jean Monnet Chairs, Centres, Modules, and TT.

Kazi Kutubuddin Sayyad Liyakat has completed his B.E., M.E., and Ph.D. in E&TC Engineering and is nowadays working as a Professor & Head of Department, E&TC Engineering Department and was Dean R&D. He is Post-Doctoral Fellow working on "IoT in Healthcare Applications". His area of Interest is IoT, AI and ML. He has published more than 120+ papers in various Journals. Also published 11 books in the field of Engineering. He has published 15 Indian Patents, 2 South African Grant Patent, 2 Indian Copyright Patents and 8 UK Grant Patent. He worked as a Reviewer for Scopus Conferences and Journal. Also work as Editorial Board Member for various Journals. He got 2 Best Researcher Award, Best Faculty Award and Appreciation Letter from MoE's Innovation Cell, Govt. of India.

Anwar Khan is an Assistant Professor in the Department of Management Sciences and Psychology at the Khushal Khan Khattak University, Karak, Pakistan. Previously, he held the position of a Postdoctoral Fellow at the Universiti Tun Hussein Onn Malaysia, Malaysia. Anwar Khan has over a decade of university teaching and research experience. His specialties include Human Factors, Occupational Health Psychology, and Psychometrics. He is currently focusing on the diagnosis and treatment of mental health problems, with a special emphasis on Post-Traumatic Stress Disorder, Major Depressive Disorder, and Generalized Anxiety Disorder. He has over thirty peer-reviewed research papers published in international peer reviewed journals.

P. Krishnamoorthy, an esteemed academician, currently serves as an Associate Professor in the Department of Computer Science and Engineering at Sasi Institute of Technology & Engineering, located in West Godavari District, Tadepalligudem, Andhra Pradesh, India. With over 13 years of dedicated teaching experience, he has made significant contributions to the field of Computer Science education. Mr. Krishnamoorthy is currently pursuing his Ph.D. at SRM University, Kattankulathur, Chennai. He holds an M.Tech in Computer Science and Engineering from PRIST University, Thanjavur, where he graduated with First Class honors. He also earned his B.E. in Computer Science and Engineering with First Class distinction from Anna University, Chennai. His academic journey is marked by excellence and a deep commitment to fostering knowledge. A prolific researcher and author, Mr. Krishnamoorthy has published 29 research papers and authored 8 textbooks in the domains of Computer Science and Information Technology. His research interests encompass cutting-edge fields such as Artificial Intelligence, Cloud Computing, the Internet of Things, Machine Learning, and Quantum Computing.

Satheesh Kumar received the MCA Post Graduate degree from the Anna University and currently pursuing Ph.D. in Visvesvaraya Technological University, Karnataka, India. Currently working as an Assistant Professor & Coordinator in Department of Computer Science, School of Applied Sciences, REVA University with 15 years of teaching experience. He is the author or coauthor of many papers in international refereed journals, Book chapters and many conference contributions. His research interests cover several aspects across Network security, Data Mining, Data Security and mainly Internet of Things (IoT). He is the reviewer for many reputed journals.

Amalia Madihie holds the position of Dean in the Faculty of Cognitive Sciences and Human Development at the Universiti Malaysia Sarawak, Malaysia. She is a counselor educator within the Counselling Programme at the Universiti Malaysia Sarawak, Malaysia. Amalia bt Madihie is actively involved in her research pursuits, particularly in the field of Counselling, Psychotherapy, and Resilience Studies. Her significant contributions include her dedication to disseminating her research findings in international peer-reviewed journals and books. Additionally, she excels in innovating and commercializing her research endeavors. Particularly, she is the founder of the Resilient Therapy Intervention, which focuses on enhancing self-concept in individuals, and the Resilience Assessment Tool (RAT-43). These instruments have gained widespread utilization within the Malaysian context. Furthermore, Amalia bt Madihie is a licensed and registered counselor in Malaysia. She practices counseling services at a private clinic, specializing in providing support to children, adolescents, and families.

Atti MangaDevi is currently working as Assistant Professor in IT Department of Pragati Engineering College, Surampalem. She has research interest in Cyber Security, ML, AI, Soft computing..

Yamuna Mundru currently working as Assistant Professor in CSE-AI&ML Department of Pragati Engineering College (A), Surampalem has a teaching experience of more than 8 Years. She has published over 22 papers in various National and International journals including Scopus indexed journals. Her area of research interest includes AR-VR, Machine Learning and Artificial intelligence. She has published 4 book chapters and has published a patent in the area of cyber security.

Anjali Raghav is a legal professional and accomplished academic, currently a Research Scholar at the Sharda School of Law, Sharda University, Greater Noida, India. With a solid educational foundation, she holds a Master in Law from Sharda School of Law, where she cultivated her expertise in Criminal Law, Intellectual Property Rights, Artificial Intelligence, Machine Learning, Blockchain Technology, Sustainable Energy, etc. Her three years of experience as a criminal practicing lawyer have equipped her with practical legal insights that she seamlessly integrates into her academic and editorial endeavors. She has a robust portfolio of publications in esteemed journals and books, reflecting her dedication to contributing to the body of knowledge in her fields of interest. Her research has been recognized on various platforms, as evidenced by her participation in national and international conferences, seminars, webinars, and symposiums. Also, in her academic and research pursuits, Anjali is a skilled editor, having successfully overseen the editorial process of several publications.

Wasswa Shafik (Member, IEEE) received a Bachelor of Science degree in information technology from Ndejje University, Uganda, a Master of Engineering degree in Information Technology (Computer and Communication Networks) from Yazd University, Iran, and a PhD in Computer Science with the School of Digital Science, Universiti Brunei Darussalam, Brunei Darussalam. He is also the Founder and Research Director of the Dig Connectivity Research Laboratory (DCRLab) after serving as a Research Associate at the Network Interconnectivity Research Laboratory at Yazd University. Prior to this, he worked as a Community Data Analyst at Population Services International (PSI-Uganda), a Community Data Officer at the Programme for Accessible Health Communication (PACE-Uganda), a Research Assistant at the Socio-Economic Data Centre (SEDC-Uganda), Uganda, an Assistant Data Officer at TechnoServe, Kampala, IT Support at Thurayya Islam Media, Uganda, and Asmaah Charity Organization. He has hundreds of publications with renowned publishers. His research interests include Computer Vision, Explainable AI, Smart Agriculture, Health and ecological informatics, Security and Privacy.

Zuber Shaikh has has 16 years of Research Experience in Drug Discovery, Personalized Medicine, Synthetic Chemistry and Medicinal Chemistry of AntiTB Agents, Research Methodologies, Preclinical Pharmacology and in Academia. The Author has Research Experience in Preclinical Pharmacology and in Academia. Research interests include Synthetic Chemistry, Research Design, Research Approaches, Biopharmaceutics of Nanoparticles, Drug Permeability Studies. Drug Targetting. Author compiles Publications in Pharmacology.

Bhupinder Singh is working as Professor at Sharda University, India. Also, Honorary Professor in University of South Wales UK and Santo Tomas University Tunja, Colombia. His areas of publications as Smart Healthcare, Medicines, fuzzy logics, artificial intelligence, robotics, machine learning, deep learning, federated learning, IoT, PV Glasses, metaverse and many more. He has 3 books, 139 paper publications, 163 paper presentations in international/national conferences and seminars, participated in more than 40 workshops/FDP's/QIP's, 25 courses from international universities of repute, organized more than 59 events with international and national academicians and industry people's, editor-in-chief and co-editor in journals, developed new courses. He has given talks at international universities, resource person in international conferences such as in Nanyang Technological University Singapore, Tashkent State University of Law Uzbekistan; KIMEP University Kazakhstan, All'ah meh Tabatabi University Iran, the Iranian Association of International Criminal law, Iran and Hague Center for International Law and Investment, The Netherlands, Northumbria University Newcastle UK,

Muhammad Usman Tariq has more than 17+ year's experience in industry and academia. He has authored more than 200+ research articles, 110+ case studies, 120+ book chapters and several books other than 4 patents. He is founder and CEO of The Case HQ, a unique repository for courses, narrative and video case studies. He has been working as a consultant and trainer for industries representing six sigma, quality, health and safety, environmental systems, project management, and information security standards. His work has encompassed sectors in aviation, manufacturing, food, hospitality, education, finance, research, software and transportation. He has diverse and significant experience working with accreditation agencies of ABET, ACBSP, AACSB, WASC, CAA, EFQM and NCEAC. Additionally, Dr. Tariq has operational experience in incubators, research labs, government research projects, private sector startups, program creation and management at various industrial and academic levels. He is Certified Higher Education Teacher from Harvard University, USA, Certified Online Educator from HMBSU, Certified Six Sigma Master Black Belt and has been awarded PFHEA, SMIEEE, and CMBE.

Vidya Rajasekhara Reddy Tetala, a healthcare IT expert, excels in data engineering, cloud technologies, and AI/ML. Raja's innovative strategies optimize healthcare operations, reduce costs, and enhance patient outcomes, establishing him as a transformative leader driving impactful advancements in healthcare technology and data-driven solutions.

Rakesh Thoppaen Suresh Babu is a Senior Technical Architect specializing in Data Science at Hexaware Technologies in the USA. With 13 years of industry experience, he is a Senior IEEE Member recognized for his expertise in data science, Industrial IoT, and cybersecurity. Rakesh has successfully led data-driven transformation programs utilizing deep learning, OCR, and generative AI to enhance profitability, optimize efficiency, streamline analytics operations, form analytics teams, and develop analytics infrastructure strategies. He holds a Master of Science in Computer Science, specializing in unstructured data analysis and object detection. Rakesh has spearheaded the establishment of an AI Center of Excellence (COE) for a major semiconductor client and has assisted numerous clients in identifying, developing, and productionizing AI use cases and capabilities. As a co-founder of BayofTech Pvt Ltd, he has contributed to creating Industry 4.0 solutions for manufacturing companies, focusing on IIoT and AI-based hardware.In addition to his professional achievements, Rakesh has served as a judge in various technology forums and peer-reviewed publications such as TheSciPub. He holds a pending US patent for an innovative authentication process designed to mitigate vulnerabilities caused by HID. His research interests encompass AI-computer vision, IIoT, and Cybersecurity.

Rehman Ullah Khan is working as a Senior Lecturer in the Faculty of Cognitive Sciences and Human Development at the Universiti Malaysia Sarawak, Malaysia. He holds a Ph. D in Cognitive Sciences with a specialization in Intelligent Systems (Mobile Augmented Reality). His research interests are Artificial Intelligence, Computer Vision, Augmented Reality, Virtual Reality, Advanced Databases, and Computational Linguistics. Rehman Ullah Khan has more than twelve years of teaching and research experience at the university level. He has more than twenty-two research publications in internationally peer-reviewed journals. Rehman Ullah Khan possesses a dedicated interest in harnessing the capabilities of digital technologies to the field of mental health science. His passion lies in exploring innovative computer-based solutions for the diagnosis and treatment of mental health problems.

V. Muthukumaran was born in Vellore, Tamilnadu, India, in 1988. He received the B.Sc. degree in Mathematics from the Thiruvalluvar University Serkkadu, Vellore, India, in 2009, and the M. Sc. degrees in Mathematics from the Thiruvalluvar University Serkkadu, Vellore, India, in 2012. The M. Phil. Mathematics from the Thiruvalluvar University Serkkadu, Vellore, India, in 2014 and Ph.D. degrees in Mathematics from the School of Advanced Sciences, Vellore Institute of Technology, Vellore in 2019. He has 4 years of teaching experience and 8 years of research experience, and he has published various research papers in high-quality journals Springer, Elsevier, IGI Global, Emerald, River, etc. At present, he has a working Assistant Professor in the Department of Mathematics, REVA University Bangalore, India. His current research interests include Algebraic cryptography, Fuzzy Image Processing, Machine learning, and Data mining. His current research interests include Fuzzy Algebra, Fuzzy Image Processing, Data Mining, and Cryptography. Dr. V. Muthukumaran is a Fellow of the International Association for Cryptologic Research (IACR), India; He is a Life Member of the IEEE. He has publishe

Varun G. is a final-year B.Tech student specializing in Cyber Security and IoT. He has demonstrated exceptional academic and research capabilities, having published numerous papers in reputed journals. Varun is actively involved in various research activities, contributing to the advancement of knowledge in his field. His dedication to cybersecurity and IoT is evident through his active participation in research and his consistent efforts to stay at the forefront of technological innovations.

Manu Y. M. received the B.E., M.Tech. and Ph.D degree in Computer Science and Engineering. He is currently working as Associate Professor in Department of Computer science and Engineering, BGS Institute of Technology-Adichunchanagiri University, B.G Nagara. He has 10 Years of teaching experience and his research interests include Video analytics, Machine Learning, Deep learning, Data mining and Artificial Intelligence. He is Recipient of 07 Awards. He is a member of Professional Bodies like ISTE, IEAE, IAENG, IEEE, the Indian Science Congress Association, Computer Society of India, Institute of Engineers, Institute of Scholars, Research Stars and ASR etc. He has published 30 research papers in peer reviewed /Scopus/UGC listed international/national journals and has presented and participated in 43 international/national conferences. He has filed 09 patents, he contributed as a reviewer for 32 IEEE Conferences and reviewed Papers in Q1 Springer and other international journals. He has authored 2 Books and 3 book chapters, He has Delivered Guest Lectures and Keynote Speaker for international conferences, He is session chair and track chair for international conferences and coordinators and organizing committee for conferences and FDPs.

Manas Kumar Yogi currently working as Assistant Professor in CSE Department of Pragati Engineering College (A), Surampalem has a teaching experience of more than 14 Years. With a paper publication record of over 250 papers from past 12 years, he has also published 15 book chapters and 4 patents and 3 books. His research area includes cyber security, soft computing, cyber physical systems, IoT, ML.

Index

A

Acceptance Sampling Plan 483, 484
Accuracy 6, 11, 13, 16, 18, 22, 23, 36, 37, 62, 67, 68, 70, 72, 74, 75, 77, 78, 92, 98, 99, 100, 101, 103, 113, 123, 124, 125, 127, 139, 145, 172, 173, 175, 176, 177, 178, 181, 184, 186, 187, 196, 200, 218, 221, 228, 230, 236, 237, 240, 243, 244, 245, 249, 251, 253, 257, 267, 268, 273, 274, 275, 276, 278, 280, 281, 282, 284, 285, 286, 287, 291, 293, 295, 296, 302, 305, 312, 313, 314, 315, 316, 317, 319, 323, 324, 325, 326, 328, 334, 338, 339, 341, 342, 343, 344, 345, 353, 356, 366, 367, 385, 387, 392, 397, 399, 400, 402, 403, 405, 406, 407, 421, 422, 423, 424, 425, 427, 429, 430, 431, 432, 433, 434, 435, 436, 437, 461, 462, 463, 464, 466, 467, 469, 470, 479, 488, 489, 490, 495, 498, 500, 503, 505, 507, 514, 517, 522, 535, 547, 552, 553, 555, 558, 559, 560, 561
AI Governance 11
Artificial Intelligence 1, 2, 3, 5, 7, 9, 11, 13, 15, 16, 17, 18, 19, 21, 22, 23, 24, 25, 26, 27, 28, 29, 31, 33, 34, 35, 36, 37, 40, 43, 47, 48, 49, 50, 51, 52, 55, 56, 57, 60, 62, 70, 80, 81, 90, 95, 99, 100, 101, 108, 112, 115, 116, 117, 122, 124, 125, 126, 127, 129, 130, 131, 147, 149, 168, 214, 217, 218, 220, 224, 233, 234, 236, 240, 243, 244, 246, 247, 248, 250, 251, 252, 253, 254, 255, 256, 257, 260, 261, 262, 263, 273, 287, 293, 295, 301, 320, 321, 322, 324, 341, 342, 343, 344, 345, 346, 348, 349, 350, 351, 352, 353, 354, 355, 356, 357, 358, 361, 362, 363, 364, 366, 368, 369, 370, 371, 372, 373, 375, 376, 382, 383, 384, 386, 388, 391, 408, 410, 411, 412, 413, 430, 437, 454, 456, 461, 462, 467, 473, 474, 475, 495, 497, 498, 499, 500, 506, 509, 510, 511, 512, 515, 516, 519, 521, 522, 525, 526, 528, 530, 531, 532, 533, 542, 544, 545, 546, 547, 550, 552, 553, 557, 563, 564
ASN 478
ATI 478
Attacks 48, 135, 143, 154, 155, 194, 195, 196, 200, 201, 202, 203, 214, 232, 296, 440, 441, 442, 443, 444, 445, 446, 447, 448, 449, 450, 452, 455, 456, 457, 504, 517, 518
Automated Diagnostics 95

B

Bias Mitigation 1, 4, 24
Big Data Analytics 62, 63, 64, 65, 69, 71, 74, 75, 76, 80, 81, 88, 147, 246, 259, 260, 261, 264, 342
Biosensors 35, 56, 99, 261, 343, 346, 348, 349, 350, 352, 354, 356, 358, 359, 501, 511, 563, 564

C

Chi2 184, 185
CKD 171, 172, 173, 174, 175, 176, 177, 179, 180, 181, 184, 185, 188
Cloud Computing 26, 40, 52, 88, 89, 119, 120, 128, 131, 192, 193, 196, 197, 205, 213, 239, 241, 259, 261, 263, 380, 388, 452, 512, 542, 562
Convolution 176, 189, 274, 277, 278, 280, 281, 425, 426
Cryptography 197, 296, 451
Cybersecurity 31, 32, 44, 111, 144, 153, 154, 157, 161, 162, 168, 169, 214, 246, 263, 444, 455, 458, 474, 495, 507, 508, 512, 516, 531

D

Database 37, 77, 109, 118, 119, 120, 121, 128, 132, 202, 203, 230, 236, 275, 280, 298, 299, 300, 301, 375, 385, 392, 422, 431, 447, 449, 474
Data Breaches 14, 133, 141, 146, 147, 149, 165, 191, 211, 350, 390, 391, 440, 443, 444, 469, 506, 508, 516, 528, 560
Data Privacy 2, 7, 8, 9, 13, 14, 18, 20, 21, 23, 31, 47, 50, 84, 108, 109, 111, 140, 141, 145, 148, 149, 152, 153, 164, 165, 166, 167, 220, 227, 233, 235, 238, 240, 246, 249, 253, 259, 293, 343, 350, 440, 461, 464, 465, 466, 468, 469, 471, 474, 506, 509, 517, 521, 526, 528, 533, 555, 559, 560
Data Synthesis 516, 517
Deep Learning 26, 34, 36, 37, 40, 45, 46, 47, 51, 55, 56, 57, 64, 71, 80, 81, 94, 131, 176, 177, 188, 196, 197, 226, 251, 252, 259, 260, 261, 262, 263, 265, 267, 273, 274, 275, 276, 277, 278, 287, 288, 289, 294, 321, 322, 325, 338, 340, 356, 357, 358, 359, 363, 366, 383, 384, 408, 410, 415, 417, 422, 423, 424, 425, 427, 436, 452, 454, 461, 463, 467, 471, 473, 474, 492, 493, 498, 531
Diabetes Classification 291, 292, 295
Diabetic Macular Edema 270, 419
Diabetic Retinopathy 252, 267, 269, 275, 288, 289, 290, 417, 437, 438
Diagnosis 1, 2, 5, 11, 15, 17, 20, 21, 23, 38, 40, 56, 57, 71, 74, 75, 84, 87, 88, 89, 91, 95, 101, 109, 116,

122, 130, 131, 133, 169, 173, 176, 178, 199, 217, 218, 223, 227, 236, 239, 243, 246, 247, 248, 250, 251, 252, 253, 254, 257, 260, 263, 267, 268, 269, 272, 273, 274, 275, 276, 287, 289, 295, 297, 301, 322, 324, 325, 339, 340, 341, 342, 345, 354, 356, 357, 358, 378, 392, 395, 410, 418, 420, 421, 423, 424, 430, 433, 435, 437, 447, 453, 461, 466, 469, 489, 493, 497, 498, 501, 502, 505, 506, 509, 515, 516, 517, 524, 527, 535, 544, 552, 555

Disease Screening 243, 244, 245, 246, 250, 253, 263
DL Approach 385, 392, 396, 407
Double Sampling Plan 477, 478, 479, 480, 482, 484, 485, 486, 488, 489, 490, 491, 492, 493
DR 267, 268, 269, 270, 271, 272, 273, 274, 275, 276, 277, 278, 279, 280, 281, 285, 286, 287, 379, 390, 392, 417, 418, 419, 420, 421, 422, 423, 424, 431, 432, 435, 436, 461, 477
Drug Design 57, 361, 362, 363, 364, 365, 370, 380, 382
Drug Discovery 89, 227, 228, 259, 341, 342, 343, 346, 358, 361, 362, 363, 364, 367, 371, 373, 378, 379, 380, 381, 382, 383, 384, 387, 461, 463, 464, 465, 468, 469, 470, 472, 474, 490, 499, 500, 519, 520, 528, 531, 532, 535, 536, 545, 548, 549, 555
DT 71, 74, 75, 176, 211, 291, 303, 304, 311, 313, 314, 315, 316, 317, 326, 334, 385, 395, 397, 400, 403, 407, 415

E

EHR 57, 63, 66, 131, 214, 253, 255, 256, 257, 461, 470, 472, 473
Electronic Health Record 57, 63, 257, 461
EMDR Psychotherapy 118, 129
Ensemble 175, 176, 189, 251, 291, 294, 296, 301, 302, 303, 305, 312, 313, 314, 316, 317, 319, 320, 322, 325, 340, 365, 397, 399, 437
Ethical AI 1, 4, 20, 21, 23, 24, 475, 533
Ethical Considerations 2, 5, 6, 7, 8, 11, 13, 16, 18, 19, 21, 22, 26, 44, 108, 227, 236, 244, 263, 343, 350, 430, 461, 464, 472, 507, 513, 515, 529, 537, 555, 559
Ethical Implications 5, 10, 50, 108, 262, 465, 469, 507, 520, 525, 556
Ethics in AI 473
Explainable AI 8, 10, 18, 20, 23, 237, 291, 305, 413, 526

F

F1-Score 67, 68, 73, 178, 295, 329, 427, 429, 430, 433

G

Generative AI 31, 32, 33, 34, 35, 37, 39, 40, 41, 43, 44, 45, 47, 49, 50, 51, 52, 53, 54, 83, 84, 87, 88, 89, 90, 91, 92, 94, 95, 96, 98, 99, 100, 101, 103, 104, 105, 106, 107, 108, 109, 110, 112, 113, 217, 218, 219, 220, 221, 224, 225, 226, 227, 228, 230, 231, 232, 233, 235, 236, 237, 238, 240, 262, 291, 292, 305, 319, 320, 495, 497, 499, 500, 501, 503, 504, 505, 506, 507, 508, 510, 511, 512, 513, 514, 515, 516, 517, 519, 520, 524, 525, 528, 530, 532, 535, 536, 537, 541, 543, 545, 546, 548, 549, 550, 551, 555, 556, 557, 558, 559, 560, 562
Generative Artificial Intelligence 31, 33, 35, 40, 47, 50, 51, 52, 217, 220, 224, 236, 495, 500, 509, 516, 550, 557
Genomic Analysis 341, 345
Global Health 176, 236, 238, 244, 269, 291, 321, 473, 520, 528

H

Hard Voting 291, 312
Healthcare 1, 2, 3, 4, 5, 6, 7, 8, 9, 11, 12, 13, 15, 16, 17, 18, 19, 20, 21, 22, 23, 24, 25, 26, 27, 28, 31, 32, 33, 34, 36, 37, 38, 39, 40, 41, 42, 43, 44, 45, 46, 47, 48, 49, 50, 51, 54, 55, 56, 57, 59, 60, 61, 62, 63, 64, 65, 66, 68, 69, 70, 71, 73, 74, 75, 76, 77, 78, 79, 80, 81, 82, 83, 84, 85, 86, 87, 88, 89, 90, 91, 92, 94, 95, 96, 99, 101, 103, 104, 105, 106, 107, 108, 109, 110, 111, 112, 113, 115, 116, 129, 130, 133, 134, 135, 136, 137, 138, 139, 140, 141, 142, 143, 144, 145, 148, 149, 150, 153, 154, 155, 156, 157, 158, 160, 161, 162, 163, 164, 165, 166, 167, 168, 171, 172, 174, 175, 176, 191, 192, 193, 194, 195, 196, 197, 198, 199, 201, 202, 203, 205, 211, 212, 213, 214, 215, 218, 219, 220, 221, 223, 224, 225, 227, 228, 230, 231, 232, 233, 234, 236, 237, 238, 239, 240, 241, 242, 243, 244, 245, 246, 247, 248, 249, 250, 251, 252, 253, 254, 255, 256, 257, 259, 260, 261, 262, 263, 264, 269, 270, 277, 287, 292, 293, 294, 295, 296, 297, 301, 303, 305, 320, 321, 322, 340, 341, 342, 343, 344, 345, 346, 348, 349, 350, 351, 352, 353, 354, 355, 357, 358, 359, 361, 371, 373, 375, 376, 378, 380, 381, 382, 385, 386, 387, 388, 390, 391, 392, 393, 394, 395, 396, 397, 399, 407, 409, 410, 412, 413, 414, 415, 420, 421, 424, 430, 436, 439, 440, 441, 442, 444, 445, 446, 447, 448, 449, 450, 451, 452, 453, 454, 455, 456, 457, 459, 461, 462, 463, 464, 465, 466, 467, 468, 469, 471, 472, 473, 474, 475, 478, 479,

480, 488, 489, 490, 491, 493, 495, 496, 497, 498, 499, 500, 501, 502, 503, 504, 505, 506, 507, 508, 509, 510, 511, 512, 513, 514, 515, 516, 517, 518, 519, 520, 521, 522, 523, 524, 525, 526, 527, 528, 529, 530, 531, 532, 533, 535, 536, 537, 542, 544, 546, 547, 548, 551, 555, 556, 557, 558, 559, 560, 561, 562, 563, 564

Healthcare Innovation 109, 410, 498, 556
Healthcare Transformation 213

I

Image Classification 273, 276, 278, 281, 340, 421, 424, 430, 433, 435, 436, 437
Internet of Medical Things 31, 34, 37, 38, 39, 40, 41, 42, 43, 46, 47, 49, 56, 57, 59, 86, 88, 89, 133, 139, 140, 141, 144, 149, 156, 161, 164, 166, 167, 168, 169, 192, 193, 194, 195, 196, 200, 213, 214, 215, 217, 218, 220, 221, 228, 236, 238, 245, 291, 292, 320, 321, 322, 361, 376, 384, 385, 390, 393, 395, 415, 439, 451, 454, 455, 456, 457, 458, 459, 472, 495, 498, 501, 503, 505, 507, 509, 510, 511, 513, 515, 517, 521, 523, 530, 531, 532, 536, 542, 543, 544, 554, 557, 561, 563, 564
IoMT 31, 32, 33, 38, 40, 41, 43, 44, 48, 49, 50, 51, 53, 54, 56, 57, 58, 59, 60, 61, 62, 63, 76, 77, 78, 79, 82, 83, 84, 85, 86, 87, 88, 89, 91, 92, 94, 95, 96, 98, 99, 100, 101, 103, 104, 105, 106, 107, 108, 109, 110, 111, 112, 113, 133, 134, 135, 136, 137, 138, 139, 140, 141, 142, 143, 144, 148, 149, 150, 152, 153, 154, 155, 156, 157, 158, 160, 161, 162, 163, 164, 165, 166, 167, 168, 169, 191, 192, 193, 194, 195, 196, 198, 199, 200, 201, 203, 204, 213, 214, 215, 217, 218, 219, 220, 221, 223, 224, 228, 230, 231, 232, 233, 234, 235, 236, 237, 238, 239, 240, 241, 242, 243, 245, 246, 263, 291, 292, 293, 294, 295, 296, 305, 319, 320, 321, 361, 362, 363, 376, 378, 380, 384, 385, 390, 391, 393, 395, 396, 407, 415, 439, 440, 441, 442, 443, 444, 445, 446, 447, 448, 449, 450, 451, 452, 453, 454, 455, 456, 457, 458, 472, 495, 496, 497, 498, 499, 501, 502, 503, 504, 505, 506, 507, 508, 509, 510, 511, 512, 513, 514, 515, 516, 517, 518, 519, 520, 521, 522, 523, 524, 525, 526, 527, 528, 530, 531, 532, 533, 535, 536, 537, 542, 543, 544, 545, 546, 547, 551, 552, 554, 555, 556, 557, 558, 559, 560, 561, 562, 563
IoMT (Internet of Medical Things) 218, 457
IoT 28, 31, 32, 36, 37, 39, 40, 41, 50, 51, 52, 53, 55, 56, 59, 60, 61, 62, 63, 64, 65, 69, 71, 74, 75, 76, 77, 81, 82, 88, 103, 111, 112, 137, 156, 169, 191, 192, 193, 194, 196, 197, 198, 203, 205, 211, 213, 214, 215, 217, 218, 220, 224, 228, 233, 239, 240, 241, 259, 260, 261, 262, 263, 264, 291, 292, 293, 297, 301, 302, 303, 305, 320, 321, 361, 376, 377, 378, 380, 384, 387, 388, 389, 390, 391, 392, 394, 395, 396, 397, 408, 409, 410, 411, 412, 413, 414, 415, 454, 455, 456, 457, 458, 511, 530, 532

K

KNN 172, 176, 184, 186, 187, 274, 291, 295, 311, 312, 313, 314, 315, 317, 318, 319, 323, 324, 326, 329, 331, 332, 334, 335, 336, 338, 396, 401, 423

L

Logistic Regression 175, 176, 177, 302, 303, 304, 323, 324, 326, 328, 329, 330, 332, 334, 336, 337, 369

M

Machine Learning 2, 22, 23, 24, 33, 35, 36, 37, 39, 47, 49, 53, 54, 56, 57, 59, 63, 64, 65, 67, 68, 70, 71, 73, 75, 79, 80, 81, 82, 87, 90, 92, 94, 96, 111, 122, 123, 124, 126, 127, 130, 131, 139, 144, 149, 150, 167, 171, 172, 173, 174, 175, 176, 177, 182, 184, 186, 188, 189, 196, 215, 218, 220, 224, 227, 230, 237, 239, 240, 241, 242, 244, 246, 251, 252, 255, 259, 260, 261, 262, 263, 264, 273, 274, 275, 280, 287, 291, 292, 293, 294, 295, 296, 301, 302, 303, 304, 305, 311, 319, 320, 321, 322, 323, 324, 325, 326, 328, 329, 330, 338, 339, 341, 342, 344, 346, 348, 356, 358, 361, 362, 366, 371, 375, 378, 379, 380, 382, 383, 385, 386, 387, 391, 392, 393, 394, 396, 397, 398, 402, 407, 409, 410, 413, 414, 415, 421, 422, 424, 427, 430, 431, 452, 457, 464, 474, 477, 478, 479, 480, 488, 489, 490, 491, 492, 493, 498, 499, 530, 531, 532, 538, 539, 542, 545, 553, 554, 563, 564
Machine Learning Algorithm 189, 239, 304, 366, 477, 478, 479, 480, 488, 489, 490, 491, 563
Medical Data Synthesis 516, 517
Medical Imaging 17, 37, 45, 46, 90, 133, 134, 218, 220, 227, 251, 252, 256, 265, 273, 277, 280, 340, 357, 358, 424, 435, 436, 461, 462, 463, 466, 467, 468, 469, 470, 473, 492, 503, 505, 516, 517
ML 26, 35, 36, 131, 139, 196, 274, 291, 293, 294, 305, 320, 321, 324, 325, 331, 341, 342, 346, 362, 363, 364, 365, 369, 371, 372, 378, 379, 380, 385, 386, 387, 392, 393, 394, 395, 396, 397, 398, 399, 400, 401, 402, 407, 409, 410, 411, 412, 415, 421, 430, 478, 479, 488, 489, 490, 545, 552, 554

MLIoMT 385, 392

N

Neural Network 36, 66, 90, 173, 177, 188, 197, 237, 259, 267, 275, 276, 289, 296, 302, 325, 339, 340, 365, 371, 374, 375, 379, 396, 409, 414, 417, 423, 424, 425, 427, 431, 432

O

OC 478, 484, 488
Optical Coherence Tomography 269, 271

P

Pandemic 23, 55, 61, 116, 131, 213, 215, 220, 243, 244, 346, 391, 496, 527
Patient Care 1, 5, 6, 8, 11, 15, 16, 17, 18, 19, 22, 24, 44, 48, 59, 60, 62, 63, 87, 96, 101, 104, 139, 143, 176, 177, 194, 196, 212, 214, 217, 218, 219, 221, 231, 233, 241, 251, 252, 253, 256, 274, 277, 281, 287, 292, 293, 342, 349, 353, 371, 376, 382, 388, 390, 391, 435, 436, 441, 447, 448, 449, 452, 461, 462, 465, 466, 468, 474, 496, 499, 503, 505, 513, 515, 522, 523, 528, 537
Patient Monitoring 1, 2, 16, 18, 22, 23, 31, 38, 43, 59, 60, 82, 85, 91, 96, 98, 100, 112, 137, 140, 141, 143, 164, 193, 223, 230, 232, 239, 250, 263, 292, 293, 353, 357, 388, 390, 391, 392, 439, 447, 453, 470, 472, 495, 499, 501, 503, 504, 506, 507, 509, 515, 517, 523
Personalized Medicine 18, 20, 59, 62, 69, 72, 73, 80, 81, 82, 91, 92, 112, 221, 227, 239, 249, 341, 342, 343, 344, 345, 355, 371, 375, 378, 382, 456, 462, 465, 468, 469, 470, 491, 498, 499, 507, 519, 520, 532, 535
Personalized Treatment 31, 59, 116, 139, 273, 292, 342, 371, 376, 378, 379, 387, 440, 464, 465, 466, 469, 536, 558
Pharmaceuticals 366, 468, 478, 480, 489, 491
Pooling Layers 273, 278
Precision 2, 17, 18, 29, 47, 61, 64, 67, 68, 69, 70, 72, 73, 79, 80, 82, 99, 111, 125, 130, 137, 174, 175, 176, 178, 184, 244, 252, 254, 259, 264, 275, 276, 280, 281, 282, 284, 285, 286, 287, 295, 313, 314, 315, 316, 317, 327, 328, 329, 337, 338, 342, 344, 351, 353, 355, 356, 378, 379, 385, 402, 403, 405, 406, 407, 410, 423, 424, 427, 429, 430, 431, 432, 433, 434, 435, 436, 462, 463, 465, 467, 469, 470, 472, 474, 477, 488, 489, 497, 499, 502, 505, 511, 519, 522, 531, 535, 536, 538, 545, 546, 547, 548, 549, 551, 561, 562, 563
Precision Medicine 64, 69, 79, 80, 82, 130, 252, 356, 378, 379, 465, 472, 499, 511, 535, 536, 547, 563
Prediction 34, 41, 46, 55, 60, 66, 67, 68, 70, 73, 74, 75, 76, 78, 82, 91, 94, 96, 98, 123, 124, 125, 127, 131, 139, 140, 171, 172, 174, 175, 176, 177, 178, 181, 184, 185, 186, 188, 189, 240, 250, 261, 281, 292, 295, 300, 301, 303, 321, 322, 323, 324, 325, 326, 328, 330, 334, 338, 339, 357, 364, 365, 366, 367, 368, 369, 370, 371, 372, 373, 374, 380, 383, 397, 400, 415, 421, 427, 428, 430, 434, 435, 463, 470, 473, 474, 492, 509, 511, 520, 540, 548, 550
Predictive Analytics 2, 16, 31, 36, 66, 68, 81, 92, 94, 96, 112, 117, 122, 124, 139, 149, 227, 244, 247, 248, 341, 343, 345, 359, 378, 379, 393, 394, 461, 462, 464, 465, 468, 469, 470, 471, 472, 474, 475, 495, 498, 499, 504, 507, 514, 522, 560
Privacy 1, 2, 3, 4, 5, 6, 7, 8, 9, 10, 12, 13, 14, 16, 18, 19, 20, 21, 22, 23, 24, 26, 27, 28, 29, 31, 32, 36, 43, 47, 48, 50, 55, 57, 58, 59, 63, 75, 76, 84, 106, 108, 109, 111, 127, 133, 135, 136, 139, 140, 141, 142, 143, 144, 145, 146, 147, 148, 149, 150, 152, 153, 161, 164, 165, 166, 167, 168, 169, 194, 195, 196, 201, 213, 214, 215, 220, 224, 227, 233, 235, 238, 240, 246, 248, 249, 253, 259, 262, 264, 293, 296, 342, 343, 350, 355, 386, 390, 391, 392, 423, 430, 439, 440, 441, 445, 448, 449, 450, 451, 453, 455, 456, 457, 458, 461, 464, 465, 466, 468, 469, 471, 474, 479, 495, 506, 507, 508, 509, 511, 514, 516, 517, 518, 520, 521, 526, 528, 530, 531, 533, 535, 555, 556, 557, 559, 560
Privacy Protection 6, 146, 164, 196, 214, 516, 530

R

Real-Time Data Collection 228, 391, 495, 518
Real-Time Monitoring 81, 106, 107, 112, 133, 164, 197, 242, 353, 389, 440, 447, 504, 537
Recall 50, 67, 68, 72, 73, 125, 175, 178, 184, 281, 282, 284, 285, 286, 287, 295, 313, 314, 315, 316, 317, 328, 329, 337, 338, 385, 402, 403, 405, 406, 407, 423, 427, 429, 430, 431, 432, 433, 435
ResNet-101 417, 424, 426, 427, 428, 429, 430, 433, 434, 435, 436
Responsible AI 1, 2, 3, 4, 5, 7, 8, 9, 10, 11, 13, 14, 15, 17, 18, 19, 21, 23, 25, 28
Retina 270, 271, 272, 418, 419, 420, 424, 435

S

Security 1, 2, 4, 6, 8, 13, 14, 16, 23, 24, 29, 32, 34, 43, 47, 57, 59, 63, 71, 72, 76, 77, 78, 79, 80, 108, 109, 111, 112, 119, 121, 124, 128, 132, 133, 135, 136, 139, 140, 141, 142, 143, 144, 145, 147, 148, 149, 150, 152, 153, 154, 155, 156, 157, 158, 159, 160, 161, 162, 163, 164, 165, 166, 167, 168, 169, 191, 192, 194, 195, 196, 197, 199, 200, 201, 203, 204, 205, 206, 211, 212, 213, 214, 215, 220, 221, 224, 227, 233, 234, 235, 238, 240, 241, 248, 253, 261, 264, 294, 295, 296, 320, 321, 342, 343, 350, 386, 387, 388, 390, 391, 392, 408, 413, 439, 440, 441, 442, 443, 444, 445, 446, 447, 449, 450, 451, 452, 453, 454, 455, 456, 457, 458, 464, 465, 468, 469, 471, 474, 506, 507, 508, 509, 511, 513, 514, 517, 518, 520, 521, 522, 526, 528, 530, 531, 535, 543, 546, 547, 548, 549, 550, 553, 555, 556, 557, 559, 560, 562
SelectKBest 177, 184, 185
SHAP 318
Socio-Economic Implications 524
Strategic Adoption 508
Sustainable Development 28, 57, 78
SVM 172, 173, 175, 176, 177, 182, 186, 291, 295, 296, 303, 311, 312, 313, 315, 317, 322, 367, 369, 395, 397, 398, 403, 407, 415, 423, 432, 434, 435
System Application 128
System Architecture 62, 69, 124
System Development 115, 117, 118, 121, 122, 129

T

Technological Readiness 32, 33, 37, 43, 44, 47, 49, 50, 51, 52
Telemedicine 18, 23, 37, 40, 48, 62, 88, 89, 134, 137, 349, 353, 391, 495, 497, 502, 515, 524, 525, 527, 528, 552
Treatment Personalization 461, 462

V

Vaccine 243, 244

W

Wearable Devices 18, 42, 63, 71, 78, 86, 88, 89, 95, 96, 134, 137, 143, 195, 232, 245, 292, 293, 295, 296, 301, 345, 347, 393, 470, 508, 518, 521, 523, 524

X

XGBoost 172, 180, 181, 186